Immunobiology of the Macrophage

CONTRIBUTORS

P. Alexander
Anthony C. Allison
A. Basten
Richard D. Berlin
J. D. Bernhard
J. Thomas Blake
Robert V. Blanden
Martin J. Cline
John R. David
Philip Davies
Vittorio Defendi
I. Djerassi
Peter C. Doherty
Jerrold J. Ellner
Lois B. Epstein
R. Evans
Martin H. Flax
Dirk K. Greineder
Andrew J. Hapel
O. A. Holtermann
Judith A. Kapp
R. Keller
E. Klein
Peter E. Lipsky
Marie-Luise Lohmann-Matthes
Stephan E. Mergenhagen
Judith Mitchell
Donald E. Mosier
D. S. Nelson
Janet M. Oliver
Joost J. Oppenheim
S. Parmett
Carl W. Pierce
Heinz G. Remold
David L. Rosenstreich
Alan S. Rosenthal
Robert C. Seeger
Ralph Snyderman
Mary Territo
Satvir S. Tevethia
Alvin Volkman
William S. Walker
P. C. Wilkinson
Joyce M. Zarling
Rolf M. Zinkernagel

Immunobiology of the Macrophage

Edited by

DAVID S. NELSON

Kolling Institute of Medical Research
The Royal North Shore Hospital of Sydney
St. Leonards, New South Wales, Australia

ACADEMIC PRESS

New York San Francisco London 1976

A Subsidiary of Harcourt Brace Jovanovich, Publishers

ACADEMIC PRESS, INC.
111 Fifth Avenue, New York, New York 10003

United Kingdom Edition published by
ACADEMIC PRESS, INC. (LONDON) LTD.
24/28 Oval Road, London NW1

Library of Congress Cataloging in Publication Data

Main entry under title:

Immunobiology of the macrophage.

Includes the bibliographies and index.
1. Macrophages. 2. Immunity. I. Nelson, David Selwyn. [DNLM: 1. Macrophages–Immunology. QW504 I323]
QR185.8.M3I45 599′.02′9 75-26342
ISBN 0–12–514550–0

PRINTED IN THE UNITED STATES OF AMERICA

Contents

List of Contributors .... *xi*
Preface .... *xv*
Introduction .... *xvii*

1 The Role of Macrophages in Antibody Responses *in Vitro*

Carl W. Pierce and Judith A. Kapp

I. Introduction 2
II. Antibody Responses *in Vitro* 4
III. Introductory Immunogenetics 6
IV. Requirements for Macrophages in Antibody Responses *in Vitro* 7
V. Functions of Macrophages in Antibody Responses *in Vitro* 13
VI. Immunogenetic Considerations of Macrophage Functions in Antibody Responses *in Vitro* 22
VII. Conclusions, Present State of the Art, and the Future 27
VIII. Note Added in Proof 29
References 30

2 The Role of Macrophages in the Specific Determination of Immunogenicity and Tolerogenicity

Donald E. Mosier

I. Introduction 35
II. *In Vitro* Requirements for Cell Activation by DNP-D-GL 38
III. Characteristics of an Antigen Which Does Not Require Macrophage Processing 41
IV. Macrophage Roles in Cell Activation 42
References 43

3 Role of Macrophages in T Cell–B Cell Collaboration in Antibody Production

A. Basten and Judith Mitchell

I. Introduction 45
II. Immunobiology of T Cell–B Cell Collaboration 46
III. Role of Macrophages in T Cell–B Cell Collaboration 52
IV. Mechanisms of T Cell–B Cell Collaboration 60
V. T Cell–B Cell Collaboration *in Vivo* 73
References 85

4 Functional Heterogeneity of Macrophages

William S. Walker

I. Introduction 91
II. Functional Heterogeneity of Macrophages from Different Tissues 92
III. Functional Heterogeneity of Macrophages from the Same Tissue 97
IV. Conclusions 106
References 108

5 The Role of Macrophages in the Induction of Cell-Mediated Immunity *in Vivo*

Joost J. Oppenheim and Robert C. Seeger

I. Introduction 112
II. Contribution of Macrophages to Induction of Delayed Hypersensitivity Reactions and in Priming Helper T Cells for Antibody Production 112
III. Relationship of Macrophage Presentation and Processing of Antigens to Induction of Cell-Mediated Immunity 117
IV. Regulation of Immunogenicity of Macrophage-Associated Antigens 123
V. Summary and Conclusions 127
References 129

6 Macrophage Function in Antigen Recognition by T Lymphocytes

Alan S. Rosenthal, J. Thomas Blake, Jerrold J. Ellner, Dirk K. Greineder, and Peter E. Lipsky

I. Introduction 131
II. Macrophages Are Required for Antigen Recognition by T Lymphocytes 132
III. Interaction between Macrophage and Soluble Antigen in the Immune Respones 134
IV. Genetic Regulation of Functional Macrophage–Lymphocyte Interaction 141
V. Physical Interactions between Macrophages and Lymphocytes 144
VI. Role of Macrophages in Nonantigenic Stimulation of T Lymphocytes 152
VII. Model Building for the Cellular and Molecular Events in Antigen Recognition by T Lymphocytes 155
References 158

7 The Role of Macrophages in the Activation of T and B Lymphocytes *in Vitro*

David L. Rosenstreich and Joost J. Oppenheim

I. Introduction 162
II. Mechanisms of Action of Macrophages 162
III. The Role of Macrophages in Antigen-Induced Lymphocyte Proliferative Responses *in Vitro* 167
IV. The Role of Macrophages in the Response of B and T Lymphocytes to Mitogens *in Vitro* 178
V. The Role of Macrophages in the Activation of Lymphocytes by Allogeneic Cells (MLR) 187
VI. The Role of Macrophages in the Activation of B Lymphocytes by Sheep Erythrocytes 189

VII. The Role of Macrophages in the Induction of Lymphokine Synthesis by B and T Lymphocytes 190
VIII. Summary and Conclusions 194
References 197

8 The Ability of Macrophages to Augment *in Vitro* Mitogen- and Antigen-Stimulated Production of Interferon and Other Mediators of Cellular Immunity by Lymphocytes

Lois B. Epstein

I. Introduction 202
II. The Ability of Macrophages to Augment Mitogen-Stimulated Production of Interferon by Lymphocytes 203
III. The Ability of Macrophages to Augment Bacterial and Viral Antigen-Stimulated Production of Interferon by Lymphocytes 214
IV. Macrophages and Their Relationship to the Production of Other Mediators of Cellular Immunity by Lymphocytes 219
V. Macrophages and Their Role in Affecting the Production of Viral-Induced Interferon by Leukocytes 225
VI. Summary 229
References 231

9 Nonspecific Immunoregulation by Macrophages and Their Products

D. S. Nelson

I. Introduction 235
II. Potentiation of Lymphoid Cell Responses 236
III. Inhibition of Lymphoid Cell Responses 239
IV. Mode of Action of Macrophages in Depressing Lymphocyte Responses .. 243
V. Significance of Lymphoid Cell Stimulation and Inhibition by Macrophages and Their Products 250
References 253

10 Macrophage Membranes

Janet M. Oliver and Richard D. Berlin

I. Introduction 259
II. Probes of Macrophage Surface Organization 261
III. Random Mobility of Macrophage Surface Proteins 262
IV. Organized Movement of Macrophage Surface Elements 264
V. Control of Translational Movements of Receptors and Transport Proteins within the Plane of the Membrane 266
VI. Summary 271
References 272

11 Macrophage Cell Lines and Their Uses in Immunobiology

Vittorio Defendi

I. Introduction 275
II. Growth of Primary Macrophages *in Vitro* 276
III. Permanent Lines with Properties of Macrophages 283

IV. Conclusion 288
References 289

12 Monocyte Kinetics and Their Changes in Infection

Alvin Volkman

I. Introduction 291
II. Theoretical and Methodological Background 293
III. Cell Kinetics of the Monocytes 295
IV. Cell Kinetics of Monocytes in Infection 311
V. Concluding Remarks 319
References 320

13 Chemotaxis of Macrophages

Ralph Snyderman and Stephan E. Mergenhagen

I. Introduction 323
II. Methods for Quantifying Macrophage Chemotaxis 324
III. Humoral Factors Chemotactic for Macrophages 329
IV. Lymphocyte-Derived Chemotactic Factors 333
V. Chemotactic Factors from Bacteria 337
VI. Factors Which Alter Monocyte Chemotactic Function 337
VII. Abnormalities of Monocyte Chemotaxis in Human Diseases 340
VIII. Summary and Conclusions 345
References 346

14 Cellular and Molecular Aspects of Chemotaxis of Macrophages and Monocytes

P. C. Wilkinson

I. Introduction 350
II. Locomotion of Different Types of Macrophage 350
III. Modes of Macrophage Migration 351
IV. Recognition of Chemotactic Factors at the Cell Membrane 353
V. Intracellular Events following Interaction of the Chemotactic Factor with the Cell Membrane 356
VI. Differential Effects of Bacterial Toxins on Locomotion of Neutrophils and Macrophages 358
VII. Recognition in Chemotaxis, Phagocytosis, and Other Macrophage Functions 360
VIII. Antigen-Specific Chemotaxis 361
IX. Conclusions 363
References 363

15 Lymphocyte–Macrophage Interactions and Macrophage Activation in the Expression of Antimicrobial Immunity *in Vivo*

Robert V. Blanden, Andrew J. Hapel, Peter C. Doherty, and Rolf M. Zinkernagel

I. Introduction 367
II. Generation of Effector T Cells 369

III. Mechanisms of T Cell and Macrophage-Mediated Immunity to Infection 375
IV. Conclusions 395
References 397

16 Macrophage Activation by Lymphocyte Mediators and Studies on the Interaction of Macrophage Inhibitory Factor (MIF) with Its Target Cell

John R. David and Heinz G. Remold

I. Introduction 401
II. Macrophage Activation by Lymphocyte Mediators 403
III. Interaction of MIF with the Macrophage 414
IV. Biologically Active Substances Produced by Macrophages 421
V. Conclusion 423
References 423

17 Secretion of Macrophage Enzymes in Relation to the Pathogenesis of Chronic Inflammation

Philip Davies and Anthony C. Allison

I. Introduction 428
II. The Origin and Turnover of Cells in Sites of Chronic Inflammation 428
III. *In Vitro* Studies on the Role of Macrophages in Chronic Inflammation 430
IV. What Is the Contribution of Hydrolytic Enzyme Secretion to Chronic Inflammation? 448
V. Other Products of Macrophages 451
VI. Interactions and Modulating Factors 454
References 457

18 Induction of Macrophage-Mediated Cytotoxicity

Marie-Luise Lohmann-Matthes

I. Introduction 464
II. Macrophage-Mediated Cytotoxicity in Allograft Rejection 464
III. Cytotoxic Macrophages in Syngeneic Tumor Systems 469
IV. Macrophage-Mediated Cytotoxicity Induced by Infection with Various Microorganisms 472
V. *In Vitro* Induction of Macrophage-Mediated Cytotoxicity 473
VI. Summary and Implications 481
References 484

19 Cytostatic and Cytocidal Effects of Activated Macrophages

R. Keller

I. Introduction 487
II. Nomenclature 488
III. Cytostatic Effects of Activated Macrophages 489
IV. Cytocidal Effects of Macrophages 499
V. The Biologic Relevance of the *in Vitro* Findings 503
VI. Critical Outlook 505
References 507

20 Macrophages and the Destruction of Syngeneic Virus-Induced Tumors

Satvir S. Tevethia, Joyce M. Zarling, and Martin H. Flax

I. Introduction 509
II. Antigenicity of Cells Transformed by Oncogenic Viruses 510
III. Immune Response of Syngeneic Host to Virus-Induced Tumors 512
IV. Role of Macrophages in Rejection of Virus-Induced Tumors 518
V. Steps in the Development of Cell-Mediated Immunity and the Mechanisms of Rejection of DNA Virus-Induced Tumors 527
References 531

21 Mechanisms of Extracellular Killing of Nucleated Mammalian Cells by Macrophages

R. Evans and P. Alexander

I. Introduction 536
II. Specific Macrophage Cytotoxicity 537
III. Nonspecific Macrophage Cytotoxicity 555
IV. Cytotoxic Macrophages and the Tumor Bearing Host 567
V. *In Vivo* Significance of the Nonspecifically Cytotoxic Macrophage 570
VI. Role of Macrophages in Surveillance 571
VII. Conclusion 572
References 573

22 Immunotherapeutic Approaches to Tumors Involving the Skin

O. A. Holtermann, E. Klein, I. Djerassi, J. D. Bernhard, and S. Parmett

I. Introduction 577
II. Clinical Investigations 579
III. A Primitive Surveillance Mechanism? 584
IV. Summary 587
References 589

23 Macrophages and Their Disorders in Man

Mary Territo and Martin J. Cline

I. Metabolism 594
II. Functions 596
III. Disorders of the Monocyte–Macrophage System 602
IV. Summary and Future Perspectives 611
References 612

24 Macrophages: Perspectives and Prospects

D. S. Nelson

Text 617

Index 623

List of Contributors

Numbers in parentheses indicate the pages on which the authors' contributions begin.

P. Alexander (535), Chester Beatty Research Institute, Belmont, Sutton, Surrey, England

Anthony C. Allison (427), Clinical Research Centre, Harrow, Middlesex, England

A. Basten (45), Immunology Unit, Department of Bacteriology, University of Sydney, New South Wales, Australia

Richard D. Berlin (259), Department of Physiology, University of Connecticut Health Center, School of Medicine, Farmington, Connecticut

J. D. Bernhard (577), Department of Dermatology, Roswell Park Memorial Institute, Buffalo, New York

J. Thomas Blake (131), Section on Biologic Structure, Laboratory of Clinical Investigation, National Institute of Allergy and Infectious Disease, National Institutes of Health, Bethesda, Maryland

Robert V. Blanden (367), Department of Microbiology, John Curtin School of Medical Research, The Australian National University, Canberra City, Australia

Martin J. Cline (593), Department of Medicine, University of California, Center for the Health Sciences, Los Angeles, California

John R. David (401), Department of Medicine, Harvard Medical School and Robert B. Brigham Hospital, Boston, Massachusetts

Philip Davies (427), Clinical Research Centre, Harrow, Middlesex, England

Vittorio Defendi (275), Department of Pathology, New York University School of Medicine, New York, New York

I. Djerassi (577), Department of Dermatology, Roswell Park Memorial Institute, Buffalo, New York

Peter C. Doherty (367), Department of Microbiology, John Curtin School of Medical Research, The Australian National University, Canberra City, Australia

Jerrold J. Ellner (131), Section on Biologic Structure, Laboratory of Clinical Investigation, National Institute of Allergy and Infectious Diseases, National Institutes of Health, Bethesda, Maryland

Lois B. Epstein (201), Cancer Research Institute, University of California, San Francisco, California

R. Evans (535), Chester Beatty Research Institute, Belmont, Sutton, Surrey, England

Martin H. Flax (509), Department of Pathology, Tufts University School of Medicine, Boston, Massachusetts

Dirk K. Greineder (131), Section on Biologic Structure, Laboratory of Clinical Investigation, National Institute of Allergy and Infectious Diseases, National Institutes of Health, Bethesda, Maryland

Andrew J. Hapel (367), Department of Microbiology, John Curtin School of Medical Research, The Australian National University, Canberra City, Australia

O. A. Holtermann (577), Department of Dermatology, Roswell Park Memorial Institute, Buffalo, New York

Judith A. Kapp (1), Department of Pathology, Harvard Medical School, Boston, Massachusetts

R. Keller (487), Immunobiology Research Group, Zurich, Switzerland

E. Klein (577), Department of Dermatology, Roswell Park Memorial Institute, Buffalo, New York

Peter E. Lipsky (131), Section on Biologic Structure, Laboratory of Clinical Investigation, National Institute of Allergy and Infectious Diseases, National Institutes of Health, Bethesda, Maryland

Marie-Luise Lohmann-Matthes (463), Max-Planck-Institut für Immunbiologie, Freiburg-Zähringen, Germany

Stephan E. Mergenhagen (323), Laboratory of Microbiology and Immunology, National Institute of Dental Research, National Institutes of Health, Bethesda, Maryland

Judith Mitchell (45), Immunology Unit, Department of Bacteriology, University of Sydney, Sydney, New South Wales, Australia

Donald E. Mosier (35), Laboratory of Immunology, National Institute of Allergy and Infectious Disease, National Institutes of Health, Bethesda, Maryland

D. S. Nelson (235, 617), Kolling Institute of Medical Research, The Royal North Shore Hospital of Sydney, St. Leonards, New South Wales, Australia

Janet M. Oliver (259), Departments of Physiology and Pathology, University of Connecticut Health Center, School of Medicine, Farmington, Connecticut

Joost J. Oppenheim (111, 161), Laboratory of Microbiology and Immunology, National Institute of Dental Research, National Institutes of Health, Bethesda, Maryland

S. Parmett (577), Department of Dermatology, Roswell Park Memorial Institute, Buffalo, New York

Carl W. Pierce (1), Department of Pathology, Harvard Medical School, Boston, Massachusetts

Heinz G. Remold (401), Departments of Medicine and Biological Chemistry, Harvard Medical School, and Robert B. Brigham Hospital, Boston, Massachusetts

David L. Rosenstreich (161), Cellular Immunology Section, Laboratory of Microbiology and Immunology, National Institute of Dental Research, National Institutes of Health, Bethesda, Maryland

Alan S. Rosenthal (131), Section on Biologic Structure, Laboratory of Clinical Investigation, National Institute of Allergy and Infectious Diseases, National Institutes of Health, Bethesda, Maryland

Robert C. Seeger (111), Department of Pediatrics, University of California Medical

School, Los Angeles, California

Ralph Snyderman (323), Division of Rheumatic and Genetic Diseases, Departments of Medicine and Immunology, Duke University Medical Center, Durham, North Carolina

Mary Territo (593), Department of Medicine, University of California School of Medicine and Veterans Administration Wadsworth Hospital Center, Los Angeles, California

Satvir S. Tevethia (509), Department of Pathology, and Cancer Research Center, Tufts University School of Medicine, Boston, Massachusetts

Alvin Volkman (291), Trudeau Institute, Inc., Immunobiological Research Laboratories, Saranac Lake, New York

William S. Walker (91), Division of Immunology, St. Jude Children's Research Hospital, Memphis, Tennessee

P. C. Wilkinson (349), Department of Bacteriology and Immunology, University of Glasgow (Western Infirmary), Glasgow, Scotland

Joyce M. Zarling (509), Immunobiology Research Center, University of Wisconsin, Madison, Wisconsin

Rolf M. Zinkernagel (367), Department of Microbiology, John Curtin School of Medical Research, The Australian National University, Canberra City, Australia

Preface

In recent years an improved understanding of the roles played by macrophages in the immune system has led to an increased interest in these cells by immunologists in general and, inevitably, to an increase in the volume of literature concerning them. In this book a group of immunologists of diverse scientific and geographic backgrounds present an account of the present state of knowledge of the immunobiology of the macrophage. The authors have been encouraged to give personal accounts of current developments in their special fields of interest as well as critical surveys of the backgrounds leading to these developments. Some topics have been considered from differing viewpoints in the different chapters so that the reader may sense the continuing activity in areas of controversy. We hope that this work will provide both knowledge and stimulation for further research.

Most scientists—especially those who edit books and write reviews—have a burden of gratitude to many people. Acknowledgment of all one's pastors and masters, colleagues, assistants, and critics would be well-nigh impossible (as well as being of little interest to the reader), but I cannot let the opportunity pass to thank the following people: Dr. Maurice Landy, who suggested the production of this book and who, with Drs J. J. Oppenheim and A. S. Rosenthal, helped mold its shape; the staff of Academic Press for their patient assistance; my colleagues in the Kolling Institute, especially Katherine Carson, Jean Penrose, and Cynthia Shneider, for administrative and scientific assistance and for tolerating my short temper while in literary labor; and my wife, Dr. Peggy Nelson, for her forebearance, encouragement, and support, both domestic and scientific, in this as in so many other ventures.

David S. Nelson

Introduction

Many would argue that the golden era of phagocyte biology occurred at the turn of the century. Highlighted by the discoveries of Ilya Metchinokoff and his contemporaries, this exciting period saw the process of phagocytosis placed in a broad and physiological perspective, spanning the phylogenetic tree from protozoa to man. Largely focused on infectious processes, this work progressed with the simplest of technologies and laid the groundwork for all that was to follow. Aided by the brilliance of the continental schools of organic chemistry, vital and supravital dyes were synthesized and rapidly employed by cytologists in their search for those cells which would eventually be categorized as belonging to the reticuloendothelial system. "Cytases" and intracellular digestion took their place in the medical literature, neutral red and Janus green reached their acme, chick embryo extract and Carrell flasks flourished, hosts and parasites began their struggle for dominance, and learned colleagues argued endlessly over the relative importance of humoral and cellular factors. Ferments and intermediary metabolism were rather vague notions and herd immunity and antitoxins were in vogue. But in spite of the uncertainties of biochemical and immunological knowledge, the cellular pathologists of the day, those visionaries of disease pathogenesis, were incorporating the microphages and macrophages with their enzymes and antienzymes into a framework of inflammation, tissue injury, degenerative disease, and wound repair. A framework which even today with ever increasing sophistication is current and timely.

This era passed and with it the verve and interest in the study of the phagocyte—in part, because investigators were diverted into other exciting areas of contemporary biology; in part, because of the advent of chemotherapy and the control of bacterial disease; in part, because the bright young investigators of the day became the Deans and Department Chairmen; in part, because departments of pathology, particularly experimental pathology, lost their regal and central role in the medical curriculum. In any event, in spite of a few dedicated phagists, the doldrums were upon us.

Yet, even a brief perusal of this volume indicates that the tides have turned and the fortunes of the macrophage are once again ascendant; a transition which has occurred within the last decade and one with uncertain origins. Spurred by all the tools and concepts of modern science, one could mention the tritiation of thymidine, the latency of rat liver phosphatases, the Millipore filter, the flying coverslip, buffered osmium, the sheep erythrocyte, zymosan and its humoral companions, the first and sixth carbons of grape sugar, bleaches and horseradishes, polystyrene and mayonnaise, ammonium sulfate and pepsin, beans and stalks. All played a role in the renaissance and the revisitation of Metchinkoff.

But if the zenith has not been reached, what of the future? What new insights can be obtained and how will they mesh with the new cell biology? Where do the answers lie which will elucidate the current phenomenon of chemotaxis and motility, endocytosis, immunological receptors, activation, secretory products, the containment of neoplasms, and the regulation of the immune response?

They lie in the wasteland of the plasma membrane and contractile proteins, in the discovery of new and meaningful genetic models, and in the development of a novel sociology to explain the interactions of the macrophage with its molecular and cellular neighbors. David Nelson and his gifted colleagues have set the stage.

Zanvil A. Cohn
Laboratory of Cellular Physiology and Immunology
The Rockefeller University
New York, New York

1

The Role of Macrophages in Antibody Responses *in Vitro*

Carl W. Pierce and Judith A. Kapp

I.	Introduction	2
II.	Antibody Responses *in Vitro*	4
	A. Methodology	4
	B. Advantages and Disadvantages of Tissue Culture Systems	4
III.	Introductory Immunogenetics	6
IV.	Requirements for Macrophages in Antibody Responses *in Vitro*	7
	A. Separation and Purification	7
	B. Characteristics of Macrophages	9
	C. Antibody Responses to T Cell-Dependent Antigens	10
	D. Antibody Responses to T Cell-Independent Antigens	12
V.	Functions of Macrophages in Antibody Responses *in Vitro*	13
	A. Promotion of Lymphoid Cell Viability	13
	B. Antigen Presentation	16
	C. Relationship of Viability-Promoting and Antigen Presentation Functions of Macrophages	19
	D. The Macrophage as a Focus for T Cell–B Cell Interaction?	20
VI.	Immunogenetic Considerations of Macrophage Functions in Antibody Responses *in Vitro*	22
	A. The Role of Macrophages in Antibody Responses to Antigens Controlled by *H-2*-Linked *Ir* Genes	22
	B. Lack of Genetic Restrictions for Interactions among Macrophages and Lymphoid Cells in Antibody Responses	24

C. Role of Macrophages in Suppression of Antibody Responses by Alloantisera against Leukocyte Alloantigens 26
VII. Conclusions, Present State of the Art, and the Future 27
VIII. Note Added in Proof 29
References 30

I. INTRODUCTION

During the last decade, our understanding of the cells and mechanisms involved in the development and the regulation of antibody responses has increased at an astonishing pace. Distinct pathways for the differentiation of two classes of clonally restricted, antigen-specific, immunocompetent lymphocytes from hemopoietic stem cells are now well recognized, as are the distinctive properties and functions of these lymphocytes. Although the precise pathway(s) of differentiation of the precursors of antibody-producing cells, or B cells, in mammals is still the subject of intensive investigation, the immunologic function of B cells is incontrovertible. B cells, after interaction with antigen via membrane immunoglobulin (Ig) receptors specific for that antigen, and under appropriate regulatory influences of thymus-derived lymphocytes, develop into plasma cells that secrete antibody molecules uniquely capable of combining with the antigenic moiety which initially stimulated the B cells. Thymus-derived lymphocytes, or T cells, after interaction with antigen via a still undefined membrane receptor, do not synthesize nor secrete antibody. T cells, however, are responsible for the various phenomena of cell-mediated immunity including the tissue rejection phenomena, such as graft versus host reactions and allograft and tumor rejection, and the production of a variety of biologically active molecules, "lymphokines," which are responsible for the inflammatory response and the tissue damage characteristic of delayed hypersensitivity reactions. T cell function is also critical for immunity and resistance to certain infectious microorganisms. Furthermore, from the experiments of numerous investigators, it is now clear that T cells, in addition to their function as effector cells for cell-mediated immune reactions, are the critical regulators of both B cell and T cell responses to antigen. T cells mediating positive regulatory functions are referred to as "helper cells" in antibody responses and "amplifier cells" in cell-mediated immune responses. Negative regulatory functions in both T cell and B cell responses are ascribed to "suppressor T cells." The relationships between and the mechanisms of action of the T cells mediating these opposing regulatory functions are currently under intensive investigation in numerous laboratories.

The antigens that stimulate antibody responses may be divided into two broad and probably artificial classes: T cell-dependent and T cell-independent antigens. T cell-dependent antigens are complex multideterminant antigens, such as heterologous erythrocytes and hapten–protein conjugates. The development of antibody responses to these antigens by B cells is strictly dependent on the concomitant positive regulatory influence, or helper effect, of T cells. T cell-independent antigens are generally polymeric molecules with repeating chemical subunits, such as pneumococcal polysaccharides, lipopolysaccharides, flagellin, and polyvinylpyrrolidone. These antigens are capable of stimulating antibody responses without the helper effect of T cells and thus derive their classification as T cell-independent antigens. However, in antibody responses to these types of antigens, the suppressive effects of T cells are most easily demonstrated and their classification as T cell-independent antigens becomes considerably less meaningful and valid. Several review articles are available which delve into this background material in greater detail (Katz and Benacerraf, 1972; Claman and Mosier, 1972; Gershon, 1974; Warner, 1974; Pierce and Benacerraf, 1975; Coutinho and Möller, 1975; Nossal and Schrader, 1975).

The macrophage is a third type of cell that is intimately involved in the development and expression of humoral and cell-mediated immune responses. In contrast to T cells and B cells, macrophages are neither clonally restricted nor antigen specific, but function as nonspecific accessory cells. Their functions in antigen uptake, catabolism, and presentation to T and B cells in the initiation of immune responses have been reviewed (Unanue, 1972), as have their roles as accessory effector cells in both cellular and humoral immune responses (Benacerraf and Green, 1969). Considerable attention has also been devoted to the physiology of macrophages, the mechanisms of phagocytosis and pinocytosis, and their functions in the inflammatory response (Cohn, 1968; Nelson, 1969; van Furth, 1970; Gordon and Cohn, 1973; Steinman and Cohn, 1974a; Ebert and Grant, 1974). The reader is referred to these articles and appropriate chapters of this book for detailed information on these aspects of macrophage function.

In this chapter, we will attempt to present a cogent overview of the functions of macrophages in the initiation and regulation of antibody responses *in vitro*. We realize some of our views may be controversial and biased by our experiences. However, if we succeed in acquainting the uninitiated reader with the complexities of these macrophage functions, and, at the same time, stimulate others to perform experiments to clarify those areas where controversy exists, we will have accomplished our goals.

II. ANTIBODY RESPONSES *IN VITRO*

A. Methodology

Two similar culture systems are used to study antibody responses *in vitro*. In both culture systems, dispersed, single spleen cells, or appropriate combinations of "purified" T cells, B cells, and macrophages are suspended in a completely supplemented culture medium containing selected fetal calf serum at a cell density between 10×10^6 and 20×10^6 cells/ml. In the system developed by Mishell and Dutton (1967), the cells are incubated with antigen in small plastic petri dishes at 37°C in a humidified atmosphere of 7% O_2, 10% CO_2, and 83% N_2 on a slowly rocking platform to facilitate interactions among the cells. Each culture is supplemented daily with a nutritional "cocktail" and fetal calf serum. In the system developed by Marbrook (1967), the cells and antigen are placed in a glass tube closed at the bottom with dialysis membrane. The bottom portion of the tube is immersed in culture medium contained in a larger vessel, and the apparatus is incubated stationary at 37°C in the humidified atmosphere used in the Mishell–Dutton system. The density of cells on the dialysis membrane is sufficient for required cell interactions, and the cultures do not require the daily supplementation with nutritional cocktail and fetal calf serum. After the desired incubation period, the cells are harvested and assayed for plaque-forming cells (PFC) to the stimulating antigen by one of the variations of the hemolytic plaque technique of Jerne *et al.* (1974). By employing appropriate modifications of this assay procedure (Pierce *et al.*, 1971), IgM, IgG, and IgA PFC responses can readily be measured.

In addition to heterologous erythrocytes [usually sheep erythrocytes (SRBC)], hapten–protein conjugates, bacterial proteins, polysaccharides, lipopolysaccharides, serum proteins, viruses, and synthetic polypeptide antigens, such as the random terpolymer of L-glutamic acid^{60}-L-alanine^{30}-L-tyrosine^{10} (GAT), stimulate both primary and secondary antibody responses in tissue culture systems. In these latter cases, the determinant of interest, the hapten, protein, or GAT, is coupled to the indicator erythrocyte used in the hemolytic plaque assay and, with appropriate controls, determinant-specific PFC responses can readily be measured.

B. Advantages and Disadvantages of Tissue Culture Systems

These two culture systems support the development of primary and secondary antibody responses with approximately equal efficiency. PFC responses that develop in culture are comparable in magnitude, kinetics, Ig class, and dependence on antigen dose to responses in intact animals during the first 7 days after immunization (Claman and Mosier, 1972; Pierce, 1974). This parallelism between responses *in vivo* and *in vitro* has been observed for most antigens that have been studied thoroughly. It also has been the general experience that those antigens that stimulate poor primary responses *in vivo* also stimulate poor primary responses *in vitro.* Since culture systems are closed systems and one has more precise control of the components of these systems than is possible *in vivo,* they are well suited for investigations of the critical factors in the induction of the antibody response. For example, the numbers, types, and immune reactivities of cells from the immune system that are added to the cultures and the interactions among these cells can be rather precisely controlled. The concentration and physical form of the antigen and the interaction of the various types of cells with antigen in the cultures can also be controlled. Furthermore, specifically reactive cells or reagents, such as antimetabolites, antibodies to antigen, or membrane molecules on the responding cells, can be added to the system at defined times in known numbers or concentrations (Pierce, 1974). Although antibody responses *in vitro* are comparable in many respects to *in vivo* responses, and although tissue culture systems offer many advantages in experimentation not possible *in vivo,* one must be extremely cautious when extrapolating from one system to the other, and one should avoid making dogmatic statements based on results from one system which have not been confirmed in the other.

Tissue culture systems are not without disadvantages. Spleen cells or partially purified T and B cells from mice are most commonly used in these culture systems; lymphoid cells from rabbit, rat, and chicken have been used successfully only by a few investigators. Most of the data we will discuss have been derived from cultures of mouse cells. However, even with mouse lymphoid cells, considerable strain to strain variation exists, and no amount of cajoling or uttering of incantations, friendly or hostile, can convince spleen cells from some strains of mice to respond faithfully on a regular basis. Cell survival in these cultures is not good; only approximately 25% of the initial cells survive for 5 days. Thus, we are dealing with a dying system, and the effects of products released from dead or dying cells on the surviving cells are still largely unknown. The tissue culture environment itself is artificial and may not provide optimal conditions in terms of nutrients. In addition, fetal bovine serum, not required for antibody responses *in vivo,* is a necessary ingredient of the culture medium. Fetal bovine sera vary in their capacity to support antibody responses *in vitro;* some are nonsupportive, and others are nonspecifically cytotoxic. This variability is an annoyance that could readily be done without. Also absent from tissue culture systems are the multitude of *in vivo* homeostatic mechanisms, such as the influences of circulating immunocompetent cells, the influx of virgin precursor cells from central lymphoid tissues, and the feedback regulation by other stimulated lymphocytes and previously synthesized antibodies, all of which obviously affect development and expression of antibody responses. Last, antibody responses in tissue culture systems are subject to a variety of maladies that we call, in all seriousness, gremlins (C. W. Pierce and J. A. Kapp, unpublished observations, 1975). These include the propensity of the investigator to put fingers in the cultures or to drop the cultures and various acts of God and man, such as the tides, phases of the moon, rocket launches, and the changes of the seasons. Nevertheless, tissue culture systems have been extremely useful for investigating many facets of the antibody response; the function of macrophages has been one of these facets.

III. INTRODUCTORY IMMUNOGENETICS

We will restrict our discussion of immunogenetics to the major histocompatibility, or *H-2*, complex of the mouse as it relates to antibody responses, and will not consider genetics of immunoglobulins. The *H-2* complex, a small segment of genome in the ninth linkage group on chromosome 17, has become the focus of great interest to immunologists with the recognition that this gene complex controls a variety of functions of immunological significance in addition to histocompatibility antigens. The *H-2* complex has been divided into four regions on the basis of the antigens or immunologic functions each region controls. At the two ends of the *H-2* complex are the *K* and *D* regions, which encode serologically detectable transplantation antigens. These antigens are present on membranes of macrophages, T cells, B cells, and nonlymphoid cells; these antigens not only stimulate T cells in the various tissue rejection responses but also are the membrane target antigens of the effector T cells in these responses. Inside the *H-2* complex and adjacent to the *D* region is the *S* region, which encodes serum proteins in the complement sequence, but is otherwise unrelated in function to other regions of the complex. The *I* region lies between the *S* and *K* regions and encodes a family of antigens, Ia antigens, which are on the membranes of T cells, B cells, and macrophages and are also involved in the stimulation of T cells in tissue rejection responses. Recent observations indicate that syngenicity of *I* region antigens is necessary for optimal cooperative interactions between

T cells and B cells in antibody responses to T cell-dependent antigens. Also, genes in the *I* region control the susceptibility to certain tumor viruses and immune responsiveness to certain antigens; these latter genes are called *H-2*-linked immune response genes (*Ir* genes). Excellent reviews are available for readers who may wish to pursue this topic in greater detail (Shreffler and David, 1975; Benacerraf and Katz, 1975).

Our understanding of the complex immune mechanism has been advanced by observations that inbred strains of guinea pigs and mice develop different degrees of immunity when stimulated by antigens of limited diversity, such as (1) synthetic polypeptides with limited structural heterogeneity, (2) alloantigens differing only slightly from host antigens, and (3) complex, multideterminant antigens administered in low doses where only the most immunogenic determinants are recognized (Benacerraf and Katz, 1975). The development of high levels of circulating antibody and/or cellular immunity to many of these antigens is controlled by the *H-2*-linked autosomal dominant *Ir* genes. The antibody response in mice to the synthetic random terpolymer of L-glutamic acid^{60}-L-alanine^{30}-L-tyrosine^{10} (GAT), is controlled by an *H-2*-linked *Ir* gene. Mice of the H-$2^{a,b,d,f,j,k,r,u,v}$ haplotypes behave as "responders," and synthesize specific antibody after injection of GAT. Mice of the H-$2^{n,p,q,s}$ haplotypes are "nonresponders" and synthesize no detectable antibody after injection of GAT. However, both responder and nonresponder mice produce GAT-specific antibody when immunized with GAT complexed to the carrier methylated bovine serum albumin (GAT-MBSA). This observation demonstrates that both nonresponder and responder mice have B cells capable of synthesizing GAT-specific antibody. Other studies have demonstrated that the failure of nonresponder mice to respond to GAT involves a still undefined defect in the stimulation of helper T cell functions in these strains (Benacerraf and Katz, 1975; Kapp *et al.*, 1975a). The function of macrophages in antibody responses to GAT will be discussed in Sections V,B and VI,A and B.

IV. REQUIREMENTS FOR MACROPHAGES IN ANTIBODY RESPONSES *IN VITRO*

A. Separation and Purification

Macrophages for use in the study of antibody responses *in vitro* have been obtained from spleen, peritoneal exudate, bone marrow, and lymph nodes. In many instances, it is desirable not only to deplete macrophages from suspensions of lymphocytes, but also to recover the macrophages as functionally active cells. This type of separation, first described by Mosier (1967), can readily be achieved by taking advantage of the well-known property of macrophages, but not lymphocytes, to adhere tenaciously to glass or plastic surfaces (Gordon and Cohn, 1973). Because of this property and method of separation, macrophages have been referred to as "adherent cells" and lymphocytes have been called "nonadherent cells." However, since the characteristics, properties, and functions of "adherent cells" have not been shown to our satisfaction to differ significantly from those of macrophages, we will use the more physiologically and functionally accurate term macrophages. When depletion of macrophages from lymphocyte preparations is all that is required, adherence techniques, such as passing the complex cell suspensions over columns of glass beads (Shortman *et al.*, 1970, 1971) or Sephadex G10 (Ly and Mishell, 1974) are quite satisfactory.

A somewhat less efficient means of depleting macrophages, in our experience, involves allowing macrophages to ingest carbonyl iron and then depleting these cells by passing the cell suspension through a magnetic field (Ford *et al.*, 1966; Schlossman and Hudson, 1973). A related method is to allow macrophages to ingest a dense particle, such as opsonized erythrocytes, and then to separate cells that have ingested the particle from those which have not ingested the particle by isopycnic centrifugation on a Ficoll-Hypaque or other suitable gradient (Pierce *et al.*, 1974a). These two techniques only separate phagocytic from nonphagocytic macrophages, and in many instances sufficient "nonphagocytic" macrophages remain in the lymphocyte preparation to mediate functions usually ascribed to the entire macrophage population. More sophisticated procedures involving velocity sedimentation (Miller and Phillips, 1970; Osoba, 1970; Gorczynski *et al.*, 1971) and buoyant density centrifugation (Haskill *et al.*, 1970; Mishell *et al.*, 1970) are also available for separating macrophages and lymphocytes, but these methods often result in significant contamination of both populations with the undesired cell type. One permanent method for depleting macrophages is to treat the cell suspension with specific, heterologous anti-macrophage serum and complement (Unanue, 1972).

In our experience, adherence techniques have been the most satisfactory and reliable for separating macrophages from lymphocytes. The procedure described by Mosier (1967) and modified in our laboratory (Pierce, 1973) is probably the simplest and most efficient method available. Since approximately 1% of spleen cells, 50% of normal peritoneal exudate cells, and 80% of peptone-induced peritoneal cells initially plated will remain firmly adherent to the culture dishes, graded numbers of macrophages per culture dish can be readily obtained. More exact quantitation of the macrophages can be achieved by counting adherent cells with a microscope (Pierce *et al.*, 1974a). The dishes containing the adherent macrophages can then be used as the culture vessel in the Mishell–Dutton system by adding antigen and the appropriate lymphoid cells. In the Marbrook system, the macrophages are recovered from the surface to which they adhered, usually by scraping or gentle trypsinization, and are added to the culture apparatus with antigen and lymphoid cells.

One important point that should be mentioned at this juncture, and one which will be emphasized later, is that no amount of care and technical skill will produce "pure" populations of macrophages and lymphocytes. At best, macrophage preparations can be obtained which are almost pure as monitored by phagocytosis of marker particles; however, a few "adherent" lymphocytes are always present. Further, in our experience, it is virtually impossible to obtain macrophage-free lymphocytes by any separation procedure. Also, precursors of macrophages present in the hemopoietic islands in mouse spleen adhere weakly to plastic and are therefore often retained in the lymphocyte preparation. During culture, these precursors often mature into phagocytic, adherent macrophages. Thus, we feel that one should consider lymphocyte preparations to be depleted of macrophages, but never macrophage-free.

B. Characteristics of Macrophages

Macrophages have several distinguishing characteristics that make their identification relatively easy. As already mentioned, these cells adhere firmly to glass or plastic surfaces and with time in culture will spread and send pseudopodia onto the surface of the culture vessel. These adherent macrophages are actively phagocytic and readily ingest a variety of marker particles visible in the light microscope. These cells also have the morphological characteristics ascribed to macrophages in tissue sections, but are by no means a homogeneous, single type of cell. Furthermore, histochemical methods have demonstrated that these "adherent cells" contain enzymes characteristically found in macrophages (Gordon and Cohn, 1973; Steinman and Cohn, 1974a).

Two other properties of the macrophages used in tissue culture systems are (1) their function is resistant to the effects of ionizing radiation delivered *in vivo* or *in vitro*, suggesting that cell division is not required for their function (Roseman, 1969; Osoba, 1970; Haskill *et al.*, 1970; Dutton *et al.*, 1970; Shortman *et al.*, 1970; Gorczynski *et al.*, 1971) and (2) their function *in vitro* is affected by treatments that block reticuloendothelial function *in vivo* (Unanue, 1972). Thus, the cells isolated by adherence procedures and which we are calling macrophages have the properties and characteristics usually ascribed to macrophages.

Macrophages also have membrane molecules and receptors which, while not unique for macrophages, are important when considering their functions in antibody responses. These membrane molecules include the alloantigens encoded by the *K, I,* and *D* regions of the *H-2* complex (Shreffler and David, 1975), a receptor for the C3 moiety of complement, and a receptor for the Fc portion of the IgG molecule (Unanue, 1972; Warner, 1974).

C. Antibody Responses to T Cell-Dependent Antigens

The first demonstration that macrophages are required for the development of antibody responses *in vitro* was by Mosier (1967), who separated spleen cells from unimmunized mice into adherent (macrophages) and nonadherent (lymphoid) cells by allowing macrophages to adhere to a series of plastic culture dishes. Neither population alone developed a primary IgM PFC response to SRBC whereas cultures of the recombined macrophages and lymphoid cells responded as well as unmanipulated spleen cells. These types of experiments were eventually confirmed by several laboratories for responses to SRBC (Pierce, 1969; Talmage *et al.*, 1970; Hartmann *et al.*, 1970; Haskill *et al.*, 1970; Shortman *et al.*, 1970; Shortman and Palmer, 1971; Unanue, 1972; Claman and Mosier, 1972) and have been extended to responses to other T cell-dependent antigens, such as a variety of hapten conjugates of proteins (Katz and Unanue, 1973; Feldmann and Nossal, 1972), erythrocytes (Kettman and Dutton, 1971), viruses (Bluestein and Pierce, 1973), and synthetic antigens (GAT) (Kapp *et al.*, 1973b). The T cell-dependent nature of all these antigens has been established using several experimental methods for T cell deprivation both *in vivo* and *in vitro* (Katz and Benacerraf, 1972; Claman and Mosier, 1972; Gershon, 1974). We are unaware of any T cell-dependent antigen that will stimulate primary antibody responses in cultures of macrophage-depleted T and B lymphocytes.

Further studies have demonstrated that macrophages from T cell-deprived mice (Mosier *et al.*, 1970; Munro and Hunter, 1970) or mice tolerant to SRBC (Forbes, 1969) are capable of supporting optimal antibody responses to SRBC *in vitro* by normal lymphoid cells, and that macrophages are not the precursors of or the actual PFC (Hartmann *et al.*, 1970; Shortman and Palmer, 1971; Munro and Hunter, 1970), i.e., macrophages do not produce antibody. Macrophages from normal or proteose peptone-induced peritoneal exudate, bone marrow, or lymph node support primary PFC responses to T cell-dependent antigens *in vitro* as efficiently, on a cell per cell basis, as splenic adherent cells (Hoffmann, 1970; Pierce *et al.*, 1974a; C. W. Pierce and J. A. Kapp, unpublished observations, 1975; Leserman *et al.*, 1972). When using peritoneal exudate macrophages, however, it has been consistently observed that more than 10^5 macrophages in cultures of 10^7 lymphoid cells are inhibitory (see also Section V,A). When spleen cells were fractionated by velocity sedimentation (Miller and Phillips, 1970; Osoba, 1970; Gorczynski *et al.*, 1971) or density gradient centrifugation (Haskill *et al.*, 1970; Mishell *et al.*, 1970), those cells recovered in fractions known to contain macrophages were also able to support PFC responses in cultures of lymphoid cells, but were unable to develop significant responses when cultured alone. Macrophages separated from spleen cells from immunized and virgin mice support primary IgM responses by separated lymphoid cells from virgin mice with equal efficiency, suggesting that immunization does not lead to an augmentation of macrophage function (Cosenza *et al.*, 1971). All the experiments described above have examined the requirement for macrophages for development of primary IgM PFC responses to SRBC. Macrophages are also strictly required for development of primary IgG and IgA PFC responses to SRBC (Pierce, 1973) and for primary IgG PFC responses to GAT (Kapp *et al.*, 1973b).

Although there is now general agreement that macrophages are required for primary IgM, IgG, and IgA PFC responses to T cell-dependent antigens *in vitro*, the question exists, in some quarters, whether the active cells are phagocytic macrophages, or whether other cells with similar properties, except the ability to phagocytose, may be mediating the functions ascribed to macrophages. The dendritic cell of lymphoid follicles, which is not actively phagocytic, but which "traps" antigen so efficiently *in vivo* (Nossal and Ada, 1971), is a prime candidate, as is the novel cell in mouse spleen described by Steinman and Cohn (1974b). However, this argument may be more semantic than real, and formal proof of whether or not the only active cells are phagocytic is difficult. Usually 80% or more of the splenic adherent cells, as well as macrophages obtained by other separatory procedures, can be routinely observed to ingest various marker particles and are therefore phagocytic. Furthermore, peritoneal exudate cells from which actively phagocytic macrophages have been removed are much less efficient, on a cell to cell basis, in supporting antibody responses *in vitro* than are unseparated peritoneal exudate cells (Pierce *et al.*, 1974a). Thus, it appears unlikely, but not impossible, that the only active cell is among the nonphagocytic cells in the macrophage preparation. The answer to this question awaits further experimentation.

The requirement for macrophages for development of antibody responses *in vitro* by lymphoid cells from the spleens of previously immunized mice is still not completely resolved. Early experiments showed that after priming with antigen, lymphoid cells became less dependent on macrophages for the development of secondary antibody responses. This phenomenon was not manifested by lymphoid cells until 7 to 10 days after priming, but persisted for at least 1 year after a single injection of antigen (Pierce, 1969). Other investigators have confirmed these results in part, but have stressed the importance of cell density and the shape of the culture vessel in this phenomenon (Theis and Thorbecke, 1970; Katz and Unanue, 1973). Thus, in cultures with high cell density, either in dishes or tubes, this phenomenon is easier to observe. Other studies in which macrophages were rigorously depleted by glass bead columns followed by anti-macrophage serum and complement, showed that macrophages were required for the development of secondary antibody responses by lymphoid cells from primed mice (Feldmann and Palmer, 1971). Thus, the caution raised earlier about the macrophage-free nature of lymphoid cell preparations should be applied to this experimental situation. We still feel that lymphoid cells from immunized animals are "less dependent" on some macrophage functions for development of antibody responses *in vitro* than are lymphoid cells from virgin mice. Our reasons for this belief will be detailed in Section V,C.

D. Antibody Responses to T Cell-Independent Antigens

The first demonstrations that a differential requirement for macrophages in the development of antibody responses to T cell-dependent and T cell-independent antigens *in vitro* existed were the studies of Feldmann and Palmer (1971) and Shortman and Palmer (1971). They showed that lymphoid cells depleted of macrophages, although not able to respond to SRBC, developed normal responses to polymerized flagellin (POL). Subsequent studies have shown POL to be a T cell-independent antigen (Feldmann and Nossal, 1972). Other studies using the phosphorylcholine determinant of pneumococci (Rowley *et al.*, 1973), bacterial lipopolysaccharide (LPS) (Coutinho and Möller, 1975), and the hapten conjugates of LPS (Jacobs, 1975) or polysucrose (DNP-Ficoll) (Mosier *et al.*, 1974) (all of which are T cell-independent antigens), have shown that macrophage-depleted lymphoid cells develop antibody responses comparable to those in cultures of unseparated spleen cells. Thus, it would appear that antibody responses to these types of antigens, in addition to being T cell independent, are also "macrophage independent." (The requirement for macrophages in responses to T cell-independent antigens is discussed in greater detail by Rosenstreich and Oppenheim, Chapter 7.) It does seem prudent, however, to point out again the caution that lymphoid cell preparations are not macrophage-free. Indeed, in the studies of Shortman and Palmer (1971), the rigorous procedures of glass bead column filtration plus anti-macrophage serum used to deplete macrophages did result in a substantially lower antibody response to POL by the lymphoid cells. Thus, the development of antibody responses to T cell-independent antigens may require macrophages, but many fewer macrophages, i.e., those contaminating the lymphoid cells, may be sufficient for responses to these antigens, but not for responses to T cell-dependent antigens. This aspect of macrophage function clearly requires further critical evaluation.

V. FUNCTIONS OF MACROPHAGES IN ANTIBODY RESPONSES *IN VITRO*

A. Promotion of Lymphoid Cell Viability

In many experiments investigating the requirement for macrophages in the development of primary antibody responses to T cell-dependent antigens *in vitro,* lymphoid cells not only failed to develop PFC responses, but viable cell recovery in these cultures was much lower than in cultures of macrophages and lymphoid cells. These first clues that macrophages might be influencing the survival of lymphocytes in culture were not recorded in published works. Chen and Hirsch (1972) first described the "viability-promoting function" of macrophages and showed that the sulfhydryl reagent, 2-mercaptoethanol, appeared to substitute for macrophages in responses to SRBC by splenic lymphoid cells. They noted that peritoneal exudate macrophages and 2-mercaptoethanol not only enhanced the survival of lymphoid cells but both supported development of comparable PFC responses by these cells. In confirming these experiments (Pierce *et al.*, 1974a), we noted that addition of either 2-mercaptoethanol (5×10^{-5} *M*) or 10^5 macrophages (peritoneal exudate cells or splenic adherent cells) to cultures of 10^7 lymphoid cells resulted in approximately equivalent viable cell recovery on day 5 ($\sim 1.5 \times 10^6$ to 2.5×10^6 cells per culture). In contrast, viable cell recovery from cultures not supplemented with 2-mercaptoethanol or macrophages never exceeded 0.5×10^6 cells per culture, and significant PFC responses failed to develop. Furthermore, although cultures of lymphoid cells supplemented with 2-mercaptoethanol developed significant PFC responses, these responses were never quite comparable to those in cultures of macrophages and lymphoid cells. Thus, although 2-mercaptoethanol appeared to substitute effectively for macrophages in terms of promoting the viability of the lymphocytes in culture, it was clear to us that this reagent was not substituting for all functions of macrophages. This led us to investigate the function of macrophages in presentation of antigen to lymphocytes (Section V,B).

It is tempting to speculate that the viability-promoting function of macrophages is akin to a feeder layer effect. However, in a limited number of experiments, we have been unable to duplicate this function with mouse fibroblast or human embryonic lung monolayers. Furthermore, the observation that 2-mercaptoethanol enhances the viability of lymphoid cells suggests that a soluble factor elaborated by macrophages is responsible for the viability effect. Several investigators have shown that cell-free supernatant fluids from cultures of macrophages can partially or completely replace macrophages in the development of immune responses by purified lymphoid cells (Dutton *et al.*, 1970; Hoffmann and Dutton, 1971; Bach *et al.*, 1970). These factors have not been rigorously purified and characterized, but the difficulty of some investigators in confirming these observations suggests that these supernatant factors, like 2-mercaptoethanol, might be extremely labile (Pierce *et al.*, 1974a; Cosenza *et al.*, 1971).

Nevertheless, supernatant factors derived from cultures of peritoneal exudate macrophages do deserve further comment, not necessarily in connection with the viability-promoting function of macrophages, but because of their demonstrated involvement in regulation of expression of lymphocyte function. The adherent cells from peritoneal exudates—presumably macrophages—but not those from unstimulated peritoneal cavities, can replace POL or LPS in allowing spleen cells from athymic nude mice to respond to the T cell-dependent antigen, fowl gamma-globulin (FGG) *in vitro*. A trypsin-sensitive factor was present in the supernatant fluids of cultures of peritoneal exudate macrophages which could provide a non-antigen-specific "second signal" in the triggering of the B cells that had interacted with the FGG antigen. Since peritoneal exudate macrophages from nude mice could provide this factor, T cells were not considered to be an obligatory participant in the activation of the macrophages to produce this factor (Nossal and Schrader, 1975; Schrader, 1973). Human monocytes can also produce factors that enhance antibody responses to SRBC in mouse spleen cell cultures depleted of T cells (Wood and Gaul, 1974).

Calderon *et al.* (1975 have described a similar, and probably identical, factor(s) produced by peritoneal exudate macrophages, which has a molecular weight between 15,000 and 21,000 daltons and provides a nonspecific "second signal" to both primed and virgin B cells in IgM and IgG antibody responses to T cell-dependent antigens in cultures of whole or T cell-depleted spleen cells. This factor, however, is not restricted in its activity to influencing only B cell function; it also supports thymocyte proliferative responses to phytohemagglutinin, a mitogen to which thymocytes normally respond quite poorly.

Calderon *et al.* (1974) have also described a dialyzable, nonprotein, noncyclic nucleotide factor, produced by peritoneal exudate macrophages, which inhibits tumor cell proliferation and antibody responses to SRBC *in vitro*. Several investigators have observed that greater than 10^5 peritoneal exudate macrophages in cultures of 10^7 lymphoid cells suppress antibody responses. This type of inhibition may be the result of production of significant amounts of this low molecular weight proliferation-inhibiting material by the peritoneal macrophages. Immunoregulation by products of macrophages is discussed in detail by Nelson, Chapter 9.

Whether the macrophage factors, which nonspecifically enhance B cell responses to antigen, are related to the viability-promoting function of macrophages must await further experimentation. It is, however, worthwhile to consider which cell, the T cell or the B cell, might be the target of the viability-promoting function of macrophages. First, the survival of T cells in culture is affected most by the removal of macrophages (Dutton and Jacobs, 1973), and T cell responses *in vitro,* such as proliferative responses to allogeneic cells, antigen, or mitogens, are strictly dependent on the presence of macrophages in the cultures (Unanue, 1972). In contrast, antibody responses to T cell-independent antigens are not affected significantly by depletion of macrophages (Section IV,D). Furthermore, splenic lymphoid cells from primed mice are considerably less dependent on macrophages for the generation of secondary antibody responses to the priming antigen *in vitro*. However, primary antibody responses by these same cells to a second antigen are strictly dependent on macrophages (Pierce, 1969). Immunization expands the clones of T and B cells responsive to the antigen and may also affect the capacity of these cells to survive in macrophage-depleted cultures. However, one cannot tell from this experiment whether the T cell or B cell is affected. The fact that lymphoid cells from mice primed with ΦX174 virus develop TNP-specific PFC responses to TNP-ΦX comparable to the responses of the same lymphoid cells plus macrophages (Bluestein and Pierce, 1973) further indicates that immunization with the carrier moiety of the immunogen, ΦX, affects the ability of cells to survive in culture and, in this case, clearly indicates that the T cell is most affected. From this evidence, we conclude that the T cell is most critically dependent on the viability-promoting function of macrophages and that the requirement for macrophages in an immune response may reflect, in part, the requirement for optimal T cell function in that response.

B. Antigen Presentation

The involvement of macrophages in the presentation of antigen to lymphocytes for the initiation of antibody responses *in vivo* has been appreciated for several years; excellent review articles on this subject containing detailed analyses of the handling of antigens by macrophages are available (Cohn, 1968; Unanue, 1972; Nossal and Ada, 1971). In his original study, Mosier (1967) showed that macrophages, after a brief exposure to SRBC and removal of non-cell-bound SRBC, could support development of antibody responses by lymphoid cells *in vitro*. These experiments confirmed the earlier observations that lymphocytes, after interaction with antigen-treated macrophages, could develop antibody responses in an adoptive transfer system (Ford *et al.*, 1966). However, although these experiments suggested an antigen-presentation function for macrophages, the presence and contribution of non-macrophage-associated SRBC in the reaction mixtures made absolute conclusions difficult. Mosier's experiments gave the impression that the SRBC that stimulated the antibody response were phagocytized by the macrophages. However, treatment of macrophages, which had been briefly exposed to SRBC, with ammonium chloride abolished their capacity to stimulate PFC responses by the lymphoid cells (Leserman *et al.*, 1972; Pierce, 1973). This evidence raised the possibility that the relevant SRBC antigen(s) were extracellular and that active phagocytosis and processing of the antigen may not be essential. "Soluble SRBC antigens," capable of stimulating antibody responses in cultures of macrophage-depleted lymphoid cells, can be derived from incubation of SRBC with supernatant fluids from macrophage cultures (Shortman and Palmer, 1971). These experiments suggest that macrophages release factors that solubilize SRBC into antigens capable of stimulating antibody responses that do not require participation of macrophages. However, this process is quite inefficient inasmuch as the soluble SRBC antigen was about 25-fold less immunogenic than SRBC associated with the macrophages. The significance of these observations may be questionable, when one considers that incubation of SRBC with fetal calf serum (C. W. Pierce and J. A. Kapp, unpublished observations, 1975) or sonication of SRBC (Feldmann and Palmer, 1971) results in the release of similar "soluble SRBC" antigens. Although the precise function of macrophages with relation to processing and/or presentation of SRBC for antibody responses by lymphoid cells remains to be elucidated, most investigators would concede that macrophages have an important function in this regard. However, the difficulty in obtaining conclusive results using SRBC as the antigen has led investigators to probe antigen presentation functions of macrophages using proteins or hapten–protein conjugates as antigens.

An analysis of the role of macrophage-bound hapten–protein conjugates in the stimulation of secondary anti-hapten antibody responses *in vitro* demonstrated several of the salient features of the antigen presentation functions of macrophages (Katz and Unanue, 1973). Hapten–protein conjugates were effectively bound by macrophages in a highly immunogenic form in the absence of specific antibody to either the hapten or the protein. This macrophage-bound antigen was a very effective stimulus for development of secondary antibody responses; several thousandfold more of the soluble antigen was required to stimulate responses comparable to those stimulated by macrophage-bound antigen, which clearly favored development of secondary IgG antibody responses as compared with IgM antibody responses. Antigen bound to macrophages as immune complexes had no advantage over equivalent quantities of antigen directly attached to macrophages in stimulating secondary antibody responses. The observation that macrophages bearing the protein used for the primary immunization and that the hapten conjugated to an irrelevant protein failed to stimulate a secondary anti-hapten response emphasizes the critical importance of determinant presentation of hapten–protein conjugates in the stimulation of antibody responses (Unanue and Katz, 1973). Furthermore, although the efficiency of stimulation of lymphocytes was markedly enhanced by macrophage-bound antigen, lymphocytes could respond to soluble hapten–protein conjugates in macrophage-depleted cultures, suggesting, as discussed above (Section IV,C) that the development of antibody responses by primed lymphocytes may be less macrophage-dependent than responses by virgin lymphocytes.

Katz and Unanue (1973) concluded that the increased immunogenicity of macrophage-bound antigen reflected certain crucial, but undefined, features of the antigen–cell membrane complex, and not merely a stabilization of antigenic determinants on a relatively immobile surface. The stabilization of antigenic determinants by macrophages is believed by some investigators to result in the "polymerization" and increase in epitope density of the antigenic determinants which are critical for the stimulation of B cells (Feldmann and Nossal, 1972; Feldmann, 1974; Feldmann *et al.*, 1974a, 1975). In support of this contention, antigen "polymerized" on inert beads can stimulate antibody responses in a manner analogous to antigen on macrophages (Feldmann *et al.*, 1974b). However, since this is not a universally repeatable phenomenon (Katz and Unanue, 1973), more critical evaluation of the variables involved is necessary before definitive conclusions can be drawn.

The foregoing experiments investigating the antigen presentation functions of macrophages in secondary antibody responses to hapten–protein conjugates have the theoretical drawback that responses by primed lymphoid cells are less dependent on macrophages than are responses by virgin lymphoid cells. Many investigators have attempted to stimulate primary antibody responses *in vitro* with hapten–protein conjugates or soluble proteins, but few have had long-term success in this endeavor.

One exception to this otherwise dismal experience has been experiments using GAT as the antigen (Kapp *et al.*, 1973a). These experiments will also be discussed in Section VI in the context of the role of macrophages in antibody responses to antigens controlled by *H-2*-linked *Ir* genes. The primary antibody response to GAT in cultures of spleen cells from responder strains of mice is comparable in terms of GAT dose requirements, magnitude, kinetics, and Ig class to responses in the spleen after *in vivo* immunization. This antigen stimulates only IgG GAT-specific PFC responses; no IgM PFC have been detected either *in vivo* or *in vitro* by the assay methods employed (Kapp *et al.*, 1973a). Furthermore, primary antibody responses to GAT are strictly dependent on the presence of macrophages and T cells in the cultures (Kapp *et al.*, 1973b). This antigen has been extremely useful in exploring antigen presentation functions of macrophages in the development of primary antibody responses *in vitro.*

To probe this question directly, we compared the responses stimulated by the optimal dose of soluble GAT (10 μg/culture) and macrophage-bound GAT in cultures of splenic lymphoid cells from responder strains of mice (Pierce *et al.*, 1974a). GAT, trace labeled with ^{125}I, was reacted with extensively washed peritoneal exudate macrophages in the cold for 30 minutes (100 μg GAT per 2×10^6 cells/ml). After further extensive washing, the amount of GAT bound per 7×10^4 macrophages was determined and a known amount of GAT bound to a known number of macrophages was added to the lymphoid cell cultures. In numerous experiments, these reaction conditions resulted in approximately 1.5 ng GAT per 7×10^4 macrophages. The amount of GAT bound by 7×10^4 macrophages is directly related to the concentration of GAT per 10^6 macrophages in the reaction mixture up to 50 μg GAT per 10^6 macrophages; greater than 50 μg GAT per 10^6 macrophages does not result in significantly greater uptake of GAT. The binding of GAT by macrophages at 4° and 37°C is equivalent, and the absence of serum from the reaction mixture does not affect the uptake of GAT. The optimum reaction time is 30 minutes; longer reaction times result in no increase in GAT uptake, and shorter reaction times result in less uptake.

Experiments using GAT bound to macrophages clearly demonstrated an antigen presentation function for macrophages in the development of primary antibody responses *in vitro* (Pierce *et al.*, 1974a). Macrophage-bound GAT was a significantly more efficient immunogen than soluble GAT; 10 μg of soluble GAT stimulated optimal PFC responses *in vitro*, whereas comparable responses were stimulated by 1.5 ng GAT bound to 7×10^4 macrophages (6667 times less GAT!). The detailed analyses performed by Katz and Unanue (1973) of secondary antibody responses have not been repeated compulsively for primary responses to GAT, but where such experiments have been carried out the results are comparable. Thus, the efficiency of macrophage-bound antigen in stimulating primary and secondary antibody responses *in vitro* is similar.

One parameter that has been investigated in detail, however, is the role of antigen released from macrophages in the stimulation of antibody responses (Pierce and Kapp, 1975). Briefly, macrophages are pulsed with GAT as outlined above and, after extensive washing, are incubated for 24 hours before addition to cultures of splenic lymphoid cells. These macrophages release 75 to 90% of the initially bound [^{125}I]GAT into the culture supernatant fluid; approximately 50% of the ^{125}I is still associated with GAT. However, this antigen, released from macrophages, in concentrations up to 0.1 μg per culture, does not stimulate antibody responses by separated splenic lymphoid cells or unseparated spleen cells. It is not practical to attempt to recover GAT in quantities such that more than 0.1 μg can be added to cultures. Further, 0.1 μg GAT is the lowest dose of soluble GAT that routinely stimulates antibody responses *in vitro* (Kapp *et al.*, 1973a). In contrast, the recovered macrophages, which now have only approximately 0.1 ng GAT per 7×10^4 macrophages, stimulate PFC responses by lymphoid cells which are comparable in magnitude to those stimulated by 7×10^4 freshly pulsed macrophages bearing approximately 1.5 ng GAT. Furthermore, similar results have been obtained with macrophages added to lymphoid cell cultures 7 days after pulsing with GAT. These experiments indicate that GAT released from macrophages is no more immunogenic than native GAT, but that the GAT retained by macrophages is highly immunogenic and stable for prolonged periods. These results are entirely consistent with those reported by Unanue (1972) using antigen-pulsed macrophages in *in vivo* transfer systems. The relevance of these observations will be more apparent in Section VI where genetic restrictions for interactions among macrophages and lymphoid cells will be discussed.

C. Relationship of Viability-Promoting and Antigen Presentation Functions of Macrophages

In the two preceding sections, we have discussed the evidence for a viability-promoting function and an antigen presentation function for macrophages in the development of antibody responses to T cell-dependent antigens *in vitro*. The evidence is overwhelming, to us at least, that macrophages have an antigen presentation function in both primary and secondary antibody responses *in vitro*. Also clear is the evidence for a viability-promoting function, probably for T cells, in, at the very least, the primary antibody response *in vitro*. How then does one relate these two diverse and seemingly unrelated functions of macrophages which are clearly so critical for the development of antibody responses, especially primary antibody responses?

Although 2-mercaptoethanol appears to completely replace the necessity for macrophage function in the development of primary antibody responses to T cell-dependent antigens *in vitro*, it should be emphasized again that even the most meticulously prepared splenic lymphoid cells, which develop no antibody response, are not "macrophage-free." Since nanogram quantities of macrophage-bound antigen stimulate antibody responses comparable to those stimulated by microgram quantities of soluble antigen, it is conceivable that the macrophages contaminating the lymphoid cell preparations are sufficient for the antigen presentation function, but not for the viability-promoting function. Hence, no response develops in these cultures even in the presence of optimal concentrations of antigen because a required cell, probably the T cell, does not survive long enough to carry out its functions. However, if 2-mercaptoethanol supplies the viability-promoting factor(s), then, in concert with the antigen presented by the contaminating macrophages, the appropriate milieu for development of an antibody response by the lymphoid cells is established, and the mechanism by which 2-mercaptoethanol appears to replace the need for macrophages in lymphoid cell cultures is explained. This explanation may be simplistic, but has merit when all the data are considered, including some preliminary data which directly support it. (Pierce and Kapp, 1975).

D. The Macrophage as a Focus for T Cell–B Cell Interaction?

This controversial aspect of macrophage function has received considerable attention in the literature and in this book (Basten and Mitchell, Chapter 3). At the crux of this controversy is a fundamental conceptual difference among various investigators as to the precise sequence of events in the initiation of the antibody response. One view has macrophage-bound antigen triggering specific T cells that, after activation, regulate the expression of the B cell response to the antigen (Katz and Unanue, 1973; Katz and Benacerraf, 1972; Unanue, 1972). The other view favors the concept that antigen first activates T cells that release a unique T cell immunoglobulin, IgT, which is cytophilic for macrophages. The IgT, after binding to macrophages, complexes antigen in a polymeric form that efficiently stimulates B cells (Feldmann and Nossal, 1972; Feldmann, 1974; Feldmann *et al.*, 1974a, 1975). Although the authors favor the former sequence of events, further investigation is definitely necessary to resolve this crucial issue. In this section, we will discuss the importance and nature of cell interactions and cell clusters in the development of primary antibody responses *in vitro.*

During the first 48 hours of culture, interactions among macrophages, T cells, B cells, and antigen are an absolute requirement for development of optimal antibody responses; removal of macrophages, T cells, or antigen during this interval significantly reduces antibody responses to T cell-dependent antigens such as SRBC (Feldmann, 1972; Claman and Mosier, 1972; Pierce, 1973). Furthermore, incubation of the cultures for 5 days on a stationary platform, which minimizes cell cluster formation and cell interactions, also greatly reduces the antibody response (Mishell and Dutton, 1967; Mosier, 1969; Pierce and Benacerraf, 1969; Pierce, 1973).

However, macrophages are required for only the first 48 hours of culture for the development of maximal primary IgM, IgG, and IgA antibody responses *in vitro.* Thereafter, lymphoid cells, which have been depleted of macrophages to the extent that they are incapable of developing a primary antibody response to a second antigen, develop antibody responses comparable to those in cultures from which macrophages have not been depleted. Furthermore, these separated lymphoid cells develop antibody responses in stationary cultures where cluster formation and cell interactions are greatly reduced. From these experiments, it was reasoned that after 48 hours incubation with macrophages and antigen, the lymphoid cells (and primarily the B cells) had been activated to a state where they could undergo the final cycles of cell division and differentiation into mature antibody-producing cells outside cell clusters and without the influences of macrophages (Pierce, 1973).

Cell clusters composed of lymphocytes around macrophages develop rapidly after initiation of Mishell–Dutton cultures (Mosier, 1969; Pierce and Benacerraf, 1969; Claman and Mosier, 1972; Pierce, 1973). Based on the requirements for cell interactions, it was predicted that if these cell clusters were isolated at an interval shortly after culture initiation (e.g., 24 hours) and incubated separately, the entire capability for developing a PFC response would be found in these cell clusters. Several investigators using other experimental systems have shown that clusters of macrophages and lymphocytes are critical for initiation of immune responses (Unanue, 1972; Claman and Mosier, 1972; Werdelin *et al.*, 1974; Lipsky and Rosenthal, 1975). Thus, this prediction seemed sound on both experimental and teleological grounds. However, cell clusters isolated during the first 48 hours after culture initiation and subsequently incubated separately developed only minimal PFC responses despite the presence of an adequate number of macrophages, T cells, and B cells in the clusters. The entire capability for developing PFC responses was recovered in the fraction composed of single, nonclustered cells (McIntyre and Pierce, 1973b). Thus, although interactions among macrophages, T cells, and B cells during the first 48 hours of culture are an absolute requirement for development of antibody responses, these interactions do not occur in tightly formed permanent cell clusters. Rather, these interactions appear to take place on a transient basis, with the relevant cells constantly coming and going from clusters and thus resident in the clusters for only brief periods. On days 3 and 4 after culture initiation, progressively more of the capability for developing PFC responses was recovered in the cell clusters. The fact that these cells developed PFC responses when incubated on a stationary platform after disruption of the isolated clusters suggested that residence of cells in clusters at these times was more a matter of convenience than necessity. Indeed, many of the PFC in a culture are in clusters but the majority exist as single cells. Since the PFC in clusters are not clonally restricted with respect to Ig class or antigenic specificity (McIntyre and Pierce, 1973a), these clusters appear to be nonspecific, random aggregates of cells that do not form as the result of any known specific immunologic phenomena.

From these data, it would appear that although cell interactions are essential for the development of antibody responses *in vitro*, such interactions do not occur in permanently established cell clusters, but rather occur in a highly dynamic and transient fashion among macrophages, T cells, and B cells that prefer to exist as independent isolated cells.

VI. IMMUNOGENETIC CONSIDERATIONS OF MACROPHAGE FUNCTIONS IN ANTIBODY RESPONSES *IN VITRO*

A. The Role of Macrophages in Antibody Responses to Antigens Controlled by *H-2*-Linked *Ir* Genes

We have previously introduced the concept that antibody responses to certain antigens, such as GAT, are controlled by *Ir* genes which map in the *I* region of the *H-2* complex of mice. Antibody responses to GAT by spleen cells *in vitro* follow the same genetic restrictions as serological responses in immunized mice. Spleen cells from responder strains of mice develop IgG GAT-specific PFC responses *in vitro* to both GAT and GAT-MBSA, whereas spleen cells from nonresponder strains of mice develop responses to only GAT-MBSA (Kapp *et al.*, 1973a). Thus, B cells are not the site of expression of the genetic defect, since GAT-specific PFC responses develop in cultures of nonresponder spleen cells stimulated with GAT-MSBA (Kapp *et al.,* 1973b).

We asked the question: Are macrophages the site of the genetic defect in nonresponder spleen cells? When macrophages and lymphoid cells from responder and nonresponder mice are cultured in syngeneic combinations, all cultures respond to SRBC and GAT-MBSA, but only cultures of responder cells respond to GAT. When allogeneic combinations of macrophages and lymphoid cells are used, all cultures develop responses to SRBC and GAT-MBSA, which are comparable to those in cultures of syngeneic combinations. Macrophages from responder mice do not confer the ability to develop GAT-specific PFC responses to GAT on lymphoid cells from nonresponder mice, whereas macrophages from nonresponder mice support development of normal responses to GAT by responder lymphoid cells (Kapp *et al.,* 1973b).

However, since lymphoid cell preparations are not macrophage-free, it could be argued that, in the preceding experiment, the nonresponder macrophages support the viability of the responder lymphoid cells, but the few contaminating responder macrophages actually present GAT in a manner that stimulates development of antibody responses by the responder lymphoid cells. To explore this possibility directly, we pulsed macrophages from nonresponder and responder mice with GAT. Both responder and nonresponder macrophages bearing approximately 1.5 ng GAT per 7×10^4 macrophages stimulate comparable PFC responses by responder lymphoid cells; neither type of GAT-bearing macrophage stimulate responses by nonresponder lymphoid cells. These observations make it highly unlikely that relevant GAT is transferred from nonresponder macrophages to macrophages contaminating the responder lymphoid cells to stimulate the antibody response (see also Sections V,B and VI,B). All of these data strongly indicate that responder and nonresponder macrophage function with regard to GAT is the same and that the macrophage is not the site of the genetic defect in nonresponder spleen cells (Kapp *et al.,* 1973b). Thus, responsiveness to GAT is determined by the genotype of the lymphoid cells, and, more specifically, by the genotype of the T cells (Kapp *et al.,* 1975a).

The defect in genetic nonresponder spleen cells appears to be the failure of GAT-specific T cells to provide effective helper function for responses to GAT by B cells (Kapp *et al.,* 1974, 1975a). However, GAT bound to macrophages can, in some instances, circumvent this defect; such macrophages stimulate development of GAT-specific helper T cells *in vivo* in nonresponder mice, which mediate "normal helper functions" in antibody responses to GAT-MBSA by B cells *in vitro* (Kapp, *et al.,* 1975b).

Further experiments are required to elucidate the precise mechanisms involved. However, it seems clear to us that although the T cell may be responsible for the defect in genetic nonresponder mice, the macrophage may play a crucial role in the expression of this defect, and the antigen presentation function of macrophages may be the key that opens the lock on some of the mysteries of *Ir* gene control of antibody responses.

B. Lack of Genetic Restrictions for Interactions among Macrophages and Lymphoid Cells in Antibody Responses

Recent experiments probing the mechanisms of interactions among T cells and B cells have suggested that these cells must share membrane antigens encoded by the *I* region of the *H-2* complex for efficient physiologic interactions to occur (Benacerraf and Katz, 1975). Similar genetic restrictions do not appear to be operative in regulating effective interactions among macrophages and lymphoid cells in the development of primary antibody responses *in vitro*.

Several investigators have demonstrated that lymphoid cells develop comparable antibody responses when incubated with antigen and syngeneic or allogeneic macrophages (Hartmann *et al.*, 1970; Haskill *et al.*, 1970; Shortman and Palmer, 1971; Cosenza and Leserman, 1972; Katz and Unanue, 1973; Kapp *et al.*, 1973b; Pierce *et al.*, 1974b). Allogeneic macrophages were used to support PFC responses in cultures of lymphoid cells to show that the latter population contained the precursors of the PFC (Hartmann *et al.*, 1970; Shortman and Palmer, 1971) and to determine the time requirement for macrophages in the generation of antibody responses (Cosenza and Leserman, 1972).

This question has been approached more directly by using macrophages bearing nanogram quantities of GAT. As described earlier, allogeneic, nonresponder macrophages pulsed with GAT supported development of antibody responses by responder lymphoid cells that were comparable to those which developed in the presence of syngeneic macrophages (Section VI,A).

However, at least three objections can be raised to these experiments. First, the strain combinations used shared specificities in the *I* region of the *H-2* complex and therefore were not absolutely allogeneic. These experiments have been repeated using macrophages and lymphoid cells which are not known to share any specificities in the *H-2* complex. The results were identical with previous experiments; allogeneic and syngeneic macrophages bearing GAT supported comparable responses. Second, it could be argued that antigen released from allogeneic macrophages during the first few hours of culture was transferred to the ubiquitous macrophages in the lymphoid cell population where it acted as the effective stimulating antigen. However, allogeneic macrophages (which had been pulsed with GAT, washed extensively, incubated 24 hours to allow for the release of 75% or more of the bound GAT, and washed extensively again) stimulated antibody responses in cultures of lymphoid cells which were comparable to those stimulated by identically treated or freshly pulsed syngeneic macrophages. Furthermore, allogeneic macrophages, incubated for 7 days after pulsing with GAT, were as efficient as freshly pulsed syngeneic macrophages in stimulating antibody responses. Thus, transfer of antigen from allogeneic to syngeneic macrophages does not appear to account for the pnenomenon. Third, the allogeneic macrophages could stimulate a mixed lymphocyte reaction in the lymphoid cell population resulting in the release of nonspecific stimulating products that enhance an otherwise minimal antibody response (Katz and Benacerraf, 1975). However, allogeneic and syngeneic macrophages stimulated comparable DNA synthetic responses by lymphoid cells, and experiments where allogeneic and syngeneic macrophages were mixed in varying ratios with lymphoid cells provided no evidence that a mixed lymphocyte reaction and its nonspecific stimulatory products were involved in the stimulation of antibody responses by allogeneic macrophages (Pierce and Kapp, 1975).

All the data available at this time indicate that allogeneic macrophages are as effective as syngeneic macrophages in stimulating antibody responses by mouse lymphoid cells *in vitro*. However, this does not appear to be the case in other types of immune responses; in the guinea pig, macrophages and T cells apparently must be syngeneic for successful development of DNA synthetic responses to antigen (Rosenthal and Shevach, 1973; Shevach and Rosenthal, 1973). These differences in the requirements for syngenicity of macrophages and responding lymphoid cells may depend on which type of lymphoid cell response is being measured and its sensitivity to activation. For DNA synthetic responses by T cells, it may be that macrophages and lymphoid cells must be syngeneic for optimal activation of T cells to proceed. Similarly, for antibody responses by B cells, it may be that T cells and B cells must be syngeneic for effective triggering of B cells to occur (Benacerraf and Katz, 1975; Katz and Benacerraf, 1975). However, allogeneic macrophages may be able to activate T cells sufficiently for their effective cooperation with syngeneic B cells in antibody responses, but not for development of optimal DNA synthetic responses. Resolution of these apparent differences must await the development of culture systems that support antibody responses by guinea pig lymphoid cells and DNA synthetic responses to antigen by murine T cells. However, one indication of a requirement for syngenicity between macrophages and T cells in the development of a T cell response in the mouse comes from studies of the generation of antigen-specific helper T cells *in vitro*. Apparently, in this system, helper T cells are only generated in the presence of syngeneic macrophages (Feldmann *et al.*, 1975). This crucial observation requires confirmation.

C. Role of Macrophages in Suppression of Antibody Responses by Alloantisera against Leukocyte Alloantigens

The experiments discussed in the preceding section indicate that no genetic restrictions exist for interactions among macrophages and lymphoid cells in the development of antibody response *in vitro*. That is not to say, however, that antigens encoded by the *H-2* gene complex and other histocompatibility antigens are not important in these interactions.

Antisera against leukocyte alloantigens can suppress the development of antibody responses to SRBC and GAT by mouse spleen cells *in vitro*. The suppression was not due to cytotoxicity of the alloantisera on the spleen cells or anti-immunoglobulin activity in the sera. The suppression was directly related to the amount of antiserum added to the cultures and was specific for spleen cells against which the sera were directed. The alloantisera suppressed PFC responses most effectively when present during the first 24 hours of incubation. Although not rendering the spleen cells incapable of developing PFC responses after removal of non-cell-bound antibody, the alloantisera did act by interfering with successful initiation of the PFC responses, probably by interfering with essential interactions among macrophages, T cells, and B cells (Pierce *et al.*, 1974b).

Alloantisera against the θ antigen on T cells and antigens encoded by the *D* region of the *H*-2 complex did not suppress antibody responses *in vitro*. These observations eliminated the possibility that the alloantisera suppressed PFC responses in a nonspecific manner by combining with membrane alloantigens on the responding spleen cells and producing membrane perturbations that precluded the development of an antibody response (Pierce *et al.*, 1974b). Antisera against non-H-2 antigens and antigens encoded by the *K* region of the *H-2* complex suppressed primary IgM and IgG PFC responses. These antisera act at the level of the macrophage and interfere with cell interactions, which are fundamental to the development of antibody responses of all immunoglobulin classes. In contrast, antisera against antigens encoded by the *I* region of the *H-2* complex selectively suppressed IgG antibody responses and acted on the lymphoid cells and not macrophages (Pierce *et al.*, 1974b, 1975). It is likely that these antisera are interfering in some manner, still to be defined, with effective interactions between T cells and B cells.

After brief exposure to specific alloantiserum, lymphoid cells rapidly recovered the ability to develop antibody responses, once the antiserum had been removed and a functional macrophage population was provided. In contrast, macrophages, after a brief exposure to alloantiserum, were unable to support the development of antibody responses by normal lymphoid cells. This inactivation of macrophage function was not the result of the death of macrophages, the inability of the macrophages to support lymphoid cell survival, or to bind soluble GAT. Thus, alloantiserum-treated macrophages bearing normal amounts of GAT and capable of supporting lymphoid cell survival were unable to stimulate an antibody response by lymphoid cells (Pierce *et al.*, 1974b). It is possible that the membranes of the antigen-bearing macrophages must have a "freedom of movement" to effectively stimulate the lymphoid cells and that the alloantiserum restricts freedom. It is also possible that the alloantiserum interferes with the antigen processing cycle distal to the initial uptake of the antigen. Thus, endocytosis, degradation in phagolysosomes, or the return of the antigen to the cell membrane could be affected by alloantiserum. Finally, although syngenicity between macrophages and lymphoid cells is not necessary for development of antibody responses, the alloantiserum could interfere with the sites on the macrophage where the actual interactions take place. It is clear from our current ignorance about the mechanisms involved in this phenomenon that further investigations are required.

VII. CONCLUSIONS, PRESENT STATE OF THE ART, AND THE FUTURE

In this chapter, we have reviewed the functions of macrophages in the development of antibody responses in tissue culture. Two important factors should be kept in mind when considering the functions of macrophages. First, macrophages are a heterogeneous population of cells that share morphological and functional properties, but they are by no means uniform in either of these respects. Second, although relatively pure populations of macrophages can readily be prepared, it is exceedingly difficult to obtain macrophage-free lymphocyte preparations.

The requirement for macrophages for development of primary antibody responses to complex, multideterminant, T cell-dependent antigens is now firmly established. The requirement for macrophages for development of secondary antibody responses to these antigens appears to be less than for primary responses, but this may depend on the culture system employed. Macrophages do not appear to be required for development of antibody responses to so-called T cell-independent antigens, but this observation must be confirmed with several of these antigens before it becomes a firmly established fact.

Macrophages have at least two crucial functions in the development of primary antibody responses to T cell-dependent antigens *in vitro*. One function is the presentation of antigen to the responding T cells and B cells in a manner that efficiently stimulates these cells to cooperate in the development of an antibody response. The second function is a viability-promoting function that can be duplicated by 2-mercaptoethanol. This function of macrophages is probably most crucial for T cells and enables these cells to survive the initial phases of the culture and mediate their cooperative interactions with B cells. Macrophages also release soluble products that can inhibit or enhance antibody responses *in vitro*. The characterization of these enhancing and suppressing factors and the definition of their mechanism(s) of action is, to us, one of the most exciting areas of current research on macrophage function. In the next few years, much more information about these factors should become available and a more coherent and integrated view of their contribution to macrophage function in initiation and regulation of antibody response *in vitro* should be possible. Further, macrophages may be the focus for interactions among T cells, B cells, and antigen, which are so crucial for the initiation of the antibody response. However, these crucial interactions do not occur in permanent cell clusters, but appear to transpire in small, short-lived, dynamic aggregates of cells.

Macrophages are not the site of expression of the genetic defect that is responsible for the failure of nonresponder spleen cells to develop antibody responses to antigens controlled by *H-2* linked *Ir* genes. Furthermore, although antigens encoded by the *H-2* gene complex appear to be important in mediating interactions among macrophages, T cells, and B cells, no genetic restrictions appear to exist for effective interactions between macrophages and lymphoid cells in primary antibody responses.*

Although it may appear that no questions remain to be answered in the realm of macrophage function in the development of antibody responses *in vitro*, do not be decieved and turn away, for many problems must still be solved. A definitive and foolproof, as well as idiot-proof, procedure for obtaining macrophage-free lymphocyte preparations must be perfected. The question of the requirement for macrophages in antibody responses to T cell-independent antigens must be resolved. The biochemical nature and mechanisms of action of the myriad of pharmaco-

* For a seemingly different view based on experiments with guinea pigs, see Rosenthal *et al.*, Chapter 6. Note also the *caveat*, in Section IV,A of this Chapter.—Ed.

logical agents released by macrophages remain to be clarified, as does the mechanism by which macrophages promote or sustain the viability of the lymphoid cells in culture. The details of mechanisms involved in antigen presentation by macrophages and an explanation of how macrophages function as the focus for cell interactions without formation of permanent cell clusters await a clever experimentalist. The mechanisms of successful macrophage–allogeneic lymphoid cell interaction and mechanisms by which antisera against antigens on macrophages can suppress antibody responses must still be elucidated. There are undoubtedly problems that we have not foreseen and questions that we are too ignorant even to ask, but if we continue to proceed in an orderly and logical fashion, the relevant questions will eventually be asked and the mystery of the macrophage will eventually be solved.

VIII. NOTE ADDED IN PROOF

In the brief interval since this Chapter was written, new information relevant to some aspects of macrophage function in antibody responses *in vitro,* which deserve comment, has been obtained.

Mosier *et al.* (1974; see also Chapter 2) have reported that macrophages are not required for primary antibody responses to the T cell-independent antigen, DNP–Ficoll. In experiments designed to take advantage of this observation, we have been unable to demonstrate that the antibody response to this antigen is "macrophage-independent." Rather, responses to DNP–Ficoll are less dependent on macrophages than responses to SRBC. D. E. Mosier (personal communication, see also footnotes in Chapter 2), using preparations of DNP–Ficoll other than the one used in the original studies, has had similar experiences. Thus, the discussion in Section IV,D that antibody responses to T cell-independent antigens may require fewer macrophages than responses to T cell-dependent antigens appears to be valid. Only further experimentation with several T cell-independent antigens will elucidate the role of macrophages in antibody responses to these antigens.

In Section VI,B, we discussed the lack of genetic restrictions for interactions among macrophages and lymphoid cells in the development of antibody responses by murine cells. It should be stressed that with one exception (Katz and Unanue, 1973) the experiments discussed involved primary antibody responses. However, we have recently obtained evidence that lymphoid cells from previously immunized mice develop secondary responses *in vitro* only in the presence of macrophages that were used for the primary immunization. For example, lymphoid cells from C57BL/6 mice, which have been immunized with GAT or GAT bound to C57BL/6 macrophages, develop anti-GAT PFC responses only in the presence of C57BL/6 macrophages bearing GAT. Lymphoid cells from C57BL/6 mice, which have been immunized with allogenic DBA/1 macrophages bearing GAT, develop anti-GAT antibody responses when incubated with GAT bearing DBA/1 macrophages, but not when incubated with syngeneic C57BL/6 macrophages bearing comparable amounts of GAT. Thus, in secondary antibody responses *in vitro,* genetic restrictions governing interactions among macrophages and lymphoid cells are apparent; primed lymphoid cells appear to respond only in the presence of those macrophages that presented antigen to the lymphoid cells to initiate the "priming" process. Further preliminary evidence suggests that it is the T cell, not the B cell, in the primed lymphoid cell population which is critically dependent upon stimulation by macrophages of the genotype used for priming. This restriction in secondary antibody responses *in vitro* is clearly analogous to the genetic restrictions that govern macrophage–T cell interactions in antigen-induced DNA synthetic responses by primed guinea pig lymphoid cells *in vitro* (Rosenthal *et al.*, Chapter 6). It may be a general phenomenon that primed T cells can respond only in the presence of macrophages that are genotypically similar to those that presented antigen to the T cells in the priming process. Further experimentation is necessary to define the parameters of these genetic restrictions, but such experiments should clarify many of the unresolved questions about the roles of macrophages in antibody responses.

ACKNOWLEDGMENTS

The investigations of the authors and collaborators that are cited are supported by United States Public Health Service Research Grants AI-09897 and AI-09920 from the National Institute of Allergy and Infectious Diseases. Dr. Pierce is the recipient of Research Career Development Award 5-KO4-AI-70173 from the National Institue of Allergy and Infectious Diseases. The patient and excellent secretarial assistance of Ms. Deborah Siner is greatly appreciated.

We apologize to any investigators whose contributions to our understanding of the functions of macrophages in the development of antibody responses *in vitro* have been overlooked in this chapter.

REFERENCES

Bach, F. H., Alter, B. J. Solliday, S., Zoschke, D. C., and Janis, M. (1970). *Cell. Immunol.* **1,** 219–227.

Benacerraf, B., and Green, I. (1969). *Annu. Rev. Med.* **20,** 141–155.

Benacerraf, B., and Katz, D. H. (1975). *Advan. Cancer Res.* **21**, 121–174.
Bluestein, H. G., and Pierce, C. W. (1973). *J. Immunol.* **111**, 137–143.
Calderon, J., Williams, R. T., and Unanue, E. R. (1974). *Proc. Nat. Acad. Sci. U.S.* **71**, 4273–4277.
Calderon, J., Keily, J. M., Lefko, J., and Unanue, E. R. (1975). *J. Exp. Med.* **142**, 151–164.
Chen, C., and Hirsch, J. G. (1972). *J. Exp. Med.* **136**, 604–617.
Claman, H. N., and Mosier, D. E. (1972). *Progr. Allergy* **16**, 40–80.
Cohn, Z. A. (1968). *Advan. Immunol.* **9**, 163–214.
Cosenza, H., and Leserman, L. D. (1972). *J. Immunol.* **108**, 418–424.
Cosenza, H., Leserman, L. D., and Rowley, D. A. (1971). *J. Immunol.* **107**, 414–421.
Coutinho, A., and Möller, G. (1975). *Advan. Immunol.* **21**, 114–228.
Dutton, R. W., and Jacobs, D. (1973). *Fed. Proc., Fed. Amer. Soc. Exp. Biol.* **32**, 973.
Dutton, R. W., McCarthy, M., Mishell, R. I., and Raidt, D. J. (1970). *Cell. Immunol.* **1**, 196–206.
Ebert, R. H., and Grant, L. (1974). *In* "The Inflammatory Process" (B. W. Zweifach, L. Grant, and R. T. McCluskey, eds.), 2nd ed., Vol. 1, pp. 4–52. Academic Press, New York.
Feldmann, M. (1972). *J. Exp. Med.* **134**, 1049–1058.
Feldmann, M. (1974). *Contemp. Top. Mol. Immunol.* **3**, 57–111.
Feldmann, M., and Nossal, G. J. V. (1972). *Transplant. Rev.* **13**, 3–34.
Feldmann, M., and Palmer, J. (1971). *Immunology* **21**, 685–699.
Feldmann, M., Basten, A., Boylston, A., Erb, P., Gorczynski, R., Greaves, M., Hogg, N., Kilburn, D., Kontiainen, S., Parker, D., Pepys, M., and Schrader, J. (1974a). *In* "Progress in Immunology II, Volume III, Biological Aspects II" (L. Brent and J. Holbrow, eds.), pp. 65–76. North-Holland Publ., Amsterdam.
Feldmann, M., Greaves, M. F., Parker, D. C., and Rittenberg, M. B. (1974b). *Eur. J. Immunol.* **4**, 591–597.
Feldmann, M., Gorczynski, R., Erb, P., and Desaymard, C. (1975). *In* "Immune Recognition" (A. S. Rosenthal, ed.), pp. 755–769. Academic Press, New York.
Forbes, I. J. (1969). *Immunology* **6**, 699–706.
Ford, W. L., Gowans, J. L., and McCullagh, P. J. (1966). *Thymus: Exp. Clin. Stud., Ciba Found. Symp., 1965* pp. 58–78.
Gershon, R. K. (1974). *Contemp. Top. Immunobiol.* **3**, 1–43.
Gorczynski, R. M., Miller, R. G., and Phillips, R. A. (1971). *J. Exp. Med.* **134**, 1201–1221.
Gordon, S., and Cohn, Z. A. (1973). *Int. Rev. Cytol.* **36**, 171–215.
Hartmann, K., Dutton, R. W., McCarthy, M., and Mishell, R. I. (1970). *Cell. Immunol.* **1**, 182–189.
Haskill, J. S., Byrt, P., and Marbrook, J. (1970). *J. Exp. Med.* **131**, 57–76.
Hoffmann, M. (1970). *Immunology* **18**, 791–798.
Hoffmann, M., and Dutton, R. W. (1971). *Science* **172**, 1047–1048.
Jacobs, D. (1975). *J. Immunol.* **114**, 365–370.
Jerne, N. K., Henry, C., Nordin, A. A., Fuji, H., Koros, A. M. C., and Lefkowitz, I. (1974). *Transplant. Rev.* **18**, 130–191.
Kapp, J. A., Pierce, C. W., and Benacerraf, B. (1973a). *J. Exp. Med.* **138**, 1107–1120.
Kapp, J. A., Pierce, C. W., and Benacerraf, B. (1973b). *J. Exp. Med.* **138**, 1121–1132.
Kapp, J. A., Pierce, C. W., Schlossmann, S. F., and Benacerraf, B. (1974). *J. Exp. Med.* **140**, 648–659.

Kapp, J. A., Pierce, C. W., and Benacerraf, B. (1975a). *In* "Immune Recognition" (A. S. Rosenthal, ed.), pp. 667–682. Academic Press, New York.
Kapp, J. A., Pierce, C. W., and Benacerraf, B. (1975b). *J. Exp. Med.* **142,** 50–60.
Katz, D. H., and Benacerraf, B. (1972). *Advan. Immunol.* **15,** 1–94.
Katz, D. H., and Benacerraf, B. (1975). *Transplant. Rev.* **22,** 175–195.
Katz, D. H., and Unanue, E. R. (1973). *J. Exp. Med.* **137,** 967–990.
Kettman, J., and Dutton, R. W. (1971). *Proc. Nat. Acad. Sci. U.S.* **68,** 199–203.
Leserman, L. D., Cosenza, H., and Roseman, J. M. (1972). *J. Immunol.* **109,** 587–594.
Lipsky, P. E., and Rosenthal, A. S. (1975). *J. Exp. Med.* **141,** 138–154.
Ly, I., and Mishell, R. I. (1974). *J. Immunol. Methods* **5,** 239–248.
McIntyre, J. A., and Pierce, C. W. (1973a). *J. Immunol.* **111,** 512–519.
McIntyre, J. A., and Pierce, C. W. (1973b). *J. Immunol.* **111,** 1526–1537.
Marbrook, J. (1967). *Lancet* **2,** 1279–1281.
Miller, R. G., and Phillips, R. A. (1970). *Proc. Soc. Exp. Biol. Med.* **135,** 63–67.
Mishell, R. I., and Dutton, R. W. (1967). *J. Exp. Med.* **126,** 423–442.
Mishell, R. I., Dutton, R. W., and Raidt, D. J. (1970). *Cell. Immunol.* **1,** 175–181.
Mosier, D. E. (1967). *Science* **158,** 1573–1575.
Mosier, D. E. (1969). *J. Exp. Med.* **129,** 351–362.
Mosier, D. E., Fitch, F. W., Rowley, D. A., and Davies, A. J. S. (1970). *Nature (London)* **225,** 276–277.
Mosier, D. E., Johnson, B. M., Paul, W. E., and McMaster, P. R. B. (1974). *J. Exp. Med.* **139,** 1354–1360.
Munro, A., and Hunter, P. (1970). *Nature (London)* **225,** 277–278.
Nelson, D. S. (1969) "Macrophages and Immunity." North-Holland Publ., Amsterdam.
Nossal, G. J. V., and Ada, G. L. (1971). "Antigens, Lymphoid Cells, and the Immune Response." Academic Press, New York.
Nossal, G. J. V., and Schrader, J. W. (1975). *Transplant. Rev.* **23,** 138–158.
Osoba, D. (1970). *J. Exp. Med.* **132,** 368–383.
Pierce, C. W. (1969). *J. Exp. Med.* **130,** 345–364.
Pierce, C. W. (1973). *Cell. Immunol.* **9,** 453–464.
Pierce, C. W. (1974). *In* "Allergology: Proceedings of the Eighth Congress of the International Association of Allergology" (Y. Yamamura, O. L. Frick, and Y. Horiuchi, eds.), pp. 176–194. Excerpta Med. Found., Amsterdam.
Pierce, C. W., and Kapp, J. A. (1975). In preparation.
Pierce, C. W., and Benacerraf, B. (1969). *Science* **166,** 1002–1004.
Pierce, C. W., and Benacerraf, B. (1975). *In* "Textbook of Immunopathology" (P. A. Miescher and H. J. Müller-Eberhard, eds.), Vol. II. Grune & Stratton, New York (in press).
Pierce, C. W., Johnson, B. M., Gershon, H. E., and Asofsky, R. (1971). *J. Exp. Med.* **134,** 395–416.
Pierce, C. W., Kapp, J. A., Wood, D. D., and Benacerraf, B. (1974a). *J. Immunol.* **112,** 1181–1189.
Pierce, C. W., Kapp, J. A., Solliday, S. M., Dorf, M. E., and Benacerraf, B. (1974b). *J. Exp. Med.* **140,** 921–938.
Pierce, C. W., Dorf, M. E., and Benacerraf, B. (1975). In preparation.
Roseman, J. (1969). *Science* **165,** 1125–1127.
Rosenthal, A. S., and Shevach, E. M. (1973). *J. Exp. Med.* **138,** 1194–1212.
Rowley, D. A., Fitch, F. W., Stuart, F. P., Köhler, H., and Cosenza, H. (1973). *Science* **181,** 1133–1141.

Schlossman, S. F., and Hudson, L. (1973). *J. Immunol.* **110,** 313–315.
Schrader, J. W. (1973). *J. Exp. Med.* **138,** 1466–1480.
Shevach, E. M., and Rosenthal, A. S. (1973). *J. Exp. Med.* **138,** 1213–1229.
Shortman, K., and Palmer, J. (1971). *Cell. Immunol.* **2,** 399–410.
Shortman, K., Diener, E., Russell, P., and Armstrong, W. D. (1970). *J. Exp. Med.* **131,** 461–482.
Shortman, K., Williams, N., Jackson, H., Russel, P., Byrt, P., and Diener, E. (1971). *J. Cell Biol.* **48,** 566–579.
Shreffler, D. C., and David, C. S. (1975). *Advan. Immunol.* **20,** 125–195.
Steinman, R. M., and Cohn, Z. A. (1974a). *In* "The Inflammatory Process" (B. W. Zweifach, L. Grant, and R. T. McCluskey, eds.), Vol. 1, pp. 450–510. Academic Press, New York.
Steinman, R. M., and Cohn, Z. A. (1974b). *J. Exp. Med.* **139,** 380–397.
Talmage, D. W., Radovitch, J., and Hemmingsen, H. (1970). *Advan. Immunol.* **12,** 271–282.
Theis, G. A., and Thorbecke, G. J. (1970). *J. Exp. Med.* **131,** 970–980.
Unanue, E. R. (1972). *Advan. Immunol.* **15,** 95–165.
Unanue, E. R., and Katz, D. H. (1973). *Eur. J. Immunol.* **3,** 559–563.
van Furth, R., ed. (1970). "Mononuclear Phagocytes." Blackwell, Oxford.
Warner, N. L. (1974). *Advan. Immunol.* **19,** 67–216.
Werdelin, O., Braendstrup, O., and Pederson, E. (1974). *J. Exp. Med.* **140,** 1245–1259.
Wood, D. D., and Gaul, S. L. (1974). *J. Immunol.* **113,** 925–933.

2

The Role of Macrophages in the Specific Determination of Immunogenicity and Tolerogenicity

Donald E. Mosier

I. Introduction 35
A. The Immunogenicity of Macrophage-Associated Antigen 36
B. Macrophage Function *in Vitro* 37
C. Macrophage Receptors for Antigen 37
II. *In Vitro* Requirements for Cell Activation by DNP-D-GL 38
A. Characteristics of the Culture System 39
B. Conditions for Tolerance Induction by DNP-D-GL *in Vitro* 39
C. Immunogenicity of DNP-D-GL Bound to Agarose Beads 41
III. Characteristics of an Antigen Which Does Not Require Macrophage Processing 41
IV. Macrophage Roles in Cell Activation 42
V. Note Added in Proof 43
References 44

I. INTRODUCTION

One of the most important functions performed by macrophages during the induction of an immune response may be the presentation of antigen to antibody-forming cell precursors in a molecular form appropriate for cell activation. Antigen that is poorly concentrated by macrophages is often only weakly immunogenic or may induce tolerance instead of immunity. This chapter will concentrate on the role of macrophages in making antigen more immunogenic and less tolerogenic.

A. The Immunogenicity of Macrophage-Associated Antigen

The immunogenicity of antigen taken up by macrophages has been studied extensively both *in vivo* and *in vitro*. These experiments will not be discussed in detail; rather, the conclusions drawn from them will be summarized.

Radioactively labeled antigen injected into an animal is taken up by macrophages, and most of the antigen undergoes rapid degradation. The fate of macrophage-associated antigen is not uniform, but is determined by its site of localization. Antigen trapped by dendritic macrophages within a lymphoid follicle seems to persist much longer than antigen trapped in extrafollicular sites. Antibody, and perhaps complement, is required for antigen binding to dendritic macrophages, and no binding occurs in tolerant animals. Only circumstantial evidence suggests that this antigen is important in induction of immune responses, however. The rate of degradation of antigen, or conversely, the duration of persistence, is of course related to the nature of the antigen as well as the site of localization (for review, see Nossal and Ada, 1971).

Antigens easily taken up by macrophages are, in general, more immunogenic than antigens that are poorly phagocytized. When a protein antigen (e.g., albumin) is separated into its polymeric and monomeric components, the polymeric aggregates are found to be highly immunogenic, whereas monomers are either very weakly immunogenic or tolerogenic. These types of experiments led Dresser and Mitchison (1968) to postulate that direct binding of monomeric antigen to lymphocytes was a tolerogenic signal, whereas binding of macrophage-associated antigen resulted in an immunogenic signal.

The importance of macrophages in the induction of immune responses in intact animals has been demonstrated by using reagents which interfere with macrophage function such as colloidal carbon, carageenan, or heterologous anti-macrophage serum. These substances reduce uptake of antigen by macrophages and depress the immune response, as manifested both by antibody production and by delayed hypersensitivity (reviewed in Unanue, 1972).

The most direct evidence for the importance of macrophage-associated antigen *in vivo* has been obtained from adoptive transfer experiments in which peritoneal macrophages were exposed to antigen, washed to remove free antigen, and injected into normal syngeneic recipients (Mitchison, 1969; Unanue and Askonas, 1968; Unanue, 1972). Such animals develop normal antibody responses and delayed hypersensitivity reactions, and such macrophage-associated antigen is clearly more immunogenic than free antigen. In many experiments of this general design, no instance of macrophage-bound antigen inducing tolerance has been observed.

B. Macrophage Function *in Vitro*

Macrophages clearly are required for the antibody response to some antigens *in vitro* (Mosier, 1967; Pierce, 1969; Shortman *et al.*, 1970). Thus, macrophages can be removed from mouse spleen cells on the basis of their adherence properties or buoyant density, and the resulting macrophage-depleted lymphoid cells fail to respond to thymus-dependent antigens such as sheep erythrocytes. Such macrophage-depleted cells do respond to thymus-independent antigens, such as 2,4-dinitrophenyl derivatives of polymerized flagellin (DNP-POL) (Shortman and Palmer, 1971) or polysucrose (DNP-Ficoll) (Mosier *et al.*, 1974). Macrophages have functions other than antigen processing *in vitro,* e.g., they promote the viability of lymphocytes (particularly those of thymic origin) in culture, and they serve as a focal point for lymphocyte interaction. Nevertheless, the implication is that thymus-independent antigens do not require macrophage presentation to be immunogenic and hence that thymus-independent antigens all should be capable of "self-presentation." In addition, binding of these antigens directly to precursors of antibody-forming cells is clearly not an obligatory signal for tolerance induction.

The studies of macrophage or adherent cell function *in vitro* and macrophage function *in vivo* show good correlation. That, in fact, the same cell type was being studied is strongly suggested by the experiments of Gorczynski *et al.* (1971), which showed that mice have a macrophage defect both *in vitro* and *in vivo* 3 days following X-irradiation, and that normal macrophages isolated by velocity sedimentation repaired both deficits.

Macrophages seem to be required for the *in vitro* proliferative response of lymphocytes to allogeneic cells, phytomitogens, or specific antigens. Irradiation of macrophages has no effect on their ability to augment either these proliferative responses or to support thymus-dependent antibody responses. The question of the role of macrophages in supporting proliferative responses again rests on discerning functions related to culture conditions versus antigen presentation.

C. Macrophage Receptors for Antigen

Although there is no evidence to suggest that macrophages synthesize antigen-specific molecules, cytophilic antibody binds avidly to the surface of macrophages via an Fc receptor (Boyden, 1964; Berken and Benacerraf, 1966). Antigen–antibody complexes are bound more avidly than monomeric immunoglobulin. The immunoglobulin class also determines the extent of binding to the macrophage Fc receptor. Animals previously immunized have been shown to carry specific cytophilic antibody on their macrophage surface; such macrophages will augment the proliferative response of lymphocytes to that antigen (Cohen *et al.*, 1973).

Feldmann (1972) has postulated that cytophilic antibody bound to macrophages is crucial in the induction of primary immune responses to thymus-dependent antigens. According to his hypothesis, monomeric IgM is released by thymic lymphocytes upon antigenic stimulation (yielding "IgT"), and this immunoglobulin is bound by macrophages and serves as a focal point for antigen–precursor cell interaction. That the immunoglobulin may be derived from antibody-producing cells contaminating primed thymus-derived lymphocytes does little to detract from the importance of the macrophage in the induction of antibody synthesis.

Macrophages also have a receptor for C3 on their surface (Lay and Nussenzweig, 1968). This receptor may augment uptake of antigen–antibody complexes. Antibody putatively directed against mouse C3 has been found to inhibit thymus-dependent immune responses *in vivo* and *in vitro* (Feldmann and Pepys, 1974), but since some non-thymus-derived (B) lymphocytes also have a C3 receptor, it is not clear at what level such an antiserum would interfere with immune induction.

In summary, antigen persists in a highly immunogenic form on the surface of macrophages *in vivo* and *in vitro*. Macrophages may serve to alter antigens to make them more immunogenic, to hold antigens on their surface to focus cell interaction between lymphocytes, and/or to aggregate antigens and remove potentially tolerogenic molecular species. While not excluding other important macrophage functions, only the role of the macrophage in determining immunogenicity versus tolerogenicity will be discussed in detail below.

II. *IN VITRO* REQUIREMENTS FOR CELL ACTIVATION BY DNP-D-GL

The 2,4-dinitrophenyl derivative of a random copolymer of D-glutamic acid and D-lysine (DNP-D-GL) is an antigen capable of inducing profound DNP-specific unresponsiveness both *in vivo* (Katz *et al.*, 1971) and *in vitro* (Nossal *et al.*, 1973). This tolerogenic behavior of DNP-D-GL may be due in part to its persistence in a relatively nonmetabolizable form on the surface of DNP-binding cells (Ault *et al.*, 1974). Under unusual circumstances, however, DNP-D-GL can induce a positive anti-DNP antibody response. One of these circumstances is in a mouse injected with large numbers of allogeneic cells and a small quantity (e.g., 1 μg) of antigen (Osborne and Katz, 1973). Antibody formation also is induced by DNP-D-GL *in vitro* if the antigen is associated with macrophages (Mosier, 1975; Mosier and Paul, 1975).

A. Characteristics of the Culture System

The basic protocol for inducing an *in vitro* antibody response to DNP-D-GL is as follows: mouse spleen cells are exposed to DNP-D-GL (at various concentrations) for 1 hour at 37°C, the cells are washed extensively, and then cultured for 1 hour in a small petri dish. Macrophages adhere to the dish, and other cells are vigorously washed free and discarded. This small number ($\sim 10^5$ per 960 mm^2) of DNP-D-GL pulsed macrophages are used as the source of antigen for 10×10^6 normal nonadherent (macrophage-depleted) spleen cells. Antigen presented in this way induces a substantial anti-DNP plaque forming cell (PFC) response of both IgM and IgG classes (see Fig. 1A) with the peak number of PFC apparent on the fourth day of culture. The *in vitro* response to DNP-D-GL is apparently independent of thymus-derived cells, since anti-θ serum and complement fail to diminish the response of lymphoid cells to macrophage-associated antigen. Cells from congenitally athymic nude mice also respond to DNP-D-GL presented on their own macrophages. The tolerogenicity of DNP-D-GL pulsed macrophages also was assessed using the response to the DNP derivative of Ficoll (polysucrose). The *in vitro* PFC response to DNP-Ficoll is both thymus-independent and macrophage-independent (Mosier *et al.*, 1974).* Only when macrophages were pulsed with very large doses (>100 μg/ml) of DNP-D-GL were those cells able to inhibit the anti-DNP response to DNP-Ficoll. Even this small degree of inhibition may well have been due to DNP-D-GL "leaking" from the macrophage surface. A potentially strong tolerogen thus appears to be converted to an immunogen by allowing it to interact with macrophages.

B. Conditions for Tolerance Induction by DNP-D-GL *in Vitro*

Concentrations of DNP-D-GL greater than 10^{-2} μg/ml induce DNP-specific tolerance as assessed by unresponsiveness to DNP-Ficoll or DNP-keyhole limpet hemocyanin (DNP-KLH) *in vitro*. Exposure of mouse spleen cells to 1 μg/ml DNP-D-GL for 1 hour is sufficient to reduce the subsequent response to DNP-Ficoll by more than 90%. The effect

* See Section V.

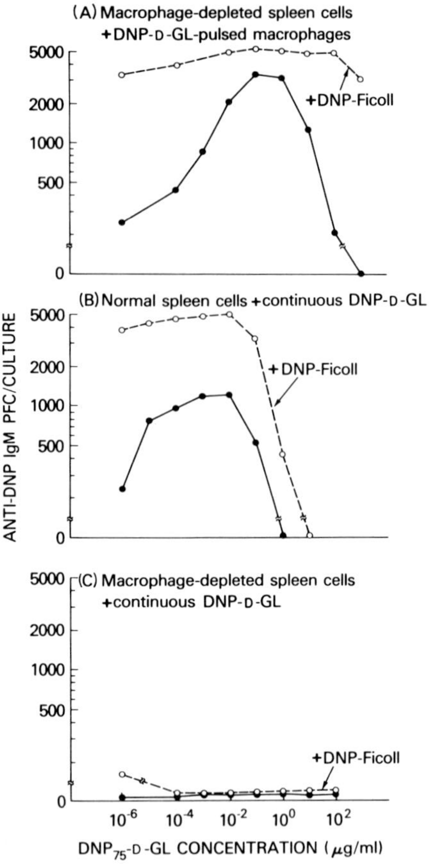

Fig. 1. The anti-DNP IgM plaque-forming cell response of BALB/c spleen cells cultured 4 days with DNP_{75}-D-GL as antigen. The ability of DNP-D-GL to act as an immunogen was assessed by the anti-DNP response without additional antigen, and its ability to induce DNP-specific tolerance was quantitated by the reduction in the concurrent response to 10 ng/ml DNP_{32}-Ficoll. (A) The anti-DNP PFC response to DNP-D-GL pulsed macrophages. Note the failure to inhibit the DNP-Ficoll response, indicating lack of tolerogenic potential. (B) The response of normal spleen cells to DNP-D-GL ± DNP-Ficoll. DNP-D-GL induces anti-DNP PFC at low concentrations but is tolerogenic at high concentrations. (C) The response of macrophage-depleted nonadherent spleen cells to DNP-D-GL ± DNP-Ficoll. Profound DNP-specific unresponsiveness is induced even at very low concentrations of DNP-D-GL.

of various concentrations of DNP-D-GL added to normal spleen cells is shown in Fig. 1B.

The effect of macrophages on tolerance induction was examined by depleting spleen cells of adherent cells, then exposing the macrophage-depleted lymphoid cells to DNP-D-GL. Tolerance induction in the absence of macrophages was rapid and complete. Concentrations of DNP-D-GL as low as 10^{-6} μg/ml caused no anti-DNP PFC response whatsoever and blocked induction of antibody synthesis by DNP-Ficoll (Fig. 1C). Exposure to DNP-D-GL for 1 hour was sufficient to induce specific unresponsiveness. Parallel PFC responses to 2,4,6-trinitrophenyl-Ficoll (TNP-Ficoll) were not inhibited significantly by the DNP-D-GL pulse. The unresponsiveness induced in nonadherent cells by a short exposure to extremely low doses of DNP-D-GL could be partially overcome by very high doses (1000 times the normal *in vitro* maximum) of DNP-Ficoll, suggesting a preferential blockade of high avidity receptors. Tolerance induction in macrophage-depleted spleen cells by DNP-D-GL is not thymus-dependent, since anti-θ and complement treatment had no effect on DNP-D-GL induced unresponsiveness. In the absence of macrophages, DNP-D-GL seems to interact directly with B lymphocytes, invariably leading to tolerance induction.

Normal spleen cells can generate an anti-DNP response when stimulated with very low concentrations of DNP-D-GL (10^{-4} μg/ml). Presumably in this situation macrophages concentrate enough antigen in an immunogenic form to overcome the tolerogenic potential of DNP-D-GL interacting directly with PFC precursors.

C. Immunogencity of DNP-D-GL Bound to Agarose Beads

Although soluble DNP-D-GL invariably induces tolerance in macrophage-depleted mouse spleen cells, DNP-D-GL insolubilized by covalent linkage to agarose beads (Affigel-10, Bio-Rad Laboratories) stimulates anti-DNP antibody formation in nonadherent as well as normal spleen cells in culture. The behavior of DNP-D-GL bound to macrophages or to agarose beads thus is indistinguishable, suggesting one crucial function of macrophages is the insolubilization of antigen and its presentation in a multivalent form. That this function can be served by agarose beads in no way diminishes the importance of the macrophage under physiological conditions.

III. CHARACTERISTICS OF AN ANTIGEN WHICH DOES NOT REQUIRE MACROPHAGE PROCESSING

The anti-DNP antibody response of cultured mouse spleen cells to DNP-Ficoll requires neither adherent cells (macrophages) nor thymus-derived lymphocytes (or so few of such cells as to escape detection) for its generation (Mosier *et al.*, 1974). The same absence of macrophage dependence has been reported for DNP-POL (Shortman and Palmer, 1971). Since DNP-Ficoll can stimulate antibody formation by purified B cells, it appears to be intrinsically immunogenic. Under no experimental circumstances studied has DNP-Ficoll induced DNP-specific tolerance.

The structure of DNP-Ficoll is therefore of great interest, since its ability to bypass macrophage uptake and presentation suggests that its intrinsic tertiary structure may resemble that of more common antigens displayed on the surface of macrophages. Ficoll is a synthetic polymer of sucrose. It consists of multiple sucrose subunits cross-linked with epichlorhydrin to form a rigid two-dimensional matrix. Ficoll behaves as a globular rather than linear molecule in solution. Haptenic DNP groups attached to Ficoll would be expected to be presented for binding in a stable, two-dimensional array. In other words, DNP groups bound to Ficoll probably have much less mobility than DNP bound to D-GL or protein molecules because of the rigidity of Ficoll. The binding of rigidly linked DNP determinants by B lymphocyte receptors is postulated to generate the induction signal for differentiation to antibody formation.

IV. MACROPHAGE ROLES IN CELL ACTIVATION

Although macrophages undoubtedly contribute to immune responsiveness in several ways, the experiments recounted above emphasize two crucial roles required for activation of antibody-forming cells. The first is the uptake of potentially tolerogenic soluble antigen, and the second is antigen expression in a cell-bound multivalent complex more suitable for immune (rather than tolerance) induction. The concept that macrophages eliminate tolerogenic molecular species is not new (see Section I,A, above), but the absolute nature of the macrophage requirement for preventing tolerance induction by DNP-D-GL *in vitro* is striking.

Since DNP-Ficoll or DNP-D-GL on agarose beads stimulate antibody formation in the virtual absence of macrophages, it will be argued by analogy that uptake of DNP-D-GL by macrophages leads to an immunogenic product that structurally resembles these antigens. The presentation of determinants to an antibody-forming cell precursor in a relatively rigid, multivalent array is postulated to be required for induction of antibody synthesis. Most antigens can achieve this form of epitope presentation only by macrophage processing and display of antigen. The exceptions, such as DNP-Ficoll, have an intrinsic structure that seems to suffice for self-presentation. This model may have general applicability, but it

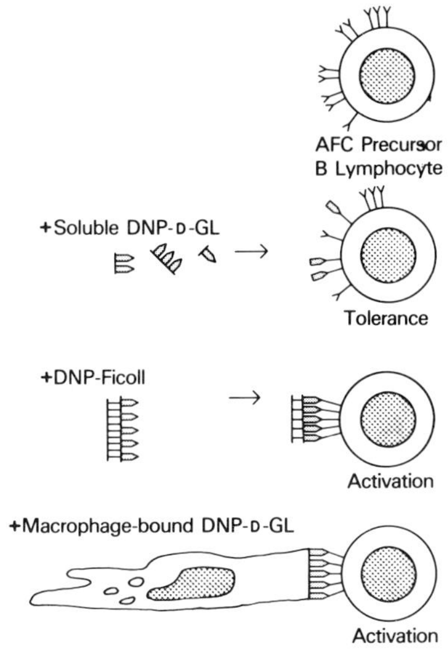

Fig. 2. A hypothetical scheme for B cell activation or tolerization in which macrophages play the crucial role of displaying antigenic determinants in a fixed, multivalent array. AFC precursor, precursor of antibody-forming cell.

should be emphasized that both DNP-D-GL and DNP-Ficoll are thymus-independent antigens. Figure 2 illustrates some aspects of this model of B cell activation.

Implicit in this model, in which macrophage-bound antigen plays such a key role, are several assumptions about the requirements for B cell activation. Activation is presumed to result from rigid cross-linking of many antigen receptors. Activation should thus be determined by antigen concentration, epitope density, the topography of epitope presentation, and the rigidity of the substrate to which epitopes are bound. Tolerance is postulated to result from either monovalent binding, a high concentration of high epitope density leading to ineffective cross-linking of receptors, or insufficient rigidity of the epitope substrate, again so that receptors are ineffectively cross-linked. Macrophages, by altering effective antigen concentration, molecular valency, and, perhaps most importantly, by providing a rigid substrate for antigen, should favor B cell activation.

V. NOTE ADDED IN PROOF

It has recently been found (Chused, Kassan, and Mosier, submitted for publication) that the immune response to DNP–Ficoll is not absolutely macrophage independent and that 99% depletion of macrophages will substantially diminish the anti-DNP response *in vitro*. Such macrophage-depleted cultures will respond when supplemented with 2-mercaptoethanol, however, suggesting that this low level of macrophage dependency may be associated with a viability-promoting effect rather than antigen presentation. Nevertheless, it is possible that antigens possess a range of macrophage dependence and that the arguments presented above should be interpreted in a quantitative rather than absolute sense.

REFERENCES

Ault, K. A., Unanue, T. R., Katz, D., and Benacerraf, B. (1974). *Proc. Nat. Acad. Sci. U.S.* **71,** 3111–3115.

Berken, A., and Benacerraf, B. (1966). *J. Exp. Med.* **123,** 119–144.

Boyden, S. V. (1964). *Immunology* **7,** 474–483.

Cohen, B. E., Rosenthal, A. S., and Paul, W. E. (1973). *J. Immunol.* **111,** 811–819.

Dresser, D. W., and Mitchison, N. A. (1968). *Advan. Immunol.* **8,** 129–181.

Feldmann, M. (1972). *J. Exp. Med.* **136,** 737–760.

Feldmann, M., and Pepys, M. B. (1974). *Nature (London)* **249,** 159–161.

Gorczynski, R. M., Miller, R. G., and Phillips, R. A. (1971). *J. Exp. Med.* **134,** 1201–1221.

Katz, D. H., Davie, J. M., Paul, W. E., and Benacerraf, B. (1971). *J. Exp. Med.* **134,** 201–223.

Lay, W. H., and Nussenzweig, V. (1968). *J. Exp. Med.* **128,** 991–1010.

Mitchison, N. A. (1969). *Immunology* **16,** 1–14.

Mosier, D. E. (1967). *Science* **151,** 1573–1575.

Mosier, D. E. (1975). *Nature (London)* **257,** 141–142.

Mosier, D. E., and Paul, W. E. (1975). *In* "Immune Recognition." (A. S. Rosenthal, ed.), pp. 133–152. Academic Press, New York.

Mosier, D. E., Johnson, B. M., Paul, W. E., and McMaster, P. R. B. (1974). *J. Exp. Med.* **139,** 1354–1360.

Nossal, G. J. V., and Ada, G. L. (1971). "Antigens, Lymphoid Cells, and the Immune Response." Academic Press, New York.

Nossal, G. J. V., Pike, B. L., and Katz, D. H. (1973). *J. Exp. Med.* **138,** 312–317.

Osborne, D. P., Jr., and Katz, D. H. (1973). *J. Exp. Med.* **137,** 991–1008.

Pierce, C. W. (1969). *J. Exp. Med.* **130,** 345–364.

Shortman, K., and Palmer, J. (1971). *Cell. Immunol.* **2,** 399–410.

Shortman, K., Diener, E., Russell, P., and Armstrong, W. D. (1970). *J. Exp. Med.* **131,** 461–482.

Unanue, E. R. (1972). *Advan. Immunol.* **15,** 95–165.

Unanue, E. R., and Askonas, B. A. (1968). *J. Exp. Med.* **127,** 915–926.

3

Role of Macrophages in T Cell-B Cell Collaboration in Antibody Production

A. Basten and Judith Mitchell

I.	Introduction	45
II.	Immunobiology of T Cell–B Cell Collaboration Components	46
III.	Role of Macrophages in T Cell–B Cell Collaboration	52
	A. Requirements for Macrophages in Antibody Production	52
	B. Relationship of Thymus Dependence to Macrophage Requirements	54
	C. Macrophage Responsiveness	55
	D. Possible Functions of Macrophages in T Cell–B Cell Collaboration	57
IV.	Mechanisms of T Cell–B Cell Collaboration	60
	A. Theories of Cell Collaboration	60
	B. Three-Cell Models of Collaboration	65
	C. Conclusions	72
V.	T Cell–B Cell Collaboration *in Vivo*	73
	A. Functional Anatomy of Lymph Nodes	74
	B. Functional Anatomy of the Spleen	79
	C. Putative Sites for Macrophage Interactions *in Vivo*	83
	References	85

I. INTRODUCTION

A role for the macrophage in antibody production took on a new dimension in the late 1960's with the discovery of the "two cell system"

(Claman and Chaperon, 1969; Miller and Mitchell, 1969; Davies, 1969). The requirement for T cells for optimal production, particularly of IgG (Miller *et al.,* 1971) and IgE (Hamaoka *et al.,* 1973) antibodies, has necessitated a reassessment of macrophage function during both induction and effector phases of the immune response. The early part of this work was well summarized a few years ago by Unanue (1972) and Claman and Mosier (1972). Since then, however, advances in understanding of regulation and genetic control have been so rapid that another review is timely. Among the most significant consequences of this burst of activity has been the establishment of various "three cell" models for T cell–B cell interaction. The principal aim of this chapter is twofold: first to examine the place of the macrophage in such models, and second to correlate the conclusions that have largely been derived from *in vitro* studies with the known facts about macrophage function *in vivo.* In so doing it is hoped that a clearer concept of the physiological significance of accessory cell function in antibody production will emerge.

II. IMMUNOBIOLOGY OF T CELL–B CELL COLLABORATION

Components

Antibody responses to the majority of multideterminant antigens appear to depend on interactions between at least three functionally distinct cell types, thymus-derived lymphocytes (T cells), non-thymus-derived lymphocytes (B cells), and accessory cells referred to collectively but somewhat loosely as adherent cells or macrophages (Unanue, 1972; Katz and Benacerraf, 1972; Claman and Mosier, 1972; Basten and Miller, 1974).

1. T Cells

The membrane and functional properties of T cells which distinguish them from B cells have been reviewed in detail elsewhere (Miller *et al.,* 1971; Katz and Benacerraf, 1972; Basten and Howard, 1973; Basten and Miller, 1974). Three characteristics do, however, need to be mentioned, since they are currently the subject of intensive investigation and are relevant to any discussion on the mechanisms of T cell–B cell cooperation.

a. Antigen Receptor. Although there is now good evidence for a specific interaction between antigen and T cells, derived in particular from *in vivo* "suicide" experiments (Basten *et al.,* 1971; Roelants and Askonas,

1971; Cooper and Ada, 1972), its precise nature remains controversial (Vitetta *et al.*, 1972; Marchalonis *et al.*, 1972). Is it an immunoglobulin-like molecule or some other non-immunoglobulin binding site that still has specificity? Recent work from several laboratories has confirmed the presence of immunoglobulin (Ig) on T cells, particularly following activation. The key questions are: Is it an integral part of the cell membrane as suggested by Marchalonis and his colleagues (Marchalonis *et al.*, 1972), or is it cytophilically bound to other sites on the T cell membrane, for example H-2 (Hudson *et al.*, 1974) or Fc receptors (Yoshida and Andersson, 1972; Playfair, 1974). Probably the most convincing evidence for the presence of Ig on specifically committed T cells comes from experiments with thoracic duct cells activated to H-2 antigens *in vivo*, usually termed T-TDL (Cone *et al.*, 1973). The Ig on the same cell has, however, been shown to be of recipient as well as of donor origin (Hudson *et al.*, 1974). Furthermore, depletion of B cells from the original thymus cell population used for production of T-TDL resulted in a marked reduction in the number of Ig-positive T cells. The simplest way of resolving this controversy was to test for immunoglobulin resynthesis after capping. When this was done with T-TDL by Pernis *et al.* (1974), the immunoglobulin was irreversibly lost. In contrast, Roelants *et al.* (1973) have found that after antigen-induced loss of T cell receptors, which they claim to consist of Ig, the receptors do indeed reappear spontaneously under similar culture conditions. Until such time as these results are confirmed, it seems that the majority of carefully performed experiments does not favor Ig as the antigen receptor on T cells. This is not, however, meant to imply that T cell Ig is unimportant. Indeed it may well play a vital role in amplification or suppression of T cell-dependent responses (see Section IV) and could possibly be offered as one explanation for the apparent broader specificity of T cell recognition. Furthermore, its presence, whether cytophilic or not, on the membrane of activated T cells could provide an efficient mechanism for interaction with Fc or C3 receptor-bearing cells, including the macrophage, during an ongoing immune response.

Recent work on genetic control of the immune response, particularly in mice, has led to the proposal that the antigen-binding site on T cells is closely linked to or is a part of the histocompatibility associated gene (*I*) complex (Benacerraf and McDevitt, 1972; Katz and Benacerraf, 1975). In other words, the antigen receptor on T cells is a new recognition system distinct from immunoglobulin and coded for by immune response (*Ir*) genes located near the *K* end of the *H-2* locus. The simplest way in which such a recognition system could operate is to assume that the T cell receptor is the *Ir* gene product. Evidence apparently in favor of this comes from the demonstration in a variety of systems of a vital role for *H-2* gene complex associated antigens in the effective operation of T cell receptors.

1. Specific antigen binding to T cells is inhibitable by anti-H-2 sera (Hämmerling and McDevitt, 1974; Katz and Benacerraf, 1975).
2. Antigen-induced suicide of T cells but not B cells can be abrogated by pretreatment with anti-H-2 fragments of appropriate specificity (Basten *et al.*, 1975a).
3. The antigen specific thymus (cell) factors described by Taussig *et al.* (1974) can be removed with anti-H-2 immunoabsorbants (Taussig and Munro, 1974).
4. The non-antigen-specific factor, "allogeneic effect factor" (AEF), can be similarly removed by immunoabsorbants prepared from appropriate anti-H-2 sera reactive against determinants at the *K* end of the *H-2* locus (Armerding *et al.*, 1974).
5. The interaction between activated T cells and antigen presented on the surface of other somatic cells (such as virus-specified antigens) occurs only when at least one set of H-2 antigen specificities is shared (Zinkernagel, 1974; Zinkernagel and Doherty, 1974).

Recently, however, antisera raised in congenic mice and specifically directed against determinants (Ia) present in the *I* region of the complex have been found to react with surface sites predominantly expressed on B cells and macrophages rather than on T cells (David *et al.*, 1973; Hauptfield *et al.*, 1973). Furthermore, the antigen-specific thymus cell factor of Taussig *et al.* (1974) when derived from responder activated T cells could switch on bone marrow cells from responder mice but not from nonresponder mice. These findings do not appear to be compatible with the concept that the *Ir* gene product is the T cell receptor, but rather to infer that the function of *Ir* genes is to control the functional capacity of the receptor molecules during cellular interactions (Bluestein, 1974; Katz and Benacerraf, 1975). If this is so, we are still faced with the problem of the precise nature of the T cell receptor for antigen. Whatever the solution, the role of the macrophage in T cell-dependent antibody responses can only be discussed in the light of the current state of knowledge concerning the nature of the antigen-binding site.

b. Fc Receptors. The second recently described feature of the T cell membrane which is relevant to the role of the macrophage is the Fc receptor. Yoshida and Andersson (1972) and Lee and Paraskevas (1972) were the first to suggest that T cells might express an Fc receptor. Their studies have been confirmed by other groups working with T cells from both mice and guinea pigs (Andersson and Grey, 1974; Van Boxel and Rosenstreich, 1974) and θ-positive lymphoma lines (Grey *et al.*, 1972). Although no evidence for such receptor sites could be found on one of the purest activated T cell preparations available, namely, T-TDL, even after capping of surface associated immunoglobulin (Basten *et al.*, 1972a, 1975b), it is now apparent that T cells at some stage in their differentiation do in fact display an Fc receptor with apparently similar properties to that expressed on B cells (Soteriades-Vlachos *et al.*, 1974; Basten *et al.*, 1975c). Thus a small percentage of murine thymus cells as well as activated T cells, particularly from the peritoneal cavity, were found to bind aggregated HGG or iodinated immune complexes. Presumably the Ig detected on T-TDL (Hudson *et al.*, 1974) represents anti-H-2 antigen complexes binding to H-2 determinants on the membrane of the activated T cell population. The capacity of other activated T cells to carry cytophilic Ig could, as previously mentioned, be one important mechanism for interaction with C3 and Fc receptor-bearing cells, including macrophages as well as B cells.

c. The Receptor for Macrophages. The existence on T cells (and B cells) from the guinea pig of a receptor for macrophages has recently been described by Rosenthal and his colleagues (Rosenthal and Shevach, 1973; Lipsky and Rosenthal, 1973). In a series of elegant experiments (see Rosenthal *et al.*, Chapter 6), they demonstrated that T cells will form rosettes around peritoneal exudate cells in the absence of antigen, the interaction in the presence of antigen resulting in activation of the T cells as measured by increased DNA synthesis provided the lymphocytes and macrophages were compatible for at least one haplotype. These findings confirm the importance of histocompatibility gene complex associated antigens in induction of T cell-dependent reactions, and in addition suggest a role for the macrophage (although indirect) in genetic control of immune responsiveness.

2. B Cells

At present there is much less controversy about antigen specific receptors on the B cell, which seem to be composed of 7 S IgM molecules synthesized by the cell itself (Vitetta *et al.*, 1972; Marchalonis *et al.*, 1972). They are distinct from C3 receptors (Lay and Nussenzweig, 1968; Parìsh and Hayward, 1974a) and possibly Fc receptors (Basten *et al.*, 1972b). However, as pointed out by Parish and Hayward (1974b) and Ramasamy *et al.* (1974), they may represent immunoglobulin on the point of secretion ("IgM-s") rather than surface Ig. Indeed recent experiments on the relationship between Ig and Fc sites by Basten *et al.* (1975c) support this conclusion. In these the Fc receptor was found to be a more integral part of the membrane than the Ig determinants. Thus B cells treated with chymotrypsin followed by actinomycin D and/or cyclohexamide were still capable of expressing Fc receptors but little or no Ig. In other words the Fc receptor may be an acceptor site for IgM-s.

A second and even more intriguing possibility is that the Fc receptor on B cells may be involved in genetic control of the immune response (Dickler and Sachs, 1974; Basten *et al.*, 1975a). The latter workers were able to block uptake of labeled immune complexes or aggregate-induced suicide of B cells by preincubation with anti-H-2 Fab fragments of appropriate specificity. Furthermore, the inhibitory effect was removed by absorption with B cells but not with thymus cells, suggesting the existence in the region of the Fc receptor of determinants distinct from those coded by the *K* or *D* end of the *H-2* complex. Dickler and Sachs (1974) have claimed similar but more specific results using an anti-Ia antibody, which they cited as strong evidence in favor of the Fc receptor being Ia itself. It is, however, apparent that some Ia antigens must be distinct from Fc receptors, since capping of the latter with immune complexes did not result in cocapping of the Ia antigen (Basten *et al.*, 1975c) and since I. F. C. McKenzie, C. R. Parish, M. Cherry, and G. D. Snell (personal communication, 1974) have demonstrated Ia on null (Ig-negative, Fc-negative) cells. Nevertheless it will be intriguing to establish whether the Ia reported to be present on macrophages (David *et al.*, 1973) has a similar steric relationship to their Fc receptors.

3. *Macrophages*

The macrophage or adherent cell has assumed an increasingly important role over the past few years in both induction and expression of the immune response. Its precise definition and behavioral characteristics in different parts of the lymphoid system are well reviewed in other chapters of this book and will not be dealt with here in detail. What is pertinent is a brief outline of those properties that may be relevant to an analysis of the mechanisms of collaboration. Since many of these properties have been extensively discussed previously (Nelson, 1969; Unanue, 1972; Gordon and Cohn, 1973) the most important have been summarized in Table I.

1. Macrophages can bind antigens either directly if sticky or indirectly if in the form of immune complexes by way of their Fc and C3 receptors.

TABLE I

Biological Properties of Macrophages Relevant to T Cell–B Cell Collaboration

Properties	Examples	References
Membrane associated antigens	Specific for macrophages, detected by anti-macrophage serum	Shortman and Palmer (1971), Holland *et al.* (1972), Gallily and Gornostansky (1972)
	Histocompatibility antigens Ia antigens	Gordon and Cohn (1973), David *et al.* (1973), Delovitch and McDevitt (1974)
Receptors	Nonspecific binding sites for protein aggregates	Steinman and Cohn (1972)
	Fc receptor for IgG	Jonas *et al.* (1965), Uhr (1965), Phillips-Quagliata *et al.* (1971), Mantovani *et al.* (1972), Arend and Mannik (1973)
	Fc receptor for monomeric IgM	Rhodes (1973),
	C3 receptor	Nelson (1965), Lay and Nussenzweig (1968), Huber *et al.* (1968)
	Lymphokine receptors (e.g., for MIF, MSF)	Fox *et al.* (1974)
	Receptors for lymphocytes (T cells and B cells)	Rosenthal and Shevach (1973)
Enzymes	Multiple, including lysosomes and C3 pro-activator	Nelson (1969), Gordon and Cohn (1973), Dukor and Hartmann (1973)
Physiological functions	Pinocytosis, phagocytosis, molecular exchange	Gordon and Cohn (1973)
Release of soluble factors	Promotors of lymphocyte activity	Hoffmann and Dutton (1971), Gery and Waksman (1972), Schrader (1973)
	Inhibitors of lymphocyte activity	Nelson (1973), Calderon *et al.* (1974)

2. Macrophages have membrane antigens against which specific antisera can be raised allowing selective depletion.

3. Macrophages display Ia antigens on their surface and are therefore capable of participating at least indirectly in regulation of immune responsiveness.

4. Macrophages carry receptors not only for B cell products (Ig) but also for T cell products (e.g., MIF) and lymphocytes themselves.

5. Macrophages can ingest and degrade antigens, thereby altering their immunogenicity in a positive or negative sense.

6. As a result of the above interactions, macrophages can release products capable either of enhancing or of suppressing an immune response or even determining the type of effector cell activated, i.e., the expression of the immune response (see Oppenheim and Seeger, Chapter 5; Nelson, Chapter 9).

III. ROLE OF MACROPHAGES IN T CELL–B CELL COLLABORATION

It is apparent from Section II,A,3 that macrophages, although nonspecific in an immunological sense, possess properties that enable them to have a profound effect on the interaction between T cells and B cells. The aim of this section is to try and answer the critical question: What is their precise function(s)? Four comments are worth making at the outset. First, the function of macrophages taken from different sources varies significantly. Second, the term adherent cells is frequently used synonymously with macrophages, but it is now known that lymphocytes, particularly some B cells and activated T cells, can stick to glass or plastic sufaces (Shortman *et al.*, 1972). Third, a large part of the relevant studies has been carried out *in vitro;* these may or may not be relevant to events occurring in the intact host, since neither the functional anatomy of lymphoid tissue nor the remarkable mobility of some lymphocytes is taken into account. Finally, even *in vitro* it is often difficult to work with sufficiently purified populations of lymphocytes or macrophages to permit the drawing of valid conclusions. Thus almost all methods of cell separations (columns, treatment with "specific" antisera, differential centrifugation) either give only 98% purity at best or may result in removal not only of unwanted cells but also of critical subpopulations of relevant cells.

A. Requirements for Macrophages in Antibody Production

The development by Mishell and Dutton (1966) and Marbrook (1967) of sensitive *in vitro* techniques for measuring antibody production led to the discovery that not only lymphocytes but also an accessory cell population were essential for an optimal immune response to many antigens. The evidence identifying the latter as macrophages has been summarized by Unanue (1972). They can adhere to glass or plastic. They can phagocytize and are affected by techniques known to induce reticuloendothelial blockade, but do not themselves synthesize antibodies. They have characteristic morphological and staining properties. They are relatively radioresistant, and they can be removed *in vitro* by treatment with specific anti-macrophage serum. Mosier's studies (1967) of *in vitro* antibody production to sheep red blood cells (SRBC) were the first to establish clearly a requirement for macrophages in the primary immune response of mouse spleen cells. Subsequently his experiments were confirmed and extended by other investigators both for SRBC (Pierce, 1969; Pierce and Benacerraf, 1969; Talmage *et al.*, 1970; Dutton *et al.*, 1970; Shortman and Palmer, 1971) and for other antigens, for example, other erythrocytes (Feldmann and Basten, 1972), monomeric flagellin (Feldmann and Basten, 1971), and hapten–protein conjugates (Feldmann, 1973; Unanue and Katz, 1973; Askonas and Roelants, 1974). Furthermore, a vital role for macrophages has been demonstrated in the *in vitro* primary response of cells from different species, including the rabbit (Theis and Thorbecke, 1970), and in the secondary response in mice both *in vivo* (Fishman and Adler, 1963; Nelson, 1969) and *in vitro* (Feldmann and Basten, 1972; Feldmann, 1972). A more detailed analysis of macrophage requirements particularly in *in vitro* collaboration is presented by Pierce and Kapp in Chapter 1.

The source of macrophages is important. Thus adherent cells from spleen and peritoneal cavity are effective in restoring the capacity of purified lymphocytes to mount an immune response *in vitro* (Claman and Mosier, 1972). In contrast, Kupffer cells and alveolar macrophages appear to lack this activity as do mononuclear cells derived from bone marrow colonies grown in liquid culture (Watson *et al.*, 1974). Nevertheless the latter cells were shown to possess many features characteristic of macrophages, including adherence to glass, phagocytosis, specific staining, and antibody-dependent cytotoxicity. These findings led the authors to suggest that another cell type may be essential for delivery of the inductive stimulus to antigen-sensitive lymphocytes, but they were unable to identify it formally (the heterogeneity of macrophages is discussed by Walker in Chapter 4). Other studies of antigen stimulation of purified lymphocytes have not been helpful in this regard, since neither fibroblasts (Hersh and Harris, 1968) nor neutrophils (Cline and Swett, 1968) were found to be capable of substituting for macrophages. Three alternative explanations for the failure of colony-forming mononuclear cells to collaborate deserve mention, particularly since they emphasize certain key features of macrophage function. First, the ratio of macrophages to lymphocytes may have been suboptimal. This is known to be a critical factor in determining whether a response will occur or not (Parkhouse and Dutton, 1966; Unanue, 1972) and may vary for macrophages from different sources. Second, macrophages, either from different sources or taken at different stages of differentiation may be heterogeneous in a functional sense. Thus they have been shown to promote (Hoffman and Dutton, 1971; Gery and Waksman, 1972) and to suppress (Nelson, 1973; Calderon *et al.*, 1974) lymphocyte activity (see Chapter 9). Finally microenvironments may play a critical role in determining whether macrophages from a particular source will exert an effect or not. Although this may not be important *in vitro,* there is evidence, although indirect, suggesting that microenvironments could be of critical importance *in vivo.* For example, macrophages situated in a pathway of lymphocyte traffic but not in sites of lymphocyte proliferation are capable of antigen trapping (see Section V). Furthermore, the specialized dendritic follicular cells found in the germinal centers may be involved in antigen presentation, but such a phenomenon cannot, by definition, be reproduced *in vitro.* In other words, to imply that certain mononuclear cells do not exert an effect *in vitro* does not necessarily exclude an important role for them *in vivo.*

The latter comment highlights the limitations of an *in vitro* assay system in determining the physiological functions of any cell, including the macrophage. This is not, however, to imply that macrophages are unimportant in the intact host. Indeed macrophage transfer experiments and histological analysis of lymphoid tissue following injection of labeled antigens strongly favor their playing vital and diverse roles. This is well illustrated by experiments correlating *in vivo* with *in vitro* requirements for splenic macrophages (Gorczynski *et al.*, 1971). Furthermore, antigen localization has been demonstrated on the processes of dendritic cells in the spleen (presumed to be a specialized form of adherent cell), and mature B (plasma) cells have been observed by some investigators (Miller and Avrameas, 1971) to cluster round macrophages in the medullary cords of lymph nodes following antigenic stimulation. A more detailed discussion of *in vivo* correlates is presented in Section V.

B. Relationship of Thymus Dependence to Macrophage Requirements

Antibody production, at least *in vitro,* to the majority of multideterminant antigens does, as already stated, depend on the presence of macrophages, a T cell influence, and B cells. In contrast, some antigens elicit an optimal immune response *in vivo* as well as *in vitro* in the apparent absence of functional T cells (reviewed by Basten and Howard, 1973). The question, therefore, arises whether such antigens can trigger B cells independently not only of T cells but also of macrophages; or to put it the other way round: Are macrophages obligatory for stimulation of helper cells? One of the best approaches to this problem has been to compare the effect of macrophage depletion on the *in vitro* response of cells in the same cultures to thymus-dependent and thymus-independent antigens. The results indicate that antibody production to the former does indeed rely on the presence of macrophages, whereas optimal responses to the latter can occur independently (Shortman and Palmer, 1971; Feldmann and Basten, 1972; Basten and Howard, 1973). In other words, helper cell function cannot be expressed in the absence of macrophages. Whether the same generalization can be applied *in vivo* remains unknown, since almost all macrophage transfer experiments and antigen tracer studies have been carried out with T-dependent antigens (see Section V).

The *in vitro* experiments described above do not indicate how the macrophage functions in rendering T-dependent antigens immunogenic. Some clue can be derived from a study of the molecular properties of T-independent antigens. They are, for example, multideterminant in nature (Feldmann and Basten, 1971) and slowly degradable (Sela *et al.*, 1972), which render them particularly well suited to cross-linking receptors on B cells in such a way as to trigger them directly. Since T-dependent antigens lack such properties, it follows that the role of the T cell-phagocyte axis may be to achieve a similar linear array of determinants capable of multipoint binding to B cells. Clearly the likely site for this to occur is on the macrophage surface, which is sticky and displays an array of receptor sites for T cell products and antigen–antibody complexes. Indeed the enhanced immunogenicity of macrophage-associated antigen (Unanue and Askonas, 1968) strongly supports this possibility. The importance of the macrophage in antigen presentation and B cell triggering will be discussed further in Section IV,B.

C. Macrophage Responsiveness

Handling of antigen by macrophages has been known for some time to differ from strain to strain (Weigle and Golub, 1969). This is manifest as a strain-dependent susceptibility to tolerance induction. In other words, mice that process antigens poorly are more readily made tolerant than are those which process antigens efficiently. More recently, Biozzi and his colleagues (1970, 1972) have bred two lines of mice (Ab/H and Ab/L) from Swiss albino stock which differ in their capacity to mount humoral but not cell-mediated immune responses (Liacopoulos-Briot *et al.*, 1972; Byfield and Howard, 1972). The responder status of these animals has now been shown to depend on macrophage rather than B cell function per se. Thus the T cell- (and macrophage-) independent antigens, levan and dextran B1355, elicited equivalent antibody responses in Ab/H and Ab/L mice (Howard *et al.*, 1974), but peritoneal cells from Ab/L mice bound antigen on their membranes much less efficiently than those from Ab/H mice (Fig. 1) (Wiener and Bandieri, 1974). Taken together the above studies indicate that the macrophage as well as the T cell and B cell may have a key role to play in the induction and expression of immune responsiveness. For example, they may, although indirectly, have an influence on determining the following.

1. Whether tolerance or immunity occurs at the level of the B cell and possibly at the level of the T cell as well. Thus, efficient antigen handlers are more likely to mount a response than poor antigen handlers.
2. Whether T cells are stimulated or not.
3. Whether immunological memory is generated (Askonas and Jarosková, 1970).
4. Whether IgM or IgG antibody is produced. In other words, they may influence both antibody class and affinity.

These functions, usually attributed exclusively to the T cell component of the collaborative response, have both pathological as well as physiological significance. Thus it can be predicted on theoretical grounds that low responder strains ought to show a greater susceptibility to certain infections requiring high affinity antibodies for their elimination. This

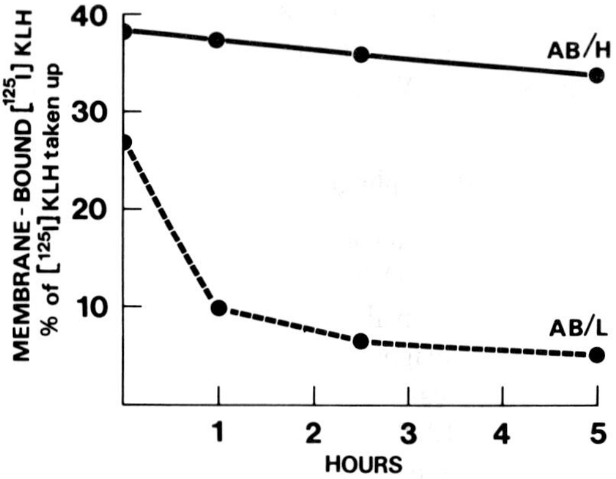

Fig. 1. Retention of membrane-bound [^{125}I]KLH after its uptake by Ab/H and Ab/L macrophages. [From Wiener and Bandieri (1974). Reproduced by courtesy of *European Journal of Immunology*.]

has indeed been shown to be so in the case, for example, of LCM virus infection (Oldstone and Dixon, 1969). Furthermore, the production of low affinity antibody in susceptible strains can result in chronic soluble immune complex disease, which further enhances morbidity (Passwell *et al.*, 1974).

D. Possible Functions of Macrophages in T Cell–B Cell Collaboration

The above sections have delineated both the requirement for and the potential importance of macrophages in collaborative responses. It now becomes relevant to discuss the precise way(s) in which their functions are carried out. A number of these have been discussed in other chapters of this book (Pierce and Kapp, Chapter 1; Mosier, Chapter 2; Walker, Chapter 4) and therefore our comments will be in the form of a summary. Basically there are two theoretical sites for macrophage involvement, namely, in antigen presentation to T cells (pre-T cell stage) and in the collaborative step itself between T cells and B cells (T cell–B cell stage).

1. Pre-T Cell Stage (Induction)

The induction phase of antibody production depends on presentation of antigen in immunogenic form. Immunogenicity in the case of a T-dependent antigen is determined not only by its chemical structure but also by its capacity to activate T cells that can then elaborate the second signal necessary for B cell triggering. Several ways can be envisaged in which macrophages may be involved in T cell stimulation and proliferation. The first is in *degradation* of particulate antigens. Thus, some experiments indicate that breakdown by macrophages of sheep red blood cells (Shortman and Palmer, 1971; Feldmann and Palmer, 1971) or *Shigella* antigens (Gallily and Feldman, 1967) may be an essential prerequisite for immune induction.

Second, macrophages probably play a key role in antigen *removal,* i.e., in determining epitope density in the microenvironment of receptors on specific lymphocytes (G. F. Mitchell, 1974). If antigen evades the macrophages then tolerance and not immunity will result (Unanue, 1972; Mosier *et al.*, 1974).

A third way in which the macrophage may be involved in the induction phase of T-dependent responses is in microenvironmental *concentration* of antigen as clearly shown by *in vivo* antigen tracer studies (Nossal and Ada, 1971). As a result of trapping, antigenic determinants can be concentrated in critical sites, for example, lymphocyte traffic areas such as the follicles and the medulla of the lymph node (Nossal and Ada, 1971), thereby optimizing the chances of contact with rare antigen reactive cells. Furthermore, once localization of previously disseminated molecules has occurred on the surface of macrophages, the resulting focus of antigen (e.g., in germinal centers) provides an efficient site for collaboration to take place (Gutman and Weissman, 1972).

Fourth, the macrophage may not only be required for rendering antigen "palatable" to T cells but also may be essential for its *presentation.* The reason for this could well be related to the poor exposure of antigen binding sites on the T cell membrane (see Section II,A,1,a). Thus, even soluble antigens, such as proteins, do not appear to trigger T cell differentiation directly. Support for this comes from the experiments of P. Erb and M. Feldmann (personal communication, 1974) and Basten *et al.* (1975). The former showed that macrophages were an obligatory requirement for *in vitro* generation of helper cells, while the latter found that "suicide" of purified T cells did not take place unless the radioactive antigen was presented on the surface of a carrier primed spleen cell population containing macrophages as well as B cells. Although B cells can play a role in antigen presentation to T cells (Miller *et al.*, 1971; S. Kirov and C. R. Parish, personal communication, 1974), the macrophage seems to be a particularly good candidate because of its sticky membrane and its array of receptors for C3, immunoglobulins, and lymphocytes including T cells (see Section II,A,3). The last receptor could well be important in the inductive phase of a primary response, and the first two in both the proliferative phase of a primary response and the inductive phase of a secondary response when antibody is already present (Mantovani *et al.*, 1972; Cohen and Paul, 1974). Whatever the precise explanation there is now persuasive evidence showing that macrophage-associated antigen is significantly more immunogenic than free antigen (Unanue and Askonas, 1968; Mitchison, 1969; Cruchaud *et al.*, 1970). Furthermore, conjugates, such as DNP-Ficoll, with a rigid structure resembling macrophage-bound antigen are apparently obligatory immunogens (Paul *et al.*, 1974).

The last way in which macrophages could contribute to T cell differentiation is by release of various *soluble factors,* although nonspecific, which may either stimulate (Hoffmann and Dutton, 1971; Pierce *et al.*, 1974; Britton, 1974; Schrader, 1973) or suppress cell proliferation (Nelson, 1973; Calderon *et al.*, 1974). Which of these effects is most vital in the intact host remains to be determined, but this in no way detracts from the potential importance of macrophages both in induction of the immune response and in its ultimate expression.

2. T Cell–B Cell Stage

The capacity of macrophages to concentrate antigens in critical sites coupled with the enhanced immunogenicity of macrophage-associated antigen strongly suggest a role for these cells in the actual interaction between T cells and B cells in T cell-dependent responses. The most direct evidence supporting this possibility comes from recent experiments by Unanue and Katz (1973) and Askonas and Roelants (1974). The former found that lymphocytes primed to a hapten carrier conjugate were stimulated by normal macrophages bearing the same conjugate. If, however, the macrophages were treated with a hapten coupled to a heterologous carrier plus the original carrier, no antibody response occurred. In other words, the need for hapten and carrier determinants to be on the same molecule (Mitchison, 1971) was confirmed, and, in addition, the macrophage surface was shown to provide the site for presentation of determinants in immunogenic form to both T cells and B cells. Askonas and Roelants (1974) extended these observations with their cloning technique. Thus the transfer of macrophages carrying only haptenic or carrier determinants, or both determinants, but on different macrophages failed to trigger B memory cells in irradiated hosts. Enhancement of antibody levels and the number of anti-hapten clones only took place if both hapten and carrier determinants were linked together on the surface of the same macrophage population. Taken together these findings point to a critical role for the macrophage as the focus of T cell–B cell interaction. Additional evidence favoring this conclusion comes from the close anatomical relationship of lymphocytes and macrophages observed *in vitro*. For example, cell clusters have been frequently reported in Mishell–Dutton culture systems (Mosier, 1967; Pierce and Benacerraf, 1969; McIntyre *et al.*, 1971). The mechanism of cluster formation is not clearly defined but could be due, in the case of B cells, to interaction of immunoglobulin receptors on B cells with the Fc receptors on macrophages (Schmidtke and Unanue, 1971), and in the case of T cells and B cells to lymphocyte receptors for macrophages (Lipsky and Rosenthal, 1973). The relationship between clusters and induction of the immune response is likewise unclear. One would have thought that the cluster ought to represent the site of antibody synthesis, but recent studies by McIntyre and Pierce (1973), which are discussed in greater detail in Chapter 1 do not support this.

A number of additional influences already mentioned in the previous section presumably play a role in the T cell–B cell stage as well. For example, lysosomal enzymes, nonspecific helper and suppressor factors, and antibody itself would be expected to exert a variety of effects within the antigen–macrophage–lymphocyte focus. These will be discussed in further detail in Section IV.

IV. MECHANISMS OF T CELL–B CELL COLLABORATION

A. Theories of Cell Collaboration

Induction of antibody synthesis by B cells is generally accepted as requiring two signals. "Signal one" is generated by binding of antigenic (haptenic) determinants to specific receptors on the B cell membrane. On its own signal one is insufficient to trigger the B cell, but rather leads to paralysis (Bretscher and Cohn, 1970; Bretscher, 1974; G. F. Mitchell, 1975). For antibody production to occur a second event ("signal two") is required. In the case of T-independent antigens their intrinsic molecular structure provides signal two (see Section III,B), whereas for T-dependent antigens it is derived from helper cells. Basically there are three possible mechanisms whereby T cells can either directly or indirectly, for example, via a macrophage, deliver signal two to the B cell. These are information transfer, antigen focusing, and soluble mediator release (Miller *et al.*, 1971; Katz and Benacerraf, 1972; Basten and Miller, 1974).

1. Transfer of Subcellular Information

In a series of provocative experiments Fishman and Adler (1963, 1970) claimed to have isolated from antigen-treated macrophages an RNA molecule that apparently could transfer allotypic specificity. The implication of the findings was that the macrophage played a key role in induction of the immune response by transferring specific immunological information to lymphocytes, at least to lymphocytes of the B cell lineage. Subsequently, however, it has become apparent that although lymphocytes do indeed interact with macrophage-associated antigen (see Section II,A,3), this process may not be essential for antibody production to all antigens, nor may it involve generation of a messenger RNA complex by the macrophage (Unanue, 1972). Furthermore, three other lines of evidence make it unnecessary to invoke transfer of subcellular information either between lymphocytes or between macrophages and lymphocytes. The first is the demonstration of specificity in both T cells and B cells (reviewed by Katz and Benacerraf, 1972; Basten and Miller, 1974). The second line of evidence is derived from experiments showing that the B cell as the direct precursor of antibody-forming cells is precommitted to synthesis of antibody of one class and one allotype (Mitchison, 1971; Lawton *et al.*, 1972). In other words, if B cells are precommitted with respect to both antigen recognition and antibody production, they must, by definition, possess the intrinsic potential to secrete specific material without transfer of genetic information from another cell such as the T cell or macrophage. Third, the affinity of antibody produced during primary and secondary anti-hapten responses has been shown to be determined by the mode and time of immunization with the hapten–carrier (Katz *et al.*, 1970). Since affinity is recognized as a marker of the variable region of the antibody molecule, these experiments again exclude a requirement for any genetic help from other cells.

2. *Antigen Focusing Hypothesis*

The discovery that the hapten–carrier system can be explained in terms of an interaction between T cells and B cells led Mitchison (1971) to propound the antigen focusing hypothesis. In this, the role of the T cell is to pick up antigen by its carrier determinant and to focus it by way of the inducing determinants (also on the same molecule) onto the corresponding receptors on B cells, thereby forming an antigen bridge. T cells would thus play a relatively passive role in cell collaboration. Although elegant in simplicity this hypothesis in its original form does not take into account the more recent experiments demonstrating the need for active participation by T cells (reviewed by Katz and Benacerraf, 1972; Basten and Miller, 1974) and for an obligatory role for macrophages (see Sections II and III) in generation of help. The macrophage can, however, be readily fitted into the hypothesis as a component of the antigen bridge. Thus, if one accepts the necessity for both hapten and carrier determinants to be on the same molecule (Unanue and Katz, 1973), which is in turn bound to the surface of the same macrophage population (Askonas and Roelants, 1974), the latter would provide a focus for interaction of T cells and B cells. This hypothesis does not necessarily require T cells and B cells to be in contact, but implies that they will at least be in close proximity. Furthermore, once interaction with macrophage-bound antigen has occurred, either one or both lymphocytes could migrate elsewhere during the effector phase of the immune response. This might account for the failure to detect antibody synthesis by cluster forming cells *in vitro* (McIntyre and Pierce, 1973) and for the difficulty in determining the site of cell collaboration *in vivo* (see Section V).

3. *Soluble Mediators*

The difficulty even with the modified antigen focusing hypothesis is that it does not account for the active role known to be played by T cells in collaboration, nor does it satisfactorily explain how rare antigen-reactive T cells and B cells could come into contact with reasonable frequency. If on the other hand, T cells proliferate with release of soluble mediators, the efficiency of interaction would be greatly enhanced. Indeed there is now a wealth of evidence favoring the existence of such factors. In general terms two basic types have been identified—one specific (Feldmann and Basten, 1972; Gorczynski *et al.*, 1973; Taussig *et al.*, 1974) and the other nonspecific (Dutton *et al.*, 1971; Schimpl and Wecker, 1972; Gisler *et al.*, 1973; Armerding and Katz, 1974; Hunter and Kettman, 1974; Britton, 1974; Pierce *et al.*, 1974).

a. Specific Mediators of Cell Collaboration. Evidence for a specific mediator was first obtained from an *in vitro* culture system in which T cells proved capable of collaborating with B cells even when separated by a cell-tight nucleopore membrane (Feldmann and Basten, 1972; Basten and Feldmann, 1972). Specificity of both cell lines was established by showing that T cells activated to a non-cross-reacting carrier collaborated much less effectively than did T cells activated to the carrier used for challenge. Furthermore, the antibody response to a second T-dependent antigen present on the B cell side of the membrane was not augmented. Subsequent studies indicated that the T cell product responsible appeared to be an "IgT–antigen complex" (Feldmann, 1972).

A number of criticisms (extensively analyzed by Miller, 1975) have been leveled at this work, particularly regarding the type of response measured and the origin of the "T cell product." Although another detailed discussion of them is irrelevant in a review of macrophage function in cell collaboration, the most important objections deserve mention. First, the *in vitro* system used only permitted measurements of low affinity IgM antibody, which is the least T cell-dependent type of B cell response. Second, the possible presence of small numbers of contaminating carrier-primed B cells and macrophages in the activated T cell population that was obtained from irradiated hosts has yet to be definitively excluded. Indeed there is now good evidence that T cells cannot be readily triggered by antigen unless it is presented on the surface of a second cell population (see Section III,D,1). Third, it has not been unequivocally shown that the IgT component of the IgT–antigen complexes is elaborated by the activated T cells. As mentioned in Section II the most readily identifiable immunoglobulin on activated T cells seems to be passively bound either to H-2 determinants or to Fc receptors. Fourth, if the T cell product does contain a specific IgT molecule that triggers B cells simply by its cytophilia for macrophages (see Section IV,B), it is hard to understand why cooperation does not occur between allogeneic T cells and B cells (Katz *et al.*, 1973) and why B cells can be triggered to produce IgG antibodies of high affinity in the absence of appropriate T cells (Klinman and Doughty, 1973). Despite these criticisms, the concept of an IgT–antigen complex provides an elegant three cell model for collaboration, which can operate in a physiological (syngeneic) situation and can be used to explain a variety of immunological phenomena including tolerance and antigenic competition.

Taussig (1974) and Taussig *et al.* (1974) have recently produced evidence for a different type of specific mediator of cell collaboration with activity *in vivo* as well as *in vitro*. Specifically activated T cells were incubated *in vitro* with the synthetic polypeptide antigen (tyrosine, glutamine)-polyalanine-polylysine [(T,G)-A-L]. Supernatants so obtained were shown to be capable of replacing T cell help in an adoptive transfer system. Production of the active components was sensitive to anti-θ serum and their activity could be absorbed by appropriate anti-H-2 antibody but not by anti-immunoglobulin. Studies with more specific alloantisera indicated that these "thymus cell factors" were coded for at the *K*-end of the *H-2* locus (Munro *et al.*, 1974) and may, as pointed out by Katz and Benacerraf (1974), contain moieties similar to or identical with the "allogeneic effect factor" (AEF). Their specificity for alloantigens expressed on the cooperating cells would therefore explain why T cells and B cells will only collaborate if they share at least one haplotype. The experimental system is, however, open to certain criticisms akin to those directed at the IgT–antigen factor model. For example, the factors, although active *in vivo*, are reported only to trigger an IgM response. Furthermore, a similar source of activated T cells obtained from irradiated hosts was used which would have been contaminated by both B cells and macrophages. Inhibition of release of the factors by anti-θ serum does at first sight appear to answer this criticism. It has, however, been shown recently that anti-θ serum treatment of mixed populations of T and B cells results in blockade of the Fc receptor on B cells (Basten *et al.*, 1975a) and macrophages (A. Basten, unpublished observations, 1974), probably due to formation of θ–anti-θ complexes in the culture fluid which bind to the B cell and macrophage membrane. Since the Fc receptors on these cells are apparently associated with Ia determinants (Dickler and Sachs, 1974) now identified as the major component of AEF, then anti-θ serum treatment might inhibit release of AEF (composed of Ia) and any other H-2 complex-linked constituents of thymus cell factors. The precise role played by the T cells themselves and the antigenic specificity of the factors therefore require elucidation, particularly as AEF by definition lacks *antigenic* specificity. This situation is rendered even more complex by the recent demonstration of cross-reactivity between (TG)-A-L and murine histocompatibility antigens (Ebringer and Davies, 1973).

b. Nonspecific Mediators of Cell Collaboration. Evidence for a nonspecific T cell influence on B cell responsiveness has been obtained in a number of different experimental situations. These have been termed the "allogeneic effect" (Katz, 1972), the "mitogen effect" (Andersson *et al.*, 1972), and the "primed B cell effect" (Miller, 1975). The key features shared by all of them is their capacity to enhance antibody production to a given antigen by activating a large number of T cells by way of an irrelevant antigenic stimulus. The first to be described was the allogeneic effect in which induction of a transient graft versus host reaction either *in vivo* (Katz, 1972; Hamilton and Miller, 1973) or *in vitro* (Dutton *et al.*, 1971; Schimpl and Wecker, 1971; Feldmann and Basten, 1972; Britton, 1974; Hunter and Kettman, 1974) obviated the requirement for carrier-specific T cells in anti-hapten antibody responses. *In vivo* allogeneic cell transfer, furthermore, can initiate an IgG response in nonresponder mice (Ordal and Grumet, 1972) and enhance the immunogenic potential of antigens, such as DNP-D-GL, which are otherwise only weakly immunogenic or tolerogenic for Bγ cells (Osborne and Katz, 1973). Similar nonspecific enhancement of T-dependent responses has been observed in serum-free tissue culture systems by the addition of mitogens, such as concanavalin A (Coutinho and Möller, 1973). Both these "effects" have, however, been criticized as being too artificial to give a valid insight into the physiological mechanisms of T cell–B cell interaction. The "primed B cell effect" on the other hand, operates *in vivo* in a syngeneic transfer system. In this, the poor anti-hapten IgG response to challenge with the hapten on an irrelevant carrier is enhanced by providing a small number of B cells primed to the irrelevant carrier (Miller, 1975). Comparable results have been obtained for IgE anti-hapten responses in another *in vivo* system (Hamaoka, *et al.*, 1973). The source of the primed B cells in the former experiment was anti-θ treated spleen cells. As pointed out in Section II, this population contains macrophages that possibly bear high affinity cytophilic antibody in addition to high affinity B cells, one or both of which seem to be essential for effective antigen interaction with T cells (Waldron *et al.*, 1973; Basten *et al.*, 1975). The primed B cell effect may therefore represent one nonspecific way of enhancing T cell triggering in *in vivo* collaborative responses.

The *in vitro* studies mentioned above have demonstrated that the T cell-dependent influence is apparently mediated by soluble factors. Different mediators have been defined in different systems, but in general they fall into two categories: dialyzable and nondialyzable. The lower molecular weight (dialyzable) component appears to be a nonspecific B cell mitogen capable of enhancing T-independent antibody responses (Feldmann and Basten, 1972; Schimpl and Wecker, 1972; Britton, 1974) and increases the number of antibody-forming cells obtained per responding B cell (Hunter and Kettman, 1974). In one system this type of factor was shown to depend on a macrophage function, which could be replaced by 2-mercaptoethanol (Gisler *et al.*, 1973). The higher molecular weight (nondialyzable) component, on the other hand, can increase the actual frequency of antibody-forming cells (Hunter and Kettman, 1974) and would therefore appear to be important during the induction rather than the effector phase of collaborative responses. The latter group of factors, increasing the frequency of antibody-forming cells, presumably contains the allogeneic effect factor (AEF) recently identified as Ia by Armerding *et al.* (1974) and possessing certain molecular features in common with the "thymus cell factors" of Munro *et al.* (1974). If this indeed proves to be the case the question of their cellular origin arises once again. Although their production is clearly T cell-dependent and *H-2* linked, the high density of Ia determinants on B cells and macrophages rather than on T cells implies that other cells like the macrophage are likely to be involved in their elaboration. Indeed there is some indirect evidence for this (Gisler *et al.*, 1973; Britton, 1974) which will be discussed in the following section.

B. Three-Cell Models of Collaboration

It is apparent from the previous discussion that a number of possible ways exist whereby T cells can either directly or indirectly provide the second signal required for B cell triggering. Various three-cell models incorporating the macrophage as well as the T cell and B cell have been proposed, which for the sake of simplicity will be discussed in turn.

1. IgT–Antigen Complex Model

This model was developed from studies on the site and mode of action of the antigen specific factor of Feldmann and Basten (1972) discussed previously. In these experiments T cells activated to the carrier keyhole limpet hemocyanin (KLH) were placed in the upper compartment of a double chamber culture flask together with DNP-KLH, and purified macrophages in the lower. After 1–3 days of incubation the macrophages were transferred to a single culture vessel containing a source of purified DNP-primed B cells without further addition of antigen. A highly significant anti-DNP response was obtained 4 days later which had specificity at the level of both T cell and B cell. The ability of macrophages to trigger hapten-primed cells in the second chamber was inhibited by trypsinization, by culturing in the presence of either anti-DNP or anti-KLH antibody, and by pretreatment with monospecific anti-Ig sera with specificity for mouse κ or μ chains (Feldmann, 1972; Basten and Feldmann, 1972). Taken together these findings suggested that cell collaboration is mediated by a T cell product containing antigenic determinants combined with Ig presumably of T cell origin. The IgT–antigen complex so formed is cytophilic (Rhodes, 1973) for the macrophage, which provides an ideal site for formation of an immunogenic complex with a surface structure resembling that of a T-independent antigen. In other words, "sensitized" macrophages provide the second signal for induction of anti-hapten antibody synthesis by B cells (Fig. 2). The concept of a specific T cell moiety of this kind is consistent with "the associative antibody" hypothesis proposed by Bretscher and Cohn (1970) and the collaborative models of Lachmann (1971), Gutman and Weissman (1972), and Gorczynski *et al.* (1973). In addition, it can be used to explain other immunological phenomena, such as tolerance and antigenic competition. Thus, if all the macrophages in a particular microenvironment in lymphoid tissue are saturated with IgT–antigen complexes the presence of excess haptenic determinants would be expected to bind directly to B cells and induce tolerance. Furthermore, the introduction of a second T-dependent antigen could not result in a response due to a lack of available macrophages required for IgT–antigen presentation to appropriate B cells (Schrader and Feldmann, 1973). The main drawbacks to general acceptance of the IgT–antigen complex model are the origin and precise nature of the IgT moiety.

2. *Cytophilic Antibody Model*

Earlier in this section the problem of the origin of IgT was raised, and it was pointed out that there is at least some evidence suggesting it could be cytophilic antibody originally derived from B cells. This raises the question of whether, even if it were cytophilic, it could still have a role to play in T cell–B cell interaction, and whether the IgT–antigen model could not, as a consequence, be reinterpreted. In this context, the requirement in cell collaboration for specific antigen would be two-fold: first to trigger T cells to release a nonspecific mediator, such as

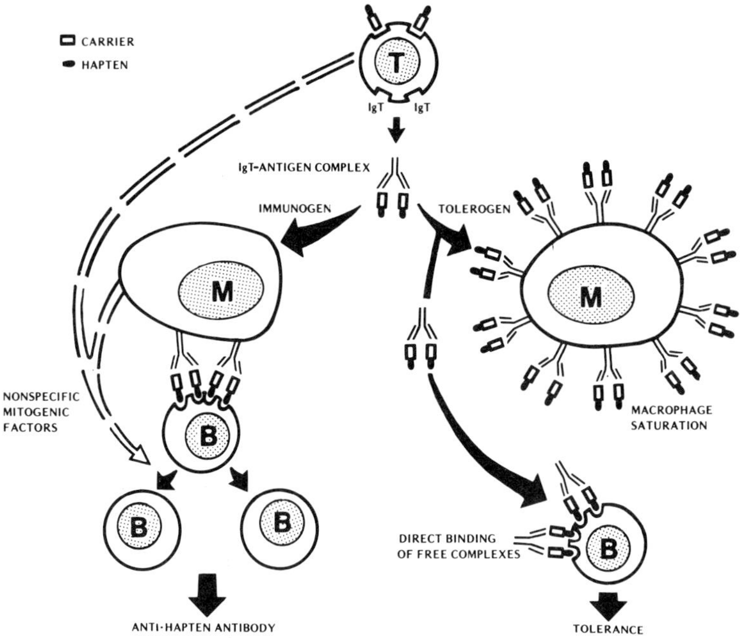

Fig. 2. Diagrammatic representation of the IgT–antigen complex model of T cell–B cell collaboration. Activated T cells (T) release a specific IgT–antigen complex cytophilic for macrophages (M). The macrophages then present the complexes to B cells (B) as an immunogenic matrix that cross-links haptenic receptors (signal 2) thereby triggering the cells into antibody production. Nonspecific factors from T cells or macrophages act at the proliferative stage of the response to increase the number of hapten-specific antibody-forming cells. If a high dose of antigen is used, the macrophage surface becomes saturated with IgT–antigen molecules allowing direct binding of free complexes to the B cell receptors which results in tolerance.

AEF, and second to generate IgM antibody from $B\mu$ cells which would directly or indirectly potentiate T cell proliferation. The presence of Fc and possibly C3 receptors (Arnaiz-Villena *et al.*, 1974) on activated T cells (Section II,A,1) would enable them to bind IgM antibody plus antigen directly, but whether this constitutes a stimulatory signal is unknown. Indeed it may instead lead to a suppressor signal as suggested by *in vitro* studies of Feldmann (1973). Alternatively antigen–IgM–C3 complexes could form and bind to the surface of macrophages, which would then interact either with the C3 receptor recently described on the T cell (Arnaiz-Villena *et al.*, 1974) or via the receptor on T cells for macrophages. The latter reaction is consistent with the data discussed previously demonstrating the importance of the macrophage in antigen presentation to T cells. Furthermore, enhancement of the immune response by

IgM (compared with IgG) antibodies is a well recognized phenomenon (Henry and Jerne, 1968). The arguments for and against a primary role for cytophilic antibody in cell collaboration have been well summarized in a recent review by Playfair (1974). Suffice it to say here that cytophilic antibody almost certainly plays a role in regulating the proliferative phase of the immune response, but it does not at this stage have to be invoked as a component of the fundamental mechanism of the inductive process (Weinbaum *et al.*, 1973). If, on the other hand, "IgT" does indeed prove to be of B cell origin and if, in addition, the Fc receptor on activated T cells is shown to be closely associated with the histocompatibility gene complex associated determinants (see Section IV,B,4) as is the case on B cells, then this conclusion may have to be revised.

3. C3 Activation Model

This model proposes that the second signal for B cell triggering is mediated by activated C3 combining with the C3 receptor sites present on the B cell membrane. Three experimental approaches favor a role for complement in B cell activation. First, *in vivo* depletion of C3 by injection of cobra venom factor was found to abrogate antibody production (Pepys, 1972) but not tolerance induction (Pepys and Taussig, 1974) to T-dependent antigens. Second, specific anti-C3 antiserum proved capable of inhibiting the *in vitro* response to the T-dependent hapten carrier conjugate, DNP-POL (Feldmann and Pepys, 1974). Third, when the C3 receptor was blocked *in vitro,* C3-containing but not C3-deficient serum enhanced the reactivity of B cells to an otherwise T cell-specific mitogen (Dukor and Hartmann, 1973). As a result of these observations the latter investigators proposed that the nonspecific diffusable factor required for collaborative responses might be activated C3. In favor of this is the finding that both proliferating thymus cells (Hirschhorn *et al.*, 1968) and macrophages (Table I) secrete lysosomal enzymes that can generate activated split products of C3 by cleavage (Hill and Ward, 1969). Since activated C3 rapidly loses its binding capacity in the fluid phase, only those B cells in close proximity to the enzyme source would be expected to bind sufficient C3 onto their C3 receptors for triggering (Fig. 3). The requirement in collaborative responses for hapten and carrier molecules to be on the same macrophage (Askonas and Roelants, 1974) would ensure such an appropriate anatomical arrangement. The hypothesis receives further support from the observation that at least some T-independent (and macrophage-independent) antigens are potent C3 activators (Götze and Müller-Eberhard, 1971; Bitter-Suermann, 1972). However, as pointed out by Feldmann and Pepys (1974), not all T-independent

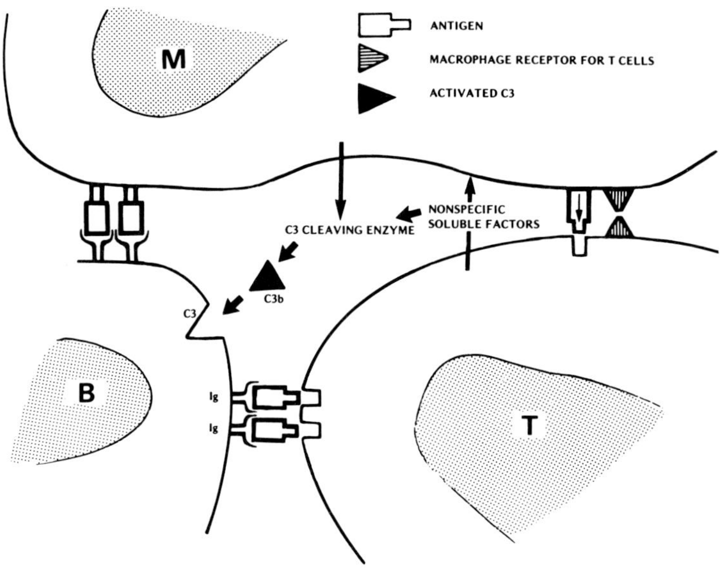

Fig. 3. Diagrammatic representation of the C3 activation model of T cell–B cell collaboration. T cells (T) activated by macrophage (M)-associated antigen release various nonspecific soluble factors including MIF, MSF, and lysosomal enzymes capable of cleaving C3 to C3b. Macrophages activated by T cell factors then release more C3-cleaving enzymes resulting in further C3 cleavage. The second signal for B cell (B) triggering is generated by the binding of C3b to the C3 receptor on B cells. The antigen bridges between the three cell types ensure close proximity of interacting cells which is necessary due to the rapid loss of binding capacity of C3b. "Tolerance" will occur if the T cell–macrophage axis is bypassed.

antigens, nor for that matter mitogens, will cleave C3 (Janossy *et al.*, 1973; Paul *et al.*, 1974). Fixed C3, on the other hand, could well be important in antigen presentation to B cells, particularly in the proliferative phase of the primary response or the inductive phase of the secondary response when antibody (IgM and IgG, respectively) would be present for binding to C3 receptors (Mantovani *et al.*, 1972).

4. *Ir–CI Gene Complex Model*

Katz and Benacerraf (1974) have put forward an hypothesis to explain cellular interactions in the light of the recent studies on histocompatibility gene complex-associated antigens. In this they proposed that the T cell has three phenotypically linked but functionally distinct surface components: the antigen binding site, the cell interaction or *CI* gene product site located in the *I* region of the histocompatibility gene complex, and the *Ir* gene product site. For an immune response to occur one or more of these components requires activation. The macrophage is envisaged as playing a key role in triggering CI sites that may well be identical to the receptors for lymphocytes described by Rosenthal and Shevach (1973). If interaction occurs only at the CI site the effect of antigen would be to induce a "suppressor" T cell, but if T cells interact with macrophages or other lymphocytes via the bimolecular complex, which is composed of both Ir and CI in the presence of antigen, a helper T cell would be generated. In the light of these suggestions, AEF may represent an Ir–CI complex, and the "thymus cell" factors of Munro *et al.* (1974) may represent an Ir–CI antigen-specific receptor complex. It might, in addition, be predicted that T cell-dependent suppression would be mediated by a macrophage-dependent lower molecular weight factor. To date there is no direct evidence for this, but recent experiments by Tada *et al.* (1973) are consistent with this idea. Furthermore, we have evidence favoring a role for an adherent cell, possibly a macrophage, in specific suppression of an anti-hapten antibody response (P. Johnson and A. Basten, in preparation).

5. *Macrophage Factor Model*

Discussion of the previous models has tended to stress the importance of T cell factors in cell collaboration, but it should be reemphasized that in several systems evidence has been produced for elaboration by macrophages either of similar factors, such as lysosomal enzymes (C3 activation model), or of different factors, such as products replacable by 2-mercaptoethanol *in vitro* (Gisler *et al.*, 1973; Pierce *et al.*, 1974). The relative frequency of macrophages compared with antigen-specific T cells makes them a more plausible source of short-range mediators that might have *in vivo* activity. Three groups of experiments can be cited in favor of this possibility. In the first, spleen cells from athymic (nu/nu) mice were shown on addition *in vitro* of peritoneal exudate cells or their supernatants to acquire the capacity to mount a primary response to the highly T-dependent antigen, fowl γ-globulin (Schrader, 1973). Since the peritoneal cells were from the same source (i.e., nu/nu mice) the macrophage, not the T cell, was apparently providing the second signal for B cell activation. Second, Britton (1974) has obtained some evidence from the *in vitro* analysis of allogeneic spleen cell mixtures to support the hypothesis that activated T cells do not provide the second signal directly, but rather by stimulating macrophages to secrete a product (as yet unidentified) that in the presence of antigen triggers the appropriate B cell. A further extension of this suggestion is discussed in Section IV,B,6. Taken in conjunction with the findings of Hunter and Kettman (1974) described previously, these observations reemphasize the possible role of macrophages in determining the type of factors operating in B cell triggering and proliferation. The third piece of evidence favoring elaboration of nonspecific factors by macrophages comes from the work of Gery and Waksmann (1972) Keller (Chapter 19), Nelson (1973 and Chapter 9), and Calderon *et al.* (1974). For example, supernatants obtained from cultures of macrophage or macrophage-containing peritoneal exudates were able to exert a cytostatic effect on various target cells, such as EL/4 leukemia cells and spleen cells undergoing a proliferative response to concanavalin A or lipopolysaccharide. In other words, macrophages may release suppressive as well as stimulatory factors, which could be important not only in inhibiting malignant cell growth but also in modifying lymphocyte proliferation in the immune response. Whether the latter proves to be true or whether any particular form of antigenic presentation will favor the release of inhibitory rather than helper factors from macrophages remains to be established.

6. Deblocking and Protection Model

The role of the macrophage in the collaborative models described to date has involved either antigen presentation or mediation or production of soluble factors. The experiments summarized by Mosier in Chapter 2, however, highlight the importance of antigen removal by macrophages in B cell activation. Thus an absolute requirement for macrophages in preventing tolerance induction to DNP-D-GL *in vitro* was observed (Mosier *et al.*, 1974; Paul *et al.*, 1974). Based on this and other observations, G. F. Mitchell (1974) has recently proposed a different model of T cell–B cell interaction termed the "deblocking and protection hypothesis." This states that, in the absence of extrinsic influences, antigen binds preferentially to high affinity B cells resulting in immobilization of receptors and tolerance (Diener and Paetkou, 1972). The function of the T cell is therefore twofold: first to release B cells from antigen blockade, thereby protecting them from tolerization, and second to promote receptor aggregation and redistribution which leads to γC_H gene expression and preferential production of high affinity IgG antibody (Fig. 4). T cells could influence antigen removal from blocked receptor sites directly by release of proteases as mentioned in the discussion of the C3 activation model. However, the absolute requirement for macrophages in T cell-dependent responses, at least *in vitro*, coupled with their relative frequency compared with specific T cells makes them a more potent source of lysosomal enzymes. T cells could therefore exert their effect indirectly by release of "lymphokines" (Anonymous, 1973) that would cause local

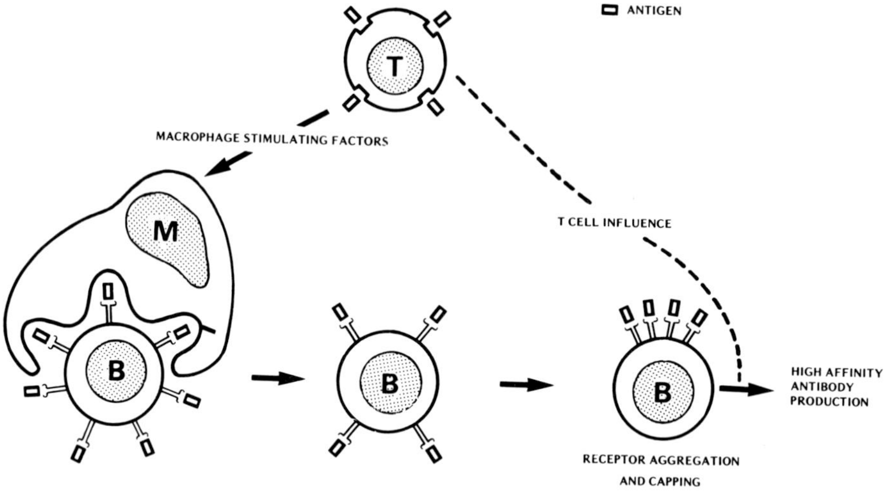

Fig. 4. Diagrammatic representation of the deblocking and protection model of T cell–B cell collaboration. Antigen binds to high affinity B cells (B) leading to a state of antigen blockade and potential tolerance. Activated T cells (T) release nonspecific factors that recruit and stimulate macrophages (M). The macrophages then release the B cells from antigen blockade by removal of excess antigenic determinants. As a result aggregation and redistribution of B cell receptors (signal 2) occurs with production of antibody-forming cells. During this process, T cells and antigen in addition effect the switch from $B\mu$ of $B\gamma$ cells. Tolerance will occur if the T cell–macrophage axis is bypassed.

activation of macrophages. Thus, the second signal for B cell triggering would be generated as a consequence of reducing the epitope density in the microenvironment of the B cell receptors. In contrast, nondegradable antigens, such as DNP-D-GL, or antigens with a rigid structure resembling macrophage-associated antigen, such as DNP-Ficoll, would block high affinity $B\gamma$ cells but stimulate low affinity $B\mu$ cells that bind antigen weakly and therefore reversibly. As a result, $B\mu$ cells would be triggered to synthesize IgM antibody essentially in the absence of T cell influence. This model is attractive, since it is consistent with current concepts of T dependence, and in addition can be readily visualized as operating *in vivo*.

C. Conclusions

The descriptions of the various models of cell collaboration is in no way meant to imply that they are mutually exclusive. Indeed more than one mechanism may be involved in the response to any particular antigen.

For example, the IgT–antigen complex and the deblocking and protection models can both be used to explain the induction phase of an immune response, while the cytophilic antibody and the C3 activation models may be involved during the proliferative phase of the same response. Furthermore, the *Ir–CI* gene complex model represents an attempt to explain events at the molecular and genetic level, which again does not exclude a contribution from C3 activation, the cytophilic antibody, or the macrophage factor models. Consideration of the models as a whole does, however, emphasize three vital facets of the immune response: First, the immune response depends in the majority of cases on the presence of macrophages, which can make a wide variety of contributions ranging from antigen presentation to release of modulating factors. Second, the macrophage apparently plays a vital role in its regulation (switch-on versus switch-off) at the cellular and possibly the genetic level. Third, the need for close contact between three cooperating cells points to a vital role for microenvironments, particularly *in vivo,* in its ultimate expression.

V. T CELL–B CELL COLLABORATION *IN VIVO*

The studies described in Sections III and IV highlight the complexity of the cellular interactions involved in antibody production. Although clearly advantageous from a teleological point of view, such diversity has meant that the majority of experiments demonstrating a requirement for macrophages in the immune response have been carried out *in vitro*. This poses very real problems in interpretation of the way(s) in which antigen–macrophage–lymphocyte interactions function *in vivo*. Thus tissue culture systems may artificially favor the operation of soluble factors. Furthermore, many of the structural features of secondary lymphoid organs cannot be reproduced or maintained *in vitro*. The physiological importance of, for example, the dendritic follicular cells found in germinal centers is therefore not amenable to this form of analysis. Conversely many of the physical aspects of cell interactions in culture, such as cluster formation, can be envisaged to occur in relatively unstructured lymphoid tissues, such as the peritoneal cavity or lung, but are much more difficult to transpose to the multiple microenvironments of lymph node and spleen. The purpose of this section is to provide a basis for interpretation of the *modus operandi* of the three cell models for collaboration *in vivo* by analyzing the anatomic relationships of the various macrophage populations found in secondary lymphoid organs with antigen and lymphocytes.

A. Functional Anatomy of Lymph Nodes

1. *Macrophages in Relations to Antigen*

The basic patterns of antigen interactions with the macrophage elements of lymph nodes have been established by radioautographic analysis of the distribution of labeled antigen. The greater part of this work was performed in the 1960's and has been reviewed in detail by several authors (Nossal and Ada, 1971; Unanue, 1972). The essential features are summarized here in relation to Fig. 5.

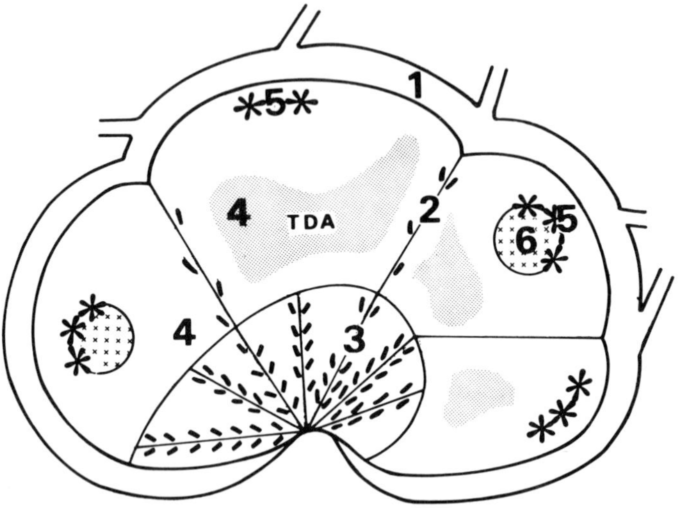

Fig. 5. Diagram of the mammalian lymph node showing locations of functionally distinct populations of macrophages. Site 1, subcapsular (outer cortical) sinus. Macrophages that phagocytize antigen are predominantly associated with the inner lining of the sinus and do not appear to be fixed. Antigen retention is transitory in this site. Site 2, cortical (trabecular) sinuses. Macrophages which appear to be fixed occur along the sinuses and phagocytize both antigen and nonantigenic particles. They appear to be similar to macrophages in site 3 (medullary sinuses). Macrophages appear to be fixed, line the sinuses, and avidly phagocytize both antigen and nonantigenic particles. This is the main site of intracellular retention of antigen over long periods. Site 4, diffuse cortex, both non-thymus-dependent and thymus-dependent (TDA). Scattered macrophages are present but show little evidence of antigen capture or sequestration. Site 5, dendritic follicular cell network of both primary and secondary lymphoid follicles. These cells (asterisks) are not typical macrophages but are included because of their antigen retaining properties. This is the major site of long-term membrane-associated display of antigen. Site 6, germinal center of the secondary lymphoid follicle. Tingible body macrophages scattered throughout the germinal centers do not usually phagocytize antigen (see text), although they engulf nonantigenic particles and lymphocytes.

When antigens are injected subcutaneously, a portion is carried very rapidly to the draining lymph node by the afferent lymph. Even as early as 3 minutes after injection, some antigen is found in association with phagocytic cells of the subcapsular sinus (site 1 in Fig. 5). The sinus appears to act as a pressure reduction system, which allows time for mixing (and possibly sorting) of monocytes, other phagocytes, and lymphocytes before they enter the more structured microenvironments of the parenchyma. The subcapsular sinus and outermost layers of the cortex, therefore, provide the first potential site for interaction among antigen, macrophages, and lymphocytes, particularly when there is a steady trickle of material draining into the node. The macrophages of the area do not constitute a permanent population responsible for prolonged retention of antigen (Nossal *et al.*, 1968a). If, however, antigen is artificially deposited in this region by emulsification in adjuvant (Humphrey *et al.*, 1967; Lind, 1968; Lamoureux *et al.*, 1968), clusters of pyroninophilic blast cells can form around microscopic droplets that on electron microscopy display antigenic particles on their surface. This phenomenon is perhaps an expression *in vivo* of the mechanism of antigen presentation proposed by Feldmann and Basten (1971) and observed in culture by Unanue *et al.* (1969).

The trabecular (inner cortical) sinuses and the more extensive medullary sinuses (sites 2 and 3 in Fig. 5) contain the majority of "fixed" macrophages, whose cytoplasmic organelles and phagocytic capacities most resemble the classical scavenger cells found in other parts of the body. These macrophages engulf and retain antigens injected into normal, immunized, or tolerant hosts, but there is little evidence from *in vivo* studies for processing of such antigen for presentation at the cell surface to lymphocytes *en passage*. There are a number of possible reasons for this. For instance, technical factors, such as the close apposition of macrophages with neighboring cells, the small areas of cell surface presented in sections, and the rigorous chemical procedures of radioautography required for electron microscopy, do not favor detection of small but possibly critical amounts of evenly distributed labeled material. Thus, although the prime function of macrophages in the lymph node cortical and medullary sinuses is one of antigen clearance and digestion (Nossal and Ada, 1971; Askonas and Jarŏsková, 1970), this by no means excludes a vital role for macrophage processed antigen in lymphocyte stimulation.

The diffuse cortex of the lymph node (site 4 in Fig. 5) likewise contains scattered cells identified morphologically as macrophages. These cells, however, display little evidence of antigen uptake, presentation, or sequestration, their precise function being unclear.

The remaining microenvironments (sites 5 and 6 in Fig. 5) where antigen is found in association with mononuclear cells are the enigmatic primary and secondary follicles which are common to lymph nodes, splenic white pulp, intestinal Peyer's patches, and many other sites. They comprise a cuff of histologically unremarkable small lymphocytes around a preexisting structure of dendritic cells that have variously been described as macrophages, reticular, reticulum, or follicular cells. Although there is still argument about the classification and nomenclature of dendritic follicular cells (Hanna and Hunter, 1971), it is now generally accepted that they are responsible for the prolonged antibody-dependent sequestration of antigen found ultrastructurally to be associated with their outer cytoplasmic membranes (J. Mitchell and Abbot, 1965). The striking contrast between the dendritic follicular cell and the true macrophage in antigen localization must be emphasized. Dendritic follicular cells are grouped with macrophages in discussions of lymphocyte–antigen interactions for historical reasons (White, 1963) and because of their antigen-localizing properties. Steinman and Cohn (1973, 1974) have recently isolated *in vitro* a "dendritic cell" present only in lymphoid organs known to contain the antigen-retaining dendritic follicular cells. The authors were unable to obtain binding of immune complexes or antibody-coated erythrocytes to their morphologically characterized "dendritic cells." It appears, therefore, that dendritic follicular cells have not yet been isolated *in vitro,* and it has proved difficult to define their role in terms of possession of surface receptors (postulated in the IgT–antigen complex, cytophilic antibody, and C3 activation models of cell collaboration, discussed in Section IV) or elaboration of enzymic or other soluble cooperating factors (C3 activation, *Ir–CI* gene complex, macrophage factor models). However, their capacity to bind antigen, predominantly via an antibody bridge linked to an Fc receptor (Herd and Ada, 1969; Nossal and Ada, 1971) has been firmly established and could be important in removal of potentially tolerogenic amounts of antigen from the binding sites on the lymphocyte membrane (deblocking and protection model). Whether the dendritic cells as well as the lymphocytes located here play a role in C3 binding (Dukor *et al.,* 1970; Mantovani *et al.,* 1972) is uncertain. Despite this, the follicular areas represent one possible site for the T cell–B cell stage of collaboration (Gutman and Weissman, 1972, 1973).

Secondary lymphoid follicles are distinguished from primary follicles by the presence of a germinal center composed of a group of cytoplasmically active lymphocytes together with tingible body macrophages (TBM) (site 6 in Fig. 5). The latter will phagocytize carbon, other nonantigenic particles (Burke and Simon, 1970), and near-mitotic lymphocytes (Fliedner, 1967). They do not, however, appear to engulf antigen presented alone or in the presence of antibody. The only time when antigen is found intracellularly in TBM is if it is associated with cell debris, as though it had been engulfed along with an antigen-labeled lymphocyte (Nossal *et al.*, 1968b; J. Mitchell, unpublished observations). Furthermore, since TBM are not found in follicles until germinal center formation has been established, a role for them in antigen processing or presentation is unlikely. It seems reasonable, on the other hand, to suggest that they may be involved in some facet of regulation of lymphocyte proliferation in germinal centers, such as "mopping up" of lymphocytes stimulated to abortive division from their contact with antigen on the dendritic follicular cells or elsewhere (T cell–B cell stage). Whether their lack of participation in antigen uptake (pre-T cell stage) represents a form of cell specialization or is merely a reflection of the absence of antigen in the area is unknown.

2. *Macrophages in Relation to Lymphocyte Traffic*

The members of the macrophage class, provisionally including dendritic follicular cells, are an essentially sessile population strategically placed in lymph nodes, while the lymphocytes of the circulating pool function as a highly mobile population obeying an apparently well-defined set of traffic rules.

Lymphocytes enter the nodes via two routes: from the blood stream through postcapillary venules (PCV, Fig. 6) which run from the outer cortex adjacent to follicles, through the paracortex, becoming typical venules near the corticomedullary junction. After entry, lymphocytes ecotax (de Sousa, 1971) either to follicular (B cell) regions (Sprent, 1973) or to the paracortical (T cell) regions (Parrott *et al.*, 1966) with little likelihood of contact with macrophages in the cortical sinuses. It is not known whether or not B cells move at random from the inner to the outer cortical areas and have a high chance of meeting the antigen-retaining dendritic cells in follicles after entry through postcapillary venules (Fig. 6).

Lymphocytes entering a node via afferent lymphatics migrate from the circular sinus into the outer cortex (Fig. 6) thereby having a much better chance of encountering antigen and macrophages in the region. This route of entry has not, however, been studied as closely as that through postcapillary venules. Thus, although B cells are known to enter the follicular cuff where they appear to migrate centrally through the areas occupied by dendritic follicular cells (Nossal *et al.*, 1968b), it has not been unequivocally established whether T cells also utilize this route. Neverthe-

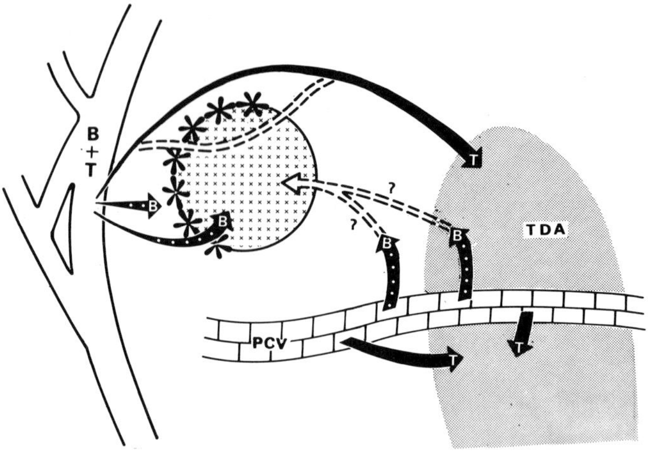

Fig. 6. Diagram of T and B lymphocyte traffic into the lymph node. Top, cells entering via afferent lymph are mixed in the subcapsular sinus where they have a high probability of contact with lymphborne antigen and macrophages. B cells move to the outer cortical regions and have a high chance of contact with antigen-retaining dendritic follicular cells. Some pass into germinal centers. T cells move to the deeper paracortical thymus-dependent area (TDA). A proportion, or a subpopulation, of them may pass through the dendritic follicular cell network of primary or secondary follicles. Bottom, blood-borne lymphocytes enter from postcapillary venules (PCV) in both non-thymus-dependent cortex and thymus-dependent cortex (TDA). After several hours B cells have localized in the former, T cells in the latter area. Whether movement from one compartment to another occurs at random is unknown. There is a low probability of contact with antigen, avid macrophages, or dendritic follicular cells on entry.

less, isolated T cells have been detected in germinal centers by an *in situ* fluorescent technique (Gutman and Weissman, 1972) that provides at least some evidence favoring antigen–macrophage–lymphocyte interaction at this site.

Circulation and exit of lymphocytes generated in the node are completed by passage from the specific T cell- or B cell-dependent microenvironments to the corticomedullary junction and then by way of the medullary cords and sinuses to the efferent lymph. The medulla, therefore, provides a second major site for circulating cells to come into physical contact with macrophages. Indeed, morphological studies of the development of plasma cells in the medullary cords have indicated that B cells can be arrested at this point in their circulation by contact with antigen possibly associated with macrophages and develop locally into antibody-forming cells (Miller and Avrameas, 1971).

The appearances of clusters of plasma cells around macrophages has been interpreted by Miller and Avrameas as evidence for cell collaboration. It should, however, be pointed out that this anatomical arrangement of the two cell types could be either coincidental or a manifestation of the scavenger properties of the medullary macrophages, which frequently contain partially digested plasmacytoid cells (Rieke *et al.*, 1963; Nossal *et al.*, 1968a). Nevertheless, it is tempting to postulate a role for the medullary cord as a microenvironment where nonspecific factors derived from T cells or macrophages might act in enhancing the proliferative phase of an ongoing immune response. The fact that the T cells as well as B cells must pass antigen-bearing macrophages provides some evidence in favor of this notion. If, on the other hand, contact between T cells and antigen leads to an inductive stimulus as well, then the T cells activated here must either migrate back to the paracortical regions of the same node or pass on in the circulation until they reach the next suitable microenvironment. Since the former proposal requires travel against the general direction of lymph and cell flow, the latter is physiologically more attractive and would be consistent with the finding of T cells in follicles (Gutman and Weissman, 1972). A definitive answer may, however, have to await development of techniques for tracing both antigen specific T cells and B cells.

B. Functional Anatomy of the Spleen

1. Macrophages in Relation to Antigen

The spleen has three major compartments, each of which contains macrophages differing both anatomically and functionally in their relation to antigen. In the first of these, the red pulp (site 1 in Fig. 7), macrophages are found particularly in association with the sinuses. But unlike their counterparts in lymph node medulla or elsewhere which both ingest carbon particles and readily bind ^{125}I labeled antigens, these macrophages label less readily with iodinated material (Nossal *et al.*, 1966; J. Mitchell and Abbot, 1971). Furthermore, nests of plasma cells occur in the splenic red pulp, but not in intimate relationship to antigen-laden macrophages as occurs in the lymph node medulla. This fact, taken together with the caution discussed earlier (Section IV,A,1) and the recent *in vitro* experiments of McIntyre and Pierce (1973) constitute evidence against the view that *in vivo* morphology shows direct macrophage–lymphocyte interaction in clusters (Miller and Avrameas, 1971). The marginal zone (site 2 in Fig. 7) is populated by macrophages, lymphocytes, a few granulocytes, and erythrocytes in a rather poorly defined network of reticulin fibers and open-ending arterioles (Weiss, 1965). The unique functional significance of this area has been emphasized by studies on the fate of intravenously injected antigen, the majority of which has been shown to localize

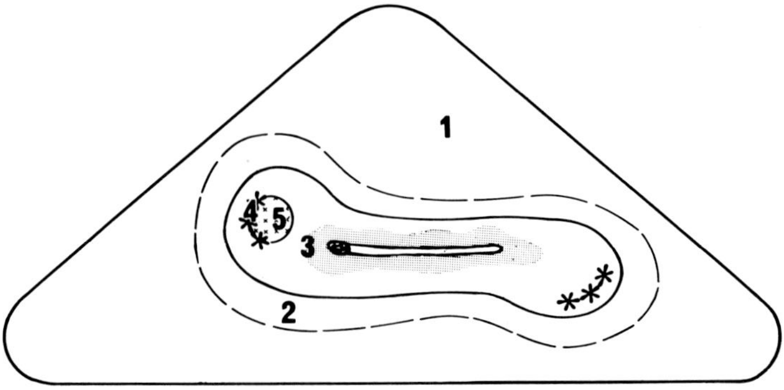

Fig. 7. Diagram of the mammalian spleen showing locations of functionally distinct populations of macrophages. Site 1, red pulp. Macrophages that phagocytize antigen and nonantigenic particles are present throughout, but these do not retain antigen for long periods and are not distributed in close relation to cords of plasma cells as in the lymph node medulla. Site 2, marginal zone containing many macrophages. Some phagocytosis of antigen and other particles occurs, but antigen localization is only transitory and frequently extracellular. Site 3, diffuse white pulp, including periarteriolar lymphocyte sheath. Scattered macrophages occur but are seldom involved in phagocytosis of antigen. Site 4, dendritic follicular cell network (asterisks) of both primary and secondary lymphoid follicles (see site 5 in Fig. 5). The only site of long-term membrane-associated display of antigen in the spleen. Site 5, germinal center of the secondary lymphoid follicle. Tingible body macrophages scattered through the germinal centers are usually not phagocytic of antigen (see site 6 in Fig. 5).

here for several hours after injection. Early work (Nossal *et al.*, 1966) suggested that macrophages played the major role not only in antigen capture but also in transport of antigen into the white pulp. The marginal zone macrophages do indeed phagocytize carbon (Burke and Simon, 1970), but it now seems that their association with antigen is more frequently membranous than phagolysosomal. This has been confirmed by recent studies of marginal zone localization of protein antigens following intraarterial injection (J. Mitchell and Abbot, 1971). In these experiments antigen shortly after injection was largely found in extracellular sites where it was associated with lymphocytoid cells. The marginal zone of the spleen, therefore, represents one potential site for macrophage–antigen–lymphocyte contact, perhaps principally at the pre-T cell stage, in the case of bloodborne antigens.

The periarteriolar lymphocyte sheath and diffuse cortex of the white pulp comprise the third compartment (site 3 in Fig. 7). They contain macrophages which will phagocytize carbon, but there is no evidence for antigen handling by these cells (Nossal *et al.*, 1966) that are therefore analogous to the scattered macrophages of the lymph node parenchyma (site 4 in Fig. 5). Scattered labeled cells do appear in the white pulp after injection of iodinated antigen, but because this is an area of active lymphocyte traffic (*vide infra*) ultrastructural studies are needed to define the cell type responsible. Indeed lymphocytes have already been more frequently implicated in antigen binding than macrophages (J. Mitchell and Abbot, 1971; J. Mitchell, 1972; Brown *et al.*, 1973).

The primary and secondary lymphoid follicles of the white pulp (sites 4 and 5 in Fig. 7) act as the major site of long-term exposition and retention of antigen in the spleen. There appears to be no differences between the follicles in the spleen and lymph nodes in their antigen retaining properties, which have been described in detail in Section V,A,1 and are a potential site for the T cell–B cell phase of the collaborative response (J. Mitchell, 1973b).

2. *Macrophage in Relation to Cell Traffic*

All cells entering the spleen are released from arterioles which terminate in the marginal zone. Here, lymphocytes have a high probability of physical contact with macrophages, which may play a role in short-term antigen retention in the region, as discussed in the preceding section. However, the duration of contact is likely to be minimal, since the marginal zone acts purely as a transit area rather than one in which lymphocytes reside. The myeloid and erythroid elements in the circulation pass from the marginal zone to the red pulp. Lymphocytes, on the other hand, have two options. A proportion pass into the red pulp, while others traverse the marginal sinus and enter the outer regions of the white pulp (Fig. 8) (Pettersen *et al.*, 1967; Ford, 1969). Sequential radioautographic studies of localization of injected cells have failed to delineate selected points of entry for T and B cells. From the few experiments that have included studies at short time intervals after injection, migrating lymphocytes of both thymic and bone marrow origin appear to spend some time in the peripheral regions where follicles (and follicular antigen-retaining dendritic cells) are located (Ford, 1969; J. Mitchell, 1972; Sprent, 1973). B cells tend to remain in these outer regions (Durkin *et al.*, 1972; Howard *et al.*, 1972; J. Mitchell, 1972), while thymus cells and thymus-derived cells localize in the central periarteriolar sheath (Parrott *et al.*, 1966).

Some doubt has been cast recently on the validity of the patterns of lymphocyte migration following intravenous injection of cell populations labeled *in vitro*. Parrott *et al.* (1974) grafted intact [^{3}H]thymidine labeled spleens into syngeneic recipients and showed that migrant cells seeding to the host spleen from this source were more frequently found in the marginal zone and red pulp than occurred after injection of a dis-

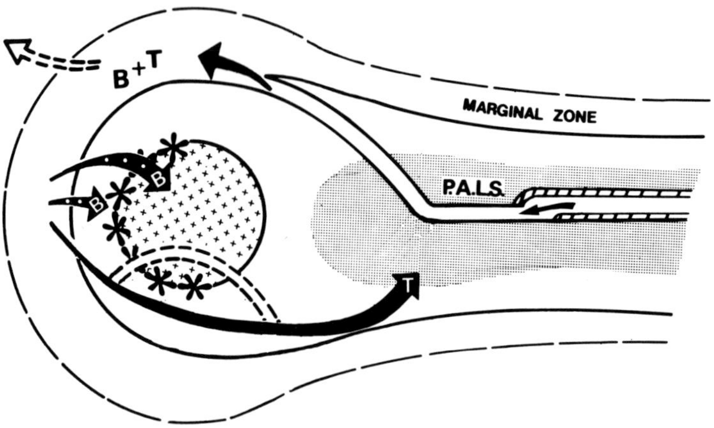

Fig. 8. Diagram of T and B lymphocyte traffic into the spleen. All lymphocytes enter from arterioles that terminate in the marginal zone. Here, T and B cells are mixed and may make contact with both antigen and macrophages. Some cells pass directly into the red pulp where they have further limited opportunity for interaction with antigen-processing macrophages. Most lymphocytes pass across a basement membrane into the white pulp. B cells tend to remain in the peripheral white pulp where they have a high chance of contact with antigen-*retaining* dendritic follicular cells represented here in a secondary follicle. Some B cells enter germinal centers. T cells pass quickly through the peripheral white pulp to the deeper periarteriolar lymphocyte sheath (P.A.L.S.). A proportion, or a subpopulation, of T cells may pass through the dendritic follicular network. No significant contact with antigen-*processing* macrophages occurs in the white pulp.

persed cell suspension. Since the earliest time studied was 24 hours after grafting, and their system was designed to follow labeled cells generated in a donor spleen undergoing a rejection response to a histoincompatible skin graft, their results may not be relevant to the initial traffic routes of lymphocytes capable of participating in collaborative antibody responses.

Lymphocytes leave the spleen mainly in the venous blood (Ford, 1969), although there is also apparently an efferent lymph flow originating from the periarteriolar regions of the white pulp (Snook, 1946; Janout and Weiss, 1972). Exit by the latter route would not involve transit through a microenvironment containing macrophages. Lymphocytes leaving the white pulp via blood would have a much higher chance of physical contact with antigen and antigen-processing macrophages, provided they migrated at random through the marginal zone into the red pulp sinuses. However, specific exit routes have recently been proposed for cells passing through or generated in the white pulp (J. Mitchell, 1973a). Should the latter prove to be correct, macrophage contact would be minimal for blood as well as lymph-borne lymphocytes during their exit from the spleen.

C. Putative Sites for Macrophage Interactions *in Vivo*

1. Pre-T Cell Stage

The principal roles of the macrophage during this stage of cell interaction consist of antigen degradation, concentration, and presentation (see Section III,D,1). Structural degradation of particulate antigens is now generally accepted as being a function of the "fixed" typical macrophages of the splenic red pulp and lymph node medulla. The problem, however, of whether or not macrophages in these sites release the products of digestion as immunogenic moieties and display them in the form of surface-localized fragments has not yet been resolved. Two facts are difficult to explain if splenic red pulp or lymph node medullary macrophages are solely responsible for antigen presentation at the pre-T cell stage. First, the major histopathological immune response is seen in either the spleen white pulp (after intravenous antigen challenge) or the cortex of the first draining lymph node (after subcutaneous challenge). Therefore, it seems probably that T-dependent antigens that require macrophage processing in the pre-T cell stage are presented to T cells before, at or shortly after, those lymphocytes arrive in the spleen or lymph node. Second, T cells reaching the splenic red pulp or the lymph node medulla are, according to cell circulation studies, in the process of leaving these organs, rather than about to enter the established sites of T cell proliferation. If immunogenic products released as a result of antigen degradation by macrophages in the splenic red pulp or lymph node medulla do indeed cause T cell stimulation, the activated T cells must subsequently migrate to the white pulp or the paracortical regions, respectively, before expressing the results of the activation process.

The factors described above point towards alternative and less obvious sites being involved in T cell activation by macrophage-processed antigen. For blood-borne antigens, most evidence points to a role for splenic marginal zone macrophages or even fixed tissue macrophages in nonlymphoid organs, such as liver or lung. For lymph-borne antigens, the peripheral tissue macrophages, or those recruited by the presence of subcutaneous antigen, may be vital in producing a local lymph node response.

The dendritic follicular cells of lymphoid follicles are unlikely to be involved in antigen processing at the pre-T cell stage. White *et al.* (1970, 1975) consider that dendrite cells in the chicken acquire antigen outside the germinal centers and later migrate into these areas. This view has not, however, gained experimental support and may not hold for other species. Until the origin of dendritic follicular cells is known, the involvement of these specialized cells cannot be entirely discounted in view of their strategic placement in areas accessible at least to some T cells.

2. *T Cell–B Cell Stage*

The possible ways in which macrophages may be involved during the actual collaborative step have been described in Section IV,A. The first priority for an *in vivo* site for T cell–B cell interaction must be the lymphoid follicles, as they represent the one microenvironment traversed by both T cells and B cells where antigen is known to be exhibited for prolonged periods on nonlymphoid cell surfaces, particularly the dendritic follicular cells. The one drawback to a strict analogy between follicles and macrophage-dependent antibody responses studied *in vitro* is the absence of local antigen-ingesting and -processing cells. Since the tingible body macrophages do not appear to subserve this function, (Section V,A,1) an extrafollicular source of processed antigen is required particularly for complex antigens. The most likely candidates are the macrophages of the marginal zone of the spleen or those of peripheral tissue, afferent lymph, or the outer cortex of the lymph node.

The preceding analysis of the functional anatomy of organized lymphoid tissue provides a basic framework on which the various three-cell models of collaboration can be discussed. In the case of the IgT–antigen complex model, the dendritic follicular cells provide a surface suitable for formation of the postulated matrix required for inductive B-cell stimulation. If IgT were isolated, this hypothesis could be tested in congenitally athymic (nu/nu) mice that possess dendritic cells capable, although with reduced efficiency (J. Mitchell *et al.*, 1972), of antigen localization in the presence of antibody. Dendritic follicular cells could also be envisaged as a focus for lymphocyte triggering in both the cytophilic antibody model and, with less supportive evidence, in the C3 activation model. Thus experimental evidence for Fc receptors on dendritic cells (Herd and Ada, 1969) may be invoked to account for binding of cytophilic antibody, which could then result in complement activation in the region. The failure of experimental approaches to isolate dendritic follicular cells *in vitro* does, however, make further analysis of the contribution of these cells to collaborative response very difficult. The way in which the other three-cell models could be related to lymphoid follicles and their antigen-stimulated germinal centers has not been extensively analyzed. When further requirements have been studied *in vitro* we should be in a better position to try to fit the pieces of the *in vitro* jigsaw onto the histological template.

Other interpretations of the three-cell models are possible in relation to the anatomic features of organized lymphoid tissue. The marginal zone of the spleen, for example, is a site where cellular interactions could occur, since macrophages are present and both T cells and B cells spend a brief time there in their circulation. Likewise, the outermost regions of the lymph node cortex could be considered if the time required for cellular interactions is very brief. All the remaining microenvironments of spleen and lymph nodes show reasonably complete compartmentation of T cells or B cells. It would, therefore, seem preferable to concentrate subsequent experimental effort on understanding the cellular interactions in sites where both lymphocyte types are mixed, rather than relying on the need to invoke extensive diffusion of soluble factors or complex routes of cell circulation between antigen stimulation and subsequent cell interaction.

ACKNOWLEDGMENTS

Some of the work referred to in this chapter was supported by grants from the National Health and Medical Research Council and the University of Sydney Cancer Research Fund. The authors thank Ms. Denyse Bartimote for typing the manuscript and the Department of Illustration at Royal Prince Alfred Hospital for preparing the figures.

REFERENCES

Andersson, C. L., and Grey, H. M. (1974). *J. Exp. Med.* **139,** 1175–1188.
Andersson, J., Sjöberg, O., and Möller, G. (1972). *Transplant. Rev.* **11,** 131-177.
Anonymous (1973). *Lancet* **1,** 1490–1491.
Arend, W. P., and Mannik, M. (1973). *J. Immunol.* **110,** 1455–1463.
Armerding, D., and Katz, D. H. (1974). *J. Exp. Med.* **140,** 19–37.
Armerding, D., and Katz, D. H. (1974). *J. Exp. Med.* **140,** 1717–1722.
Arnaiz-Villena, A., Gyöngyössy, M. I. C., and Playfair, J. H. L. (1974). *Clin. Exp. Immunol.* **18,** 177–186.
Askonas, B. A., and Jarŏsková, L. (1970). *In* "Mononuclear Phagocytes" (R. van Furth, ed.), pp. 595–612. Blackwell, Oxford.
Askonas, B. A., and Roelants, G. (1974). *Eur. J. Immunol.* **4,** 1–4.
Basten, A., and Feldmann, M. (1972). *Advan. Exp. Med. Biol.* **29,** 171–178.
Basten, A., and Howard, J. G. (1973). *Contemp. Top. Immunobiol.* **2,** 265–291.
Basten, A., and Miller, J. F. A. P. (1974). *In* "Cell Communication" (R. P. Cox, ed.), pp. 187–216. Wiley, New York.
Basten, A., Miller, J. F. A. P., Warner, N. L., and Pye, J. (1971). *Nature (London), New Biol.* **231,** 104–106.
Basten, A., Miller, J. F. A. P., Sprent, J., and Pye, J. (1972a). *J. Exp. Med.* **135,** 610–626.
Basten, A., Warner, N. L., and Mandel, T. E. (1972b). *J. Exp. Med.* **135,** 627–642.
Basten, A., Miller, J. F. A. P., and Abraham, R. (1975a). *J. Exp. Med.* **141,** 547–560.
Basten, A., Miller, J. F. A. P., Warner, N. L., and Abraham, R. (1975b). *J. Immunol.* **115,** 1159–1164.

Basten, A., Miller, J. F. A. P. Abraham, R. Gamble, J., and Chia, E. (1975c). *Int. Arch. Allergy Appl. Immunol.* in press.
Basten, A., Miller, J. F. A. P., and Johnson, P. (1975d). *Transplant Rev.* **26,** 130–169,
Benacerraf, B., and McDevitt, H. O. (1972). *Science* **175,** 273–279.
Biozzi, G., Asofsky, R., Lieberman, R., Stiffel C., Mouton, D., and Benacerraf, B. (1970). *J. Exp. Med.* **132,** 752–764.
Biozzi, G., Stiffel, C., Mouton, D., Bouthillier, Y., and Decreusefond, C. J. (1972). *J. Exp. Med.* **135,** 1071–1094.
Bitter-Suermann, D. (1972). *Klin. Wochenschr.* **50,** 277–286.
Bluestein H. G. (1974). *J. Exp. Med.* **140,** 481–493.
Bretscher, P. A. (1974). *Cell. Immunol.* **13,** 171–195.
Bretscher, P. A., and Cohn, M. (1970). *Science* **169,** 1042–1049.
Britton, S. (1974). *Scand. J. Immunol.* **3,** 433–444.
Brown J. C., Harris, G., Papamichail, M., Šljivić, V. S., and Holborow, E. J. (1973). *Immunology* **24,** 955–968.
Burke, J. S., and Simon, G. T. (1970). *Amer. J. Pathol.* **58,** 157–165.
Byfield, P. E., and Howard, J. G. (1972). *Transplantation* **14,** 133–135.
Calderon, J., Williams, R. T., and Unanue, E. R. (1974). *Proc. Nat. Acad. Sci. U.S.* **71,** 4273–4277.
Claman, H. N., and Chaperon, E. A. (1969). *Transplant. Rev.* **1,** 92–113.
Claman, H. N., and Mosier, D. E. (1972). *Progr. Allergy* **16,** 40–80.
Cline, M. J., and Swett, V. C. (1968). *J. Exp. Med.* **128,** 1309–1325.
Cohen, B. E., and Paul W. E. (1974). *J. Immunol.* **112,** 359–369.
Cone, R. E., Sprent, J., and Marchalonis, J. J. (1973). *Proc. Nat. Acad. Sci. U.S.* **69,** 2556–2560.
Cooper M. G., and Ada, G. L. (1972). *Scand. J. Immunol.* **1,** 247–253.
Coutinho, A., and Möller, G. (1973). *Eur. J. Immunol.* **3,** 531–537.
Cruchaud, A., Despont, J. P., Giraud, J. P., and Mach, B. (1970). *J. Immunol.* **104,** 1256–1261.
David, C. S., Schreffler, D. C., and Frelinger, J. A. (1973). *Proc. Nat. Acad. Sci. U.S.* **70,** 2509–2514.
Davies, A. J. S. (1969). *Transplant. Rev.* **1,** 43–91.
Delovitch, T. L., and McDevitt, H. O. (1975). *Immunogenetics* in press.
de Sousa, M. A. B. (1971). *Clin. Exp. Immunol.* **9,** 371–380.
Dickler, H. B., and Sachs, D. (1974). *J. Exp. Med.* **140,** 779–796.
Diener, E., and Paetkou, V. H. (1972). *Proc. Nat. Acad. Sci. U.S.* **69,** 2364–2368.
Dukor, P., and Hartmann, R. V. (1973). *Cell. Immunol.* **7,** 349–356.
Dukor, P., Bianco, C., and Nussenzweig, V. (1970). *Proc. Nat. Acad. Sci. U.S.* **67,** 991–997.
Durkin, H. G., Theis, G. A., and Thorbecke, G. J. (1972). *Nature (London), New Biol.* **235,** 118–119.
Dutton, R. W., McCarthy, M. M., Mishell, R. I., and Raidt, D. J. (1970). *Cell. Immunol.* **1,** 196–206.
Dutton, R. W., Falkoff, R., Hirst, J. A., Hoffmann, M., Kappler, J. W., Kettman, J. R., Lesley, J. R., and Vann, D. (1971). *In* "Progress in Immunology" (B. Amos, ed.), pp. 355–368. Academic Press, New York.
Ebringer, A., and Davies, D. A. L. (1973). *Nature (London) New Biol.* **241,** 144–147.
Feldmann, M. (1972). *J. Exp. Med.* **136,** 737–760.
Feldmann, M. (1973). *Nature (London), New Biol.* **242,** 82–84.

Feldmann, M., and Basten, A. (1971). *J. Exp. Med.* **134,** 103–119.
Feldmann, M., and Basten, A. (1972). *J. Exp. Med.* **136,** 722–736.
Feldmann, M., and Palmer, J. (1971). *Immunology* **21,** 685–699.
Feldmann, M., and Pepys, M. B. (1974). *Nature (London)* **249,** 159–161.
Fishman, M., and Adler, F. L. (1963). *J. Exp. Med.* **117,** 595–602.
Fishman, M., and Adler, F. L. (1970). *In* "Mononuclear Phagocytes" (R. van Furth, ed.), pp. 581–592. Blackwell, Oxford.
Fliedner, T. M. (1967). *In* "Germinal Centers in Immune Responses" (H. Cottier *et al.*, eds.), pp. 218–222. Springer-Verlag, Berlin and New York.
Ford, W. L. (1969). *Brit. J. Exp. Pathol.* **50,** 257–269.
Fox, R. A., Gregory, D. S. and Feldman, J. D. (1974). *J. Immunol.* **112,** 1867–1872.
Gallily, R., and Feldman, J. (1967). *Immunology* **12,** 197–206.
Gallily, R., and Gornostansky, M. (1972). *Immunology* **22,** 431–439.
Gery, I., and Waksman, B. H. (1972). *J. Exp. Med.* **136,** 143–155.
Gisler, R. H., Staber, F., Rüde, E., and Dukor, P. (1973). *Eur. J. Immunol.* **3,** 650–652.
Gorczynski, R. M., Miller, R. G., and Phillips, R. A. (1971). *J. Exp. Med.* **134,** 1201–1221.
Gorczynski, R. M., Miller, R. G., and Phillips, R. A. (1973). *J. Immunol.* **111,** 900–903.
Gordon, S., and Cohn, Z. A. (1973) *Int. Rev. Cytol.* **36,** 171–214.
Götze, T., and Müller-Eberhard, H. J. (1971). *J. Exp. Med.* **134,** 90S–108S.
Grey, H. M., Kubo, R. T., and Cerottini, J.-C. (1972). *J. Exp. Med.* **136,** 1323–1328.
Gutman, G. A., and Weissman, I. L. (1972). *Immunology* **23,** 465–479.
Gutman, G. A., and Weissman, I. L. (1973). *Transplantation* **16,** 621–629.
Hamaoka, T., Katz, D. H., and Benacerraf, B. (1973). *J. Exp. Med.* **138,** 538–556.
Hamilton, J. A., and Miller, J. F. A. P. (1973). *J. Exp. Med.* **138,** 1009–1014.
Hämmerling, G. J., and McDevitt, H. O. (1974). *J. Immunol.* **112,** 1734–1740.
Hanna, M. G., and Hunter, R. L. (1971). *Advan. Exp. Med. Biol.* **12,** 257–279
Hauptfield, V. D., Klein, D., and Klein, J. (1973). *Science* **181,** 167–169.
Henry, C., and Jerne, N. K. (1968). *J. Exp. Med.* **128,** 133–152.
Herd, Z. L., and Ada, G. L. (1969). *Aust. J. Exp. Biol. Med. Sci.* **47,** 73–80.
Hersh, E. H., and Harris, J. E. (1968). *J. Immunol.* **100,** 1184–1194.
Hill, J. H., and Ward, P. A. (1969). *J. Exp. Med.* **130,** 505–518.
Hirschhorn, R., Brittinger, G., Hirschhorn, K., and Weissmann, G. (1968). *J. Cell Biol.* **37,** 412–423.
Hoffmann, M., and Dutton, R. W. (1971). *Science* **172,** 1047–1048.
Holland, P., Holland, N. H., and Cohn, Z. A. (1972). *J. Exp. Med.* **135,** 458–475.
Howard, J. G., Hunt, S. V., and Gowans, J. L. (1972). *J. Exp. Med.* **135,** 200–219.
Howard, J. G., Courtenay, B. M., and Desaymard, C. (1974). *Eur. J. Immunol.* **4,** 453–457.
Huber, H., Polley, M. J., Linscott, W. D., Fudenberg, H. H., and Müller-Eberhard, H. J. (1968). *Science* **162,** 1281–1283.
Hudson, L., Sprent, J., Miller, J. F. A. P., and Playfair, J. H. L. (1974). *Nature (London)* **251,** 60–62.
Humphrey, J. H., Askonas, B. A., Auzins, I., Schechter, I., and Sela, M. (1967). *Immunology* **13,** 71–86.
Hunter, P., and Kettman, J. R., (1974). *Proc. Nat. Acad. Sci. U.S.* **71,** 512–516.
Janossy, G., Humphrey, J. H., Pepys, M. B., and Greaves, M. F. (1973). *Nature (London), New Biol.* **245,** 108–112.

Janout, V., and Weiss, L. (1972). *Anat. Rec.* **172,** 197–219.
Jonas, W. E., Gurner, B. W., Nelson, D. S., and Coombs, R. R. A. (1965). *Int. Arch. Allergy Appl. Immunol.* **28,** 86–104.
Katz, D. H. (1972). *Transplant. Rev.* **12,** 141–179.
Katz, D. H., and Benacerraf, B. (1972). *Advan. Immunol.* **15,** 1–94.
Katz, D. H. and Benacerraf, B. (1975). *Transplant. Rev.* **22,** 175–195.
Katz, D. H., and Unanue, E. R. (1973). *J. Exp. Med.* **137,** 967–990.
Katz, D. H., Paul, W. E., Goidl, A. E., and Benacerraf, B. (1970). *J. Exp. Med.* **132,** 261–282.
Katz, D. H., Hamaoka, T., and Benacerraf, B. (1973). *J. Exp. Med.* **137,** 1405–1418.
Klinman, N., and Doughty, R. A. (1973). *J. Exp. Med.* **138,** 473–478.
Lachmann, P. (1971). *Proc. Roy. Soc. B* **176,** 425–426.
Lamoreux, G., McPherson, T. A., Carnegie, P. R., and Mackay, I. R. (1968). *Clin. Exp. Immunol.* **3,** 25–35.
Lawton, A. R., Asofsky, R., Hylton, M. B., and Cooper, M. D. (1972). *J. Exp. Med.* **135,** 277–297.
Lay, W. H., and Nussenzweig, V. (1968). *J. Exp. Med.* **128,** 991–1009.
Lee, S. T., and Paraskevas, F. (1972). *J. Immunol.* **109,** 1262–1271.
Liacopoulos-Briot, M., Bouthillier, Y., Mouton, D., Lambert, F., Decreuseford, C., Stiffel, C., and Biozzi, G. (1972). *Transplantation* **14,** 590–596.
Lind, P. E. (1968). *Aust. J. Exp. Biol. Med. Sci.* **46,** 189–208.
Lipsky, P. E., and Rosenthal, A. S. (1973). *J. Exp. Med.* **138,** 900–924.
McIntyre, J. A., and Pierce, C. W. (1973). *J. Immunol.* **111,** 1526–1537.
McIntyre, J. A., Niblack, G D., Prater, T. F. K., and LaVia, M. F. (1971). *Fed. Proc., Fed. Amer. Soc. Exp. Biol.* **30,** 649 (abstr.).
Mantovani, B., Rabinovitch, M., and Nussenzweig, V. (1972). *J. Exp. Med.* **135,** 780–792.
Marbrook, J. (1967). *Lancet* **2,** 1279–1281.
Marchalonis, J. J., Cone, R. E., and Atwell, J. L. (1972). *J. Exp. Med.* **135,** 956–971.
Miller, H. R. P., and Avrameas, S. (1971). *Nature (London), New Biol.* **229,** 184–185.
Miller, J. F. A. P. (1975). *Ann. N.Y. Acad. Sci.* (in press).
Miller, J. F. A. P., and Mitchell, G. F. (1969). *Transplant. Rev.* **1,** 3–42.
Miller, J. F. A. P., Basten, A., Sprent, J., and Cheers, C. (1971). *Cell. Immunol.* **2,** 469–495.
Mishell, R. I., and Dutton, R. W. (1966). *Science* **153,** 1004–1006.
Mitchell, G. F. (1974). *Progr. Immunol.* **II,** (3), 89–98.
Mitchell, J. (1972). *Immunology* **22,** 231–245.
Mitchell, J. (1973a). *Immunology* **24,** 93–107.
Mitchell, J. (1973b). *Advan. Exp. Med. Biol.* **29,** 49–53.
Mitchell, J., and Abbot, A. (1965). *Nature (London)* **208,** 500–502.
Mitchell, J., and Abbot, A. (1971). *Immunology* **21,** 207–224.
Mitchell, J., Holmes, M. C., Pye, J., and Nossal, G. J. V. (1972). *Aust. J. Exp. Biol. Med. Sci.* **50,** 637–650.
Mitchison, N. A. (1969). *Immunology* **16,** 1–14.
Mitchison, N. A. (1971). *Eur. J. Immunol.* **1,** 18–27.
Mosier, D. E. (1967). *Science* **158,** 1573–1575.
Mosier, D. E. (1969). *J. Exp. Med.* **129,** 351–362.
Mosier, D. E., Johnson, B. M., Paul, W. E., and McMaster, P. R. B. (1974). *J. Exp. Med.* **139,** 1354–1360.

Munro, A. J., Taussig, M. J., Campbell, R., Williams, H., and Lawson, Y. (1974). *J. Exp. Med.* **140**, 1579–1587.
Nelson, D. S. (1965). *Complement, Ciba Found. Symp., 1964* pp. 222–237.
Nelson, D. S. (1969). "Macrophages and Immunity." North-Holland Publ. Amsterdam.
Nelson, D. S. (1973). *Nature (London)* **246**, 306–307.
Nossal, G. J. V., and Ada, G. L. (1971). "Antigens, Lymphoid Cells, and the Immune Response." Academic Press, New York.
Nossal, G. J. V., Austin, C. M., Pye, J., and Mitchell, J. (1966). *Int. Arch. Allergy Appl. Immunol.* **29**, 368–383.
Nossal, G. J. V., Abbot, A., and Mitchell, J. (1968a). *J. Exp. Med.* **127**, 263–276.
Nossal, G. J. V., Abbot, A., Mitchell, J., and Lummus, Z. (1968b). *J. Exp. Med.* **127**, 277–290.
Oldstone, M. B. A., and Dixon, F. J. (1969). *J. Exp. Med.* **129**, 483–499.
Ordal, J. C., and Grumet, F. C. (1972). *J. Exp. Med.* **136**, 1195–1206.
Osborne, D. P., and Katz, D. H. (1973). *J. Exp. Med.* **137**, 991–1008.
Parish, C. R., and Hayward, J. A. (1974a). *Proc. Roy. Soc., Ser B* **187**, 47–63.
Parish, C. R., and Hayward, J. A. (1974b). *Proc. Roy. Soc., Ser. B* **187**, 65–81.
Parkhouse, R. M. E., and Dutton, R. W. (1966). *J. Immunol.* **97**, 663–669.
Parrott, D. M. V., de Sousa, M. A. B., and East, J. (1966). *J. Exp. Med.* **123**, 191–203.
Parrott, D. M. V., Tilney, N. L., and Sless, F. R. (1975). *Clin. Exp. Immunol.* in press.
Passwell, J. H., Steward, M. W., and Soothill, J. F. (1974). *Clin. Exp. Immunol.* **17**, 159–167.
Paul, W. E., Karpf, M., and Mosier, D. (1974). *In* "Immunological Tolerance: Mechanisms and Potential Therapeutic Application" (D. H. Katz and B. Benacerraf, eds.), pp. 141–158. Academic Press, New York.
Pepys, M. B. (1972). *Nature (London), New Biol.* **237**, 157–159.
Pepys, M. B., and Taussig, M. J. (1974). *Eur. J. Immunol.* **4**, 349–352.
Pernis, B., Miller, J. F. A. P., Forni, L., and Sprent, J. (1974). *Cell. Immunol.* **10**, 476–482.
Pettersen, J. C., Borgen, D. F., and Graupner, K. C. (1967). *Amer. J. Anat.* **121**, 305–317.
Phillips-Quagliata, J. M., Levine, B. B., Quagliata, F., and Uhr, J. W. (1971). *J. Exp. Med.* **133**, 589–601.
Pierce, C. W. (1969). *J. Exp. Med.* **130**, 345–364.
Pierce, C. W., and Benacerraf, B. (1969). *Science* **166**, 1002–1004.
Pierce, C. W., Kapp, J. A., Wood, D. D., and Benacerraf, B. (1974). *J. Immunol.* **112**, 1181–1189.
Playfair, J. H. L. (1974). *Clin. Exp. Immunol.* **17**, 1–8.
Ramasamy, R., Munro, A. J., and Milstein, C. (1974). *Nature (London)* **249**, 573–574.
Rhodes, J. (1973). *Nature (London)* **243**, 527–528.
Rieke, W. O., Caffrey, R. W., and Everett, N. B. (1963). *Blood* **22**, 674–689.
Roelants, G. E., and Askonas, B. A. (1971). *Eur. J. Immunol.* **1**, 151–157.
Roelants, G. E., Forni, L., and Pernis, B. (1973). *J. Exp. Med.* **137**, 1060–1077.
Rosenthal, A. S., and Shevach, E. M. (1973). *J. Exp. Med.* **138**, 1194–1212.
Schimpl, A., and Wecker, E. (1971). *Eur. J. Immunol.* **1**, 304–306.
Schimpl, A., and Wecker, E. (1972). *Nature (London) New Biol.* **237**, 15–17.

Schmidkte, J., and Unanue, E. R. (1971). *Nature (London) New Biol.* **233,** 84–86.
Schrader, J. W. (1973). *J. Exp. Med.* **138,** 1466–1480.
Schrader, J. W., and Feldmann, M. (1973). *Eur. J. Immunol.* **3,** 711–717.
Sela, M., Mozes, E., and Shearer, G. M. (1972). *Proc. Nat. Acad. Sci. U.S.* **69,** 2696–2700.
Shortman, K., and Palmer, J. (1971). *Cell. Immunol.* **2,** 399–410.
Shortman, K., Byrd, W., Williams, N., Brunner, K. T., and Cerottini J.-C. (1972) *Aust. J. Exp. Biol. Med. Sci.* **50,** 323–336.
Snook, T. (1946). *Anat. Rec.* **94,** 43–55.
Soteraides-Vlachos, C., Gyöngyössy, M. I. C., and Playfair, J. H. L. (1974). *Clin. Exp. Immunol.* **18,** 187–192.
Sprent, J. (1973). *Cell. Immunol.* **7,** 10–39.
Steinman, R. M., and Cohn, Z. A. (1972). *J. Cell Biol.* **55,** 616–634.
Steinman, R. M., and Cohn, Z. A. (1973). *J. Exp. Med.* **137,** 1142–1162.
Steinman, R. M., and Cohn, Z. A. (1974). *J. Exp. Med.* **139,** 380–397.
Tada, T., Okumura, K., and Taniguchi, M. (1973). *J. Immunol.* **111,** 952–961.
Talmage, D. W., Radovich, J., and Hemmingsen, H. (1970). *Advan. Immunol.* **12,** 271–282.
Taussig, M. J. (1974). *Nature (London)* **248,** 234–236.
Taussig, M. J., and Munro, A. J. (1974). *Nature (London)* **251,** 63–65.
Taussig, M. J., Mozes, E., and Isaac, R. (1974). *J. Exp. Med.* **140,** 301–312.
Theis, G. A., and Thorbecke, G. J. (1970). *J. Exp. Med.* **131,** 970–980.
Uhr, J. W. (1965). *Proc. Nat. Acad. Sci. U.S.* **54,** 1599–1606.
Unanue E. R. (1972). *Advan. Immunol.* **15,** 95–165.
Unanue, E. R., and Askonas, B. A. (1968). *J. Exp. Med.* **127,** 915–926.
Unanue, E. R., and Cerottini, J.-C. (1970). *Semin. Hematol.* **7,** 225–248.
Unanue, E. R., and Katz, D. H. (1973). *Eur. J. Immunol.* **3,** 559–563.
Unanue, E. R., Cerottini, J.-C., and Bedford. M. (1969). *Nature (London)* **222,** 1193–1195.
Van Boxel, J. A., and Rosenstreich, D. L. (1974). *J. Exp. Med.* **139,** 1002–1012.
Vitetta, E. S., Bianco, C., Nussenzweig, V., and Uhr, J. W. (1972). *J. Exp. Med.* **136,** 81–93.
Waldron, J. A., Jr., Honn, R. H., and Rosenthal, A. S. (1973). *J. Immunol.* **111,** 58–64.
Watson, J., Thomas, M., Ralph, P., and Trenkner, E. (1974). *J. Immunol.* **112,** 1873–1883.
Weigle, W. O., and Golub, E. (1969). *In* "Immunological Tolerance" (M. Landy and W. Braun, eds.), pp. 210–213. Academic Press, New York.
Weinbaum, F. I., Gilmour, D. G., and Thorbecke, G. J. (1973). *J. Immunol.* **110,** 1434–1436.
Weiss, L. (1965). *Semin. Hematol.* **2,** 205–228.
White, R. G. (1963). *Ciba Found. Study Group* **16,** 6–16.
White, R. G., French, V. I., and Stark, J. M. (1970). *J. Med. Microbiol.* **3,** 65–83.
White, R. G., Henderson, D. C., Eslami, M. B., and Nielsen, K. H. (1975). *Immunology* **28,** 1–21.
Wiener, E., and Bandieri, A. (1974). *Eur. J. Immunol.* **4,** 457–463.
Yoshida, T. O., and Andersson, B. (1972). *Scand. J. Immunol.* **1,** 401–408.
Zinkernagel, R. M. (1974). *Nature (London)* **251,** 230–232.
Zinkernagel, R. M., and Doherty, P. C. (1974). *Nature (London)* **251,** 547–548.

4

Functional Heterogeneity of Macrophages

William S. Walker

I. Introduction 91
II. Functional Heterogeneity of Macrophages from Different Tissues 92
A. Alveolar and Peritoneal Macrophages 92
B. Splenic and Liver Macrophages 95
III. Functional Heterogeneity of Macrophages from the Same Tissue 97
A. Spleen and Lymph Nodes 97
B. Alveolar Macrophages 98
C. Peritoneal Macrophages 99
IV. Conclusions 106
References 108

I. INTRODUCTION

In the traditional view, the function of macrophages has been limited to the removal of foreign substances and damaged or effete cells from host tissues. In recent years, however, this view has become much too narrow to accommodate the functional diversity of the mononuclear phagocytes. Especially troublesome is the inconsistency between accepted notions of macrophage function and the diverse activities more recently ascribed to these cells in acquired immunity. On the one hand, macrophages are thought to have a supportive position in the induction of acquired immunity. Their function, according to one view, is solely to engulf and degrade antigen (Perkins and Makinodan, 1965; Ehrenreich and Cohn, 1967), thereby protecting the immune apparatus from antigen overdose (Burnet, 1959). Others have reported that macrophages release nutrient factors that provide the necessary environmental conditions for optimal immune induction (Hoffmann and Dutton, 1971; Chen and Hirsch, 1972). On the other hand, others again have shown that macrophages concentrate and maintain antigen on or near their surfaces, and then either preserve it (Unanue and Cerottini, 1970) or present it to lymphocytes in a manner conducive to immune induction (Mitchison, 1969). Also suggested is a more direct role that promotes macrophages as "antigen processors," a function believed to precede antibody formation in response to some (Adler and Fishman, 1969) but not all antigens (Shortman *et al.*, 1970). The macrophage has been cast in a similar but more general role as a possible regulatory cell involved in the control of humoral as well as cell-mediated immunity (Parish, 1972; Oppenheim and Seeger, Chapter 5; Nelson, Chapter 9). Finally, some macrophages, or cells with certain properties in common with macrophages, are reported to have the ability to synthesize and secrete antibody (Bussard, 1966; Noltenius and Chattin, 1969; Holub and Hauser, 1969; Teplitz *et al.*, 1973).

At present, the most attractive explanation for the functional diversity assigned to macrophages in acquired immunity is that populations of cells belonging to the mononuclear phagocyte system (MPS) (Langevoort *et al.*, 1970) are not homogeneous but vary from site to site and within a given site as well. In this chapter, I shall point out some functional distinctions between macrophages at different sites and, in more detail, review evidence showing that macrophages from a single tissue can be separated into subclasses of cells that are functionally distinct. These distinctions, the latter in particular, should help reconcile the conflicting views of macrophage function in the induction of acquired immunity.

II. FUNCTIONAL HETEROGENEITY OF MACROPHAGES FROM DIFFERENT TISSUES

Macrophages are found in every tissue in the body and exhibit regional differences in their biochemistry, morphology, and function, depending on the tissue in which they are located. These properties have been extensively compared between alveolar and peritoneal macrophages because of the ease with which large numbers of such "free" macrophages can be obtained from the lungs and peritoneum.

A. Alveolar and Peritoneal Macrophages

Alveolar macrophages differ metabolically from peritoneal macrophages, relying primarily upon oxidative metabolism rather than glycolysis (Leake *et al.*, 1964; Karnovsky *et al.*, 1970). These two populations are morphologically distinct (Bennett, 1966; Leake and Heise, 1967), and the lysosomal enzyme content of alveolar macrophages is generally higher than that of peritoneal macrophages (Pavillard and Rowley, 1962; Cohn and Wiener, 1963). Details of these morphological and biochemical differences have been fully described by Pearsall and Weiser (1970), Vernon-Roberts (1972), and Carr (1973) and will not be dealt with in this review.

1. Bactericidal Activity

Alveolar and peritoneal macrophages differ in their capacity to ingest and kill bacteria. Pavillard and Rowley (1962) and Pavillard (1963) showed that despite their higher content of lysosomal enzymes, alveolar macrophages do not destroy bacteria as readily as do peritoneal macrophages. Leake and Myrvik (1966), in confirming these observations, suggested that the apparent discrepancy in function is related to the ability of the two cell types to discharge the contents of their lysosomes into phagosomes, rather than to any quantitative differences in enzyme content. However, since the functional capacities of macrophages are related to their metabolic activities, the apparent capacity of alveolar macrophages to kill ingested bacteria may depend more upon physiological conditions *in vitro* than upon any inherent inability to kill ingested bacteria (Kilburn, 1974).

2. Responses to Chemotactic Stimuli

Alveolar and peritoneal macrophages also differ in ability to respond to chemotactic agents. Keller and Sorkin (1967) and Ward (1968) showed that polymorphonuclear leukocytes (PMN) and cells of the MPS respond to separate chemotactic agents. Ward (1968) further demonstrated that rabbit alveolar macrophages do not respond to any agent with chemotactic activity for peritoneal macrophages or PMN's, an observation confirmed by Sorkin and associates (1970). The reason for this difference is not clear, but it may be related to a membrane-associated serine esterase which appears necessary for migrational responses (Becker and Henson, 1973; Snyderman and Mergenhagen, Chapter 13; Wilkinson, Chapter 14).

3. Responses to Migration Inhibition Factor

Leu and associates (1972) reported that whereas peritoneal macrophages were responsive to the migration inhibition factor (MIF), alveolar macrophages were not. The basis for this difference appeared to be the lack of a surface receptor for MIF on the alveolar macrophage. More recent studies by others (Warr and Martin, 1973; Reynolds *et al.*, 1974; Moore and Myrvik, 1974) have failed to confirm the unresponsiveness of the alveolar macrophage to MIF.

4. The Fc Receptor for Cytophilic Antibody

Mononuclear phagocytes possess surface receptor sites for the Fc portion of cytophilic antibodies (Nelson, 1969). Rhodes (1975) recently showed that alveolar and peritoneal macrophages differed from one another in the avidity of the Fc receptor for immune complexes. Normal (noninduced) peritoneal macrophages possessed a threefold greater mean avidity for sensitized erythrocytes than did normal alveolar macrophages, but the latter showed a greater range of receptor avidities than peritoneal macrophages (see Section II,B,1). Both macrophage populations responded to the stimulus of *in vitro* culturing, i.e, they increased their Fc receptor activities until the populations were essentially homogeneous in this regard. This finding is consistent with observations that *in vitro* culture conditions provide the stimuli by which the functional properties of macrophages can be altered (Cohn and Benson, 1965; Blanden, 1968).

It is not clear at present whether reported differences in the expression of Fc receptors between normal alveolar and peritoneal macrophages represent a dissimilarity in the maturation stage of the cells (Leake and Heise, 1967) or in local tissue environments. An additional possibility is that the alveolar population consists of cells of a hematological (blood monocyte) origin as well as cells whose immediate precursors are within the lung itself (Pinkett *et al.*, 1966). It may be that macrophages of recent blood monocyte origin represent a less functionally mature and more heterogeneous population than macrophages derived from within the lung. It may be this former population which, upon stimulation *in vitro,* rapidly matures with regard to Fc receptors.

5. Immunogenicity of Endocytized Antigen

Cohn (1964) observed that alveolar macrophages and PMN's were more active in the breakdown of bacterial antigens and less able to render such antigens immunogenic than were peritoneal macrophages. These data suggested that the rabbit contains at least three functionally distinct populations of phagocytes: PMN's, alveolar macrophages, and peritoneal macrophages.

Further evidence of functional differences between these populations may be found in the work of Fishman on the formation of immunogenic

RNA–antigen complexes and informational RNA derived from macrophages (for reviews, see Fishman, 1969). After ingestion and "processing" of antigen, peritoneal macrophages yielded RNA preparations with immunogenic activity, while alveolar macrophages and PMN's consistently failed to form active preparations. These findings have been confirmed by Gottlieb (1968).

6. *Differences in Macrophage-Specific Antigens*

Macrophages appear to possess a cell-specific surface antigen(s) that can be detected with anti-macrophage sera. Montfort and Tamayo (1971) reported that certain rabbit anti-rat alveolar macrophage antisera discriminated between the "free" macrophages of the alveoli and peritoneum and the "fixed" macrophages of liver and spleen, suggesting that these two populations were antigenically distinct. Feldman and associates (1972) failed to detect any organ specificity in guinea pigs using rabbit antisera prepared against the surface-adherent peritoneal exudate population. However, Dressler and Skornik (1974) were able to prepare antisera specific for either rat alveolar or peritoneal macrophages by immunizing rabbits with the appropriate cell type. The injection of anti-alveolar serum was reported to reduce the recoverable lung macrophage content by approximately 70%. Similar specificities were reported for a "natural" complement-dependent antibody from rabbits that was cytotoxic to alveolar but not to peritoneal macrophages (Godleski *et al.*, 1974). However, the apparent specificity of these antisera may be directed against inhaled antigens that are bound only to the surfaces of alveolar macrophages. Clearly, more detailed studies are required to resolve the important question of organ-specific macrophage antigens.

The comparative activities of alveolar and peritoneal macrophages are summarized in Table I, which suggests that the latter are functionally more "mature" than the former (Leake and Heise, 1967).

Present evidence on the life history of macrophages supports the view that most of these cells, regardless of their eventual tissue location, have as their precursor the promonocyte in the bone marrow (van Furth, 1970). This would indicate that differences observed between alveolar and peritoneal macrophages are a reflection of regional environmental adaptations that affect the immune potential of these populations in distinct and as yet unknown ways.

B. Splenic and Liver Macrophages

The liver contains more macrophages (Kupffer cells) than any other organ and is the major phagocytic barrier of the host. Although splenic

TABLE I

Comparison of Selected Activities between Alveolar and Peritoneal Macrophages

Activity[a]	Macrophage population: Alveolar	Macrophage population: Peritoneal	Reference
Bactericidal	+	+++	Pavillard, 1963
Chemotaxis	−	+	Ward, 1968
Response to MIF	+(?)	+	Leu *et al.*, 1972 Moore and Myrvik, 1974
Fc receptor activity	+	+++	Rhodes, 1975
Immunogenicity of ingested antigen	−	+	Cohn, 1964
Formation of immunogenic RNA's	−	+	Fishman and Adler, 1970

[a] Activities are expressed as either present (+) or absent (−); where appropriate, a relative degree of activity is indicated.

and peritoneal macrophages clearly participate in immune induction, the significance of Kupffer cells in such reactions remains undetermined (Howard, 1970). The early findings of Askonas and White (1956) that liver produced little if any immunoglobulin (see, however, Garvey and Campbell, 1973) does not rule out the possibility that this organ may serve as an antigen depot (Garvey and Campbell, 1957).

Immunogenicity of Endocytized Antigen

Macrophages from the spleen and liver interact in distinct ways with antigens that affect the immunogenic potential of the antigen. Franzl (1962) compared the subcellular lysosomal fractions of spleen and liver from mice injected with sheep erythrocytes for their ability to elicit a secondary response in primed animals. Liver fractions consistently failed to elicit a response, while comparable fractions from spleens were active. Similar results were obtained by Inchley (1969) using cell transfer techniques. Mouse Kupffer cells, although engulfing up to 12 times more antigen than splenic macrophages, failed to induce significant levels of antibody upon transfer to syngeneic recipients. Inchley and Howard (1969) also found that Kupffer cells were unable to functionally replace splenic macrophages in splenectomized mice that had received sufficient lymphocytes to compensate otherwise for the loss of their spleens. The failure of Kupffer cells to restore splenic macrophage function in the mouse is consistent with observations in man suggesting that liver sequesters but does not process antigen for immune induction (Bjørneboe *et al.*, 1972; Triger *et al.*, 1972). Thus, even though both liver and splenic macrophages appear to be derived from a common precursor cell, their functional expressions may depend on local environmental factors (Howard, 1970).

The rapid uptake and lysosomal localization of antigen by liver cells was also reported by Uhr and Weissmann (1965) for rabbits and guinea pigs. In contrast with results obtained with the mouse, liver fractions from these animals were immunogenic for up to 48 hours following antigen injection. This difference in function between mouse Kupffer cells, on the one hand, and rabbit and guinea pig cells, on the other, illustrates that macrophage properties differ not only from tissue to tissue within the same animal, but also from species to species.

III. FUNCTIONAL HETEROGENEITY OF MACROPHAGES FROM THE SAME TISSUE

The presence of functionally distinct macrophage populations in different tissues is insufficient to account for the diverse and often mutually exclusive roles assigned to these cells. Indications that macrophage populations are functionally diverse within a single tissue site furnish a promising lead toward the clarification of macrophage functions in acquired immunity (Fishman and Adler, 1970).

A. Spleen and Lymph Nodes

The established lymphatic system provides an efficient tissue network where antigen and immunologically relevant cells can meet and initiate the induction of immunity. Macrophages within thse tissues exhibit morphological and functional differences depending upon their location and associations with other cell types.

Antigen-Trapping

The detailed studies of Ada, Nossal, and co-workers (see Nossal and Ada, 1971, for review) and those of Hanna and Szakal (1968) have delineated the sequence of events in lymph nodes and spleens following the entry of antigen. Using ^{125}I-labeled flagellar antigens from *Salmonella*, Ada and associates found that antigen entering rat lymph nodes almost immediately became associated with the macrophages in the medullary sinuses, where it was retained for extended periods of time.

Later, and possibly dependent upon antibody, antigen appeared in the follicles of the cortex associated with a distinct type of cell that has been variously referred to as the "antigen-retaining reticulum cell" or the "dendritic macrophage" (White, 1963). Antigen was localized on or near the surfaces of these cells, where the dendritic processes were in close association with bone marrow-derived lymphocytes (B cells) (Durkin *et al.*, 1971).

A similar situation was observed in the spleen where, again, antigen was first associated with macrophages of the red pulp and later appeared in the dendritic cells of the follicles (Hanna and Szakal, 1968). The dendritic cells were easily differentiated from the "tingible body" macrophage, which appeared to have no active role in lymphocyte stimulation (Mitchell and Abbot, 1965).

These studies raised an important question: Are the dendritic cells macrophages? Such cells were excluded from the reclassification of macrophages into the mononuclear phagocyte system (MPS) on the basis that they were not highly phagocytic (Langevoort *et al.*, 1970) and contained few lysosomes (Nossal *et al.*, 1968). However, the demonstration that dendritic cells posses receptors for immunoglobulins (Lang and Ada, 1967), together with evidence that macrophages are heterogeneous in their phagocyte properties (Walker, 1974a; Rice and Fishman, 1974), makes this exclusion questionable.

B. Alveolar Macrophages

Fc Receptors for Cytophilic Antibodies

Arend and Mannik (1973) showed that the ability of rabbit alveolar macrophages to bind soluble immune complexes depended upon both the numbers of IgG receptors per cell and their average association constant. Injection of Freund's complete adjuvant resulted in populations with marked increases in both the numbers of Fc receptors and their average avidities. These data represented average values for the population and did not take into account the possible lack of functional uniformity between macrophages. More recent studies on the single cell level have demonstrated that normal guinea pig macrophages are functionally heterogeneous with regard to Fc receptor activity (Rhodes, 1975). Rhodes observed that the percentage of normal guinea pig macrophages that formed rosettes with sensitized erythrocytes was dependent upon the concentration of IgG used to coat the indicator cells as well as on the state of macrophage activation.

These results, with those of Arend and Mannik (1973), indicate that normal alveolar macrophage populations exist as a heterogeneous group of cells that, in response to stimuli, differentiate into a population possessing functional uniformity with enhanced Fc receptor activity.

C. Peritoneal Macrophages

1. Bactericidal Activity

Mackaness (1960) and Jenkin and Benacerraf (1960) observed that within the peritoneal macrophage population some cells were less able than others to ingest and kill bacteria. The lack of functional uniformity within this population was overcome either by specific immunization or by nonspecifically stimulating the animals with agents such as BCG. These procedures resulted in marked morphological and enzymatic changes concomitant with the development of a more functionally homogeneous population of cells (Blanden, 1968), a situation comparable to that found with alveolar macrophages (Arend and Mannik, 1973; Rhodes, 1975). McIntyre and associates (1967) confirmed heterogeneity at the single cell level by showing that not all macrophages were able to phagocytize bacteria even in the presence of specific antibody. Cooper and Houston (1964) concluded that approximately 40% of the normal peritoneal macrophage population was capable of immediate phagocytosis and that functional changes were required in the rest of the cells before they could become active.

Further evidence of heterogeneity at the single cell level was obtained by Perkins and Leonard (1963), who showed that mouse peritoneal macrophages had phagocytic preferences for different species of erythrocytes. When incubated simultaneously with two different types of red cells, some macrophages engulfed one species to the complete exclusion of the second.

An additional demonstration of functional heterogeneity among mouse peritoneal macrophages suggests that differences between the stability of surface-associated immunoglobulins and the binding of lectins vary depending upon the size of the macrophages (Loor and Roelants, 1974). Small- and medium-sized macrophages were reported to maintain their surface immunoglobulins for extended periods of time in culture (at least 96 hours), while larger macrophages lost such molecules within 48 hours, presumably by a capping reaction. It was further reported that small macrophages were less active in binding and retaining antigen both on and in the cells than were larger macrophages.

Just how a macrophage's size, as well as its stability of surface-bound immunoglobulins, phagocytosis, and antigen binding relate to its possible functions in immune induction is unknown at present. The recent application of cell separation techniques based upon differences in cell density

(Walker, 1974a; Rice and Fishman, 1974) may provide the means by which to approach such problems.

2. *Immunogenic RNA*

Fishman and Adler (1963) showed that RNA from antigenically stimulated macrophages is immunogenic *in vitro*. The characterization of immunogenic RNA's led to the postulation that the peritoneal macrophage population consisted of at least three functionally distinct subclasses of cells (Fishman, 1969): (1) The majority of macrophages act as classical scavenger cells and engulf and degrade antigen into immunologically nonreactive products. (2) A second population, consisting of less than 1 cell per 1000, forms but does not necessarily secrete, immunoglobulin and preferentially binds antigen to its surface possibly through surface-associated antibody. This cell responds by synthesizing informational RNA (iRNA) which elicits IgM antibody carrying the allotypic specificity of the macrophage donor (Adler *et al.*, 1966). (3) The third type of macrophage reacts with antigen and gives rise to the RNA–antigen complex, which is responsible for the induction of IgG antibody carrying the allotype markers of the lymphocyte donor (Fishman, 1969).

These studies have raised a number of questions with regard to the cellular origin and biological relevance of the immunogenic RNA species. Is it the peritoneal cell that forms iRNA a macrophage or a lymphocyte, or is it a cell possessing some properties in common with both cell types? Is iRNA solely a laboratory artifact of little biological relevance, as has been suggested by some (Lefkovits, 1974), or is it a means by which the immune response is rapidly amplified without the requirement of cell replication (Tannenberg and Malaviya, 1968; Bussard, 1966; Kolodny *et al.*, 1972)? Is the RNA–antigen complex the means by which immune induction occurs (Gottlieb and Schwartz, 1972), or are such RNA–antigen complexes an artifact of the RNA extraction procedures employed (Roelants and Goodman, 1969)?

The first step in answering these and other questions was the direct testing of the hypothesis that peritoneal exudate cells were functionally heterogeneous. Table II summarizes data obtained when rabbit peritoneal exudates, rich in macrophages (70–80%), were incubated with antigen (bacteriophage T2) and separated into density subclasses on discontinuous gradients of Ficoll (Walker, 1971). RNA's were extracted from the subclasses and tested for the ability to induce antibody formation in cultures of normal rabbit spleen cells. It is evident that the peritoneal exudate cells were heterogeneous in both their density and ability to bind radiolabeled antigen (^{125}I-labeled T2). Furthermore, the immunogenic

TABLE II

Antigen-Binding and Immunogenic RNA Activities of Rabbit Peritoneal Exudate Cells Exposed to Phage T2 and Separated on Discontinuous Ficoll Gradients[a,b]

Macrophage subclass	% of cells	% of macrophages	^{125}I-labeled T2 bound	Immunogenic RNA	Ig class of anti-T2 antibody
0–5	10–15	>95	4+	variable	IgM, IgG
5–8	30–40	>90	2+	yes	IgM
8–9	10–20	70–80	1+	yes	IgG
9–10	10–20	60–65	1+	no	None
10–pellet	20–30	50	2–3+	no	None

[a] Data modified from Walker (1971) with permission of Macmillan Journals.
[b] The binding of labeled antigen is summarized on a scale of 1+ to 4+. Peritoneal exudate cells were incubated with phage T2 for 30 minutes at 37°C and separated on gradients of Ficoll. RNA was extracted and 100 μg were added to cultures of normal rabbit spleen cells. The anti-phage activity was assayed on days 3 and 7 of culture and the antibody class determined by 2-mercaptoethanol and the distribution of phage neutralization activity on linear sucrose gradients.

RNA responsible for IgM antibody formation was obtained from cells isolated primarily at the 5–8% Ficoll interface (90% macrophages, hereafter referred to as the 5–8 subclass), which contained between 30 and 40% of the cells applied to the gradients. In contrast, cells isolated at the 8–9% interface (approximately 75% macrophages) yielded RNA that induced IgG antibody and represented up to 20% of the total cell population. Cells isolated from the uppermost interface (0–5%) gave rise to a mixture of RNA's that induced both IgM and IgG, but such activity was only rarely observed. This latter subclass contained numerous cells that had engulfed oil and was thus an artifact of the exudate induction procedure (Walker, 1974a; Rice and Fishman, 1974). These data provided direct experimental support for the hypothesis of functional heterogeneity among peritoneal macrophages, both in antigen-binding activity and the yielding of immunogenic RNA's.

Rice and Fishman (1974), by refining the gradient separation procedure, improved these results by limiting the percentage of cells responsible for formation of immunogenic RNA's to 15% of the total peritoneal exudate cell population. This minor population of cells could be further separated into one population that yielded RNA that induced IgM antibody, and another that induced IgG. In addition, they observed that the subclass responsible for iRNA was enriched up to 40% with a morphologically distinct type of mononuclear cell they termed "A" cells. These cells, representing approximately 1% of the total peritoneal exudate population, were weakly phagocytic, attached firmly to the surfaces of culture dishes, and tended to send out cytoplasmic processes more rapidly than typical macrophages. The question of whether or not "A" cells are the source of the iRNA has yet to be answered. Further, the relationships, if any, of "A" cells to other atypical mononuclear leukocytes recently described (Allison, 1972; Steinman and Cohn, 1973) or to transitional cells in the maturation of promonocytes to macrophages is unknown at present (Cline and Sumner, 1972).

3. *Fc Receptors*

Recent studies have shown that peritoneal macrophage subclasses obtained on Ficoll gradients differ in their surface receptors for immunoglobulin (Walker, 1974a). For these studies the surface-adherent population from rabbit exudates was used as a source of macrophages in order to reduce to a minimum lymphocyte contamination of the density subclasses.

Evidence suggestive of heterogeneity in Fc receptors was obtained by studying the effects of specific antibody on antigen uptake by cells of the different subclasses (Table III). Two subclasses (8–9 and 9–10) responded to a greater degree with enhanced antigen uptake than did cells

TABLE III

Antigen-Binding Activities of Macrophage Density Subclasses[a,b]

Macrophage subclass	Antigen-binding without antibody	Percentage of macrophages	Enhanced uptake with antibody	Ig receptor (rosettes)
0–5	4+	>95	1+	1+
5–8	3+	>95	1+	1+
8–9	1+	90–95	2–3+	2+
9–10	1+	90–95	4+	4+
10–Pellet	2+	70–80	1+	1+

[a] Data from Walker (1974a) with permission of Blackwell Scientific Publications, Ltd.

[b] The activities are expressed on an increasing scale of 1+ to 4+ for macrophage subclasses prepared from a 24-hour surface-adherent population of rabbit peritoneal exudates.

from the other subclasses. When the macrophage–erythrocyte rosette technique (Berken and Benacerraf, 1966) was used to test for Fc receptor activity by the subclasses, the same two groups, 8–9 and 9–10, formed more rosettes than the others, furnishing direct evidence of heterogeneity in Fc receptors. Rhodes (1975) has reported a similar distinction for guinea pig macrophages.

4. *Subcellular Distribution of Endocytized Antigen*

Kölsch and Mitchison (1968) found that most of the antigen (approximately 90%) engulfed by mouse peritoneal macrophages quickly entered a lysosomal compartment of density 1.19 gm/cm^3, where it was rapidly degraded. The remaining antigen became associated with a high density (1.26 gm/cm^3) "storage" compartment, where it remained intact for a number of hours. Although Kölsch and Mitchison were unable to demonstrate that this latter compartment was immunogenic, they did suggest that it may be relevant to the immunological role of the macrophage in immune induction.

If certain macrophages are, in fact, distinct in their ability to react with and subsequently provide to lymphocytes antigen in an immunogenically enhanced form, then one would predict that such cells would compartmentalize antigen in a manner different from that of macrophages that do not productively interact with lymphocytes. In an attempt to correlate the localization of endocytized antigen with other properties of macrophage subclasses, we have begun to compare the subcellular distribution of radiolabeled bovine serum albumin ([^{125}I]BSA) within selected subclasses of cells obtained from Ficoll gradients (Walker, 1974b).

Macrophage suspensions prepared by removing the 24-hour surface-adherent populations of rabbit peritoneal exudates from plastic culture dishes with a rubber policeman were incubated with antigen and separated into density subclasses (Walker, 1974a). A constant number of cells (5×10^6) from each subclass tested (5–8, 8–9, and 9–10) were homogenized and centrifuged in isopycnic sucrose gradients (Kölsch and Mitchison, 1968). Comparison of the gradient distribution patterns revealed both quantitative and qualitative differences in antigen distribution in the cells from the different subclasses (Fig. 1). First, the total gradient-associated radioactivity reflected the differential capacity of the cells to bind antigen. As previously shown (Table II), the 5–8 subclass was more active in binding antigen than either the 8–9 or 9–10 subclasses, the latter two being about equal in this regard. Second, the subclasses differed in the subcellular compartmentalization of ingested antigen after a 30-min-

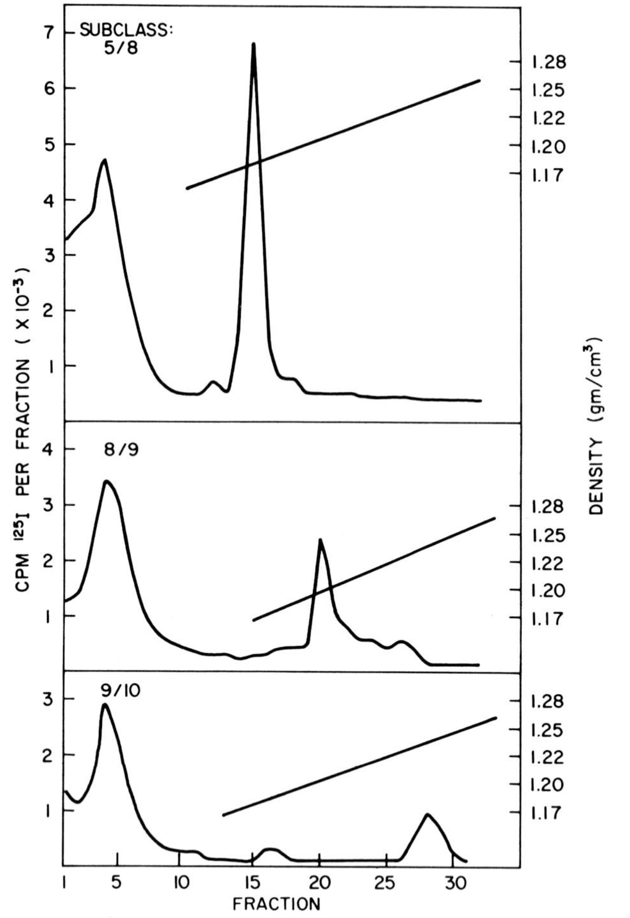

Fig. 1. The subcellular isopycnic distribution of [^{125}I]BSA in cells from the indicated macrophage subclasses. Homogenized cells were layered over 30–70% (w/v) sucrose gradients and centrifuged for 16 hours at 4°C in a Spinco SW 27.1 rotor at 18,000 rpm. The top of the gradients is on the left. The total distribution of radioactivity is presented and the density was calculated from the refractive index of sucrose in each fraction.

ute incubation period. This time period was chosen because Fishman (1969) observed that a minimum incubation period of 20–30 minutes with antigen was necessary before peritoneal macrophages yielded active RNA preparations. It was reasoned that if distinct subcellular antigen compartments were to be detected and eventually correlated with the immunopotential of the cells, then such compartments would be more readily detected after a short incubation period rather than an extended one.

The 5–8 subclass localized approximately 25% of the total gradient-associated radioactivity within a compartment of density 1.18 gm/cm^3, which contained acid phosphatase and a modest amount of β-glucuronidase activity. The majority of radioactivity associated with the 1.18 compartment (approximately 60–70%) precipitated with trichloroacetic acid (TCA), and to a lesser extent (approximately 50%) with a potent anti-BSA antiserum in the presence of carrier protein.

The 8–9 subclass localized about 15% of the total radioactivity in the gradient into a density compartment of 1.20 gm/cm^3, and to a lesser extent into a slightly higher density region. Approximately 80% of the radioactivity in the 1.20 compartment was precipitated with TCA and to a lesser degree with antiserum (50–60%).

The 9–10 subclass did not deposit any label in the 1.20 region of the gradients, and only a trace amount in the 1.18 compartment, which contained very little acid phosphatase activity. However, approximately 10% of the total radioactivity in the gradients was found in a high density compartment of 1.24 gm/cm^3, which appeared to be unique to this subclass. All the radioactivity in this compartment was precipitated with either TCA or antiserum, indicating that antigen was not being rapidly degraded. This latter compartment appears to be similar to the 1.26 antigen "storage" compartment described by Kölsch and Mitchison (1968) for mouse peritoneal macrophages.

These data, although preliminary, suggest that peritoneal macrophages differ in the subcellular localization of antigen, and agree with the electron microscopic observations of Fishman and associates (1964) and Catanzaro and co-workers (1969) on the subcellular localization of antigen in macrophages. These authors showed that some macrophages did not concentrate antigen in lysosomes, but rather antigen was found in the perinuclear region of the cells where it remained intact. The 1.26 compartment described by Kölsch and Mitchison appears to be the perinuclear fraction because it was associated with nuclei and could be solubilized from this particulate fraction with the detergent sodium dodecyl sulfate. The 1.24 compartment described here for the 9–10 macrophage subclass also appears to be the perinuclear compartment.

The relationships between the subcellular localization of antigen, the presence or absence of high Fc receptor activity, and the ability of a given subclass to form either species of immunogenic RNA is unclear at present. The density subclasses of macrophages obtained with the adherent-purified population from peritoneal exudates have yet to be tested for their ability to yield immunogenic RNA. This is because of the difficulty of obtaining cells from the subclasses in high enough numbers to extract sufficient amounts of RNA for testing. Nevertheless, the data show that those macrophages possessing a high level of phagocytosis (5–8 subclass) primarily concentrated ingested BSA into a lysosomal compartment where antigen was rapidly degraded. In contrast, those macrophages that are weakly phagocytic but possess high Fc receptor activity (9–10 subclass) located a small amount of antigen into an extra-lysosomal compartment of high density where antigen was not rapidly degraded. The relationships between these antigen compartments and the ability of the subclasses to interact productively with lymphocytes in the induction of immunity is currently under study.

IV. CONCLUSIONS

This chapter has not only drawn attention to the functional diversity of macrophages from different tissues but also has attempted to show that this functional heterogeneity extends to macrophages from the same tissue site. Clearly, the primary activity of macrophages is the removal and degradation of foreign substances from host tissues. It is equally clear, however, that many antigens, by virtue of their association with macrophages, are markedly enhanced in their immunogenicity (reviewed by Unanue, 1972).

Implicit in the hypothesis of macrophage functional heterogeneity is the idea that antigen reacts with a distinct macrophage subclass in order to be rendered optimally immunogenic. There exists some circumstantial evidence to support this view. For example, Mosier and Coppleson (1968) concluded that in mice no more than 1–10 cells per 10,000 splenic macrophages cooperated with lymphocytes in the *in vitro* induction of antibody synthesis. This ratio is similar to that reported by Fishman and associates (Fishman *et al.*, 1965) for that portion of the total peritoneal macrophage population responsible for the formation of the immunogenic iRNA species. In addition, several studies have demonstrated that the ratio of macrophages to lymphocytes is critical for immune induction: macrophage-to-lymphocyte ratios of less than 1:1000 are usually suboptimal for induction, whereas ratios in excess of 1:100 are inhibitory (Hoffmann, 1970; Shortman and Palmer, 1971; Feldmann, 1972; for review, see Claman and Mosier, 1972). Thus, the ability of a population of macrophages to interact productively with antigen and lymphocytes in a manner conducive to optimal immune induction apparently depends more upon the proportion and activity of a distinct subclass of macrophages than on the population as a whole.

Wiener and Bandieri (1974) recently reported striking differences in the peritoneal macrophage populations of two strains of mice differing in their ability to form antibodies to certain antigens. Compared with macrophages from normal responder mice, the macrophages from low responder animals were characterized by an altered morphology, elevated levels of lysosomal enzymes, increased phagocytic activity, and rapid loss of surface-bound antigen, suggesting that the basis of low responsiveness was at the level of the macrophage and not the lymphocyte (Howard *et al.*, 1974). It may be that the weakly responsive animals lacked the necessary subclass of macrophages required for optimal induction, so that comparison of density subclasses of macrophages from these two strains of mice might allow one to detect either the physical or functional loss of the requisite subclass.

Is the functional uniqueness of the proposed subclass of macrophages because they are being derived from a precursor cell distinct from that of the classic macrophage, or are the activities of the subclasses related to various stages of differentiation or maturation of cells possessing a common precursor? It is well established that macrophages respond to various stimuli by increasing existing activities (Blanden, 1968; Rhodes, 1975) and by acquiring additional ones, such as the selective release of lysosomal enzymes (Page *et al.*, 1974) and the development of cytotoxic activities toward target cells (Alexander and Evans, 1971; Keller, 1973; Hibbs, 1974). Thus, while the origin of cells in the various distinct subclasses remains unknown, most current evidence indicates that at least some of the observed functional heterogeneity is the result of the maturation of a single lineage of cells possessing a common precursor.

Many questions remain, such as the cellular origin of the immunogenic RNA species that transfers to lymphocytes the information for both allotype and antigen-combining site specificity for IgM antibody (Adler *et al.*, 1966). Furthermore, is the development of cell-mediated and humoral immunity regulated by separate macrophage subclasses, possibly differing in their numbers or avidities of Fc receptors (Liew and Parish, 1972; Zembala *et al.*, 1974)? Are the macrophages that participate in the inductive events of acquired immunity the same macrophages that assume an effector function against target cells (Greenberg *et al.*, 1973)?

Only further work will answer these and other questions, but the recognition that macrophage populations are functionally heterogeneous and the availability of well-defined macrophage subclasses should permit more precise definitions of macrophage functions in the induction and expression of acquired immunity.

ACKNOWLEDGMENTS

The author's work was supported by Childhood Cancer Research Center Grant CA-08480 from the National Cancer Institute, a Brown–Hazen grant from the Research Corporation of America, an institutional grant from the American Cancer Society, the Ruth Estrin Goldberg Memorial for Cancer Research, grant DRG-1282 from the Damon Runyon-Walter Winchell Cancer Fund, and by ALSAC. The assistance of Mr. John Gilbert during the preparation of the manuscript is gratefully acknowledged.

REFERENCES

Adler, F. L., and Fishman, M. (1969). *Develop. Biol., Suppl.* **3,** 112–132.
Adler, F. L., Fishman, M., and Dray, S. (1966). *J. Immunol.* **97,** 554–558.
Alexander, P., and Evans, R. (1971). *Nature (London), New Biol.* **232,** 76–78.
Allison, A. C. (1972). *Ann. Inst. Pasteur, Paris* **123,** 585–608.
Arend, W. P., and Mannik, M. (1973). *J. Immunol.* **110,** 1455–1463.
Askonas, B. A., and White, R. G. (1956). *Brit. J. Exp. Pathol.* **37,** 61–74.
Becker, E. L., and Henson, P. M. (1973). *Advan. Immunol.* **17,** 93–193.
Bennett, B. (1966). *Amer. J. Pathol.* **48,** 165–181.
Berken, A., and Benacerraf, B. (1966). *J. Exp. Med.* **123,** 119–144.
Bjørneboe, M., Prytz, H., and Ørskov, F. (1972). *Lancet* **1,** 58–60.
Blanden, R. V. (1968). *J. Reticuloendothel. Soc.* **5,** 179–202.
Burnet, F. M. (1959). *Brit. Med. J.* **2,** 645–650.
Bussard, A. E. (1966). *Science* **153,** 887–888.
Carr, I. (1973). "The Macrophage." Academic Press, New York.
Catanzaro, P. J., Graham, R. C., Jr., and Schwartz, H. J. (1969). *J. Immunol.* **103,** 618–621.
Chen, C., and Hirsch, J. G. (1972). *Science* **176,** 60–61.
Claman, H. N., and Mosier, D. E. (1972). *Progr. Allergy* **16,** 40–80.
Cline, M. J., and Sumner, M. A. (1972). *Blood* **40,** 62–69.
Cohn, Z. A. (1964). *J. Exp.* Med. **120,** 869–883.
Cohn, Z. A., and Benson, B. (1965). *J. Exp. Med.* **122,** 455–466.
Cohn, Z. A., and Wiener, E. (1963). *J. Exp. Med.* **118,** 991–1008.
Cooper, G. N., and Houston, B. (1964). *Aust. J. Exp. Biol. Med. Sci.* **42,** 429–442.
Dressler, D. P., and Skornik, W. A. (1974). *J. Reticuloendothel. Soc.* **15,** 55a, (abstr.).
Durkin, H. G., Theis, G. A., and Thorbecke, G. J. (1971). *Advan. Exp. Med. Biol.* **12,** 119–128.
Ehrenreich, B. A., and Cohn, Z. A. (1967). *J. Exp. Med.* **126,** 941–958.
Feldman, J. D., Tubergen, D. G., Pollock, E. M., and Unanue, E. R. (1972). *Cell. Immunol.* **5,** 325–337.
Feldmann, M. (1972). *J. Exp. Med.* **135,** 1049–1058.
Fishman, M. (1969). *Annu. Rev. Microbiol.* **23,** 199–222.
Fishman, M., and Adler, F. L. (1963). *J. Exp. Med.* **117,** 595–602.
Fishman, M., and Adler, F. L. (1970). *In* "Mononuclear Phagocytes" (R. van Furth, ed.), pp. 581–592. Blackwell, Oxford.
Fishman, M., Adler, F. L, van Rood, J. J., and Binet, J. L. (1964). *Proc. Int. Symp. Reticulo-Endothelial Soc., 4th, 1963* pp. 229–237.
Fishman, M., van Rood, J. J., and Adler, F. L. (1965). *In* "Molecular and Cellular Basis of Antibody Formation" (J. Sterzl, ed.), pp. 491–498. Academic Press, New York.
Franzl, R. E. (1962). *Nature (London)* **195,** 457–458.
Garvey, J. S., and Campbell, D. H. (1957). *J. Exp. Med.* **105,** 361–372.
Garvey, J. S., and Campbell, D. H. (1973). *Ann. N.Y. Acad. Sci.* **207,** 258–278.

Godleski, J. J., Brain, J. D., and Coffin, D. L. (1974). *J. Reticuloendothel. Soc.* **15**, 54a (abstr.).
Gottlieb, A. A. (1968). *In* "Nucleic Acids in Immunology" (O. J. Plescia and W. Braun, eds.), pp. 471–482. Springer-Verlag, Berlin and New York.
Gottlieb, A. A., and Schwartz, R. H. (1972). *Cell. Immunol.* **5**, 341–362.
Greenberg, A. H., Shen, L., and Roitt, I. M. (1973). *Clin. Exp. Immunol.* **15**, 251–259.
Hanna, M. G., Jr., and Szakal, A. K. (1968). *J. Immunol.* **101**, 949–962.
Hibbs, J. B., Jr. (1974). *Science* **184**, 468–471.
Hoffmann, M. (1970). *Immunology* **18**, 791–797.
Hoffmann, M., and Dutton, R. W. (1971). *Science* **172**, 1047–1048.
Holub, M., and Hauser, R. E. (1969). *Immunology* **17**, 207–226.
Howard, J. G. (1970). *In* "Mononuclear Phagocytes" (R. van Furth, ed.), pp. 178–199. Blackwell, Oxford.
Howard, J. G., Courtenay, B. M., and Desaymard, C. (1974). *Eur. J. Immunol.* **4**, 453–457.
Inchley, C. J. (1969). *Clin. Exp. Immunol.* **5**, 173–187.
Inchley, C. J., and Howard, J. G. (1969). *Clin. Exp. Immunol.* **5**, 189–198.
Jenkin, C., and Benacerraf, B. (1960). *J. Exp. Med.* **112**, 403–417.
Karnovsky, M. L., Simmons, S., Glass, E. A., Shafer, A. W., and Hart, P. D. (1970). *In* "Mononuclear Phagocytes" (R. van Furth, ed.), pp. 110–117. Blackwell, Oxford.
Keller, H. U., and Sorkin, E. (1967). *Int. Arch. Allergy Appl. Immunol.* **31**, 575–586.
Keller, R. (1973). *J. Exp. Med.* **138**, 625–644.
Kilburn, K. H. (1974). *Int. Rev. Cytol.* **37**, 153–270.
Kolodny, G. M., Culp, L. A., and Rosenthal, L. J. (1972). *Exp. Cell Res.* **73**, 65–72.
Kölsch, E., and Mitchison, N. A. (1968). *J. Exp. Med.* **128**, 1059–1079.
Lang, P. G., and Ada, G. L. (1967). *Immunology* **13**, 523–534.
Langevoort, H. L., Cohn, Z. A., Hirsch, J. G., Humphrey, J. H., Spector, W. G., and van Furth, R. (1970). *In* "Mononuclear Phagocytes" (R. van Furth, ed.), pp. 1–6. Blackwell, Oxford.
Leake, E. S., and Heise, E. R. (1967). *Advan. Exp. Med. Biol.* **1**, 133–146.
Leake, E. S., and Myrvik, Q. N. (1966). *J. Reticuloendothel. Soc.* **3**, 83–100.
Leake, E. S., Gonzalez-Ojeda, D., and Myrvik, Q. N. (1964). *Exp. Cell Res.* **33**, 553–561.
Lefkovitz, I. (1974). *Curr. Top. Microbiol. Immunol.* **65**, 21–58.
Leu, R. W., Eddleston, A. L. W. F., Hadden, J. W., and Good, R. A. (1972). *J. Exp. Med.* **136**, 589–603.
Liew, F. Y., and Parish, C. R. (1972). *Cell. Immunol.* **4**, 66–85.
Loor, F., and Roelants, G. E. (1974). *Eur. J. Immunol.* **4**, 649–660.
McIntyre, J., Rowley, D., and Jenkin, C. R. (1967). *Aust. J. Exp. Biol. Med. Sci.* **45**, 675–680.
Mackaness, G. (1960). *J. Exp. Med.* **112**, 35–53.
Mitchell, J., and Abbot, A. (1965). *Nature (London)* **208**, 501–502.
Mitchison, N. A. (1969). *Immunology* **16**, 1–14.
Montfort, I., and Tamayo, R. P. (1971). *Proc. Soc. Exp. Biol. Med.* **138**, 204–207.
Moore, V. L., and Myrvik, Q. N. (1974). *J. Reticuloendothel. Soc.* **16**, 21–26.
Mosier, D. W., and Coppleson, L. W. (1968). *Proc. Nat. Acad. Sci. U.S.* **61**, 542–547.
Nelson, D. S. (1969). "Macrophages and Immunity." North-Holland Publ., Amsterdam.
Noltenius, H., and Chattin, M. (1969). *Experientia* **25**, 401.

Nossal, G. J. V., and Ada, G. L. (1971). "Antigen, Lymphoid Cells, and the Immune Response." Academic Press, New York.

Nossal, G. J. V., Abbot, A., Mitchell, J., and Lummus, Z. (1968). *J. Exp. Med.* **127**, 277–290.

Page, R. C., Davies, P., and Allison, A. C. (1974). *J. Reticuloendothel. Soc.* **15**, 413–438.

Parish, C. R. (1972). *Transplant. Rev.* **13**, 35–66.

Pavillard, E. R. J. (1963). *Aust. J. Exp. Biol. Med. Sci.* **41**, 265–274.

Pavillard, E. R. J., and Rowley, D. (1962). *Aust. J. Exp. Biol. Med. Sci.* **40**, 207–214.

Pearsall, N. N., and Weiser, R. S. (1970). "The Macrophage." Lea & Febiger, Philadelphia, Pennyslvania.

Perkins, E. H., and Leonard, M. R. (1963). *J. Immunol.* **90**, 228–237.

Perkins, E. H., and Makinodan, T. (1965). *J. Immunol.* **94**, 765–777.

Pinkett, M. O., Cowdrey, C. R., and Nowell, P. C. (1966). *Amer. J. Pathol.* **48**, 859–867.

Reynolds, H. Y., Thompson, R. E., and Devlin, H. B. (1974). *J. Clin. Invest.* **53**, 1351–1358.

Rhodes, J. R. (1975). *J. Immunol.* **114**, 976–981.

Rice, S. G., and Fishman, M. (1974). *Cell. Immunol.* **11**, 130–145.

Roelants, G. E., and Goodman, J. W. (1969). *J. Exp. Med.* **130**, 557–574.

Shortman, K., and Palmer, J. (1971). *Cell. Immunol.* **2**, 399–410.

Shortman, K., Diener, E., Russell, P., and Armstrong, W. D. (1970). *J. Exp. Med.* **131**, 461–482.

Sorkin, E., Borel, J. F., and Stecher, V. J. (1970). *In* "Mononuclear Phagocytes" (R. van Furth, ed.), pp. 397–418. Blackwell, Oxford.

Steinman, R. M., and Cohn, Z. A. (1973). *J. Exp. Med.* **137**, 1142–1162.

Tannenberg, W. J. K., and Malaviya, A. N. (1968). *J. Exp. Med.* **128**, 895–925.

Teplitz, R. L., Mazie, J. C., Arnaud, D., Lowy, I., and Bussard, A. (1973). *Advan. Exp. Med. Biol.* **29**, 247–256.

Triger, D. R., Alp, M. H., and Wright, R. (1972). *Lancet* **1**, 60–62.

Uhr, J. W., and Weissmann G. (1965). *J. Immunol.* **94**, 544–550.

Unanue, E. R. (1972). *Advan. Immunol.* **15**, 95–165.

Unanue, E. R., and Cerottini, J. C. (1970). *J. Exp. Med.* **131**, 711–725.

van Furth, R. (1970). *In* "Mononuclear Phagocytes" (R. van Furth, ed.), pp. 151–165 Blackwell, Oxford.

Vernon-Roberts, B. (1972). "The Macrophage." Cambridge Univ. Press, London and New York.

Walker, W. S. (1971). *Nature (London), New Biol.* **229**, 211–212.

Walker, W. S. (1974a). *Immunology* **26**, 1025–1037.

Walker, W. S. (1974b). *J. Reticuloendothel. Soc.* **15**, 45a (abstr.).

Ward, P. A. (1968). *J. Exp. Med.* **128**, 1201–1221.

Warr, G. A., and Martin, R. R. (1973). *Infec. Immunity* **8**, 222–227.

White, R. G. (1963). *Ciba Found. Study Group* **16**, 6–16.

Wiener, E., and Bandieri, A. (1974). *Eur. J. Immunol.* **4**, 457–463.

Zembala, M., Ptak, W., and Hanczakowska, M. (1974). *Immunology* **26**, 465–476.

5

The Role of Macrophages in the Induction of Cell-Mediated Immunity *in Vivo*

Joost J. Oppenheim and Robert C. Seeger

I. Introduction 112
II. Contribution of Macrophages to Induction of Delayed Hypersensitivity Reactions and in Priming Helper T Cells for Antibody Production ... 112
A. Effect of *in Vivo* Suppression of Macrophages ... 112
B. Macrophage Interaction with Hapten–Carrier Conjugates 113
C. Effect of Sensitization with Macrophage-Associated Antigens 114
III. Relationship of Macrophage Presentation and Processing of Antigens to Induction of Cell-Mediated Immunity 117
A. Unique Capacity of Macrophages to Induce CMI 117
B. Requirement for Macrophage Viability 119
C. Role of Surface and Intracellular Compartments 119
D. Effects of Antigen Degradation 121
IV. Regulation of Immunogenicity of Macrophage-Associated Antigens 123
A. Effect of Soluble Antigens 124
B. Effect of Humoral Antibodies 124
V. Summary and Conclusions 127
References 129

I. INTRODUCTION

Macrophages are important participants in both the afferent and efferent limbs of the immune response. This review will be limited to considering the afferent role of macrophages in inducing *in vivo* T cell-mediated immunity (CMI). The voluminous evidence that macrophages enhance *in vitro* T cell proliferation and mediator production will be reviewed elsewhere in this volume. We will concentrate much of our discussion on the role of macrophage-associated antigens (m-Ag) in inducing cutaneous delayed hypersensitivity (DH), since it provides the most readily accessible and most thoroughly studied manifestation of *in vivo* CMI. We will also discuss the data concerning the contribution of m-Ag to priming T helper cells to enhance antibody production, since such antibody production in response to thymus-dependent antigens associated with macrophages provides another indicator of activation of T cells.

Until 1970 the view that macrophages just enhanced the *in vivo* production of antibodies predominated. These studies of the enhancement of both *in vivo* and *in vitro* antibody production by macrophages have been thoroughly reviewed by Unanue (1972). The observations of Mitchison (1969) and Unanue and Askonas (1968a) indicated that immunization of mice with a single dose of m-Ag results in low or no antibody production. However, m-Ag primed the mice very effectively, since subsequent boosts with subimmunogenic doses of soluble antigen induced considerable antibody production. Furthermore, m-Ag failed to prime thymectomized mice (Unanue, 1970). In retrospect, since thymus-dependent antigens were used in these studies, it is probable that these findings were actually based on m-Ag activation of T helper cells rather than direct m-Ag activation or antibody producing bone marrow derived (B) cells.

II. CONTRIBUTION OF MACROPHAGES TO INDUCTION OF DELAYED HYPERSENSITIVITY REACTIONS AND IN PRIMING HELPER T CELLS FOR ANTIBODY PRODUCTION

A. Effect of *in Vivo* Suppression of Macrophages

There are several lines of evidence that substances which are toxic for macrophages interfere with cutaneous DH reactions. For example, it has been observed that carrageenan is selectively toxic to macrophages. Administration of antigen simultaneously with carrageenan to guinea pigs temporarily suppresses their delayed hypersensitivity (DH) (Schwartz and Leskowitz, 1969). Specific anti-macrophage antisera (AMS) administered 2 days after antigen also suppress DH of guinea pigs more consistently and to a greater extent than antibody production (Unanue, 1972). However, from these studies one cannot determine whether these inhibitors interfere with the requirement for macrophages in the expression of DH or interfere at the level of induction of immunity. The experiment of Feldman and Unanue (1971), which showed that the capacity of lymph node or bone marrow cells to transfer DH to irradiated nonimmune syngeneic guinea pigs, is reduced by AMS, whereas AMS did not inhibit cutaneous DH of immune guinea pigs, suggests that macrophages may be involved in the induction of DH.

B. Macrophage Interaction with Hapten–Carrier Conjugates

Kunin *et al.* (1972) have used another approach to study the relationship among macrophages and T and B cells which takes advantage of the principle that T cells react predominantly with the carrier and B cells with the hapten components of antigens. They utilized thymectomized, irradiated mice that were then restored with thymocytes and bone marrow (BM) cells. The spleen cells of such mice were primed equally well to make antibody *in vitro* to the hapten component of a hapten–carrier conjugate within 8 days when immunized with either Freund's complete adjuvant (FCA) or peritoneal exudate cells (PEC) mixed with the carrier component of the antigen. *In vitro* antibody production was obtained even when such mice were given PEC-Ag and thymocytes followed by BM cells 8 days later. However, when the PEC-Ag were given together with BM cells and followed by thymocytes (T cells) 8 days later, no antibody was made. Thus, it was concluded that T cells were the targets for priming by PEC-Ag followed by interaction with BM precursors of antibody producing cells. Presumably m-Ag could not directly activate B cells in the absence of T cells. Thus, three cell types that cooperate in sequence, PEC → T → B, are necessary for antibody production to a thymus-dependent hapten–carrier conjugate. Askonas and Roelants (1974) using similar approaches also concluded that macrophages were essential for T cell–B cell collaboration.

Recently Klaus (1974) using a double cell transfer system found that m-Ag was 3 logs more effective than soluble antigen in priming T cells. He injected lethally irradiated mice with hydrocortisone-resistant thymocytes and m-carrier antigen. Five days later their spleens which presumably contained educated T cells were transferred to secondary, irradiated mice together with hapten–carrier and 2×10^7 spleen cells from mice immunized to the hapten on an unrelated carrier. These secondary irradiated mice made considerable antibody, whereas those that had received spleen T cells primed by soluble carrier failed to do so. Although these studies indicate that macrophages apparently activate T cells, they do not preclude additional macrophage–B cell interactions.

C. Effect of Sensitization with Macrophage-Associated Antigens

The most direct and dramatic demonstration that m-Ag induces CMI comes from studies that show that immunization with m-Ag induces cutaneous DH and primes T helper cells. Generally in such experiments adherent macrophages from nonimmune donors are incubated with antigen for a period of time (usually 1–2 hours) sufficient for maximal antigen uptake. They are then washed (4 or more times) to remove nonadherent soluble antigen, and injected together with the associated antigen (usually less than 5% of the total amount of antigen to which they were exposed) into unimmunized syngeneic adult recipients.

In 1960, Bloch and Nordin reported that immunization of guinea pigs with macrophages associated with purified protein derivative (PPD) provided a particularly effective means of inducing only cutaneous DH and not antibody reactions to PPD. In contrast, similar doses of soluble PPD induced only antibody production. Unanue and Feldman (1971) reported that m-Ag was as effective in inducing DH in rats as soluble antigens but not as effective as a mixture of antigen and CFA. In addition, m-Ag was more effective than soluble Ag in stimulating antibody production. These experiments indicate that the nature and quantity of antigen and/or species used significantly influences the effect of sensitization with m-Ag.

The duration of exposure of antigen to macrophages has also been found to have an important influence on the effect of m-Ag. Pearson and Raffel (1971) found that guinea pigs sensitized with sheep red blood cells (SRBC) that had been exposed to macrophages for only 1 hour produced only antibodies. In contrast, sensitization with SRBC that had been preincubated for 7–24 hours with macrophages induced DH. This suggests that in 1 hour macrophages may "process" and liberate soluble antigens from SRBC which directly stimulate B cell antibody production, whereas longer "processing" leads to m-sRBC fragments that are more capable of inducing T cell-mediated DH.

According to Zembala *et al.* (1974) another factor that influences the immunogenicity of m-Ag is cytophilic antibody. They observed that the ability of macrophage-associated SRBC (m-SRBC) to induce DH is increased in the presence of cytophilic anti-SRBC, whereas it depressed antibody production. This suggests that the anti-SRBC antibodies may increase the rate of "processing" of SRBC by macrophages, thus leading to the earlier appearance of antigenic fragments that induce DH rather than antibody. Liew and Parish (1972) also had found that small amounts of passively administered antibody inhibited production of antibody but enhanced DH in rats that had received sensitized peritoneal exudate cells. However, higher concentrations of antibody inhibited both antibody production and DH.

Clear-cut differences between the effects of m-Ag and soluble Ag have been obtained by performing these types of studies using small doses of antigen in syngeneic guinea pigs. DH is easily studied in this species, and when small doses of antigen are used less of it presumably dissociates from the macrophages (Seeger and Oppenheim, 1972a). Either intradermal or even intracardiac injections of very small doses of tetanus toxoid (0.03–0.6 μg) or of dinitrophenylated ovalbumin (DNP-OA, 1–2.5 μg) when associated with macrophages induce DH but no detectable humoral antibodies in 3 weeks (Table I). By contrast, comparable amounts of soluble antigens produced only immediate Arthus (4–6 hours) reactions. Guinea pigs given two sequential doses of m-Ag manifested still more DH, but still no antibody production. Only after they were given three consecutive doses of m-Ag did the guinea pigs show some Arthus as well as delayed reactions and low titers of antibody. In contrast, guinea pigs that were primed with m-Ag and boosted 1 week later by a skin test with soluble antigen (4.5 μg) showed only DH at day 7, but 2 weeks later had less DH, some Arthus reaction, and high titers of antibody. Guinea pigs primed with soluble antigen and boosted with a skin test manifested no DH at 1 week and developed an Arthus reaction and considerable antibody titers by 3 weeks. These observations indicate that low doses of m-Ag selectively produce DH. Several boosts with m-Ag enhance the degree of DH, but produce only a little antibody. In contrast, after boosting with soluble antigen considerable antibody production ensues. Thus our experiments indicated that m-Ag activates *in vivo* T cell-mediated DH and presumably T helper cells that enhance antibody responses to thymus-dependent antigens. Soluble antigens induce little DH but prime well for antibody production, perhaps because resident *in vivo* macrophages take up sufficient antigen to prime T helper cells, but insufficient antigen to induce DH.

In contrast with our findings with low doses of antigens, Asherson *et al.* (1972) have observed that after single intraperitoneal injections of high doses of m-Ag, guinea pigs develop both more DH and antibody production than those given soluble antigen. It has been observed (Unanue and Askonas, 1968b; Mitchison, 1969) that high doses of antigens are capable of directly stimulating B cells without the help of macro-

TABLE I

Effect on Cutaneous Reactions and Antibody Production of Immunizing Guinea Pigs with Varying Doses of Macrophage-Associated Tetanus Toxoid (m-Tet) and/or Soluble Tetanus Toxoid (s-Tet)

Time and type of immunization			Cutaneous reaction[a] at 21 days (radius)^2		Antibody titer[b] at 21 days (ln)	
day 0	day 7	day 14	4–6 hours Arthus reaction	24 hours DH	Hemagglutinating	Antigen binding
m-Tet (0.51 μg)	0	0	1	29 ± 14	0	0
s-Tet (0.231 μg)	0	0	74 ± 6	8 ± 3	0	0
—	m-Tet (0.51 μg)	m-Tet (0.51 μg)	1	77 ± 24	0.5	0
—	s-Tet (0.51 μg)	s-Tet (0.51 μg)	1	39 ± 14	0	0
m-Tet (0.51 μg)	m-Tet (0.51 μg)	m-Tet (0.51 μg)	27 ± 2	87 ± 15	1.7 ± 0.9	3.3 ± 0.3
m-Tet (0.03–0.3 μg)	s-Tet (4500 μg)	0	27 ± 2	33 ± 6	6.1 ± 0.3	6.7 ± 0.5
s-Tet (0.03–0.3 μg)	s-Tet (4500 μg)	0	26 ± 7	18 ± 5	2 ± 0.7	4.4 ± 0.9

[a] Mean ± SEM of (radius)^2 of erythematous area in millimeters.
[b] Mean ± SEM of ln of titer.

phages. In addition, there is the observation that thymus-independent antigens, such as polymerized flagellin (Miller *et al.*, 1971a), *Escherichia coli* lipopolysaccharide, and polyvinylpyrrolidone (Anderson and Blomgren, 1971), also activate B cells directly in the absence of either T cell or macrophage helper cells. Thus, when high doses of an Ag are used sufficient antigen may dissociate from the macrophages to emulate thymic independent antigens and activate B cells directly. Alternatively the longer *in vivo* persistence of higher doses of antigen may provide the equivalent of a booster dose of soluble antigen.

III. RELATIONSHIP OF MACROPHAGE PRESENTATION AND PROCESSING OF ANTIGENS TO INDUCTION OF CELL-MEDIATED IMMUNITY

The mechanism by which macrophages enhance activation of T cells remains unclear. Macrophages may just passively concentrate and focus antigen and increase its ability to bind and activate lymphocytes. They may produce factors that can enhance lymphocyte reactions. There is indirect evidence that macrophages may also actively process the antigens and either increase or decrease their immunogenicity. Their contribution to immunogenicity is unique; it requires viable metabolizing macrophages. Immunogenic antigen can be found intracellularly as well as on their surface, and they degrade antigens.

A. Unique Capacity of Macrophages to Induce CMI

Macrophages are much more effective than other cell types in inducing DH and priming T cells that enhance antibody production. Seeger and Oppenheim (1972b) compared the ability of antigens associated with various cell types, namely, lymphocytes, thymocytes, hepatoma cells, and macrophages, to induce DH (Table II). We observed that under similar conditions macrophages take up 4 to 37 times more antigen than the other cell types. When we administered equal cell numbers, only macrophages, which had taken up considerably more antigen than the other cell types, induced delayed hypersensitivity (DH). We, therefore, administered equal doses of antigen that had been taken up by the various cell types. Even though this meant that considerably fewer macrophages were administered than other cell types, macrophages still induced much more DH and primed more effectively for antibody. Only lymphocytes induced a little DH and antibody production, which did not differ significantly from the effect of the same dose of soluble antigen. Therefore even this effect may have involved antigen transfer to resident *in vivo* macro-

TABLE II

Comparison of Uptake and Immunogenicity of Cell-Associated ^{125}I-Labeled Tetanus Toxoid (Tet)

				Day 9 (radius)[2]		Antibody titer (ln) on day 21	
Cell type	% of ^{125}I associated with 10^8 cells	Tet per 10^6 cells (pg)	No. cells ($\times 10^6$) with 150 pg Tet	4–6 hours Arthus reaction	24 hours DH	Hemagglutination	Antigen binding
Macrophages	0.05	31.8	4.7	15	68	6.4	5.1
Lymphocyte	0.74	5.1	29.4	6	25	2.9	2.8
Thymocyte	0.02	2.0	75.0	3	3	2.4	1.6
Hepatoma cells	0.18	6.6	22.7	3	3	0.5	1.3
Soluble Tet	—	—	—	4	17	1.5	2.4

phages. However, it has been reported that thoracic duct lymphocytes when coated with anti-lymphocyte globulin or antigen–antibody complexes are capable of activating T helper cells directly and can also induce production of antibody by B cells (Miller *et al.*, 1971b). Furthermore, haptens, such as DNP, if coupled to lymphocytes are very effective inducers of contact hypersensitivity to DNFP (Baumgarten and Geczy, 1970). Thus, under some circumstances lymphocyte-associated antigen appeared capable of activating T cells. However, the participation of macrophages has not been excluded in these studies and may therefore be contributing to the immunogenicity of lymphocyte-associated antigens.

B. Requirement for Macrophage Viability

It is clear from *in vitro* studies that macrophage–lymphocyte interactions occur only when actively metabolizing macrophages are used. It is therefore surprising that both Pearson and Raffel (1971) and Seeger and Oppenheim (1972a) have observed that emulsified or frozen-thawed macrophage-associated antigens were as effective as viable macrophages in inducing *in vivo* immune responses. However, if the macrophages were killed before exposure to the antigens, they failed to enhance the immunogenicity of the antigen. These observations suggest that prior to being lysed or disrupted these macrophages may modify the antigens by some metabolically dependent process. These modified antigens may then be picked up by the recipient's viable macrophages for presentation to lymphocytes.

C. Role of Surface and Intercellular Compartments

Considerable evidence has been presented that immunogenic antigen resides predominantly on the surface of the macrophage (Unanue, 1972). It is known that antigens aggregated by heating are phagocytized and degraded more readily by macrophages (Schmidtke and Unanue, 1971). We have observed that aggregated antigens associated with macrophages are also more effective in inducing DH. Therefore macrophages may just concentrate and present a more dense array of antigens on their surface in a configuration that is particularly effective in binding to and activating T cells. This has been supported by the observation that trypsinization frequently abrogates the ability of m-Ag to induce antibody production (Cruchaud and Unanue, 1971). We have, therefore, tested the effect of trypsinization on the ability of m-Ag to induce DH. We have also found that this reduces both the amount of antigen associated with the macrophages and the immunogenicity of the m-Ag (Table III). However,

TABLE III

Effect of Trypsinization on Immunogencity of Macrophage-Associated Antigens

Preimmunization procedure	Cutaneous reactions (radius)[2]				Antibody titers (ln) 21 days	
	7 days		21 days			
	4–6 hours	24 hours	4–6 hours	24 hours	Hemagglutination	Antigen binding
Incubated macrophages at 37°C for 90 minutes with DNP-OA	4 ± 2	34 ± 6	41 ± 11	25 ± 5	5 ± 0.5	2.5 ± 0.5
Trypsinize m-DNP-OA[a]	18 ± 2	39 ± 3	36 ± 0.5	23 ± 7	4.5 ± 1.5	2
Trypsinize macrophage then incubate them at 37°C for 90 minutes with DNP-OA	12	30	30	24	4	2
Incubated macrophages at 37°C for 90 minutes with tetanus toxoid	13 ± 0.5	58 ± 5	22 ± 5	19 ± 4	ND[b]	ND
Trypsinized m-Tet[a]	7 ± 3	40 ± 6	24 ± 4	20 ± 3	ND	ND
Trypsinized macrophages then reincubated them at 37°C for 90 minutes with tetanus toxoid	8 ± 1	46 ± 15	28 ± 7	26 ± 6	ND	ND

[a] The amount of antigen associated with macrophages was reduced by 50–70% by trypsinization. In order to inject equal doses of m-Ag 2 to 3 times more trypsinized macrophages were injected.

[b] Not done.

when the residual, presumably intracellular, m-Ag was reconcentrated, it was capable of inducing DH. Thus, provided the trypsin removed all the surface antigen, as has been observed by A. Rosenthal (personal communication, 1974), one must agree with Kölsch and Mitchison (1968) and Calderon and Unanue (1974) that intracellular antigen can also be immunogenic.

The nature of both the surface and intracellular antigen remains unclear. The presence or persistence of an antigen on the surface of the macrophage does not preclude it from having been modified, as suggested by the studies of Fishman and Adler (1967).

D. Effects of Antigen Degradation

As has already been indicated (Section II,C) the immunogenicity of SRBC changes dramatically with increasing exposure to macrophages. Furthermore, antibodies to hidden determinants on subunits of the antigen appear after exposure of soluble antigen to macrophages (Unanue, 1969).

TABLE IV

In Vitro Degradation of [^{125}I]DNP-OA by Macrophages

Duration of incubation (hours)	Mean % [^{125}I]DNP-OA adhering to 10^6 macrophages	Mean % increase in free ^{125}I[d]
1.5[a]	0.61	0.38
3[b]	0.42	0.73
24	0.37	1.10
48	0.28	4.25
72	0.22	9.50
72 ± 1.5[c]	0.80	5.40

[a] Macrophages usually were exposed to antigen for 90 minutes at 37°C and then washed four times to remove nonabsorbed antigen and the cpm of absorbed [^{125}I]DNP-OA determined.

[b] The macrophages were reincubated for an additional period before assay of cpm.

[c] After 72 hours of *in vitro* incubation they were repulsed for 90 minutes at 37°C to ensure that they were still functionally capable of adsorbing antigen.

[d] cpm in nonprecipitable supernatant of suspension of macrophages after treatment with 10% trichloroacetic acid.

TABLE V

Effect of Duration of Prior Incubation on Induction of Immunity with Macrophage-Associated Antigen

Immunization	Dose (μg)	No. of macro-phages	Cutaneous reactions (radius)[2]: 7 days, 24 hours	Cutaneous reactions (radius)[2]: 18 days, 4–6 hours	Cutaneous reactions (radius)[2]: 18 days, 24 hours	Antibody titer at 23 days: Hemagglu-tination	Antibody titer at 23 days: Antigen binding
m-Tet[a] preincubated 1½ hours	0.09	1.1×10^6	83 ± 28	33 ± 2	20 ± 9	9 ± 0.3	6 ± 0.3
m-Tet preincubated 44 hours	0.09	2×10^6	0.5 ± 0.5	11 ± 2	31 ± 3	6 ± 0	3 ± 0.5
m-Tet preincubated 68 hours	0.09	2.5×10^6	1 ± 0	43 ± 35	103 ± 54	7 ± 0.5	2 ± 2
Soluble tetanus toxoid	0.09	—	18 ± 2	64 ± 22	14 ± 7	8	6 ± 5
Cutaneous dose of tetanus toxoid on day 7	3	—	0	46 ± 10	99 ± 57	0	0

[a] m-Tet, macrophage-associated tetanus toxoid.

TABLE VI

Effect of Duration of Incubation on Induction of Delayed Hypersensitivity with Macrophage-Associated DNP-OA

Duration of preincubation (hours)	Dose (μg)	No. of macrophages (10^6)	7 days, 24 hours	Cutaneous reaction (radius)[2] 21 days	
				4–6 hours	24 hours
1.5	1	18.9	9 ± 4	40 ± 2	38 ± 4
6	1	26.4	0.7 ± 0.4	3 ± 2	10 ± 7
24	1	22.8	2 ± 0.4	1 ± 0.9	3 ± 2
48	1	26.4	0.3 ± 0.3	0.3 ± 0.3	0.3 ± 0.3
72	1	26.4	0.3 ± 0.3	2 ± 0.9	17 ± 3

Thus, degradation of antigens by macrophages may represent a prominent role for these cells. We, therefore, studied the effect of prolonged incubation of antigen with macrophages on their ability to induce CMI. In these experiments macrophages were incubated for 90 minutes with antigen and the supernatant soluble antigen washed off as usual. The m-Ag was then incubated for longer periods and the amount of residual cell-associated, as well as nonprecipitable, free ^{125}I appearing in the supernatant was determined (Table IV). There was a decrease in the amount of macrophage-associated ^{125}I with time, which was inversely related to the increase in free ^{125}I appearing in the medium presumably due to degradation of antigen. Since macrophages after 72 hours of incubation were still capable of taking up more antigen, these results are not due to impairment of macrophage function. The immunogenicity of the m-Ag that had been incubated for longer periods was then tested (Tables V and VI). As expected the ability of m-Ag to induce DH and to a lesser degree antibody production decreased with longer incubation of m-Ag. This occurred despite the administration of equal doses of m-Ag. Therefore, the residual antigen remaining with macrophages for longer periods of time is no longer as immunogenic as originally. Presumably the cell-associated antigen has also been partly degraded. Thus macrophages exert a biphasic effect on the immunogenicity of antigens. Initially they enhance and subsequently they reduce the efficacy of antigens.

IV. REGULATION OF IMMUNOGENICITY MACROPHAGE-ASSOCIATED ANTIGENS

In addition to degradation of antigen by macrophages, both soluble antigen and antibodies may interfere with the immunogenicity of m-Ag. As has been observed (Section II,C) DH induced by m-Ag at 3 weeks

TABLE VII

Effect of Soluble Antigen on Immunogenicity of Macrophage-Associated Antigen

Immunization	Dose (μg)	Cutaneous reaction (radius)^2: 7 days, 4–6 hours	Cutaneous reaction (radius)^2: 7 days, 24 hours	Cutaneous reaction (radius)^2: 21 days, 4–6 hours	Cutaneous reaction (radius)^2: 21 days, 24 hours	Titer of antigen binding (ln) 21 days
m-Tet[a]	0.075	23 ± 2	78 ± 3	23 ± 2	29 ± 3	4
Macrophages + soluble tetanus toxoid	— 120	5 ± 4	7 ± 3	14 ± 0.5	8 ± 2	7
m-Tet + soluble tetanus toxoid	0.075 120	1	9	14	12	7
m-DNP-OA[b]	2	11 ± 2	55 ± 5	37 ± 7	57 ± 6	4 ± 0.6
m-DNP-OA + soluble DNP-OA	2 800	7 ± 3	15 ± 5	105 ± 41	30 ± 2	4 ± 0.5

[a] m-Tet, macrophage-associated tetanus toxoid.
[b] m-DNP-OA, macrophage-associated dinitrophenylated ovalbumin.

is reduced whereas antibody production and Arthus reactions are increased when soluble antigen was administered in the form of skin tests on the seventh day. Thus soluble antigen and/or subsequently induced antibodies may inhibit DH.

A. Effect of Soluble Antigens

We tested the effect of administering m-Ag in the presence or absence of excess soluble antigen. We found that injection of a mixture of soluble Ag and m-Ag induced less DH at 7 days but the same amount of antibody production at 3 weeks as m-Ag by itself (Table VII). Since no antibody is detectable by 7 days this inhibition of DH is presumably mediated by soluble antigen and not by antibodies. As such, it resembles "split tolerance" or "immune deviation" in which soluble antigens presumably selectively directly inactivate some of the T but not B cells.

B. Effect of Humoral Antibodies

The addition of antisera to immunizing doses of m-Ag at times interfered with the induction of DH and less often with production of antibodies (Table VIII). Such inhibition was observed when the antibody

TABLE VIII

Effect of Antibodies on the Immunogenicity of Macrophage Antigen

Immunization	Cutaneous reaction (radius)[2]				Antibody titer (ln) 21 days	
	7 days		21 days			
	4–6 hours	24 hours	4–6 hours	24 hours	Hemagglutination	Antigen binding
m-Tet	2.2 ± 1	43 ± 13	25 ± 3	26 ± 7	5.3 ± 0.9	4 ± 0.6
m-Tet + anti-Tet[a]	88 ± 17	133 ± 20	26 ± 13	5 ± 3	3.3 ± 0.7	0.7 + 0.7
m-DNP-OA	2 ± 0.3	9 ± 3	9 ± 8	15 ± 5	0	0
m-DNP-OA + anti-DNP-OA[a]	2 ± 1	1 ± 0.5	0.8 ± 0.3	1 ± .5	0	0

[a] Unfractionated high titer antisera obtained from hyperimmunized guinea pigs after repeated injections with antigen. m-Tet, macrophage-associated tetanus toxoid; m-DNP-OA, macrophage-associated dinitrophenylated ovalbumin.

was mixed with preformed m-Ag prior to injection. It was also obtained when the macrophages were first exposed to the antiserum, then washed (leaving only the cytophilic antibodies on the cells), incubated with antigen as usual (90 minutes at 37°C), and injected (Table IX). However, in the case of the latter experiment considerably more antigen was "associated" with the antibody-coated macrophages. Therefore, after equalization of doses of m-Ag, relatively small numbers of macrophages were administered which may provide a trivial cause for the decrease in immunogenicity under these circumstances. Liew and Parish (1972) report that antigens associated with cytophilic antibodies on macrophages may enhance expression of DH but induce less antibody production. Thus different classes of antibody may have opposing effects on immunological responses.

Finally, in an effort to understand the effect of antibodies, we tested the effect of antibodies on m-Ag incubated for longer periods *in vitro*. We found that the presence of antibody increased the rate and degree of degradation of antigens (Table X). This presumably is mediated by the increase in opsonization of antigen–antibody complexes by macrophages. Thus antibodies may influence the immunogenicity of antigens by several mechanisms, such as by increasing the sequestration of antigen and increasing its rate of degradation. Antibodies produced by B cells, therefore, provide an important regulatory feedback control of activation

TABLE IX

Effect of "Cytophilic" Antibody (AT) on Macrophage-Associated Tetanus Toxoid

Immunization[a]	Day 10 skin reaction (radius)^2 24 hours	Day 21 antibody titer (ln) Farr assay
m-Tet pulsed with GPS	85[b]	4[c]
m-Tet pulsed with AT	22	0
Macrophage pulsed with GPS then tetanus toxoid	76[b]	4[c]
Macrophage pulsed with AT then tetanus toxoid	8	0.8

[a] m-Tet, macrophage-associated tetanus toxoid; GPS, normal guinea pig serum.

[b] $p < 0.01$.

[c] $p < 0.05$.

TABLE X

Effect of Antibodies on Degradation of Macrophage-Associated Antigen

Duration of incubation (hours)	μg[^{125}I]DNP-OA per 10^6 macrophages in	
	Normal guinea pig serum	Anti-DNP-OA
1.5[a]	0.267	—
6[b]	0.106	0.105
24	0.056	0.048
48	0.137	0.070
72	0.079	0.040
72 ± 1.5[c]	0.274	0.277

[a] Macrophages usually were exposed to antigen for 90 minutes at 37°C and then washed four times to remove nonadsorbed antigen and the cpm of the adsorbed [^{125}I]DNP-OA determined.

[b] The macrophages were reincubated for an additional period before assay of cpm.

[c] After 72 hours of *in vitro* incubation the macrophages were repulsed for 90 minutes at 37°C to ensure that they were still functionally capable of adsorbing antigen.

of T cells to participate in DH, which operates at the level of the macrophage.

V. SUMMARY AND CONCLUSIONS

The evidence that macrophages are crucial participants in inflammatory reactions is incontrovertible. They are chemotactically attracted to the site of inflammation by cell products including lymphokines and serum complement components. They are concentrated there by migration inhibitory factors (MIF) and activated by macrophage activation factors (MAF). They secrete hydrolytic enzymes and phagocytize and digest debris as well as foreign antigens. In addition, they contribute to the activation of immunological responses. In this chapter, we have collated the available data documenting the role of immunological activation in amplifying inflammatory responses. This role of the macrophage is difficult to separate from their scavenger role in ongoing immunological reactions in which their behavior resembles that of a reverberating circuit. By studying the requirement for purified macrophages in the activation of the early stages of the immune response, their crucial role in activating lymphocytes, whose products in turn attract, arrest, and activate macrophages, becomes apparent.

There is now considerable evidence that antigens associated with macrophages selectively induce *in vivo* cell-mediated immunological reactions, such as delayed hypersensitivity and the priming of T helper cells involved in facilitating antibody production. Since macrophages also enhance T cell reactions *in vitro,* the *in vivo* effects are unlikely to be merely due to the rerouting and delivery of antigen by macrophages to sites rich in T rather than B cells. Presumably macrophages are intimately involved in antigen binding and activation of T cells. *In vitro* rather than *in vivo* studies will be more effective in elucidating the nature of the macrophage–lymphocyte interaction.

Any approach that is capable of selectively inducing cell-mediated immunity has potential applicability to tumor immunology. Sensitization with macrophage-associated tumor antigens should activate T cells without inducing blocking antibodies. Indeed we obtained limited DH and minimal protection against hepatomas in guinea pigs that were sensitized with macrophages exposed to solubilized tumor antigens (J. Oppenheim, R. C. Seeger, and M. Meltzer, unpublished data). Perhaps more dramatic results can be obtained with this type of approach in other systems.

Although soluble thymus-dependent antigens are not usually effective in inducing DH, they presumably always associate with macrophages sufficiently to activate helper T cells. This is supported by the observations of Frei *et al.* (1965) that "biologically filtered" antigens, which have been made totally macrophage independent, also are no longer immunogenic, but become tolerogenic because macrophages sequestered the immunogenic fraction of antigen.

There are many unresolved problems that require further studies.

1. Do the helper T cells belong to the same or a different population of T cells involved in expressing DH?
2. Our studies do not exclude the possibility that macrophages may also directly interact with B cells.
3. Although macrophages are known to reveal new antigenic sites in the process of digesting larger antigens and may contribute an immunogenic RNA component to the antigen, the actual mechanism of antigen "processing" by macrophages remains to be elucidated.
4. Immunologists have naturally concentrated their investigations on the activation aspect of immunological reactions, but the regulatory role

of macrophages in reducing immunological responses are just beginning to be defined. Macrophages not only reduce reactions to antigens by degrading them, but also produce factors which inhibit proliferation of lymphocytes (Kirchner *et al.*, 1974; Owen and Seeger, 1973; Nelson, Chapter 9).

5. Finally, the effects of mediators of CMI, such as the macrophage product "lymphocyte activating factor" (LAF) as well as the lymphokines, MIF, and MAF, on macrophage–lymphocytes interaction need to be explored.

ACKNOWLEDGMENT

We are grateful to the excellent technical assistance of Mrs. S. Dougherty.

REFERENCES

Anderson, B., and Blomgren, H. (1971). *Cell. Immunol.* **2**, 411–424.
Asherson, G. L., Allison, A. C., and Zembala, M. (1972). *Immunology* **22**, 465–473.
Askonas, B. A., and Roelants, G. E. (1974). *Eur. J. Immunol.* **4**, 1–4.
Baumgarten, A., and Geczy, A. F. (1970). *Immunology* **19**, 205–217.
Bloch, H., and Nordin, A. A. (1960). *Nature (London)* **187**, 434–435.
Calderon, J., and Unanue, E. R. (1974). *J. Immunol.* **112**, 1804–1814.
Cruchaud, G. A., and Unanue, E. R. (1971). *J. Immunol.* **107**, 1329–1340.
Feldman, J. D., and Unanue, E. R. (1971). *Cell. Immunol.* **2**, 275–281.
Fishman, M., and Adler, F. L. (1967). *Cold Spring Harbor Symp. Quant. Biol.* **32**, 343–348.
Frei, C. P., Benacerraf, B., and Thorbecke, G. J. (1965). *Proc. Nat. Acad. Sci. U.S.* **53**, 20–24.
Kirchner, H., Chused, T. M., Herberman, R. B., Holden, H. T., and Lavrin, D. H. (1974). *J. Exp. Med.* **159**, 1473–1487.
Klaus, G. G. B. (1974). *Cell. Immunol.* **10**, 483–488.
Kölsch, E., and Mitchison, N. A. (1968). *J. Exp. Med.* **128**, 1059–1079.
Kunin, S., Shearer, G. M., Globerson, A., and Feldman, M. (1972). *Cell. Immunol.* **5**, 288–295.
Liew, F. Y., and Parish, C. R. (1972). *Cell. Immunol.* **5**, 520–535.
Miller, J. F. A. P., Basten, A., Sprent, J., and Cheers, C. (1971a). *Cell. Immunol.* **2**, 469–495.
Miller, J. F. A. P., Sprent, J., Basten, A., Warner, N. L., Breitner, J. C. S., Rowland, G., Hamilton, J., Silver, H., and Martin, W. J. (1971b). *J. Exp. Med.* **134**, 1266–1284.
Mitchison, N. A. (1969). *Immunology* **16**, 1–14.
Owen, J. J. T., and Seeger, R. C. (1973). *Brit. J. Cancer* **28**, 526–534.
Pearson, M. N., and Raffel, S. (1971). *J. Exp. Med.* **133**, 494–505.
Schmidtke, J. R., and Unanue, E. R. (1971). *J. Immunol.* **107**, 331–338.
Schwartz, H. J., and Leskowitz, S. (1969). *J. Immunol.* **103**, 87–91.
Seeger, R. C., and Oppenheim, J. J. (1972a). *J. Immunol.* **109**, 244–254.
Seeger, R. C., and Oppenheim. J. J. (1972b). *J. Immunol.* **109**, 255–261.

Unanue, E. R. (1969). *J. Immunol.* **102,** 893–898.
Unanue, E. R. (1970). *J. Immunol.* **105,** 1339–1343.
Unanue, E. R. (1972). *Advan. Immunol.* **15,** 95–165.
Unanue, E. R., and Askonas, B. A. (1968a). *Immunology* **15,** 287–296.
Unanue, E. R., and Askonas, B. A. (1968b). *J. Exp. Med.* **127,** 915–926.
Unanue, E. R., and Feldman, J. D. (1971). *Cell. Immunol.* **2,** 269–274.
Zembala, M., Ptak, W., and Hanczakowska, M. (1974). *Immunology* **26,** 465–476.

6

Macrophage Function in Antigen Recognition by T Lymphocytes

Alan S. Rosenthal, J. Thomas Blake, Jerrold J. Ellner, Dirk K. Greineder, and Peter E. Lipsky

I. Introduction 131
II. Macrophages Are Required for Antigen Recognition by T Lymphocytes 132
III. Interaction between Macrophage and Soluble Antigen in the Immune Response 134
IV. Genetic Regulation of Functional Macrophage-Lymphocyte Interaction 141
V. Physical Interactions between Macrophages and Lymphocytes 144
VI. Role of Macrophages in Nonantigenic Stimulation of T Lymphocytes 152
A. Mitogens 152
B. Alloantigens 153
C. Aldehyde-Induced Proliferation 154
VII. Model Building for the Cellular and Molecular Events in Antigen Recognition by T Lymphocytes 155
References 158

I. INTRODUCTION

It is now generally accepted that macrophages are required for optimal expression of *in vitro* antigen-induced T lymphocyte proliferation and mediator production, T and B lymphocyte collaboration, and maintenance of cell viability. The mechanisms by which such complex physiologic functions are carried out remain for the most part poorly understood.

This chapter will emphasize data obtained in the guinea pig and other species which relate to the role of the macrophage in antigen recognition by T lymphocytes. We will first consider the evidence that macrophages are required for the initial uptake and presentation of soluble protein antigens. Then, the handling of antigen by macrophages and the functional and physical correlates of macrophage–lymphocyte interaction will be explored in detail. On the basis of these data we will propose a model for describing the cellular events that underlie the process of signal transduction. In that model, the macrophage is envisaged as playing a central role both in antigen presentation and in the modulation and genetic control of the immune response.

II. MACROPHAGES ARE REQUIRED FOR ANTIGEN RECOGNITION BY T LYMPHOCYTES

The guinea pig T lymphocyte lacks easily detectable surface membrane immunoglobulin or antigen-binding capacity (Rosenthal *et al.*, 1972). The chemical nature of its antigen-specific receptor, immunoglobulin or otherwise, has not been defined. This contrasts with the B lymphocyte, which binds antigen directly via a specific membrane-associated immunoglobulin receptor (Davie and Paul, 1974). Antigen-specific activation of T lymphocytes occurs as the result of the cooperation of antigen-bearing macrophages with an immunologically committed lymphocyte (Waldron *et al.*, 1973). The biologic constraints implicit in two cell immunogenic unit are the chief concern of this chapter.

One experimentally useful *in vitro* technique that provides a sensitive assay system for evaluating macrophage function in antigen recognition is the induction of immune lymphocyte proliferation on exposure to specific antigen. This is most simply assessed by measurement of [^{3}H]thymidine incorporation into new DNA after 48–96 hours of culture. In both man (Hersh and Harris, 1968) and guinea pig (Seeger and Oppenheim, 1970) it has been demonstrated that this response can be depressed by removal of glass-adherent cells and restored specifically by readdition of phagocytic mononuclear-adherent cells. Moreover, the macrophages used to reconstitute the lymphocyte proliferative response need not come from animals immune to that antigen. Lymphocytes, polymorphonuclear leukocytes, and fibroblasts (Oppenheim *et al.*, 1968) cannot substitute for macrophages in this function (Rosenstreich and Rosenthal, 1973). However, such experiments do not establish whether macrophages are serving as accessory cells supporting lymphocyte viability and/or whether they function more specifically to present antigen to the lymphocyte in some favorable configuration. In either case, the efficiency of nonimmune macrophages as accessory cells indicates that the role for these cells is not predicated upon or restricted by the immune state of the animal from which the mononuclear phagocyte component of the immunogenic T cell recognition unit is derived (Rosenstreich and Rosenthal, 1974).

Recent studies from our laboratory have employed inbred strain 2 and 13 guinea pigs to analyze further the role of the macrophage in the *in vitro* proliferative assay. We have found that the initial antigen-binding cell in lymphoid populations enriched in T cells is an adherent, phagocytic, radioresistant cell with all of the generally accepted morphologic features of a macrophage (Rosenstreich and Rosenthal, 1974; Waldron *et al.*, 1973).

The functional significance of this initial uptake of antigen by macrophages is readily demonstrable. When macrophages are briefly exposed to soluble protein antigens (15–60 minutes, 37°C), washed, and mixed with immune lymphocytes, they induce proliferation to a degree far in excess of that predicted when concentrations of antigen equivalent to that carried by the pulsed macrophage are added continuously to cultures of macrophages and lymphocytes (Rosenstreich and Rosenthal, 1973). Moreover, lymphocytes that are pulse-exposed to antigen in a similar fashion do not proliferate even when macrophages are added back to them prior to culture (Table I). This latter experiment is of some impor-

TABLE I

Evidence That T Lymphocyte Activation Requires Macrophage Presentation of Antigen[a]

Additions	$[^3H]$TdR incorporation (mean cpm $\times 10^{-3}/10^6$ cells) lymph node lymphocytes: Control	Antigen pulsed
None	0.6 ± 0.1	0.8 ± 0.1
Macrophages	1.4 ± 0.3	2.4 ± 0.2
Antigen-pulsed macrophages	10.1 ± 0.1	10.8 ± 0.9

[a] Macrophages and lymphocytes were pulsed (37°C for 60 minutes) with 10 μg/ml purified protein derivative (PPD) of tuberculin washed and mixed with appropriate pulsed or nonpulsed lymphocytes. DNA synthesis was assessed at 48 hours of culture following an overnight addition of 1 μCi $[^3H]$thymidine.

tance, as it excludes the possibility that macrophages function in this response solely to maintain cell viability. However, what has not been excluded in this experiment is that the direct interaction of antigen with a putative T lymphocyte receptor produced a state of tolerance. To evaluate the latter possibility, antigen-pulsed macrophages were added to control lymphocytes and lymphocytes previously exposed to antigen; equivalent degrees of new DNA synthesis were observed with both lymphocyte populations, indicating that direct antigen exposure under our experimental conditions did not render the lymphocyte unresponsive.

Having defined a function for macrophages in antigen presentation does not exclude their participation in the maintenance of more optimal *in vitro* culture conditions. Indeed, in the mouse, macrophages play a critical role in maintaining lymphocyte viability in Mishell–Dutton cultures (Chen and Hirsch, 1972) and in the mixed leukocyte reaction (Bevan *et al.*, 1974). This trephocytic function can be replaced in part by reducing compounds, such as 2-mercaptoethanol (2-ME). However, in the guinea pig, 2-ME does not replace the macrophage requirement for the T cell proliferative response to soluble antigen (Lipsky *et al.*, 1976).

III. INTERACTION BETWEEN MACROPHAGE AND SOLUBLE ANTIGEN IN THE IMMUNE RESPONSE

We have already pointed out that the immunologic activity of antigen-pulsed macrophages (Harris, 1965; Unanue and Askonas, 1968; Schecter and McFarland, 1970; Katz and Unanue, 1973; Waldron *et al.*, 1973, 1974) and the absence of antigen-binding T cells indicates a critical role for the macrophage in the processing and effective presentation of immunologically active moieties to the T lymphocyte. In this section, we will explore the relationship between uptake and degradation of soluble antigens by the macrophages and the immunogenicity of macrophage-associated antigen.

The lack of differences in the uptake and degradation of autologous and heterologous proteins by macrophages (Schmidtke and Unanue, 1971) implies that variation in physical properties as opposed to foreigness per se determines the nature of the interaction of antigenic proteins with the macrophage. Soluble proteins are taken up by macrophage by macro- and micropinocytosis (Gordon and Cohn, 1974). The rate and extent of uptake varies as a function of the magnitude of protein binding to the cell prior to internalization. For example, the binding of the hapten–protein conjugate dinitrophenyl guinea pig albumin

(DNP–GPA) to guinea pig macrophages appears to involve a high avidity saturable interaction site presumably mediated by the lipophilic hapten. As a result approximately 0.6% of the exposed antigen is bound by 10^6 macrophages from nonimmunized animals in 1 hour at 4°C (Fig. 1). The increment in uptake available via preliminary binding of such an antigen to macrophages, in the absence of cytophilic antibody, contrasts with the relatively meager uptake of horseradish peroxidase, which occurs

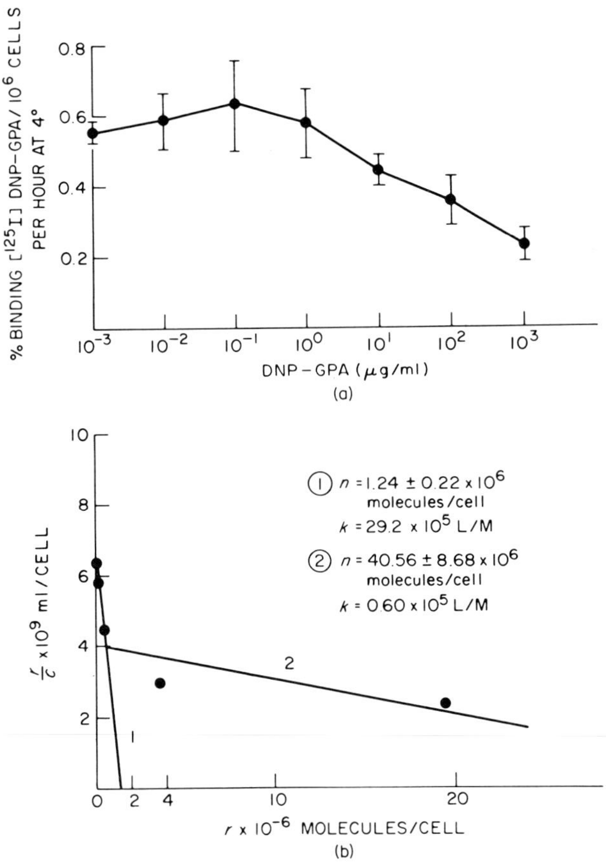

Fig. 1. Binding of DNP-GPA to the macrophage surface. (a) 15×10^6 strain 13 macrophages were pulsed with serial dilutions of [^{125}I]DNP-GPA at 4°C for 1 hour. The cells were washed at 4°C and transferred for determination of ^{125}I content. The data is expressed as percent of pulsed [^{125}I]DNP-GPA bound per 10^6 cells and represents the mean ± SEM of five experiments. (b) Standard Skatchard plot of the data indicating (1) high affinity, readily saturable interaction of DNP-GPA with surface constituents and (2) lower affinity, relatively unsaturable interaction(s).

principally by fluid phase pinocytosis (without antecedent binding) at a rate of 0.0025%/10^6 cells/hour at 37°C in mouse macrophages (Steinman and Cohn, 1972a). Furthermore, macrophages from immune animals which bear specific cytophilic antibody on their surface have an additional mechanism for high avidity surface binding (Cohen *et al.*, 1973).

In addition to differences in uptake, the intracellular fate of antigenic proteins also varies with respect to the particular molecular species under consideration. Most iodinated proteins, including mouse serum albumin (Schmidtke and Unanue, 1971), bovine γ-globulin (Ehrenreich and Cohn, 1967), keyhole-limpet hemocyanin (Unanue and Cerottini, 1970), and DNP-GPA (Ellner and Rosenthal, 1975), undergo extensive early catabolism with release of 75–90% of the initially cell bound radiolabel, predominantly as monoiodotyrosine (Gordon and Cohn, 1974) within the first 24 hours of culture. Thereafter, residual macrophage-bound protein remains relatively stable both qualitatively and quantitatively (Ellner and Rosenthal, 1975) (Fig. 2, lower panel). There are several exceptions. Human serum albumin and hemoglobin appear to undergo continued although slow degradation following the initial catabolic burst (Ehreneich and Cohn, 1967, 1968), and horseradish peroxidase is slowly but totally degraded at a constant rate with a half-life of 20–30 hours (Steinman and Cohn, 1972a,b). Moreover, some of those protein molecules that resist initial catabolism appear to reside in a stable macromolecular surface-associated pool that comprises 20–30% of the residual noncatabolized protein. Retained intracellular antigen, which accounts for 70–80% of the total stable material, also appears to be macromolecular (Ellner and Rosenthal, 1975). Studies by Kölsch and Mitchison (1968) have partially defined such intracellular *subsurface* storage compartments.

The relationship between macrophage–protein interaction and resultant immunogenicity has been most extensively defined with the mouse transfer system, which assesses the extent to which macrophage-associated antigen will prime a syngeneic recipient for antibody production. Preliminary *in vitro* culture of macrophage-bound *Maia squinado* hemocyanin (Unanue and Askonas, 1968) did not affect its immunogenicity on transfer. However, removal of the surface compartment with trypsin or EDTA or covering it with specific antibody significantly decreased the resultant antibody response on transfer (Unanue and Cerottini, 1970). These studies suggest that the physically and functionally stable macromolecular surface pool of antigen has major relevance in the complicated intracellular dynamics involved in antibody synthesis.

Recently, the proliferative response of thymus-derived lymphocytes to soluble antigen has been employed to study the immunogenic correlates of guinea pig macrophage handling of DNP-GPA (Ellner and Rosenthal,

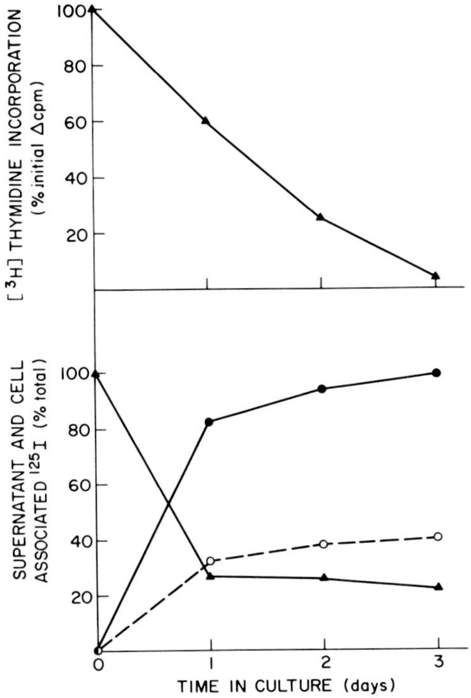

Fig. 2. Comparison of the macrophage-handling of DNP-GPA with immunogenicity of macrophage-associated antigen. Upper panel: Strain 13 peritoneal exudate cells were pulsed with 1.0 μg/ml DNP-GPA for 1 hour at 37°C, washed, cultured 0–3 days, and washed again. Then antigen-pulsed or control PEC's were added back to a single population of immune peritoneal exudate lymphocytes. [^{3}H]Thymidine incorporation is expressed as percent of that obtained with pulsed, uncultured macrophages. Lower panel: In parallel experiments, macrophages were pulsed with [^{125}I]DNP-GPA under the same conditions and residual cell-associated antigen (▲——▲), total supernatant antigen (●——●), and TCA-precipitable antigen (○---○) were determined at the appropriate culture interval.

1975). In this system, antigen-pulsed macrophages are cultured 1 to 3 days, washed, and then mixed with immune lymphocytes for an additional 72 hours at which time DNA synthesis is assessed. These data indicate that preliminary culture of macrophages briefly exposed to antigens (60 minutes) prior to determination of [^{3}H]thymidine incorporation into immune lymphocytes resulted in progressive decrease in immunogenicity (Fig. 2, upper panel). This decline reflected neither the rapid catabolic phase of antigen handling nor the ensuing antigen stability (Fig. 2, lower panel), but rather may have resulted from a decrease in the efficiency of presentation of antigen to the responding lymphocyte, whether due to macrophage aging or sequestration of antigen. Moreover, trypsinization removed 20% of the total residual cell-associated DNP-GPA but did not further diminish the immune response (Fig. 3). Studies with ^{125}I-labeled Fab'$_2$ anti-DNP-GPA confirmed the loss of the surface component following trypsinization. These data suggest that the stable surface pool was neither the sole nor, in this case (the proliferative response of T lymphocytes to soluble antigen), the critical site of antigen retention.

Morphologic studies using a horseradish peroxidase conjugate of DNP-GPA were carried out at the light and electron microscopic level. Localization of the cytochemical reaction product at 24 hours of culture at

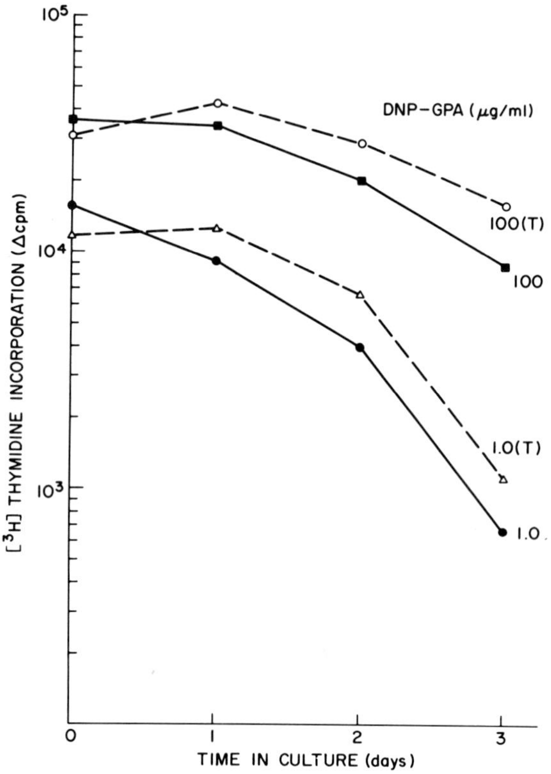

Fig. 3. Effect of trypsinization on the immunogenicity of macrophage-associated DNP-GPA. Strain 13 peritoneal exudate macrophages were pulsed with 1.0 or 100 μg/ml DNP-GPA and cultured as described in the Fig. 1. At the end of the appropriate periods of culture, aliquots of the pulsed and control cells were trypsinized. Then [^{3}H]thymidine incorporation was determined 72 hours after macrophages were added back to DNP-GPA immune peritoneal exudate lymphocytes. The results represent the mean of five experiments.

37°C was restricted to cytoplasmic sites. To overcome the objection of a possible dissociation of the enzymatic probe from the antigen molecules, confirmatory experiments were carried out with [^{3}H]DNP-GPA (Fig. 4). These studies of 1 μm sections of plastic embedded macrophages failed to indicate the presence of significant amounts of membrane-associated [^{3}H]DNP-GPA after trypsinization and culture. It appears that although macrophage surface-associated antigen may have major relevance in the *in vivo* antibody response in the mouse, an intracellular pool retains full activity as regards *in vitro* T cell proliferation in the guinea pig. Although it would be theoretically possible for trypsinization of surface antigen from macrophages to be followed by generalized return of such material to the cell surface with restoration of the surface compenent, in fact this has not been noted to occur spontaneously (Unanue *et al.*, 1969; Ellner and Rosenthal, 1975) nor is it apparent when the macrophages are incubated with immune lymphocytes (A. S. Rosenthal, unpublished observation). Thus the manner in which intracellular antigen becomes available for T lymphocyte interaction is unclear. Exocytosis of antigen either occurring spontaneously (Calderon and Unanue, 1974)

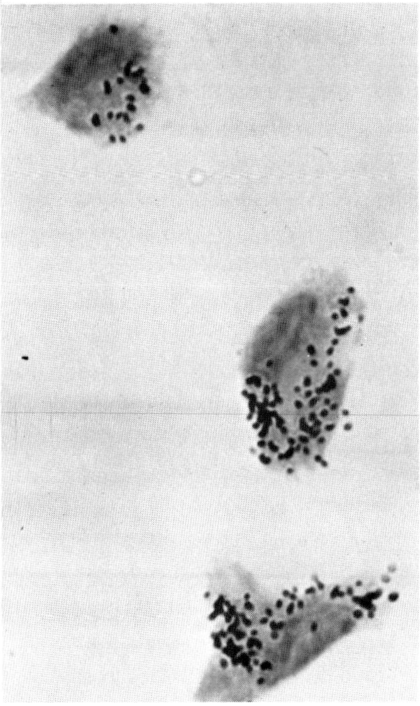

Fig. 4. Autoradiographs of 1 μm sections of plastic-embedded macrophages pulsed with [^{3}H]DNP-GPA at 37°C for 60 minutes and cultured for 24 hours before fixation. ×1200.

or induced by the physical interaction between macrophage and lymphocyte remains an attractive possibility.

Other studies have addressed the question of whether the nature of macrophage uptake and degradation of protein antigen may, in part, define the antigenicity of substances or the degree to which the immune response to them is under genetic control. Clearly, the presence of specific cytophilic antibody or immune complexes markedly enhances the association of protein antigens with macrophages (Cohen *et al.*, 1973; Steinman and Cohn, 1972b). Cohen and colleagues (1973) have demonstrated that immune macrophages have a definite advantage in the presentation of antigen for T lymphocyte proliferation at limiting concentrations of antigen. In addition, antigens, such as DNP-GPA, which bind avidly to the nonimmune macrophage, are highly immunogenic following pulse exposure even at low concentrations. Ryan and Lee (1970) found that the antibody response following priming with most soluble proteins correlated with the stability of the antigens during exposure to cell-free lysosomal cathepsins. That is, those substances which resisted catabolism were more antigenic.

The study of differential handling of antigens by macrophages from high and low responder strains of mice and guinea pigs has yielded conflicting results. No differences in the degradability of hapten-conjugated poly-L-lysine were observed between spleen extracts from responder nonresponder guinea pigs (Levine and Benacerraf, 1964). However, TG-Pro-L was taken up and degraded more by responder than nonresponder mouse macrophages (Gallily and Eliahu, 1974). In contrast, keyhole limpet hemocyanin (KLH) was both taken up and degraded less well by macrophages from responder than by macrophages from nonresponder Biozzi mice (Wiener and Bandieri, 1974).

Another issue that will require further definition is the physical alteration in the immunogenic moiety by macrophages. The relevance of extracts, subcellular fractions, and particularly antigen–RNA complexes remain unestablished in immune phenomena requiring intact, viable macrophages (Pearson and Raffel, 1971; Cohn, 1962; Uhr and Weissman, 1965; Franzel, 1962; Unanue, 1972). Both the stable surface and intracellular antigen pools resisting initial catabolism appear to be macromolecular (Ellner and Rosenthal, 1975; Unanue and Cerottini, 1970). However, at least as regards the macrophage handling of sheep red blood cells, progressive digestion is required for optimal generation of delayed hypersensitivity. Finally, the constraints on macrophage–lymphocyte interaction discussed in Section IV suggest that antigen may be directly or conformationally coupled to serologically defined histocompatibility and/or *Ir* gene products.

Although knowledge of the cellular biology of the macrophage is extensive, certain crucial issues on the relationship between the handling of immunogenic proteins and their immunologic activity when associated with macrophages require further study. These include (1) the basis for the maintenance of surface and intracellular pools of antigen resistant to lysosomal degradation, (2) the relative contribution of these compartment to lymphocyte activation during cellular interactions (3) the mechanisms of access of the lymphocyte to intracellular macrophage-associated antigen, and (4) the physical and conformational state of immunologically relevant antigen, particularly as regards potential association with histocompatibility antigens and/or *Ir* gene products.

IV. GENETIC REGULATION OF FUNCTIONAL MACROPHAGE–LYMPHOCYTE INTERACTION

In the guinea pig, activation of T lymphocyte DNA synthesis by macrophages bearing complex protein antigens requires identity of histocompatibility-linked gene products on both macrophage and lymphocyte (Rosenthal and Shevach, 1973) (Table II). The failure of allogeneic antigen-bearing macrophages to initiate effectively proliferation of T lymphocytes immune to that antigen does not result from the presence of

TABLE II

Requirement for Histocompatible Macrophages in Antigen-Mediated DNA Synthesis in Immune Guinea Pig Lymph Node Lymphocytes[a]

Macrophage		$[^3H]$TdR incorporation (cpm × 10^{-3}) lymphocyte DNA synthesis		
Strain	Antigen Pulse	Strain 2	Strain 13	(2 × 13) F_1
2	0	0.92 ± 0.28	5.68 ± 1.08	1.60 ± 0.30
2	+	26.38 ± 8.27	8.61 ± 2.08	6.98 ± 0.80
13	0	4.63 ± 1.86	1.66 ± 0.37	1.78 ± 0.47
13	+	3.12 ± 0.67	19.89 ± 4.47	7.81 ± 1.75
(2 × 13) F_1	0	1.91 ± 0.99	4.27 ± 0.34	1.66 ± 0.53
(2 × 13) F_1	+	12.42 ± 3.19	11.81 ± 1.98	12.57 ± 2.33

[a] Macrophages (1.0 × 10^6 cells) were pulsed with 100 μg/ml PPD for 60 minutes at 37°C, washed, and mixed with an equal number of syngeneic, allogeneic, or (2 × 13) F_1 lymph node lymphocytes from animals immunized to Freund's complete adjuvant. Lymphocyte proliferation was assessed at 72 hours of culture; $[^3H]$thymidine (1 μCi) was added the last 18 hours.

an inhibitor of blastogenesis released in mixtures of allogeneic cells or differing kinetics of activation. In other studies, functional cooperation between macrophages bearing antigen and lymphocytes immune to that antigen was blocked by specific alloantisera when directed against determinants present on both macrophage and lymphocyte. One objection that can be raised to studies of the effect not only of alloantisera but also of inhibitors in general is that in the proliferation assay, the response (i.e., [^{3}H]thymidine incorporation) is separated from the initial signal (addition of antigen-bearing macrophages) by periods in excess of 48–72 hours. The macrophage migration inhibitory factor (MIF) assay has the distinct advantage that it can be assessed as early as 18 hours following the mixing of antigen-bearing macrophages and lymphocytes. Ben-Sasson and colleagues (Ben-Sasson *et al.*, 1974) overcame these objections to some extent by confirming that syngeneic macrophages are required for production of MIF and further showing that MIF synthesis induced by antigen-bearing macrophages was inhibited by alloantisera.

It has been suggested that the main function of the products of immune response (*Ir*) genes (reviewed by Benacerraf and Katz, 1975) is in antigen recognition. Functional interactions between macrophages and lymphocytes are apparently controlled by genes linked to the main histocompatibility complex. We therefore began studies exploring these interactions using antigens under unigenic control, such as the random copolymer of L-glutamic acid-L-tyrosine (GT) (strain 13 responder; strain 2 non-responder) and L-glutamic acid-L-lysine (GL) (strain 2 responder; strain 13 non-responder), and F_1 (nonresponder $\times$ responder) animals that respond to both artificial copolymers (Shevach and Rosenthal, 1973). Parental macrophages pulsed with an antigen, the response to which is controlled by an *Ir* gene lacking in that parent, will not stimulate F_1 (responder) T lymphocyte DNA synthesis. By contrast, parental macrophages pulsed with antigens controlled by *Ir* genes which they possess or with antigens not under unigenic control will initiate F_1 T lymphocyte proliferation. These studies do not define whether or not genes controlling macrophage T lymphocyte cooperation are identical or separate from classically defined immune response genes.

Shevach *et al.* (1975) have recently examined this question in studies using phenotypically characterized outbred guinea pigs that have been classified both by their serologically defined histocompatibility determinants as well as by their response to antigen, such as GT, known to be under genetic control. They found, for example, that mixing macrophages from a 13^+, GT^- outbred guinea pig pulsed with GT would not induce proliferation of lymphocytes from inbred strain 13 guinea pigs immune to GT, but would induce inbred strain 13 lymphocyte proliferation to another antigen to which both were responders, such as PPD. In a series of experiments, Shevach *et al.* found that macrophages bearing genetically controlled antigens do not initiate proliferation in lymphocytes from immunized animals unless both possess identical *Ir* and serologically defined histocompatibility products. Thus, functional cooperation between macrophages bearing antigens and lymphocytes requires the presence in both of products of the *Ir* gene as well as of products of separate genes linked to the seriologically definable histocompatibility loci.

It is reasonable to ask at this time whether these observations have general applicability to other animal models, such as the mouse, whose genetic makeup has been more extensively characterized and is therefore more amenable to analysis than that of the guinea pig. Initial studies by Katz and Unanue (1973) appeared to suggest that such genetic restriction of macrophage–T lymphocyte interaction did not operate in the mouse. They employed an *in vitro* assay of the secondary antibody responses to hapten–protein conjugates. It is unclear at this time whether their assay required antigen presentation to T lymphocytes or only to B lymphocytes. In addition it was not known whether the strain combinations purporting allogeneic collaboration differed at those loci that determined cellular interaction. More recent studies indicate that T lymphocyte antigen recognition in the mouse exhibits histocompatibility linked constraints on antigen presentation by macrophages which parallel those of the guinea pig (Schwartz and Paul, 1975). Schwartz and Paul have employed a proliferative assay using peritoneal exudate lymphocytes from mice immunized to soluble protein antigens, such as DNP_5-ovalbumin and T,G--A--L. This response was shown to be the result of T lymphocyte proliferation because it was eliminated by treatment with anti-θ serum plus complement. In addition, the system exhibited carrier specificity. Table III shows a dose response curve for C57BL/10Sn immune lymphocytes when stimulated by antigen on varying numbers of syngeneic (B10) or allogeneic (B10.A) macrophages. It can be seen that at every dose tested, antigen on syngeneic macrophages resulted in greater proliferation than antigen on allogeneic macrophages. Moreover the inefficiency of allogeneic macrophage presentation of antigen was shown not to be the result of kinetic differences in proliferation as both syngeneic and allogeneic macrophages, as well as continuous antigen, showed similar kinetics.

Additional support for making a generalization of allogeneic restriction in cellular cooperation is found in the recent studies in the mouse by Erb and Feldmann (1975) who have shown that syngeneic macrophages are more efficient than allogeneic macrophages in the induction of antigen-specific T helper activity.

TABLE III

Antigen Presentation by Syngeneic and Allogeneic Murine Peritoneal Exudate Macrophages[a]

Number of macrophages added ($\times 10^4$)	Syngeneic B10 macrophages (Δ cpm)[b]	Allogeneic B10.A macrophages (Δ cpm)[b]
1	42,600	10,500
2	39,100	7,200
4	70,400	8,400
10	57,500	7,100
20	9,000	200

[a] From Schwartz and Paul, 1975.

[b] Incorporation of [^{3}H]thymidine by 2×10^5 C57BL/10Sn (B10) peritoneal exudate lymphocytes 5 days after presentation of DNA-OA bound to macrophages (Δ cpm).

V. PHYSICAL INTERACTIONS BETWEEN MACROPHAGES AND LYMPHOCYTES

The development of physical approximations between lymphocytes and macrophages seems to be a central biological phenomenon necessary for the efficient expression of a wide variety of the physiologic functions of lymphoid cells, such as the maintenance of lymphocyte viability (Chen and Hirsch, 1972) and the promotion of functional maturation and differentiation of thymocytes (Mosier and Pierce, 1972). The role of macrophage–lymphocyte interaction in the development of a variety of *in vitro* immune responses has also been described. Clustering of lymphocytes about macrophages, presumably bearing an antigenic signal, has been observed during cultivation of lymphoid cells from mouse (Mosier, 1969), rabbit (Sharp and Burwell, 1960), guinea pig (Salvin *et al.*, 1971), and man (McFarland *et al.*, 1966). Clustering of lymphocytes about blast-like cells has also been described (Sulitzeanu *et al.*, 1971; Werdelin *et al.*, 1974), but both the nature of the central blast-like cell and the functional significance of these particular cellular interactions remains unclear. More detailed investigation has indicated the importance of interaction between macrophages and lymphocytes for the *in vitro* induction of primary (Mosier, 1969) and secondary (Katz and Unanue, 1973) antibody responses as well as the antigen-mediated *in vitro* initiation of immune lymphocyte proliferation (Cline and Swett, 1968). In these systems, macrophages, as indicated above, are thought to interact initially with antigen, handling it such a way as to maintain its immunological potential (Unanue, 1972). Macrophage–lymphocyte interaction would thus serve to provide an efficient mechanism for the presentation of immunologically relevant antigen to immune lymphocytes. Even in situations in which physiological activities have been demonstrated to be mediated by supernatant factors, these factors can often be seen to function most efficiently when direct cell to cell contact develops between macrophages and lymphocytes. Thus the enhancement of the bactericidal capacity of macrophages by antigenically stimulated lymphocyte supernatants is accomplished most effectively when actual physical approximation develops between lymphocytes and macrophages (Simon and Sheagren, 1972).

Lipsky and Rosenthal (1973, 1975a) have characterized and quantitated the physical interactions between macrophages and lymphocytes. Initially, the physical interaction that developed in the absence of antigen between macrophages and lymphocytes was studied. A scanning electron micrograph of thymocytes bound to a guinea pig macrophage is shown in Fig. 5. Tranmission electron microscopy revealed extremely broad

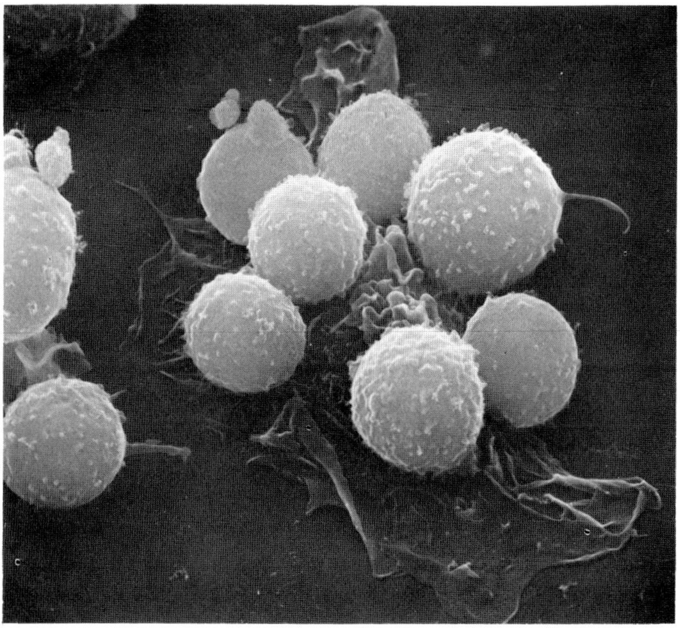

Fig. 5. Scanning electron micrograph of guinea pig macrophages binding thymocytes. ×2000. Courtesy of Dr. T. Triche.

areas of closely opposed surface membranes but no evidence of cytoplasmic contact or specialization of the submembrane architecture in the areas adjacent to cell–cell contact (Lipsky and Rosenthal, 1973).

Different populations of glass-adherent macrophages, namely, peritoneal exudate, resident peritoneal, splenic, and alveolar macrophages bound thymocytes to a greater extent than either polymorphonuclear leukocytes or fibroblasts. Likewise, thymocytes and lymph node lymphocytes were bound by macrophages in numbers significantly greater than either L_2C leukemia cells, homologous erythrocytes, or heterologous (mouse) thymocytes. Thus, there is specificity for each of the participant cell types, suggesting the existence of a unique cellular recognition mechanism. No selectivity for T or B lymphocytes were observed, and they were bound to macrophages in proportion to their frequency in the added population.

Data obtained using heat-killed cells and metabolic inhibitors indicated that the interaction required viable, metabolically intact macrophages. The role of the lymphocyte, however, was passive in that heat-killed or metabolically poisoned lymphocytes exhibited no decreased binding. The *in vitro* characteristics of the antigen-independent binding of thymocytes or lymphocytes by macrophages are summarized in Table IV. Note that the binding of lymphocytes by macrophages has *in vitro* physiologic parameters different from those of binding of various other particles by macrophages. It is, therefore, likely that the macrophage binding of lymphocytes is mediated by a distinct receptor mechanism and not the one previously described as mediating the macrophage binding of 7 S or 19 S coated erythrocytes, antibody and complement-coated red cells, or aldehyde-treated red cells (Lay and Nussenzweig, 1968; Rabinovitch, 1968).

Another feature of antigen-independent macrophage–lymphocyte interaction is its dynamic nature. When thymocytes are added to macrophages, the maximal degree of observed binding is reached after a 60

TABLE IV

Characteristics of Antigen-Independent Binding of Lymphocytes by Macrophages

Dependent on active macrophage but not lymphocyte metabolism
Abolished by trypsinization of macrophage but not lymphocyte
Temperature dependent
Dependent on divalent cations
Cannot distinguish T from B cells
Binding is not inhibited by excess immunoglobulin
"Reversible"

minute incubation, with further incubation leading to no increased binding. This plateau in macrophage–thymocyte interaction is interpreted as indicating that a dynamic equilibrium has been reached with cellular association equivalent numerically to cellular dissociation. The existence of such a steady state is supported by experiments using radiolabeled thymocytes in which it was demonstrated that macrophage monolayers exchanged unlabeled thymocytes for isotopically labeled cells without a significant change in the total number of macrophage-bound thymocytes. These studies on the dynamic nature of macrophage–lymphocyte interaction are consonant with the microcinematographic studies reported by Salvin *et al.* (1971).

Thus, macrophages have the unique ability to recognize and reversibly bind thymocytes and lymphocytes in the absence of antigen by means of a trypsin-digestible, temperature-sensitive, divalent cation-dependent receptor mechanism. We next examined whether the presence of immune lymphocytes and specific antigen would affect the degree of observed macrophage–lymphocyte interaction. For these experiments, antigen was introduced into the cultures by exposing the established glass-adherent macrophages to soluble antigens for 60 minutes at 37°C and washing prior to the addition of lymphocytes. Lymphocytes for study were obtained from the lymph nodes of guinea pigs previously immunized with either Freund's complete adjuvant (CFA) alone or soluble antigens emulsified in CFA. The lymphocytes were passed over nylon wool/glass bead adherence columns to deplete both macrophages and B lymphocytes before use.

Initial studies showed that after a standard 1 hour incubation, the degree of macrophage–lymphocyte interaction observed was not affected by the presence of specific antigen. However, when incubations were prolonged beyond the 1 hour period routinely used to assay antigen–independent interaction, differences between the binding manifested by antigen-bearing macrophages and control macrophages became evident (Lipsky and Rosenthal, 1975b). In the absence of antigen, there was a steady decline in the degree of macrophage–lymphocyte interaction as culture was prolonged, while in cultures containing antigen-bearing macrophages no such decline occurred. A significant difference between the binding exhibited by antigen-bearing and control macrophages was seen by 8 hours and was maximal by around 20 hours (Table V). The development of this phenomenon was found to be dependent on the coincidence in cultures of macrophages bearing specific antigen with lymphocytes obtained from animals immune to that antigen. The immune status of the animal from which the macrophages were obtained was found to be irrelevant. Brief direct exposure of the lymphocytes to antigen did not result in the

TABLE V

Effect of Prolongation of Culture on Macrophage–Lymphocyte Interaction[a]

Length of incubation (hours)	Macrophage exposure (lymphocytes bound/100 macrophages)	
	Control	Antigen
1	73 ± 2	76 ± 3
2	69 ± 2	66 ± 4
4	62 ± 4	67 ± 8
8	48 ± 5	80 ± 3
20	21 ± 3	89 ± 5

[a] The binding of lymph node lymphocytes obtained from PPD immune animals to syngeneic macrophages as a function of the length of time the two cell types were incubated together in standard fashion. The macrophages had previously been exposed to either PPD (100 μg/ml) in PBS or PBS alone for 60 minutes at 37°C and washed four times prior to use. Each term represents the mean ±SEM of four replicate experiments.

development of antigen-mediated interaction when they were added to control macrophages, and it did not block the development of antigen-dependent interactions when these antigen-pulsed lymphocytes were cultured with antigen-bearing macrophages. Finally, antigen-dependent binding was found to be principally carrier- or conjugate-specific rather than hapten-specific when hapten–protein conjugates were used as antigens.

When incubations were prolonged beyond 20 hours, greater binding of immune lymphocytes by antigen-bearing macrophages compared to control continued for at least 72 hours in culture (Fig. 6). The functional significance of antigen-dependent binding is shown by assessing macrophage-bound and unbound lymphocytes autoradiographically for the incorporation of tritiated thymidine after various periods of culture. [^{3}H]Thymidine incorporation is manifested by macrophage-bound lymphocytes after 48 hours in culture, while significant numbers of unbound lymphocytes are not found to be undergoing DNA synthesis until 72 hours of culture (Fig. 7). These data suggest that DNA synthesis occurs while the lymphocytes are macrophage-bound (Fig. 8).

Two lines of evidence suggest that antigen-mediated binding precedes

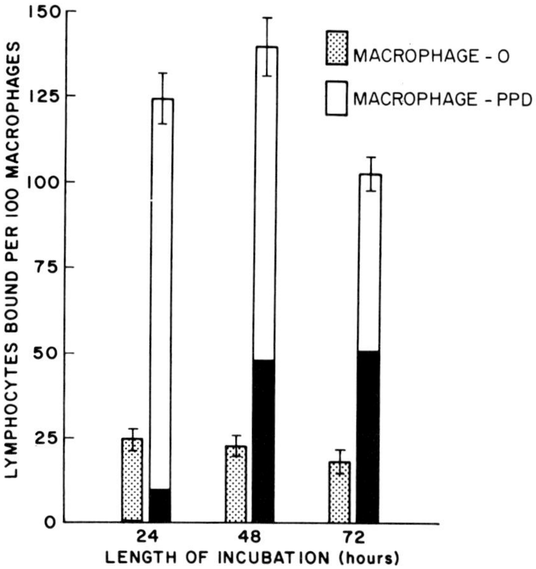

Fig. 6. The binding of lymph node lymphocytes from PPD immune guinea pigs to syngeneic macrophages during prolonged incubation. The macrophage had previously been exposed to either 100 μg/ml of PPD in PBS (macrophage-PPD) or to PBS alone (macrophage-0) for 60 minutes at 37°C and washed four times prior to use. Each point represents the mean ± SEM of three replicate experiments. Shaded areas of the bars indicate the number of macrophage-bound lymph node leukocytes that were detected autoradiographically to be incorporating tritiated thymidine.

lymphocyte activation and is not dependent on the initiation of DNA synthesis or its occurrence. First, immune lymphocytes, which have been treated with mitomycin C and thus do not exhibit a DNA synthetic response to antigen-bearing macrophages, participate in antigen-dependent macrophage–lymphocyte interaction as well as control, untreated lymphocytes. Second, when immune lymphocytes are exposed to both antigen-bearing macrophages and control macrophages simultaneously in the same culture chamber, antigen-mediated binding involves only those macrophages actually bearing antigen. The observation that control macrophages in these cultures manifest no enhanced binding as a result of being cultured with antigen-bearing macrophages and immune lymphocytes suggests that antigen-mediated binding is a primary event that develops between an immune lymphocyte and an antigen-bearing macrophage, and does not represent a nonspecific event that results from lymphocyte activation.

Finally the role of histocompatibility-linked determinants in the de-

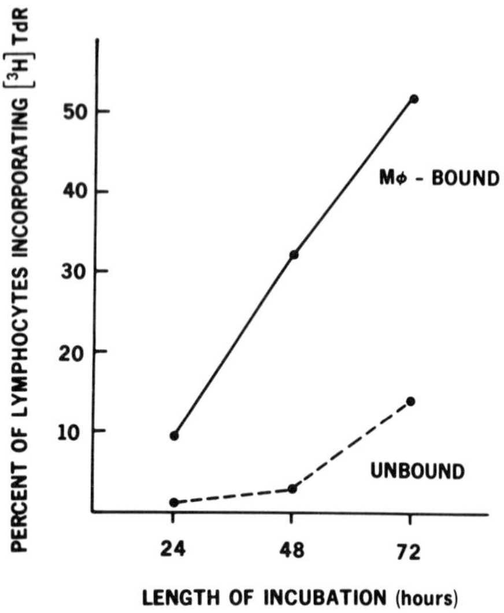

Fig. 7. Lymph node lymphocytes from PPD immune guinea pigs were incubated with syngeneic PPD-bearing macrophages. [^{3}H]TdR (2 μCi) was added to each culture for the last 18 hours of incubation. At the termination of cultures, autoradiographs were prepared to evaluate the incorporation of tritiated thymidine by the lymphocytes bound to the macrophages. Lymphocytes that were not bound by macrophages were also harvested and similarly evaluated for uptake of [^{3}H]TdR.

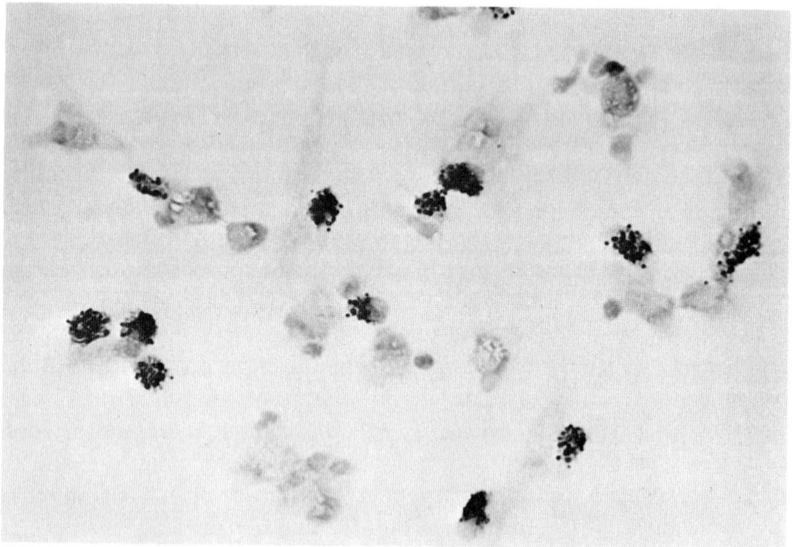

Fig. 8. Autoradiograph of [^{3}H]thymidine incorporation into clusters of antigen-pulsed macrophages and syngeneic lymphocytes from immunized guinea pigs at 3 days of culture.

velopment of both antigen-independent and antigen-mediated macrophage lymphocyte interaction was examined. Table VI indicates that no significant differences were noted in the ability of either strain 2 or 13 macrophages to bind syngeneic or allogeneic lymphocytes in the absence of antigen. Furthermore, prolonged cultures of allogeneic combinations of lymphocytes and macrophages in the absence of antigen resulted in binding that was numerically similar to that observed for syngeneic cells. The development of antigen-mediated macrophage–lymphocyte interaction by contrast was found to require that lymphocytes and macrophages share histocompatibility-linked identity. These findings parallel the observation that the functional recognition of soluble protein antigens by immune guinea pig thymus-derived lymphocytes requires the presentation of antigen by histocompatible macrophages.

These observations indicate that physical interaction between macrophages and lymphocytes plays an important role in antigen initiated proliferation of immune lymphocytes. Furthermore, these studies suggest the possibility that physical events may proceed sequentially from antigen-independent reversible binding of lymphocytes by macrophages to antigen-independent reversible binding of lymphocytes by macrophages to antigen-stablized specific interactions. The first step could bring together lymphocytes and macrophages without regard to their immunological

TABLE VI

***Macrophage–Lymphocyte Interaction: Histocompatibility Requirement*[a]**

Strain		Macrophage exposure to antigen	Lymphocytes bound/100 macrophages length of incubation	
Macrophage	Lymphocyte		1 hour	20 hours
2	2	0	75 ± 6	19 ± 6
		+	—	112 ± 12
2	13	0	66 ± 5	18 ± 7
		+	—	25 ± 7
13	13	0	70 ± 3	17 ± 44
		+	—	100 ± 11
13	2	0	77 ± 8	21 ± 5
		+	—	33 ± 6

[a] Data express the binding observed when 5×10^6 lymph node lymphocytes obtained from either strain 2 or 13 PPD immune guinea pigs are added to antigen exposed (PPD, 100 μg/ml) or control macrophage monolayers and incubated in standard fashion for 1 or 20 hours. Each term represents the mean ±SEM of four replicate experiments.

commitment or previous exposure to antigen. When this step has brought specifically immune lymphocytes into apposition with antigen-bearing macrophages, antigen-mediated interaction will result, eventuating in immune lymphocyte proliferation if lymphocyte and macrophage share gene products linked to the major histocompatibility complex.

VI. ROLE OF MACROPHAGES IN NONANTIGENIC STIMULATION OF T LYMPHOCYTES

The preceding discussion has focused on the *in vitro* secondary response of immune T lymphocytes to soluble protein antigens. Several other modes of T lymphocyte activation have been studied with respect to their macrophage requirement.

A. Mitogens

The role of macrophages in mitogen-induced T lymphocyte proliferation remains controversial. Macrophages have been reported to potentiate phytohemaglutinin-induced (PHA-induced) lymphocyte proliferation (Alter and Bach, 1970; Levis and Robbins, 1970; Lohrmann *et al.*, 1974). However, other investigators have found that macrophages inhibit (Walker and Fowler, 1965) or have no effect (Waldron *et al.*, 1973) on PHA-induced lymphocyte proliferation. Some of these conflicting observations are likely to be the result of the degree of macrophage depletion achieved in various studies and of the use of optimal or suboptimal doses of mitogen. Thus, with suboptimal doses of PHA, macrophages facilitate the PHA response (Lohrmann *et al.*, 1974; Oppenheim *et al.*, 1968), suggesting that macrophages are able to "concentrate" or "focus" PHA for more efficient presentation to T lymphocytes. It is clear that, if macrophages are indeed required for PHA-induced proliferation of T lymphocytes, the number necessary is far less than that required for soluble protein antigen or allogeneic leukocyte-induced proliferation in the mixed lymphocyte culture (MLC) (Waldron *et al.*, 1973; Lohrmann *et al.*, 1974). However, it should be noted that extensive depletion of adherent cells may interfere with T lymphocytes viability in *in vitro* culture. Such studies, therefore, cannot be interpreted as indicating that this represents an obligatory pathway. It is of interest that in contrast to the situation with macrophage bound antigen-induced T lymphocyte proliferation, induction of lymphocyte proliferation by macrophage-bound PHA does not require that the macrophage and lymphocyte share identity of some histocompatibility-linked gene product (Rosenthal and Shevach, 1973).

B. Alloantigens

The role of macrophages in allogeneic T cell activation has not been extensively studied in the MLC. Early observations suggested that macrophage-depleted lymphocyte populations lost MLC reactivity in parallel with soluble antigen reactivity and that both responses were restored by the addition of macrophages (Oppenheim *et al.*, 1968). When these populations were studied in undirectional MLC reactions (i.e., one donor's lymphocytes X-irradiated or mitomycin C treated), it appeared that macrophages of either stimulator or responder origin could equally restore the response, suggesting a nonspecific role (Alter and Bach, 1970; Twomey *et al.*, 1970). However, more recent studies have shown that human or guinea pig macrophages are 10–80 times more effective stimulators of allogeneic T lymphocyte DNA synthesis than are purified lymphocytes (Rode and Gordon, 1974; Greineder and Rosenthal, 1975). Such findings suggest that one important role of macrophages in the MLC is to induce allogeneic lymphocyte proliferation directly (Table VII). In the guinea pig MLC, little stimulatory activity can be attributed to lymphocytes (Greineder and Rosenthal, 1975). However, in the mouse, considerable stimulatory activity has been demonstrated with both B and T lymphocytes (von Boehmer, 1974; Harrison, 1973; Fathman *et al.*, 1974). Since the role of the macrophage has not been studied in the murine MLC, it is difficult at this time to reconcile these findings fully.

TABLE VII

Relative Ability of Allogeneic Macrophages and Lymphocytes to Initiate Strain 13 Lymphocyte Proliferation[a]

Strain 2 stimulators			Strain 13 lymphocyte proliferation
Cell type	Number ($\times 10^{-5}$)	B cells (%)	(Δ cpm $\times 10^{-3}$/culture)
Macrophages	0.08	—	6.99 ± 1.32
	0.4	—	46.69 ± 6.02
	0.8	—	69.02 ± 6.53
Lymph node lymphocytes	0.4	30	0.03 ± 0.01
	1.2	30	0.15 ± 0.10
	2.4	30	1.52 ± 0.98

[a] 2.4×10^5 strain 13 lymph node lymphocytes were incubated for 6 days with the indicated number of mitomycin C-treated strain 2 or 13 macrophages or lymphocytes. Tritiated thymidine was added 18 hours prior to cell harvest. Results are expressed as the mean ±SEM of the difference in cpm between syngeneic and allogeneic cultures.

In the guinea pig, these observations can be compared with the cellular mechanisms of T lymphocyte activation by macrophage-bound protein antigen. In both cases, the macrophage appears to have a preferred ability to interact with T lymphocytes and induce lymphocyte DNA synthesis. However, as we have discussed, soluble protein antigens can be presented to T lymphocytes only by histocompatible macrophages; whereas in the MLC it is the *histoincompatible* macrophages that stimulate T lymphocyte proliferation. It is intriguing to speculate that the critical difference between the two processes may lie in the physical characteristics of alloantigen display as contrasted with less accessible macrophage-bound soluble antigen.

C. Aldehyde-Induced Proliferation

Novogrodsky and his co-workers (Novogrodsky and Katchalski, 1972, 1973; Novogrodsky, 1975) have described the efficient induction of T lymphocyte proliferation by treatment with sodium metaperiodate ($NaIO_4$) or neuraminidase and galactose oxidase (NG). The optimal conditions for this activation are such as to suggest that in either case an aldehyde moiety is generated in the same molecule but on different sugar residues (on sialic acid when $NaIO_4$ is used and on galactose when NG is used) (Novogrodsky and Katchalski, 1973).

We have investigated the macrophage requirement for this response and found that (1) extensively macrophage depleted lymphocytes fail to proliferate after $NaIO_4$ or NG treatment, (2) addition of untreated macrophages to treated lymphocytes restores the response, (3) mitomycin C blocked and $NaIO_4$- or NG-treated macrophages are the most efficient inducers of lymphocyte proliferation obtained by this method, (4) mitomycin C blocked and $NaIO_4$- or NG-treated lymphocytes fail to induce proliferation in untreated lymphocytes, and (5) the $NaIO_4$- or NG-treated macrophages do not demonstrate a histocompatibility requirement for lymphocyte activation (Table VIII). These results indicate a macrophage requirement for aldehyde-induced T lymphocyte proliferation and demonstrate that treated macrophages are efficient stimulators of this response (Greineder and Rosenthal, 1975b).

In summary, in all three of the above mechanisms of T lymphocyte activation, macrophages are required and are the most efficient inducers of lymphocyte proliferation (i.e., macrophage–PHA, allogeneic macrophage, macrophage–aldehyde). Additional studies of the morphologic correlations of mitogen- and aldehyde-stimulated lymphocyte proliferation have revealed marked clustering of lymphocytes about aldehyde-modified and PHA-pulsed macrophages during *in vitro* culture.

TABLE VIII

Proliferative Response of Lymphocytes to Oxidized Syngeneic or Allogeneic Macrophages[a]

Macrophage strain	Treatment	Strain 13 lymph node lymphocytes DNA synthesis [^{3}H]TdR incorporation (cpm × 10^{-3})
13	0	0.74 ± 0.05
13	NG	101.42 ± 6.49
13	IO_4	87.46 ± 5.86
2	0	7.46 ± 0.32
2	NG	132.12 ± 6.51
2	IO_4	93.14 ± 0.61

[a] Monolayer purified macrophages and adherence column purified lymph node lymphocytes were treated with mitomycin C (40 μg/ml, 30 minutes at 37°C), washed, and then incubated with (NG) neuraminidase (50 units/ml) + galactose oxidase (0.5 units/ml) for 30 minutes at 37°C or (IO_4) sodium metaperiodate (10^{-3} *M*, 10 minutes at 22°C). 1.2 × 10^5 stimulator cells were incubated with 2.4 × 10^5 untreated lymph node lymphocytes for 3 days. Tritiated thymidine was added 18 hours prior to harvest.

VII. MODEL BUILDING FOR THE CELLULAR AND MOLECULAR EVENTS IN ANTIGEN RECOGNITION BY T LYMPHOCYTES

Recognition of antigen is a cooperative event between the immunospecific T lymphocyte and an antigen-bearing macrophage. Detection of the antigenic signal requires (1) an antigen-specific receptor on the lymphocyte; (2) a functionally defined, genetically determined cellular interaction structure on both macrophage and lymphocyte linked to a serologically detectable component of the major histocompatibility complex; (3) antigen bound to metabolically intact macrophages in a form resistant to proteolytic treatment and located in a cellular site whose display on the macrophage surface is restricted; (4) an auxiliary antigen recognition molecule, presumably an *Ir* gene product, on either or both macrophage and lymphocyte; and (5) a macrophage-associated nonspecific membrane trigger site or secretory product.

For the purposes of this discussion, definitive knowledge of the specific molecular character of the T cell antigen receptor is not required. However the reader should note that the integrity of this model demands that antigen not be presented on the macrophage membrane in an unrestricted fashion. Thus either *H*-linked gene products involved in cellular interaction regulate its presentation or the *Ir* gene product modulates the accessibility of antigen to the lymphocyte receptor. Such modulation could occur by either enzymatic or conformational changes in either the antigen itself or in the antigen presentation process.

Viewed dynamically (Fig. 9), macrophage-associated antigen initiation of T lymphocyte proliferation proceeds via an initial antigen-independent phase of binding of the immune lymphocytes to macrophages. This initial macrophage–lymphocyte interaction is followed by a period of antigen-dependent lymphocyte binding to the macrophage and DNA synthesis if and only if (1) both macrophage and lymphocyte share identity of membrane determinants coded for by *H*-linked loci and (2) the macrophage bears the appropriate antigen for which the lymphocyte has an immunospecific receptor. Thus, antigen-independent binding serves to approximate or focus lymphocytes on the macrophage without conveying immune specificity; a subsequent antigen- and histocompatibility-dependent physical and functional phase of interaction conveys specificity, and an "auxiliary receptor" or *Ir* gene product regulates genetically controlled immune responses.

Support for a model in which the *Ir* gene product is not itself the antigen-specific receptor is found in the studies of Hämmerling and McDevitt (1974), who find equivalent numbers of antigen binding T and B lymphocytes in nonresponder as well as responder mice, and in the studies of Kapp *et al.* (1974) using the terpolymer L-glutamic acid-L-alanine-L-tyrosine in which immunized nonresponder mice develop suppressor rather than helper T cells.

To what extent are these events either sufficient or necessary for signal transduction during the recognition process? The data presented in this chapter lead one to consider the possibility that the macrophage possesses a specialized region of surface membrane or secretes a product that acts as a nonspecific trigger for initiation of T lymphocyte proliferation under a variety of experimental conditions. At least in the guinea pig, initiation of cell proliferation by either soluble antigenic proteins, cell-bound alloantigen, or aldehydes on carbohydrates results morphologically in extended stabilization of the binding of the lymphocyte to the macrophage membrane. Is the induction of lymphocyte proliferation thus the consequence of stabilization of the lymphocyte on the macrophage membrane, although in some ordered relationship? Is this hypothetical nonspecific triggering event, enzymatic, ionic, or electrical? This last possibility must be considered in view of our recent demonstration that the

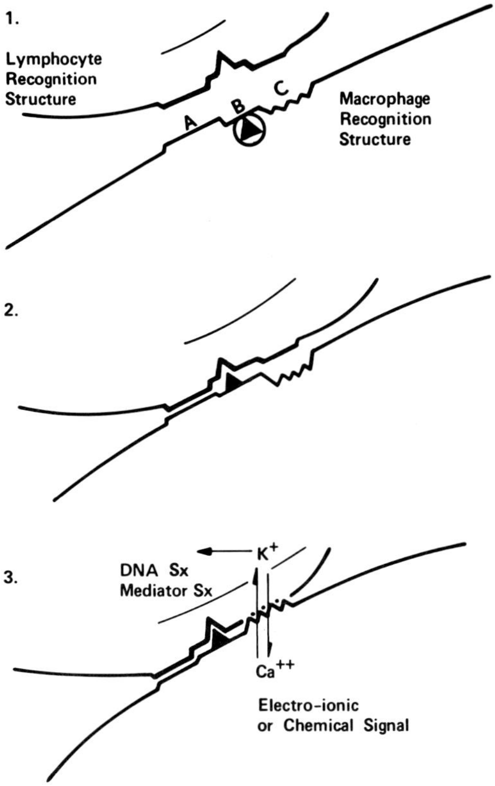

Fig. 9. Schematic diagram of macrophage–lymphocyte interaction in antigen recognition. (A) Site of antigen-independent macrophage–lymphocyte interaction (B) Antigen-dependent, histocompatibility-linked interaction site. (C) Hypothetical trigger site. Step 1: Metabolic-dependent uptake of soluble protein antigens by macrophage into immunologically relevant cell compartment. Step 2: Antigen-independent, reversible macrophage–lymphocyte interaction between allogeneic or syngeneic lymphocytes and macrophages. This step may serve to facilitate alloantigen presentation step in MLC between strain 2 and 13 guinea pigs or aldehyde-modified surface activation of lymphocyte proliferation. Blocked by cytochalasin B. Step 3: Antigen-dependent, "irreversible" macrophage–lymphocyte interaction. This requires the presence of macrophage-bound antigen (solid triangle) and an antigen-specific receptor on the T lymphocyte. Stabilization is blocked specifically by alloantisera against *H*-linked gene products and presumably regulated by an *Ir* gene product. Hypothetical trigger step: Transduction of signal may involve chemical or electrotonic events at cell surface which modify or perturb the lymphocyte surface as does mitogen. In this model antigen serves only to select which clone of lymphocytes is expanded; antigen interaction with receptor need not be the trigger event itself.

macrophage is an electrically active cell exhibiting spontaneous hyperpolarizing currents across its plasma membrane (Gallin *et al.*, 1975).

The basic similarity between this model and that for T cell–B cell collaboration supports the importance of cellular cooperation in a variety of immune phenomenon. The existence of other macrophage-dependent pathways for T lymphocyte antigen recognition which do not require direct physical interaction but instead are mediated by soluble macrophage or lymphocyte products has not been excluded, and indeed seems highly likely to occur.

We consider this model a reasonable alternative recognition system to that in which interaction between antigen and a receptor on the surface membrane is a sufficient antigenic signal. Perhaps its greatest value is that it is subject to direct experimental verification at both a morphological and functional level.

ACKNOWLEDGMENTS

The authors wish to acknowledge Mrs. Kerstin Cehrs for her expert technical assistance during the course of these studies and Drs. R. Schwartz and W. E. Paul for their generous permission to present their data concerning allogeneic restriction in recognition of macrophage-associated antigen by mouse T lymphocytes.

REFERENCES

Alter, B. J., and Bach, F. H. (1970). *Cell. Immunol.* **1,** 207–218.
Benacerraf, B., and Katz, D. H. (1975). *Advan. Cancer Res.* (in press).
Ben-Sasson, S. Z., Shevach, E. M., Green, I., and Paul, W. E. (1974). *J. Exp. Med.* **140,** 383–395.
Bevan, M. J., Epstein, R., and Cohn, M. (1974). *J. Exp. Med.* **139,** 1025–1030.
Calderon, J., and Unanue, E. R. (1974). *J. Immunol.* **112,** 1804–1814.
Chen, C., and Hirsch, J. G. (1972). *J. Exp. Med.* **136,** 604–617.
Cline, M. J., and Swett, V. C. (1968). *J. Exp. Med.* **128,** 1309–1324.
Cohen, B. E., Rosenthal, A. S., and Paul, W. E. (1973). *J. Immunol.* **111,** 820–828.
Cohn, Z. A. (1962). *Nature* (*London*) **196,** 1066–1068.
Davie, J. M., and Paul, W. E. (1974). *Contemp. Top. Immunobiol.* **3,** 171–192.
Ehrenreich, B. A., and Cohn, Z. A. (1967). *J. Exp. Med.* **126,** 941–958.
Ehrenreich, B. A., and Cohn, Z. A. (1968). *J. Cell Biol.* **38,** 244–248.
Ellner, J. J., and Rosenthal, A. S. (1975). *J. Immunol.* **114,** 1563–1568.
Erb, P., and Feldmann, M. (1975). *J. Exp. Med.* **42,** 460–472.
Fathman, C. G., Handwerger, B. S., and Sachs, D. H. (1974). *J. Exp. Med.* **140,** 853–858.
Franzel, R. E. (1962). *Nature* (*London*) **195,** 457–458.
Gallily, R., and Eliahu, H. (1974). *Immunology* **26,** 603–612.
Gallin, E. H., Wiederhold, M. L., Lipsky, P. E., and Rosenthal, A. S. (1975). Submitted for publication.
Greineder, D. K. and Rosenthal, A. S. (1975a). *J. Immunol.* **115,** 932–938.

Greineder, D. K., and Rosenthal, A. S. (1975b). *J. Immunol.* **114,** 1541–1547.
Gordon, S., and Cohn, Z. A. (1974). *Int. Rev. Cytol.* **36,** 171–214.
Hämmerling, G., and McDevitt, H. O. (1974). *J. Immunol.* **112,** 1734–1740.
Harris, G. (1965). *Immunology* **9,** 529–541.
Harrison, M. R. (1973). *J. Immunol.* **111,** 1270–1273.
Hersh, E. M., and Harris, J. E. (1968). *J. Immunol.* **100,** 1184–1194.
Kapp, J. A., Pierce, C. W., and Benacerraf, B. (1974). *J. Exp. Med.* **140,** 172–184.
Katz, D. H , and Benacerraf, B. (1975). *Transplant. Rev.* **22,** 175–195.
Katz, D. H., and Unanue, E. R. (1973). *J. Exp. Med.* **137,** 967–990.
Kölsch, E., and Mitchison, N. A. (1968). *J. Exp. Med.* **128,** 1059–1079.
Lay, W. H., and Nussenzweig, V. (1968). *J. Exp. Med.* **128,** 991–1009.
Levine, B. B., and Benacerraf, B. (1964). *J. Exp. Med.* **120,** 955–965.
Levis, W. R., and Robbins, J. H. (1970). *Exp. Cell Res.* **61,** 153–158.
Lipsky, P. E., and Rosenthal, A. S. (1973). *J. Exp. Med.* **138,** 900–924.
Lipsky, P. E. and Rosenthal, A. S. (1975a). *J. Immunol.* **115,** 440–445.
Lipsky, P. E., and Rosenthal, A. S. (1975b). *J. Exp. Med.* **141,** 138–154.
Lipsky, P. E., Ellner, J. J., and Rosenthal, A. S. (1976). *Proc. Leukocyte Cult. Conf., 10th 1975* (V. Eijsvoegel, ed.) Academic Press, N.Y., in press.
Lohrmann, H. P., Novikovs, L., and Graw, R. G. (1974). *J. Exp. Med.* **139,** 1553–1567.
McFarland, W., Heilman, D. H., and Moorhead, J. F. (1966). *J. Exp. Med.* **124,** 851–858.
Mosier, D. E. (1969). *J. Exp. Med.* **129,** 351–362.
Mosier, D. E., and Pierce, C. W. (1972). *J. Exp. Med.* **136,** 1484–1500.
Novogrodsky, A., and Katchalski, E. (1972). *Proc. Nat. Acad. Sci. U.S.* **69,** 3207–3210.
Novogrodsky, A., and Katchalski, E. (1973). *Proc. Nat. Acad. Sci. U.S.* **70,** 1824–1827.
Novogrodsky, A. (1975). *In* "Immune Recognition" (A. S. Rosenthal, ed.), pp. 43–61. Academic Press, New York.
Oppenheim, J. J., Levinthal, B. G., and Hersh, E. M. (1968). *J. Immunol.* **101,** 262–270.
Pearson, M. N., and Raffel, S. (1971). *J Exp. Med.* **133,** 494–505.
Rabinovitch, M. (1968). *Semin. Hematol.* **5,** 134–155.
Rosenstreich, D. L., and Rosenthal, A. S. (1973). *J. Immunol.* **110,** 934–942.
Rosenstreich, D. L., and Rosenthal, A. S. (1974). *J. Immunol.* **112,** 1085–1093.
Rode, H. N., and Gordon, J. (1974). *Cell. Immunol.* **13,** 87–94.
Rosenthal, A. S., and Shevach, E. M. (1973). *J. Exp. Med.* **138,** 1194–1212.
Rosenthal, A. S., Davie, J. M., Rosenstreich, D. L., and Blake, J. T. (1972). *J. Immunol.* **108,** 279–281.
Ryan, W. L., and Lee, J. W. (1970). *Immunochemistry* **7,** 251–256.
Salvin, S. B., Sell, S., and Nishio, J. (1971). *J. Immunol.* **107,** 655–662.
Schecter, G. P., and McFarland, W. (1970). *J. Immunol.* **105,** 661–669.
Schmidtke, J. R., and Unanue, E. R. (1971). *J. Immunol.* **107,** 331–338.
Schwartz, R., and Paul, W. E. (1975). Submitted for publication.
Seeger, R. C., and Oppenheim, J. J. (1970). *J. Exp. Med.* **132,** 44–65.
Sharp, J. A., and Burwell, R. G. (1960). *Nature (London)* **188,** 474–475.
Shevach, E. M., and Rosenthal, A. S. (1973). *J. Exp. Med.* **138,** 1213–1229.
Shevach, E. M., Lee, L., and Ben-Sasson, S. Z. (1975). *In* "Immune Recognition" (A. S. Rosenthal, ed.). pp. 627–649. Academic Press, New York.
Simon, H. B., and Sheagren, J. N. (1972). *Infec. Immunity* **6,** 101–103.
Steinman, R. M., and Cohn, Z. A. (1972a). *J. Cell Biol.* **55,** 186–204.
Steinman, R. M., and Cohn, Z. A. (1972b). *J. Cell Biol.* **55,** 616–634.

Sulitzeanu, D., Kleinman, R., Benezra, D., and Gery, I. (1971). *Nature (London) New Biol.* **229,** 254–255.
Twomey, J. J., Sharkey, O., Brown, J. A., Laughter, A. H., and Jordan, P. H. (1970). *J. Immunol.* **104,** 845–853.
Uhr, J. W., and Weissman, G. (1965). *J. Immunol.* **94,** 544–550.
Unanue, E. R. (1972). *Advan. Immunol.* **15,** 95–165.
Unanue, E. R., and Askonas, B. A. (1968). *Immunology* **15,** 287–296.
Unanue, E. R., and Cerottini, J. C. (1970). *J. Exp. Med.* **131,** 711–725.
Unanue, E. R., Cerottini, J. C., and Bedford, M. (1969). *Nature (London), New Biol.* **272,** 1193–1195.
von Boehmer, H. (1974). *J. Immunol.* **112,** 70–78.
Waldron, J. A., Horn, R. G., and Rosenthal, A. S. (1973). *J. Immunol.* **111,** 58–64.
Waldron, J. A., Horn, R. G., and Rosenthal, A. S. (1974). *J. Immunol.* **112,** 746–755.
Walker, R. I., and Fowler, I. (1965). *Exp. Cell Res.* **38,** 379–385.
Werdelin, O., Braendstrup, O., and Pedersen, E. (1974). *J. Exp. Med.* **140,** 1245–1259.
Wiener, E., and Bandieri, A. (1974). *Eur. J. Immunol.* **4,** 457–463.

7

The Role of Macrophages in the Activation of T and B Lymphocytes *in Vitro*

David L. Rosenstreich and Joost J. Oppenheim

I. Introduction 162
II. Mechanisms of Action of Macrophages 162
A. "Handling" of Antigens and Mitogens by Macrophages 162
B. Macrophage-Derived Soluble Factors and Synthetic Compounds That Replace Macrophages 163
III. The Role of Macrophages in Antigen-Induced Lymphocyte Proliferative Responses *in Vitro* 167
A. Macrophage Dependence of Antigen-Induced T Lymphocyte Proliferation *in Vitro* 169
B. Macrophage Dependence of B Lymphocytes for Proliferation Induced by Thymus-Dependent Antigens 172
C. Mechanisms of Macrophage Action in Antigen-Induced Proliferation of T and B Lymphocytes 175
IV. The Role of Macrophages in the Response of B and T Lymphocytes to Mitogens *in Vitro* 178
A. Macrophage Independence of B Cell Mitogens and Thymus-Independent Antigens 178
B. Macrophage Dependence of T Cell Mitogens 181
V. The Role of Macrophages in the Activation of Lymphocytes by Allogeneic Cells (MLR) 187
VI. The Role of Macrophages in the Activation of B Lymphocytes by Sheep Erythrocytes 189
VII. The Role of Macrophages in the Induction of Lymphokine Synthesis by B and T Lymphocytes 190
VIII. Summary and Conclusions 194
References 197

I. INTRODUCTION

Unlike bone marrow-derived (B) or thymus-derived (T) lymphocytes, the macrophage does not by itself possess immunological specificity. Nevertheless, it is now known that activation of both B and T cells by most types of stimuli requires the participation of an additional cell, the macrophage. Evidence from a variety of sources suggests that macrophages play a pivotal role in both the initiation and regulation of the immune response *in vivo* as well as *in vitro*.

The ways in which macrophages function to help activate lymphocytes are complex, and are only recently starting to be understood. For the sake of simplicity, however, the nature of macrophage help can be divided into two major categories. First, macrophages "take up" antigens and "present" them to lymphocytes in a stimulatory fashion. The second major mechanism of macrophage help is via the elaboration of soluble substances.

Because of these dual functions, some confusion has arisen as to the nature of macrophage help in the immune response. Thus, if macrophages are required to bind and present antigen, why can they be replaced by a soluble factor or 2-mercaptoethanol (2-ME)? Similarly, if macrophage help merely consists of elaborating soluble factors, why is macrophage antigen binding and direct macrophage–lymphocyte contact necessary?

The answer to these questions clearly lies in the dual nature of macrophage function. Furthermore, the exact type of help furnished by macrophages in any given immune response depends on two factors: (1) the nature of the responding lymphocyte, i.e., T or B and (2) the nature of the activating agent, i.e., antigen or mitogen.

In this chapter, we will analyze lymphocyte activation *in vitro* in terms of the cells involved and the nature of the stimulating agents. In each case we will attempt to describe the nature of the macrophage requirement or lack of it and try to analyze how the known mechanisms of macrophage function explain the observed phenomena.

II. MECHANISMS OF ACTION OF MACROPHAGES

A. "Handling" of Antigens and Mitogens by Macrophages

It is well accepted that one way in which macrophages operate in the immune response is by binding and processing certain antigens and mitogens and subsequently "presenting" them to lymphocytes in such a fashion so as to induce lymphocyte activation. This mode of action appears to require direct contact between the macrophage and lymphocyte, and is certainly the easiest to conceptualize. The topic of macrophage "handling" of antigen is covered in detail elsewhere in this book (see Rosenthal *et al.*, Chapter 6). Nevertheless, there are several points that should be emphasized. First, macrophage–lymphocyte interaction is also necessary for response to nonspecific mitogens as well as for antigens. Some T-cell mitogens such as phytohemagglutinin (PHA) (Rosenthal and Shevach, 1973) and sodium periodate (Biniaminov *et al.*, 1974) can also be presented to lymphocytes by macrophages in a manner analogous to the way in which macrophages present antigens to lymphocytes. Second, the presence of an antigen on or within macrophages does not ensure that lymphocyte activation by that agent is macrophage-dependent. The best example of this phenomenon is the thymus-independent antigen and B cell mitogen, endotoxin (LPS) which is taken up by macrophages (Bona *et al.*, 1973), but, at least *in vitro,* is a macrophage-independent stimulus (see Section IV). Finally, even though a macrophage-dependent activating agent may be taken up by macrophages, the mechanism of action of the macrophage may not depend on presentation at all. The best example of this phenomenon is with lymphocyte activation produced by sheep erythrocytes (SRBC) a thymus-dependent antigen, where macrophages can be replaced by soluble factors even though macrophages also take up this antigen (Mosier, 1969).

B. Macrophage-Derived Soluble Factors and Synthetic Compounds That Replace Macrophages

The second major mechanism of macrophage action in lymphocyte activation is via the elaboration of soluble substances. At present there appears to be a multiplicity of these factors with different names, depending on the assay system in which they were first described. Nevertheless, they all share the property of being able to replace the need for macrophages in lymphocyte cultures, and they can be roughly organized into two groups: (1) macrophage-derived soluble factors that act on the reactive lymphocyte and (2) macrophage-derived soluble factors that act on the antigen. In addition, there are some synthetic compounds that can replace macrophages.

1. Conditioned-Medium Reconstituting Factor (CMRF) and Lymphocyte Activating Factor (LAF)

The first type of soluble factors are those that act on the reactive lymphocyte directly. Bach *et al.* (1970), were the first to note that supernatants from cultured macrophages would at times reconstitute the mixed lymphocyte reaction (MLR) of macrophage-depleted lymphocytes, and they named this factor "conditioned-medium reconstituting factor" (CMRF). More recently, Gery and Waksman (1972) found that a soluble factor derived from cultured macrophages, which they termed "lymphocyte activating factor" (LAF), would greatly enhance the response of mouse thymocytes or macrophage-depleted spleen cells to the T cell mitogens, PHA and concanavalin A (Con A). LAF has also been found to enhance the response of thymocytes to another T cell mitogen, sodium periodate (Novogrodsky and Gery, 1972), and to the antigen, PPD (Havemann and Schmidt, 1973). Thus, this macrophage factor or factors, is operative in the activation of lymphocytes by a variety of different stimuli. Furthermore, it is likely that CMRF and LAF are the same, since their methods of preparation and modes of action are so similar. This, however, remains to be established.

Some work has been done to examine the nature and mode of action of LAF. The release of LAF from macrophages can be increased by a variety of stimuli that generally increase the metabolic activity of macrophages, including PHA, endotoxin, and X-irradiation *in vivo* (but not *in vitro*) (Geiger *et al.*, 1973). It is a low molecular weight (5000–15,000 daltons), heat-labile, nondialyzable compound (Gery and Handschumacher, 1974). To date, efforts to characterize this compound further have been hampered by its relative instability.

Some information about the cell target of LAF can be inferred from the reactions in which it functions. It clearly acts on T lymphocytes, since the MLR (Lohrmann *et al.*, 1974) and the mitogenic response to PHA, Con A (Rosenstreich *et al.*, 1973), and periodate (Thurman *et al.*, 1974) are all T lymphocyte reactions. LAF does not enhance B cell activation by LPS, but the *in vitro* growth and proliferation of a B cell line can be enhanced by macrophage culture supernatants (Namba and Hanaoka, 1972).

The mechanism of action of LAF remains for the present in the realm of speculation. Observations on similar factors (Namba and Hanaoka, 1972) or certain synthetic compounds such as 2-ME (Chen and Hirsch, 1972a;b) suggest that at least one action of LAF is to enhance cell viability in culture. However, it is certainly possible that it possesses other properties as well. It may act during the initial induction of lymphocyte activation, functioning as a "second signal" that is essential for cell activation. Lymphocyte activation may occur in the absence of LAF, but macrophage factors might be required to make this activation an irreversible step or even allow the cell to differentiate.

2. *Sheep Red Blood Cell Solubilization Factor*

A second type of macrophage-derived soluble factor acts on the stimulating antigen rather than on the reactive lymphocyte. This factor has so far been found to function only in the response of B lymphocytes to SRBC. Hoffmann and Dutton (1971) first reported that supernatants of cultured macrophages would restore the PFC response of macrophage-depleted spleen cells. However, it is clear that this factor was functionally different from LAF, since SRBC that were incubated with this factor and then washed free could then themselves activate macrophage-depleted spleen cells in the absence of additional supernatant or macrophages. Similar work by other groups have confirmed these findings, and in addition demonstrated that macrophage supernatant acted by "solubilizing" antigen from SRBC and thereby rendering it directly immunogenic for lymphocytes in the absence of macrophages (Calkins and Golub, 1972; Shortman and Palmer, 1971; Wood and Gaul, 1974). This concept was further substantiated by the work of Feldmann and Palmer (1971), who found that solubilized SRBC prepared by sonication were macrophage- as well as thymus-independent.

The only work that may shed any light on the nature of this macrophage "solubilization factor" has been done by Munder and Madolell (1973), who reported that most common adjuvants (with the notable exception of endotoxin) activated macrophage phospholipase A, which in turn caused the release of lysolecithin into the culture medium. These workers also found that lysolecithin itself was a potent adjuvant *in vivo* and, in addition, could enhance the plaque-forming cell (PFC) response to SRBC *in vitro* (Munder *et al.*, 1970). It is noteworthy that lysolecithin is a highly membrane active substance, and this could possibly account for the "solubilization" of SRBC noted in macrophage supernatants. However, lysolecithin itself has not yet been tested on macrophage-depleted T or B cell populations so that this hypothesis remains unproven.

3. *Synthetic Compounds That Can Replace Macrophages*

It is now known that in addition to macrophage-derived factors, certain synthetic compounds, such as 2-mercaptoethanol (2-ME), can substitute for macrophages in the enhancement of lymphocyte activation *in vitro*. This observation has been of great importance in this area for two reasons. First, these synthetic compounds are easy to obtain and stable, in comparison to macrophage-derived factors. Second, knowledge of the properties of these relatively simple compounds should shed some light on both the nature and mode of action of the macrophage-derived factors. Click *et al.* (1972) reported that the reducing agent 2-mercaptoethanol (2-ME) would enhance the primary *in vitro* mouse spleen cell PFC to SRBC. Chen and Hirsch (1972a,b) extended these observations and showed that the response of macrophage-depleted mouse spleen cell cultures to SRBC could be completely restored by 2-ME. They found that 2-ME had to be present for the entire culture period to restore an optimal response. Furthermore, the addition of small numbers of macrophages along with 2-ME did not increase the response, suggesting that the 2-ME was totally replacing the function of macrophages in these cultures.

Some work has been done on the mechanism of action of 2-ME. It seems to mimic the action of LAF because its primary action is on the reactive lymphocyte rather than the antigen. In the case of SRBC antigens, Chen and Hirsch (1972b) suggest that 2-ME is acting directly on the B lymphocyte by promoting cell viability and enhancing cell reactivity, since they in fact found that 2-ME did enhance the viability of their macrophage-depleted cultures. Furthermore, there is other evidence that 2-ME does promote cell viability, since Broome and Jeng (1973) found that the growth of several lymphoid tumor cell lines was enhanced in the presence of reducing agents such as 2-ME. However, since the response to SRBC requires both T and B lymphocytes, it is not possible to be certain which cell type (or both) 2-ME is acting on. In fact, it is conceivable that the effect of 2-ME on B cells may be mediated indirectly through its action on T cells.

2-Mercaptoethanol has also been found to enhance T cell responses. Thus, Fanger *et al.* (1970) found that 2-ME would enhance the response of human and rabbit peripheral lymphocytes to T cell mitogens. Furthermore, the mouse MLR is also greatly enhanced by 2-ME (Heber-Katz and Click, 1972). However, there is no evidence as yet that 2-ME can replace macrophages completely in these responses. In fact, recent work has shown that 2-ME would not replace the need for macrophages for guinea pig T-cell activation by mitogens (Rosenstreich and Wilton, 1975). Therefore, it is clear that either 2-ME is not an analog for LAF, or alternatively there may be several different macrophage factors necessary for T cell activation, and 2-ME only replaces one of these factors.

Finally, in addition to 2-ME and related sulfhydryl-containing compounds, a natural reducing agent, vitamin E, has recently been shown to be able to replace macrophages in the response of macrophage-depleted spleen cells to SRBC (Campbell *et al.*, 1974). The demonstration that a natural reducing agent, vitamin E, can also replace macrophages, suggests that it is possible that LAF may also be a natural reducing agent and act via a mechanism similar to 2-ME or vitamin E. Presumably, the reduction of cellular sulfhydryl groups may be the common denominator that somehow promotes cell survival and growth.

III. THE ROLE OF MACROPHAGES IN ANTIGEN-INDUCED LYMPHOCYTE PROLIFERATIVE RESPONSES *IN VITRO*

There is considerable evidence that viable intact macrophages directly interact with lymphocytes and thus play an important role in antigen presentation. Historically, the importance of macrophages for lymphocyte activation was first noted when it was found that macrophage-depleted lymphocyte cultures would no longer transform in response to antigens. Oppenheim *et al.* (1966) found that human lymphocytes would not undergo blast transformation when exposed to antigens, such as streptolysin-O, PPD, or vaccinia vaccine after passage over a glass-bead column which removed adherent cells. That this was due to a macrophage deficiency was suggested by the fact that Thorotrast, a compound that is toxic for phagocytic cells, also blocked antigen-induced proliferation. Furthermore, it was later found that autologous adherent monocytes would restore antigen responsiveness to column-passaged lymphocytes (Hersh and Harris, 1968). The macrophage-dependence of antigen-induced proliferation has also been described in several other species, such as rabbit (Harris, 1965; Theis and Thorbecke, 1970), guinea pigs (Seeger and Oppenheim, 1970), and rats (Yoshinaga *et al.*, 1972).

The mechanisms by which macrophages act in this response are only partially understood. It is clear that macrophages bind antigens and preserve them in some protected site in a form that remains immunogenic (Rosenthal *et al.*, Chapter 6). It is equally clear that these macrophages that have bound antigens are able in turn to activate lymphocytes from immune donors. This was first shown by Cline and Swett (1968) in the human and subsequently confirmed in the guinea pig by a number of other workers (Seeger and Oppenheim, 1972; Rosenstreich and Rosenthal, 1973; Waldron *et al.*, 1973).

It is unlikely that the only function of macrophages in antigen-induced lymphocyte proliferation is simply to present antigen to the immune lymphocyte. Nevertheless, on the basis of this known mechanism, it is possible to explain many of the observations related to this phenomenon. First, as would be expected, this response requires direct contact between the lymphocyte and the macrophage. Thus, Hersh and Harris (1968) found that macrophages would not restore responsiveness to depleted lymphocyte cultures when they were separated from the lymphocytes by a Millipore filter. Second, it is known that the macrophage does not possess immune specificity in this response (Levis and Robbins, 1970c) and that normal macrophages (Seeger and Oppenheim, 1970; Rosenstreich and Rosenthal, 1973) and macrophages from tolerant donors (Harris, 1965) function as well as immune macrophages. This is consistent with the finding that macrophages bind antigen through a nonimmune, nonspecific mechanism. However, it is also clear that immune macrophages can bind antigen via specific cytophilic antibody, and under conditions where antigen is limited (low concentrations), immune macrophages will function much better than normal macrophages (Cohen *et al.*, 1973). These workers suggest that *in vivo*, under physiological conditions, antigen concentrations are normally low, and, therefore, macrophage antigen binding via cytophilic antibody is probably more important than nonspecific binding. While this may very well be the case, antigen bound to macrophages *in vitro* in both ways appears to be equally effective in activating lymphocytes.

It has been observed that syngeneic macrophages and lymphocytes interact more effectively than do allogeneic cells, indicating that more than antigen presentation is involved in the interaction. Using inbred guinea pigs and antigens, which were under strict genetic control, Rosenthal and Shevach (1973) found that there had to be histocompatability between macrophages and lymphocytes in order to obtain lymphocyte activation. This observation supports the idea that direct macrophage–lymphocyte contact is required for activation. However, it also suggests that there are more sophisticated requirements for activation beyond a passive presentation of antigen by macrophages so that the lymphocyte must recognize additional determinants on the macrophage surface in addition to antigen. On the other hand, under other experimental conditions using other antigens, this strict requirement for histocompatibility is not always observed. Blaese *et al.* (1972) found that allogeneic macrophages would restore human lymphocyte responsiveness to several antigens although not as well as autologous macrophages. Possible reasons for this apparent discrepancy are that since humans are genetically heterogeneous, allogeneic human cells which are not strictly histocompatible, are not totally histoincompatible, so that lymphocyte–macrophage cooperation is effected via those determinants that are similar. Actually, a similar partial cooperation of lymphocytes and macrophages is also seen in guinea pigs using F_1 hybrids or outbred guinea pigs (Rosenthal and Shevach, 1973). Alternatively, the lack of an absolute histocompatibility requirement for any given antigen may be an indication that antigen presentation may not be the mechanism by which macrophages function for that antigen. This seems to be the case in the

MLR, where allogeneic macrophages can restore the responsiveness of lymphocytes in this response as well as do autologous macrophages (Levis and Robbins, 1970b,c; Alter and Bach, 1970). As will be discussed later, it is clear that macrophages function in the MLR via the elaboration of a soluble factor and not via antigen presentation, therefore making a histocompatibility requirement unnecessary.

There also remain a variety of unanswered questions in regard to the function of macrophages in antigen-induced blastogenesis. One of the most difficult questions to resolve is whether there is an absolute requirement for lymphocyte activation by macrophages or whether there is some degree of direct activation of lymphocytes by antigens. Most workers have found that even highly macrophage-depleted lymphocyte populations will manifest some degree of proliferation in response to higher concentrations of antigen (Waldron *et al.*, 1973). It is theoretically impossible to determine whether this reflects direct lymphocyte activation or merely the effect of a few contaminating macrophages, since no single technique can remove all macrophages and very few macrophages ($<0.1\%$) can produce activation of lymphocytes (Rosenstreich and Rosenthal, 1974). Second, there certainly exist subpopulations of both T and B lymphocytes, and it is therefore possible that some lymphocyte subpopulations vary greatly in the macrophage dependence of their responses (Rosenstreich and Wilton, 1975).

Finally, the exact cell specificity of antigen-induced blastogenesis and the lymphocyte that is the target cell for macrophage action is also not known. Thus, it has not been clear if macrophages help only T cells or B cells or perhaps help both. In the remainder of this section and in later sections we will present experimental data that bears on some of these problems.

A. Macrophage Dependence of Antigen-Induced T Lymphocyte Proliferation *in Vitro*

For many years, antigen-induced proliferation *in vitro* was thought to be purely a T cell function, and, therefore, it was also assumed that the phenomenon of macrophage dependence reflected only T cell requirements for activation. More recently, it has been found that in mixed populations of B and T cells, B lymphocytes would proliferate in response to antigens in the guinea pig (Elfenbein *et al.*, 1973; Oppenheim *et al.*, 1975) and in humans (Geha *et al.*, 1973). In light of this finding, it has been necessary to reevaluate the target cell specificity of the macrophage *in vitro*.

When the macrophage requirements of enriched or purified T cell populations have been studied, it has been found that T lymphocytes are macrophage-dependent for activation by antigens. Thus, Waldron *et al.* (1973) found that column-passaged guinea pig lymph node lymphocytes, which are 80–90% T cells (Rosenthal *et al.*, 1972b), required macrophages to proliferate in response to antigen. Similarly, guinea pig peritoneal exudate lymphocytes (PEL's), which are virtually a pure T lymphocyte population (Rosenthal *et al.*, 1972a), although it is much more difficult to deplete macrophages from this cell population, can also be shown to require macrophages to proliferate in response to antigen (Rosenstreich and Rosenthal, 1974).

More recently, we have developed techniques to obtain macrophage-depleted, purified T lymphocyte populations from peripheral (spleen or lymph node) lymphocyte populations in the guinea pig. Guinea pig T

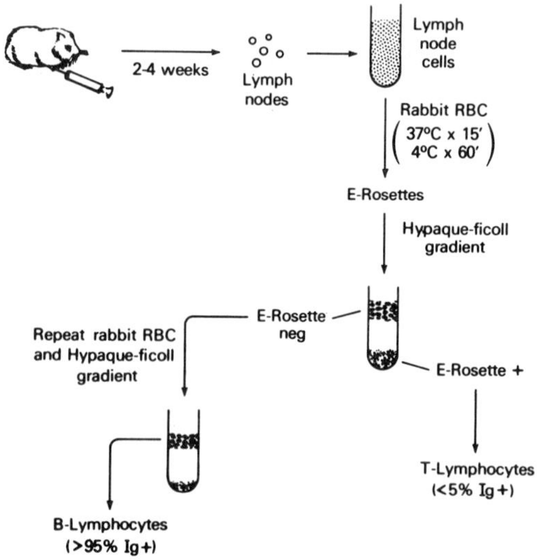

Fig. 1. Technique of preparing purified populations of B and T lymphocytes in the guinea pig by selective depletion of E-rosette + (T) cells. Guinea pigs were immunized with DNP-OA in Freund's complete adjuvant divided between the four footpads (50 μg DNP-OA/guinea pig). 2–4 weeks later the draining lymph nodes or spleen were collected and single cell suspensions prepared. These cells were incubated with prewashed rabbit red blood cells (E) for 15 minutes at room temperature, spun into a pellet, and allowed to stand at 4°C for 60 additional minutes. The cell suspension was gently resuspended and the rosetted cells (T) separated from the nonrosetted cells (B) by centrifugation over a Hypaque-Ficoll gradient (200 *g* for 20 minutes at room temperature). The rosetted cells were used as T lymphocytes. To prepare highly purified B cells, the nonrosetted cells were reincubated with rabbit E and reseparated by gradient centrifugation. The nonrosetted cells from this second purification were used as B cells.

lymphocytes will form spontaneous rosettes with rabbit erythrocytes (RRBC), while B lymphocytes and macrophages will not (Wilson and Coombs, 1973). It is therefore possible to allow a mixed cell population to form rosettes with RRBC, separate the rosetted T lymphocytes from the nonrosetted B lymphocytes and macrophages by differential gradient centrifugation, and obtain a highly purified (>95%) T lymphocyte population. This method is outlined schematically in Fig. 1.

This purified T lymphocyte population was cultured in the presence of various stimuli and lymphocyte proliferation determined by the incorporation of $[^3H]$TdR into new DNA (Table I). The functional purity of this population is demonstrated by the fact that it no longer responds to the B cell mitogen, lipopolysaccharide (LPS), but still responds to the T cell mitogen, phytohemagglutinin (PHA). Furthermore, the response to two antigens, purified protein derivative (PPD) and DNP-ovalbumin (DNP-OA) to which the lymphocyte donors had been immunized, is also very poor. When these T lymphocytes are reconstituted

TABLE I

Effect of Macrophages on the Proliferative Response of Highly Purified T Cells to Antigens and Mitogens

Stimulant	Concentration (μg/ml)	Lymphocyte proliferative response[a] (cpm $[^3H]$TdR incorporated): T	T + macrophage[b]
None		140	384
DNP-OVA	10	567	3,265
PPD	50	195	5,534
LPS	100	476	586
PHA	2	8,139	73,308

[a] Strain 13 guinea pig lymphocytes were cultured for 3 days in RPMI 1640 containing penicillin, streptomycin, L-glutamine, and 5% heat-inactivated fetal calf serum. After 72 hours they were labeled with 0.5 μCi of $[^3H]$TdR (6.0 Ci/mmole) for 4 hours, harvested on an automated cell harvesting apparatus, and counted in a Packard Tri-Carb scintillation counter (for details of method, see Oppenheim *et al.*, 1975). T lymphocytes were prepared by separating E-rosette + cells as outlined in Fig. 1.

[b] Oil-induced peritoneal exudate cells from strain 13 guinea pigs, that received 2500 R irradiation and were added back at a macrophage:lymphocyte ratio of 1:4.

with 20% X-irradiated, syngeneic macrophages, it is clear that there is a marked enhancement in the response to both antigens as well as to the mitogen, PHA. However, the cells still do not respond to LPS. Thus, it is clear that antigen-induced proliferation of these T lymphocytes is absolutely macrophage-dependent but does not require B cells. Furthermore, the marked enhancement of the PHA response suggests that T lymphocyte activation by mitogens may be macrophage-dependent as well. This point will be dealt with in greater detail in Section IV.

B. Macrophage Dependence of B Lymphocytes for Proliferation Induced by Thymus-Dependent Antigens

1. The in Vitro Proliferative Response of Purified B Lymphocytes

We undertook a series of experiments to evaluate the role of macrophages in B lymphocyte activation *in vitro*. The first question we sought to answer was whether macrophages helped purified B lymphocytes respond to antigens or mitogens in a fashion similar to T cells. In order to answer this question we prepared purified B lymphocytes from the draining lymph nodes of guinea pigs immunized to DNP-OA in Freund's complete adjuvant (FCA). The procedure that we followed was a modification of the technique outlined in Fig. 1. By allowing the cells to form rosettes with RRBC and then removing the rosetted cells, it is possible to deplete T lymphocytes and enrich B lymphocytes. When this procedure is repeated twice as in Fig. 1, one obtains a highly enriched (>95%) B lymphocyte population.

These purified B lymphocytes were cultured in the presence of various stimuli, and their proliferative response was again measured by assaying incorporation of [^{3}H]TdR (Table II). In contrast to T cells, these B lymphocytes respond very well to the B cell mitogen LPS, while they do not respond at all to the T cell mitogen, PHA. Thus, they exhibit functional as well as morphological purity. However, their response to antigen is even more interesting. They respond poorly to DNP-OA but respond quite well to PPD.

When these purified B lymphocytes are reconstituted with 20% X-irradiated, syngeneic macrophages, a pattern entirely different from that of T cells is seen. They still do not respond to PHA, confirming their B cell purity, but their response to LPS is decreased rather than increased by the addition of macrophages. Furthermore, unlike T cells, the response of these B cells to the antigen DNP-OA is not enhanced by macrophages and their response to another antigen, PPD, is decreased in a manner similar to LPS.

TABLE II

Effect of Macrophages on the Proliferative Response of Highly Purified B Lymphocytes to Antigens and Mitogens

Stimulant	Concentration (μg/ml)	Lymphocyte proliferative response[a] (cpm [^{3}H]TdR incorporated): B	B + macrophage
None		383	454
DNP-OVA	10	1,012	805
PPD	50	4,343	1,861
LPS	100	10,132	4,124
PHA	2	887	706

[a] For culture details see footnote *a* and *b* of Table I. Guinea pig B lymphocytes were prepared by selective depletion of T lymphocytes (E-rosette + cells) as outlined in Fig. 1.

Based on these and other experiments, it is possible to make several observations. First, B cells will respond to the mitogen LPS directly and in the absence of macrophages. Second, since pure B cells respond to PPD in the absence of T cells, PPD by definition is a thymus-independent mitogen or antigen. B cells appear to respond directly to this thymus-independent stimulant also without the help of macrophages. Third, in the absence of T cells, B cells do not respond to the thymus-dependent antigen, DNP-OVA, either with or without macrophages, thus suggesting that T cell cooperation is required for B cell proliferation *in vitro* as well as for antibody formation. Finally, in contrast to T cells, macrophages appear to depress rather than enhance the response of purified B cells to antigens or mitogens. Thus, it is clear that macrophages do not help B cells in exactly the same fashion that they help T cells.

2. *The Role of Macrophages in the Activation of B Lymphocytes in the Presence of T Cells*

Since T cells are required for B lymphocytes to proliferate in response to thymus-dependent antigens, it was necessary to use a technique that would identify the nature of a dividing cell in a mixed cell population. Since only B and not T lymphocytes possess a receptor for the third component of complement (C3), it is possible to identify B cells by allowing them to form rosettes with sheep erythrocytes coated with antibody and complement (EAC). If a proliferating cell population is labeled with [^{3}H]TdR, allowed to form rosettes with EAC, and then autoradiography of the population performed, it is possible to identify each dividing cell in a population and characterize it as either a B cell (EAC-positive) or a T cell (EAC-negative). This technique was first developed by Elfenbein *et al.* (1973).

Using this technique, we asked the following questions: First, given the presence of T cells, would macrophages also enhance B cell proliferation or did macrophages truly help only T cells? Second, if macrophages did enhance B cell proliferation to antigens, would macrophage-bound antigen also trigger B cells, or was macrophage-bound antigen stimulatory only for T cells while B cells were triggered by non-macrophage-bound soluble antigen?

In order to answer these questions, lymph node cells from guinea pigs sensitized to DNP-OA in Freund's complete adjuvant were obtained, passed over glass bead columns to partially purify them (Rosenstreich and Rosenthal, 1973), and cultured with various stimulants. The percentage of B cells dividing was determined by the technique of simultaneous EAC rosetting and autoradiography (Table III).

Both the antigens, DNP-OA and PPD, and the B cell mitogen, LPS, induced good proliferative responses in these lymph node lymphocytes (LNL). In response to DNP-OA, mostly T lymphocytes proliferated, although the B lymphocyte component was significant (18%) especially in view of the fact that only 28% of the cells in this population were B lymphocytes. In response to PPD, however, there was much more B lymphocyte proliferation (41%). As expected, the proliferative response to the B cell mitogen, LPS was due almost entirely to B lymphocytes (90%) confirming the specificity of this technique.

When 20% syngeneic, X-irradiated macrophages were added, there was an enhanced proliferative response to both antigens. In both cases, a good proportion of the response was by B cells (21–31%), demonstrating that in the presence of T cells, macrophages will help B cells as well as T cells. However, as was seen with the purified B cell population, macrophages completely suppressed the B cell response to the mitogen, LPS.

Finally, when the LNL were stimulated by macrophage-bound antigens, the same picture emerges. There is a good proliferative response to both antigens, and again a significant proportion of both responses is due to B cell proliferation (26%). Therefore, it is clear that macrophage-bound stimuli will trigger B cell proliferation as well as T cell proliferation. As expected, macrophage-bound LPS was nonstimulatory.

Thus, these data demonstrate that in the presence of T cells, macrophages will enhance antigen-induced proliferation of B lymphocytes in

TABLE III

Effect of Macrophages and Macrophage-Bound Stimulants on B and T Cell Proliferation in Vitro

Cells	Stimulants	Lymphocyte proliferative response[b] (Δcpm[^{3}H]TdR incorporated)	Radioautographs[c]: Total B lymphocytes (% EAC-positive)	Radioautographs[c]: Dividing B lymphocytes (% of ^{3}H-labeled cells that were EAC-positive)
Lymph node lymphocytes alone	DNP-OVA[a]	19,300	27.8	17.7
	PPD	18,800	25.8	40.7
	LPS	21,450	39.0	90.0
Lymph node lymphocytes + macrophages	DNP-OVA	24,943	25.0	31.0
	PPD	49,645	19.0	21.0
	LPS	150	20.0	82.0
Lymph node lymphocytes alone	Macrophage-DNP-OVA[d]	48,389	35.1	26.0
	Macrophage-PPD	63,276	28.0	26.0
	Macrophage-LPS	N.S.[e]	—	—

[a] Stimulant concentrations: DNP-OVA, 10 μg/ml; PPD, 50 μg/ml; LPS, 100 μg/ml.

[b] See footnotes *a* and *b* of Table I for details of method. Unstimulated LNL usually incorporated <500 cpm, and the majority of the few labeled cells were T cells.

[c] For details of technique of simultaneous EAC rosetting and autoradiography, see Elfenbein *et al.* (1973).

[d] X-irradiated peritoneal exudate cells were incubated with DNP-OVA, PPD, or LPS all at 100 μg/ml for 1 hour at 37°C, washed four times, and added to lymphocytes at a macrophage:lymphocyte ratio of 1:4.

[e] N.S., not significant.

response to thymus-dependent antigens. Furthermore, they show that stimulation of a mixed cell population with macrophage-bound antigens results in B cell as well as T cell proliferation.

C. Mechanisms of Macrophage Action in Antigen-Induced Proliferation of T and B Lymphocytes

It is clear from some data presented here and from work of many other laboratories, that macrophages help activate T lymphocytes to divide in response to antigen, and that this involves direct presentation of antigen by macrophages to T lymphocytes. It is likely that a soluble factor derived from macrophages, such as lymphocyte activating factor (LAF), is also required. Observations with the antigen, PPD, suggest that LAF is indeed involved (Havemann and Schmidt, 1973). If this is so, then we can predict that triggering of T lymphocytes by antigen requires two distinct signals both of which are derived from macrophages (Fig. 2). The first signal would be the interaction of macrophage-bound antigen with the antigen-specific receptors of the T cell. The second signal would be the interaction of LAF or a related compound with the T cell, which would complete the inductive signal and initiate lymphocyte activation.

Why T lymphocytes require antigen to be presented by macrophages is not known. However, it is very likely that this is related to the nature of the T cell antigen receptor, which is much harder to detect than its B cell counterpart. For many years, T cells were not thought to possess detectable surface antigen receptors (Rosenthal *et al.*, 1972b). However, more recent data demonstrate that T cells do possess receptors capable of binding soluble protein antigens. Thus, Hämmerling and McDevitt (1974) have analyzed the binding of the radiolabeled synthetic antigen (tyrosine, glutamine)-polyalanine-polylysine (TGAL) to mouse cells. They made the following observations: First, T cells did possess antigen-specific receptors but only one-fifth the number of receptors possessed by B cells. Second, they found that T cell antigen binding, in contrast to that of B cells, was temperature-dependent and required active T cell metabolism. Finally, they found that antigen binding by T cells was not blocked by anti-immunoglobulin (in contrast with B cells) but that it could be blocked completely by anti-H_2 antisera and partially by anti-IgM. Findings similar to these have also been reported by Engers and Unanue (1974). T cell antigen receptors are therefore fewer, more

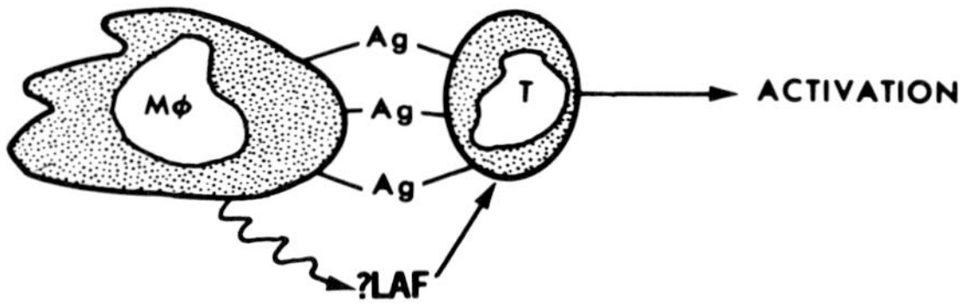

Fig. 2. The mechanism of action of macrophages in the activation of T lymphocytes by soluble protein antigens. Macrophages (Mϕ) bind antigen (Ag) and "present" it to the immune T lymphocyte in a form that is able to stimulate and produce a first "signal" for activation. The necessary second "signal" may be supplied by the soluble factor, LAF.

labile, and possibly consist of a different molecular species than those of B cells. Furthermore, T cells appear to shed their surface receptors spontaneously (Ramseier, **1974**). Therefore, macrophages may be required to enhance the binding of antigens to the less avid T cell receptors, or they may function by stabilizing these receptors and prevent their being shed. Possibly T cells may not even recognize free antigen, but their receptor specificity may be directed toward antigens in combination with some component of the macrophage cell surface. Certainly, the data on the requirement for histocompatibility between macrophages and lymphocytes suggest that the lymphocyte recognizes more than just the antigen that is bound to the macrophage surface.

Since macrophages do not appear to trigger purified B lymphocytes directly, it is even more difficult to understand with any certainty the mechanism of action of macrophages in antigen-induced B lymphocyte proliferation. In those cases where macrophage-bound antigen did trigger B lymphocytes (Table III) it is possible that macrophages were activating only the T lymphocytes, and the T lymphocytes were in turn activating the B lymphocytes in a secondary fashion. However, there are data from other systems that do suggest that B lymphocytes may also be recognizing and responding to macrophage-bound antigen. Katz and Unanue (**1973**), using mice, demonstrated that macrophage-bound protein antigens would induce the formation of antibody-forming cells (PFC) *in vitro*. Since, in this case, the PFC were producing antibody specifically for the antigen that had been bound to the macrophages, it is certain that the B cells must have been triggered by the macrophage-bound antigen directly. If the B cells had been triggered secondarily and nonspecifically by the T cells, then the PFC should have been directed against a variety of other antigens, which they were not. Hamaoka *et al.* (**1971**) found that macrophage-bound antigen would directly activate B cells *in vivo* as well. On the other hand, it is necessary to point out that although macrophage-bound antigen may be able to trigger B cells, it may in fact activate T lymphocytes preferentially. Thus, Seeger and Oppenheim (**1972**) found that macrophage-bound antigen would induce only delayed hypersensitivity and not antibody formation when given *in vivo*. The reasons for this phenomenon are not yet understood (see Oppenheim and Seeger, Chapter 5).

Whether B cells also require the presence of soluble factors from macrophages is not known. The data showing that LAF did not enhance the response of B cells to LPS suggest that they do not (Gery and Waksman, **1972**). However, since LPS does not even require macrophages to activate B cells, the data cannot be so interpreted.

IV. THE ROLE OF MACROPHAGES IN THE RESPONSE OF B AND T LYMPHOCYTES TO MITOGENS *IN VITRO*

It is well accepted that macrophages are involved in the activation of both B and T lymphocytes by antigens. On the other hand, whether or not macrophages are required for lymphocyte activation by mitogens remains controversial. Nevertheless, as we will discuss in Sections IV,A and IV,B, most of the recently available data suggest that T lymphocyte activation induced by mitogens is completely macrophage-dependent, while mitogen-induced B lymphocyte activation appears in most cases to be macrophage-independent.

The essential difference between mitogens and antigens is that mitogens will activate lymphocytes from nonimmune donors, i.e., that have had no previous exposure to the mitogen. This ability to interact directly with receptors on many nonsensitized lymphocytes and produce activation has made mitogens extremely valuable tools in studying the process of immune activation. By studying the mechanisms by which mitogens activate lymphocytes it is possible to delineate the simplest but still essential steps that are necessary for activation. For example, one would assume that a compound such as PHA, which binds avidly to cells, would not require macrophage presentation if the function of macrophages was only to stabilize cell receptors or to enhance binding of stimulants to cell receptors. If on the other hand, PHA-induced activation of T cells also required macrophage presentation as did antigen, this would suggest that the role of direct lymphocyte–macrophage contact might be important in cell activation for reasons other than enhancement of stimulant binding to the cell. Similarly, the fact that B cell mitogens such as LPS require neither macrophage nor T cell help to activate B cells suggests that B lymphocyte triggering may be entirely different from that of T lymphocytes. In Sections IV,A and IV,B we will analyze the macrophage requirements of T or B cell mitogens and try to correlate this with the known properties of the various mitogens and their known mechanisms of activation.

A. Macrophage Independence of B Cell Mitogens and Thymus-Independent Antigens

It is clear from our data (Table II and III) that activation of B lymphocytes in the guinea pig by LPS is macrophage-independent. Not only do additional macrophages suppress the response to LPS, but macrophage-bound LPS is also nonstimulatory, in contrast to stimulation of

B lymphocytes by macrophage-bound antigens (Table III). This phenomenon has been confirmed in other species as well. In the rat, Yoshinaga *et al.* (1972), found that removal of macrophages enhanced reactivity to LPS while readdition of macrophages suppressed the LPS response. The same is true in the mouse. If mouse spleen cells are depleted of macrophages by incubation on a rayon-wool adherence column (Rosenstreich *et al.*, 1971), the response to LPS is doubled, while the response to the T cell mitogens, Con A and PHA, remains the same or decreases slightly (Table IV). As in the rat, addition of small numbers of normal peritoneal cells to mouse spleen cells markedly decreases their response to LPS (Table V).

The unequivocal interpretation of these findings is difficult. It is hard to deplete B cells of macrophages completely, since those techniques usually used to remove macrophages (i.e., surface adherence) also remove B cells. Since in most systems studied, excess macrophages (>5%) seem to suppress the response of B cells to mitogens, it is therefore difficult to rule out the possibility that small numbers of macrophages may in fact be required for B cell activation by mitogens, while large numbers suppress activation.

There are supporting data on the macrophage independence of B cell mitogens derived from studies with thymus-independent antigens rather than mitogens. Since there appears to be a close correlation between these

TABLE IV

Effect of Macrophage Removal on the Response of Mouse Spleen Cells to Endotoxin

Stimulant	Dose (μg/ml)	Lymphocyte proliferative response[a] (E/C): Spleen cells	Lymphocyte proliferative response[a] (E/C): Macrophage-depleted spleen cells[b]
Con A	1	38.5 ± 1.6	37.8 ± 2.0
PHA	2	27.8 ± 0.4	24.4 ± 1.7
E. coli K235 LPS	10	8.7 ± 0.4	17.4 ± 0.3
E. coli 0111:B4 LPS	10	6.9 ± 0.4	16.3 ± 0.5

[a] For details of cell culture, see Rosenstreich *et al.* (1974). Stimulation ratio (E/C) is calculated as the mean cpm[^{3}H]TdR incorporated by stimulated cultures divided by the mean cpm of control cultures ± SEM.

[b] Macrophage depletion was performed by incubation of spleen cells on a rayon-wool adherence column (Rosenstreich *et al.*, 1971).

TABLE V

Suppression of Response of Mouse Spleen Cells to Endotoxin by Normal Peritoneal Macrophages

	Lymphocyte proliferative response[a] (E/C)	
% Added peritoneal cells[b]	+ LPS[c]	% Decrease
0	53.0 ± 2.7	—
0.1	27.8 ± 1.7	47.5
1.0	17.7 ± 2.1	66.6
10	7.4 ± 0.3	86.0

[a] For details of cell culture, see Rosenstreich *et al.* (1974) and footnote *a* Table IV.

[b] Peritoneal cells were obtained by rinsing the peritoneal cavity of C3H/HEN female mice with warm medium.

[c] LPS, *E. coli* 0114:B4 lipopolysaccharide (10 μg/ml).

two properties (Coutinho and Möller, 1973), observations made in one system may apply to the other. The basic observation is that any antigen that is thymus-independent is also macrophage-independent (Feldmann, 1972; Shortman *et al.*, 1970). Thus, using careful techniques to remove macrophages, such as adherence column depletion coupled with anti-macrophage serum, Feldmann (1972) was able to demonstrate that B cell activation by the thymus-independent antigen, polymerized flagellin (POL), was completely macrophage-independent. POL has been found to be a B cell mitogen as well (Coutinho and Möller, 1973). This relationship between thymus independence and macrophage independence has been confirmed with other antigens. Thus, when SRBC which are thymus-dependent are "solubilized" by sonication, they become both T cell- and macrophage-independent (Feldmann and Palmer, 1971). Sonicated SRBC also possess B cell mitogenic activity (Rosenstreich, 1975). Likewise, a hapten–carrier conjugate can be rendered T cell and macrophage independent by coupling the protein to Sepharose beads (Feldmann, 1974).

There are two special cases where this macrophage independence of B cell mitogens does not appear to bear up. First, the response of cells from Peyer's patch of nu/nu mice to endotoxin has been found to require both T cells and macrophages (Kagnoff *et al.*, 1974). However, since endotoxin is thymus-dependent in this somewhat unusual situation, these findings are still consistent with the observation that agents that are thymus-independent are also macrophage-independent. The second case is in the response to the thymus-independent antigen, DNP-D-GL, which is the DNP derivative of a random copolymer of D-glutamic acid and D-lysine. This compound is stimulatory *only* in the presence of macrophages. However, DNP-D-GL is a potent tolerogen when directly exposed to lymphocytes so that this also appears to be a special case (see Mosier, Chapter 2).

What are the shared characteristics of B cell mitogens and thymus-independent antigens that make them macrophage-independent, and what does the nature of these compounds tell us about the activation requirements of B cells by thymus-dependent antigens? As a group, these compounds are all macromolecular, polymeric compounds with multiple repeating epitopes. Therefore, the interaction of a B lymphocyte surface at multiple points with a relatively rigid molecule may be the minimal essential stimulus required to initiate activation of B cells. Feldmann (1972) has speculated that it is the role of the macrophage in B lymphocyte activation by thymus-dependent antigens to convert small or monomeric compounds to a large polymeric form by binding these small molecules to the macrophage surface, thus simulating the physicochemical structure of a B cell mitogen that is stimulatory for B lymphocytes.

It has also been postulated that B lymphocytes require two distinct signals for activation, the binding and cross-linking of surface immunoglobulin receptors by antigenic determinants and some type of activating "second signal" (Watson *et al.*, 1973). Presumably, B cell mitogens possess both of these "signals" within their molecular structure. By analogy, the macrophage may function to convert thymus-dependent antigens to a polymeric form, while the second "signal" may be a T cell-derived soluble factor (TRF). Indeed, Feldmann (1972) suggests that a T cell factor plus antigen on macrophages is necessary for B cell activation.

B. Macrophage Dependence of T Cell Mitogens

Almost all of the available evidence suggests that B cell mitogens can activate B lymphocytes without macrophage help. Presumably, this is because they somehow interact directly with B cells, and their molecular configuration is such that it delivers a strong enough signal to cause activation. Similarly in the case of T cells, it is known that a variety of mitogens bind very tightly to their cell surface. Therefore, one might expect that these agents would be able to activate T cells without macrophage help. Indeed, many authors have observed that macrophage-depleted lymphocytes were fully capable of responding to mitogens (Shortman *et al.*, 1970; Waldron *et al.*, 1973). However, others have found that macrophage-depleted lymphocytes had a reduced but not absent response to PHA, and that this response could be markedly enhanced by readdition of macrophages (Lohrmann *et al.*, 1974). Similarly, Oppenheim *et al.* (1968) observed that responses of purified lymphocytes to two mitogens, staphylococcal filtrate and suboptimal doses of PHA, were significantly lower than those of unpurified lymphocytes.

These inconclusive findings could be attributed to incomplete removal of macrophages because Levis and Robbins (1970a) demonstrated a marked reduction in blastogenesis with all doses of PHA when adherent cells were sequentially removed, first on columns containing nylon, and then by incubation on a large glass surface. They were able to restore the lymphocyte reactions by readdition of either autologous or allogeneic macrophages. Our own observations in the guinea pig also suggest that macrophage-depleted T lymphocytes had a decreased response to PHA that could be restored by macrophages (Table I). For that reason, we decided to further study the macrophage dependence of the PHA response using more highly purified T lymphocytes.

Purified T lymphocytes were prepared as outlined in Fig. 3. Lymph node cells were obtained from previously immunized guinea pigs and partially purified over an adherence column of nylon wool and fine glass beads (Rosenstreich and Rosenthal, 1973). The nonadherent cells from this column, referred to as lymph node lymphocytes (LNL), were then further purified by passage over an adherence column of packed nylon wool (Julius *et al.*, 1973). T lymphocytes were obtained by slow elution off this column. The B cell and macrophage contamination of this population was quantitated through the use of a variety of markers (Table VI). There were only 0.3% macrophages as tested for by the ability to phagocytize latex beads or by the presence of a cytoplasmic esterase, which is also a macrophage marker (Yam *et al.*, 1971). There were less than 2% B cells as determined by the presence of easily detectable surface immunoglobulin or the receptor for C3 which are B cell markers.

These purified T cells were cultured with Con A or PHA and tested for activation using the uptake of [^{3}H]TdR (Table VII). Surprisingly, there was virtually no detectable response in this population to the mitogens, Con A and PHA. When these T cells were reconstituted with 20% syngeneic, X-irradiated macrophages, however, they exhibited a striking response to both mitogens and antigens. These data establish beyond a doubt that mitogen-induced activation of T lymphocytes in the guinea pig is macrophage-dependent.

Since mitogen stimulation was so clearly macrophage-dependent, it was possible that mitogens may have had the same type of macrophage requirements as antigens. That is, that a mitogen bound directly to a T lymphocyte would be nonstimulatory, while mitogen bound to a macro-

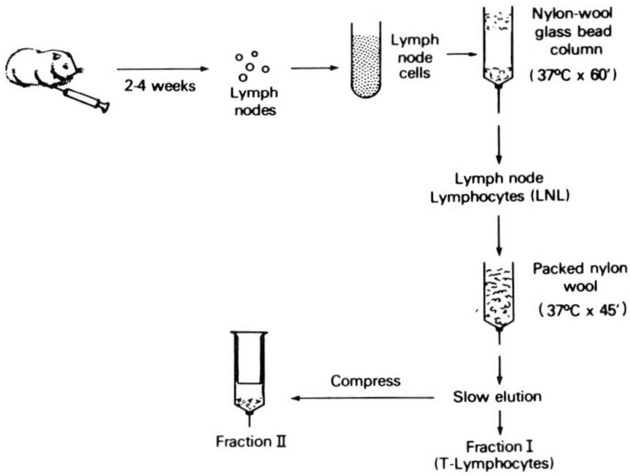

Fig. 3. Preparation of highly macrophage-depleted T lymphocyte populations in the guinea pig by passage over a nylon wool column. Lymph node cells were prepared as in Fig. 1. The cell suspension, in 5 ml of pure fetal calf serum was allowed to incubate for 60 minutes at 37°C on an adherence column of nylon wool and fine glass beads (Rosenstreich and Rosenthal, 1973), and the nonadherent lymph node lymphocytes (LNL) were slowly eluted with warm media with 10% fetal calf serum. LNL (100×10^6 in 1 ml) in media with 10% fetal calf serum were then placed on a column of packed nylon wool (Julius *et al.*, 1973) and incubated at 37°C for 45 minutes. To obtain purified T lymphocytes, the column was washed with 20 ml of warm media with 10% fetal calf serum added dropwise. To obtain the fraction II population, the column was rapidly washed with 50 ml of warm media and fetal calf serum and the effluent discarded. Then 10 ml of warm media + 10% fetal calf serum was added and the nylon wool rapidly compressed with the sterile syringe barrel. This compression was repeated twice, and the eluted enriched B cells pooled, washed, and counted.

phage and then presented to a T lymphocyte would be stimulatory. In order to evaluate this question, either purified T lymphocytes or macrophages were exposed to PHA for 1 hour at 37°C, washed free of unbound PHA, and then cultured (Table VIII).

Macrophage-bound PHA was an effective stimulant for these T lymphocytes, demonstrating that macrophages can bind and present mitogens to T cells just as they do with antigens. As expected, PHA-pulsed T lymphocytes by themselves did not respond. However, when these pulsed lymphocytes were reconstituted with fresh, nonpulsed macrophages, they exhibited a large proliferative response. Thus, in contrast to what is seen with antigens, PHA will directly bind to the surface of a T cell. However, activation still required an additional signal that is contributed by the macrophage.

TABLE VI

Characterization of Nylon Column Passaged Lymph Node Lymphocyte (LNL) Subpopulations[a]

Parameter	% Positive	
	LNL	Nylon fraction I (T)
Viability	>95	>95
Phagocytosis (latex)	<0.1	<0.1
Esterase	0.7	0.3
Surface IG	6.3 ± 0.7	0.25 ± 0.1
C3 receptor	7.3 ± 0.3	1.8 ± 0.3

[a] Guinea pig T lymphocytes prepared as outlined in the text and Fig. 2. Marker studies were performed by the following techniques: phagocytosis of latex beads (Rosenstreich *et al.*, 1971), esterase (Yam *et al.*, 1971), surface IG and C3 (Van Boxel and Rosenstreich, 1974), viability by trypan blue dye exclusion.

The next series of experiments were performed to determine if this signal was mediated via a soluble factor from macrophages or if this phenomenon required lymphocyte–macrophage contact. Nonirradiated guinea pig peritoneal exudate cells were cultured in glass petri dishes and the

TABLE VII

Absolute Macrophage Dependence of T Lymphocytes for Activation by Mitogens

Cell population	No. of experiments	Mean lymphocyte proliferative response (cpm[^{3}H]TdR incorporated per 2 × 10^5 cells)[a]		
		0	Con A	PHA
LNL	4[b]	327 ± 187	5,734 ± 1,317	20,699 ± 6,383
LNL + macrophage	4	294 ± 125	42,841 ± 4,584	69,173 ± 12,177
T lymphocytes (fraction I)	9	70 ± 23	155 ± 32	770 ± 286
T lymphocytes + macrophage[c]	9	104 ± 14	10,835 ± 3,999	35,227 ± 9,287

[a] Guinea pig lymphocytes were cultured using the same conditions as outlined in Table I, using disposable plastic microtrays (Rosenstreich *et al.*, 1974).
[b] Results are the arithmetic means ± SEM of the number of experiments indicated.
[c] 20% syngeneic, X-irradiated oil-induced guinea pig peritoneal exudate cells.

TABLE VIII

Macrophage Dependence of Response When PHA Is Directly Bound to Surface of T Lymphocyte[a]

Cell population	Treatment	Mean lymphocyte proliferative response (cpm[^{3}H]TdR incorporated per 2×10^5 cells)		
		Add back	+ 0	+ PHA
T lymphocytes	None	0	142	1,509
		Macrophage	256	104,624
		Macrophage-PHA	36,251	125,672
T lymphocytes	PHA-pulsed	0	607	630
		Macrophage	32,091	24,563

[a] For details of culture technique and method of PHA exposure see Table I and text.

supernatants collected after 24 hours. The pooled supernatants were dialyzed overnight against two changes of medium to remove any low molecular weight suppressive factors, and then tested for their ability to reconstitute the response of macrophage-depleted T lymphocytes to

TABLE IX

Reconstitution of the Proliferative Response of PHA-Pulsed T Lymphocytes by a Macrophage Soluble Factor (LAF)

Cell population	Mean lymphocyte proliferative response[a] (cpm[^{3}H]TdR incorporated per 2×10^5 cells)		
	Add back	+0	+PHA
T lymphocytes	0	96 ± 14	342 ± 61
	Macrophage	320 ± 13	13,572 ± 938
	LAF	170 ± 35	15,990 ± 156
PHA-pulsed[b] T lymphocytes	0	915 ± 138	928 ± 70
	Macrophage	31,330 ± 1,256	38,177 ± 1,788
	LAF	7,468 ± 787	7,853 ± 660

[a] Guinea pig cells were cultured as outlined in Table I. Results represent the arithmetic means ± SEM.

[b] Lymphocytes were cultured with PHA (10 μg/ml) for 60 minutes at 37°C, then washed 4 times, and cultured. Macrophages are 20% irradiated, syngeneic guinea pig peritoneal exudate cells. Supernatants of cultured, nonstimulated PEC were used as a source of LAF (see text for details).

PHA (Table IX). T lymphocytes by themselves did not respond to PHA. However, when cultured in the presence of the macrophage supernatant (referred to as LAF), they responded well to PHA. This reconstitution was as great as that seen with intact macrophages. PHA-pulsed T lymphocytes again did not proliferate when cultured by themselves. However, when cultured in the presence of the lymphocyte activating factor- (LAF) rich supernatant, they proliferated well without the further addition of PHA.

Thus, these data demonstrate that there are two essential requirements for T lymphocyte activation by mitogens. The first is binding of the mitogen to the T cell surface, and the second is a signal delivered via a soluble factor, LAF, derived from macrophages.

Data obtained by others using another nonlectin T cell mitogen, sodium periodate, support our findings with PHA. Periodate is a T cell mitogen (Thurman *et al.*, 1974) that acts by oxidizing certain surface glycoproteins (Novogrodsky and Katchalski, 1971). One would expect that because this mitogen acts directly on the cell, it would activate T cells without additional cells or factors very much like a B cell mitogen. Nevertheless, it is clear that like antigens and lectin mitogens, periodate stimulation is macrophage-dependent and can be enhanced by LAF (Novogrodsky and Gery, 1972). Furthermore, it is even more interesting to note that periodate-treated macrophages will activate lymphocytes in a manner analogous to macrophages that have bound PHA (Biniaminov *et al.*, 1974). Whether this totally unexpected phenomenon represents oxidation of glycoproteins on the lymphocyte surface by already oxidized macrophage surface components, or some other mechanism, is yet to be explained.

Based on the available data, it is possible to make the following generalizations about the mechanism of T cell activation. First, unlike the phenomenon observed with B cells where certain mitogens by themselves can directly activate the cell, T cells appear to require macrophage help even under conditions where the stimulant binds directly to the cell surface. Second, under conditions where a stimulant does bind to the T cell, macrophage presentation is not necessary, and the only function of the macrophage in this situation is to elaborate a soluble factor that acts as a "second signal." Therefore, there appear to be two ways that T lymphocytes can be activated by PHA, Con A, and probably periodate as well (Fig. 4). The mitogen can interact directly with the lymphocyte producing one signal, while the second signal is delivered via LAF. Alternatively, the mitogen can be presented to the T cell by a macrophage. Presumably, this method of activation also requires a second signal that is produced by LAF, although this has not yet been proved.

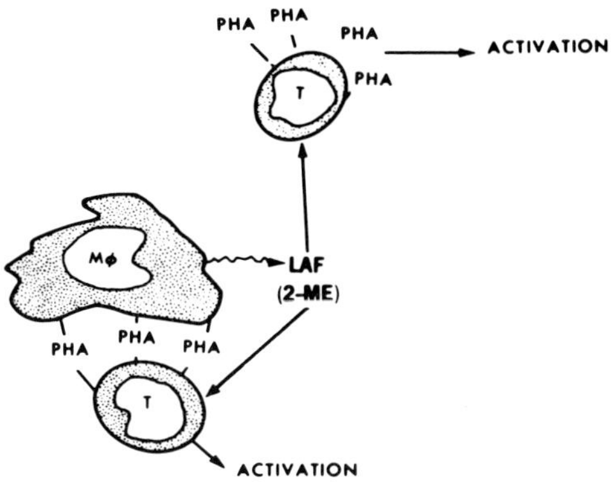

Fig. 4. The mechanism of action of macrophages in the activation of T lymphocytes by soluble protein antigens. There are two pathways by which T lymphocytes are activated by mitogens, both of which require macrophages. The first pathway involves binding of PHA directly to the T lymphocyte. Activation occurs only after the interaction of a macrophage-derived soluble factor or factors (LAF) with the PHA-treated T cell (T). In the second pathway, macrophages (Mϕ) first bind PHA and "present" it to the T cell. This pathway probably also depends on soluble macrophage factors to activate the T cell. 2-Mercaptoethanol (2-ME) can substitute for some macrophage functions in this response, but it clearly cannot totally replace macrophages.

V. THE ROLE OF MACROPHAGES IN THE ACTIVATION OF LYMPHOCYTES BY ALLOGENEIC CELLS (MLR)

The proliferative response of lymphocytes to allogeneic lymphocytes has also been found to be macrophage-dependent (Alter and Bach, 1970). It is interesting to analyze the nature of the macrophage requirement for this response, since it possibly represents a more direct means of T cell activation then do either mitogens or antigens.

T cells are able to bind allogeneic cells directly to their surface (Golstein *et al.,* 1971). Therefore, based on the observations made with mitogens, one would predict that macrophages should not be required for binding and presentation of allogeneic cells, but only as a source of soluble factor. That this is the case was shown by Bach *et al.* (1970) who found that the MLR of macrophage-depleted cultures could be restored with a soluble factor from macrophages (see Section II). 2-Mercaptoethanol (2-ME) has been found to enhance the mixed lymphocyte reaction (MLR) (Heber-Katz and Click, 1972). However, as was previously discussed, 2-ME probably does not completely replace macrophages in this system.

The fact that macrophage presentation is not required in the MLR also helps explain certain other observations. Thus, most workers have found that allogeneic macrophages function as well as autologous macrophages in reconstituting this response (Alter and Bach, 1970; Twomey *et al.*, 1970), which is perfectly understandable in light of the fact that the MLR does not require macrophage–lymphocyte contact. Furthermore, macrophages may play an additional role in the MLR, that of a stimulator cell (Rode and Gordon, 1974). Finally, recent work by Rosenthal and his co-workers (see Chapter 6) suggests that macrophages are the most potent stimulators of the MLR in the guinea pig. Whether this is due to their additional ability to produce LAF or due to an increased amount of the appropriate cell-surface histocompatability antigens is not known. A schematic model illustrating the two signal hypotheses and the role of macrophages in the MLR is shown in Fig. 5. In this case, there is direct binding of the stimulant (allogeneic cells) to the T lymphocyte, which furnishes one signal. The second signal for activation is again delivered via a macrophage-produced soluble factor (LAF). There is no evidence at all that suggests a role for macrophage "presentation" of the stimulator cell in this system.

The fact that T lymphocytes can bind allogeneic cells to their surface and do not require macrophage antigen "presentation" suggests that one function of macrophages may be to convert soluble protein antigens to a cellular configuration that promotes binding. One would predict, therefore, that if antigens were artificially coupled to intact cells, they would no longer require macrophage presentation. There is some evidence that supports this hypothesis.

Lymphocytes from guinea pigs or patients contact-sensitized to dinitrochlorobenzene react *in vitro* to DNP-coated lymphocytes (Baumgarten and Geczy, 1970; Levis *et al.*, 1973). In these experiments viable lymphocytes are required, and autologous cells were more stimulatory than homologous cells, which is very much like the requirements for macro-

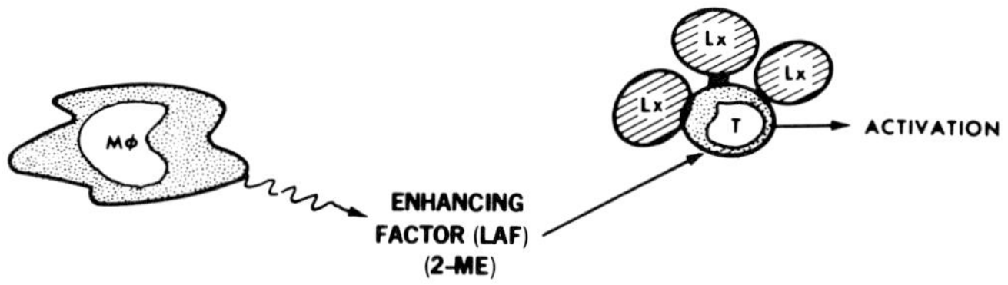

Fig. 5. The mechanism of action of macrophages in the activation of T lymphocytes by allogeneic cells (MLR). The first signal for cell activation is produced by the direct binding of the foreign cell to the T lymphocyte. The macrophage (Mϕ) supplies the "second signal" in the form of a soluble factor (LAF). As with mitogen stimulation of T-cells (T), 2-mercaptoethanol (2-ME) can enhance MLR reactivity but cannot completely replace macrophages on this response.

phage presentation of antigen. Moreover, Spengler *et al.* (1974) found that viable lymphocytes coated with penicilloyl determinants would activate primed human or guinea pig T lymphocytes even after macrophage depletion. W. R. Levis (personal communication) also finds that the addition of LAF enhances the activation of lymphocytes by DNP-coated lymphocytes. These experiments emphasize the important role of cell surface antigen configuration in the activation of T lymphocytes.

VI. THE ROLE OF MACROPHAGES IN THE ACTIVATION OF B LYMPHOCYTES BY SHEEP ERYTHROCYTES

The activation of B lymphocytes to produce antibody against SRBC *in vitro* was one of the first responses noted to be macrophage-dependent (Mosier, 1967). Since that time a great deal of work has been done to evaluate the nature of this macrophage requirement. Surprisingly, some of the data in this particular field have been contradictory. However, it is still possible to construct a general model for B cell activation by SRBC that reconciles most of the published observations. This model suggests that there are two distinct pathways for activation of B cells by sheep erythrocytes (SRBC), both of which involve the macrophage. It seems clear that the macrophage requirement in this response can be replaced completely by 2-ME (Chen and Hirsch, 1972b). Therefore, it is fair to assume that macrophage soluble factors, and not macrophage "presentation" is involved. This response also requires the presence of T cells, which presumably must also be activated. Since we know from other systems (MLR) that T cell activation requires the interaction of the T lymphocyte with the foreign cell plus a second signal derived from macrophages, it is fair to assume that the first stage of this response involves T cell activation by SRBC in combination with 2-ME or LAF. This T cell activation would result in the production of TRF, the soluble T cell factor (Watson, 1973). B cells would then be activated by the interaction of two distinct signals, the binding of SRBC to B cell surface receptors and the action of TRF.

The earliest postulated mechanism of action of macrophages in the antibody response to SRBC was that macrophages actually "presented" the SRBC to the B cell (Mosier, 1967). This hypothesis was based on the observation of macrophage–lymphocyte clusters in culture and the fact that macrophages could bind SRBC and trigger B cells (Mosier, 1969). Furthermore, there was also evidence that integrity of these clusters was essential for B cell activation (Pierce and Benacerraf, 1969). However, whether macrophages actually function to "present" antigens in this response is doubtful. Thus, in addition to the observation that

2-ME can replace macrophage function, Calkins and Golub (1972) found that the primary response to SRBC would occur even if the B cells and macrophages were separated by a Millipore filter. Furthermore, they found that only the SRBC and not the macrophage had to be in contact with B cells.

Finally, the fact that macrophage soluble factors rather than "presentation" are involved in this response is consistent with the observation that allogeneic macrophages reconstitute this response as well as do autologous macrophages (Cosenza and Leserman, 1972). Therefore, it is more likely that the importance of macrophage–lymphocyte contact in this response may be related to the more efficient delivery of macrophage soluble factors to B or T cells engendered by their proximity, rather than to any need for actual antigen presentation.

The second major pathway of B cell activation in contrast with the above involves a soluble factor from macrophages, that "solubilizes" SRBC. As was discussed in Section IV,A, B cell mitogens and thymus-independent antigens can directly activate B lymphocytes without macrophage or T cell help. Most of these agents are macromolecular, polymeric structures. Therefore, one would predict that if an antigen was converted to this form it would also become T cell- and macrophage-independent, which is exactly what seems to occur with SRBC. When SRBC are broken into polymeric fragments ("solubilized") by the process of sonication, they became T cell and macrophage-independent B cell stimulants (Feldmann and Palmer, 1971). Furthermore, it is clear that supernatant factors from macrophages can also "solubilize" SRBC and render them T cell- and macrophage-independent (see Section II,B,2).

Finally, activated T cells also release a macrophage activating factor (MAF) (Wilton *et al.*, 1975), and supernatants of activated T cells will induce enzyme release from macrophages (S. M. Wahl *et al.*, 1975). Therefore, since the response to SRBC is thymus-dependent, it is likely that T cells could be indirectly involved in this second pathway also, by enhancing the solubilization of the SRBC by macrophages even though its end-product appears to be a thymus-independent stimulant. (For an extended discussion of the role of macrophages in T cell–B cell collaboration, see Basten and Mitchell, Chapter 3.)

VII. THE ROLE OF MACROPHAGES IN THE INDUCTION OF LYMPHOKINE SYNTHESIS BY B AND T LYMPHOCYTES

Both of the commonly employed assays that have been used to demonstrate a requirement for macrophages (lymphocyte proliferation and induction of PFC) depend on measurements made relatively long after the initiation of cell culture (48–144 hours) and presumably long after the initiation of lymphocyte activation has occurred. Thus, it is equally plausible that macrophages may not be required for the initiation of lymphocyte activation, but only for the prolongation or amplification of the response. That is, macrophage-bound antigen may merely be a nontolerogenic source of antigen that can produce the continuous restimulation of each new lymphocyte generation that is essential to obtain a measurable proliferative response *in vitro*. Similarly, it is also possible that macrophage soluble factors may also only be required to enhance cell viability or promote cell differentiation.

In order to determine if and how macrophages play a role in the early activation of lymphocytes, it is necessary to be able to measure accurately changes that occur early after the initiation of lymphocyte activation. One such response that is widely used is the elaboration of lymphokines such as macrophage migration inhibition factor (MIF) or monocyte chemotactic factor (MNL-CTX) by activated lymphocytes. Lymphokine synthesis has been detected in significant amounts as soon as 4 hours after activation (Wahl *et al.*, 1974a). Therefore, an analysis of the role of macrophages in lymphokine synthesis should shed some light on whether macrophages are indeed involved in the initiation of lymphocyte activation.

Macrophages are required for the production of two lymphokines by PHA-stimulated human peripheral blood lymphocytes, interferon (see Epstein, Chapter 8) and osteoclast-activating factor (Horton *et al.*, 1974). In the rat, lymphotoxin synthesis induced by antigens is macrophage-dependent (Yoshinaga and Waksman, 1973). In the guinea pig, macrophages are also required for the production of two other lymphokines, MAF and MNL-CTX, induced by antigens (Wahl *et al.*, 1975). Furthermore, this response requires viable macrophages, and macrophage-bound antigens will also trigger lymphokine synthesis. Thus, the macrophage requirements for lymphokine synthesis are very similar to the requirements for lymphocyte proliferation. Moreover, they support the idea that macrophages are involved in the early events of lymphocyte activation rather than just the later events.

Until recently, lymphokine synthesis has been thought of as a specific T cell function. However, recent data from several laboratories demonstrates that when appropriately stimulated, B cells can produce lymphokines that are similar to those produced by T cells. It was observed that lymphoid cell lines bearing surface immunoglobulins and/or complement receptors (i.e., B cell-like) could elaborate various types of mediators including MIF (Pagageorgiou *et al.*, 1972), lymphotoxin (Granger *et al.*,

1970), and osteoclast activation factor (OAF) (Mundy *et al.,* 1974). Later it was noted that human (Epstein *et al.,* 1974) and mouse (Wallen *et al.,* 1973) B lymphocytes were capable of producing interferon. More recently, Yoshida *et al.* (1973) observed that enriched B cell populations produced MIF as well as did T cells, when cultured with either LPS or PPD. Furthermore, Wahl *et al.* (1974b) observed that purified guinea pig B lymphocytes produced MNL-CTX when stimulated with LPS, PPD, EAC, anti-immunoglobulin, or antigen–antibody complexes. Human B lymphocytes are also stimulated to make a number of mediators by the process of rosetting them with EAC (Mackler *et al.,* 1974). Finally, guinea pig B-lymphocytes also produce MAF when stimulated by endotoxin (Wilton *et al.,* 1975). Thus, there is no doubt that B lymphocytes as well as T lymphocytes produce lymphokines.

It was of great interest to determine whether the different macrophage requirements that were found for the proliferation of T or B lymphocytes held for lymphokine synthesis as well. In order to answer this question, purified B or T lymphocyte populations were prepared from the spleens of guinea pigs previously immunized with DNP-OA in CFA, using the method outlined in Fig. 1. The lymphokine measured was MNL-CTX, which was assayed in modified Boyden chambers (Wahl *et al.,* 1974a). When purified T lymphocytes were cultured by themselves, no MNL-CTX was produced in response to DNP-OA or PPD (Fig. 6). The readdition of 10% macrophages produced a great enhancement of MNL-CTX production, while nonviable macrophages (frozen and thawed) had no effect. Thus, the macrophage requirement for antigen activation of T lymphocytes to produce this lymphokine appeared to be very similar to the requirements for cell proliferation. In contrast, when purified B lymphocytes were cultured by themselves, they did produce significant amounts of lymphokine in response to LPS and to PPD (Table X), while they did not produce this lymphokine in response to DNP-OA or the T cell mitogens, Con A and PHA. The readdition of macrophages actually suppressed lymphokine synthesis to all the stimulants. Similarly, macrophage-bound stimulants did not induce lymphokine synthesis except to a limited degree in the case of LPS. The independence of B and dependence of T cell production of lymphokine on the presence of macrophages is analogous to the pattern which is observed with proliferation of purified T and B lymphocytes, suggesting very strongly that similar mechanisms are operating on these two reactions.

All these data taken together suggest very strongly that macrophages are involved in the earliest stages of T lymphocyte activation. Whether similar mechanisms of macrophage action, such as antigen presentation and elaboration of soluble factors, are involved in both early and late activation responses remains to be established.

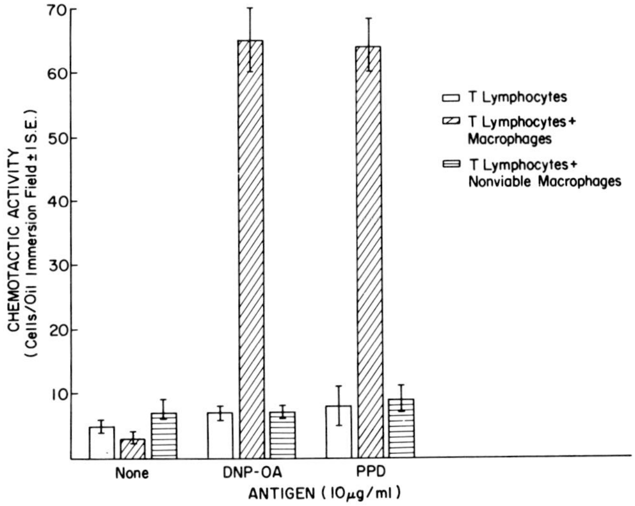

Fig. 6. Chemotactic activity measured in the 48 hour supernatants of 1×10^6 thymus-dependent (T) lymphocytes stimulated with 10 μg/ml DNP-OA or PPD in the presence or absence of 10% viable or frozen and thawed (nonviable) macrophages.

TABLE X

Effect of Macrophages on Monocyte Chemotactic Factor Production by Guinea Pig B Lymphocytes

Stimulant	B cells	Chemotactic activity: B cells + macrophages[b]	B cells + pulsed macrophages[c]
None[a]	6 ± 3	3 ± 1	2 ± 1
DNP-OA	3 ± 1	4 ± 1	3 ± 2
PPD	18 ± 2	6 ± 2	7 ± 2
Con A	6 ± 1	6 ± 2	2 ± 1
PHA	14 ± 3	5 ± 1	6 ± 4
LPS	66 ± 3	54 ± 8	15 ± 2

[a] 1×10^6 isolated B lymphocytes were cultured for 48 hours with no stimulant, 10 μg/ml DNP-OA or PPD, 1 μg/ml Con A or PHA, or 100 μg/ml LPS. The culture supernatants were then assayed for chemotactic activity, which is expressed as the mean number of migrating cells per oil immersion field ±1 SE.

[b] Oil-induced peritoneal exudate cells (macrophages) (1×10^5) were added to the B cells at the beginning of culture with the stimulants.

[c] 1×10^5 macrophages were incubated for 1 hour with 100 μg/ml antigen or mitogen, washed 4 times, and added to the B cell cultures.

VIII. SUMMARY AND CONCLUSIONS

In general, B and T lymphocytes both require two distinct signals for activation. The first involves binding of their surface receptors with stimulant that leads to cross-linkage of receptors. For B cells, the optimal form of stimulant presentation is a polymer with multiple repeating epitopes. For T cell activation by allogeneic cells or soluble protein antigens, the optimal form of stimulant presentation for both appears to be provided by a cell surface configuration. Whether this is just a matter of stimulant concentration or involves the participation of determinants or configurations that are unique to cell surfaces is not known. In contrast, the minimal essential requirement for T cell activation by mitogens involves direct binding to lymphocyte surface receptors without an apparent need for a polymeric or cell surface configuration.

Both B and T cells seem to require a second signal to be activated that is mediated either by soluble factors or by some property of the stimulant itself. The soluble factor for B cells appears to be elaborated by T cells, T cell replacing factor (TRF), while the second signal for the T lymphocyte is mediated by a soluble factor produced by macrophages, lymphocyte activating factor (LAF). Thus, macrophages have two major types of function in the immune response *in vitro*. One is to bind and "present" antigen to the lymphocyte, and the second is to produce soluble factors. The type of macrophage help that is required for any given immune reaction depends on both the nature of the stimulant and the responding cell. The mechanism of action of macrophages in any particular immune response can, therefore, be predicted by analyzing what is necessary to convert a substance to a stimulatory form and to generate the type of second signal that is appropriate for the responding lymphocyte.

In the case of soluble antigens, macrophages supply both of the signals that are necessary for T cell activation. By binding antigen, macrophages produce a cell surface coated with foreign determinants that provides an optimal stimulatory configuration for T cells. In addition, although there is as yet no available evidence on this point, lymphocyte activating factor (LAF) is produced by macrophages and may act as the necessary second signal.

In the mixed lymphocyte reaction (MLR) where the stimulant is an allogeneic cell and, therefore, already in a cell surface configuration that can bind directly to T cells, no macrophage antigen presentation is required. However, macrophages are required to deliver the second signal via LAF. Moreover, allogeneic macrophages themselves can act as potent stimulator cells in the MLR, possibly because they supply both necessary signals in a highly efficient fashion.

There are two separate pathways for T cell activation by the plant lectins, concanavalin A (Con A) and phytohemagglutinin (PHA). These compounds bind avidly to the T lymphocyte. Therefore, as predicted, the only macrophage help that is required for T cell activation by these compounds is supplied by the soluble factor LAF. In addition, although it is not obligatory, macrophages can also "present" these mitogens to the lymphocyte and thus function in a manner analogous to that with soluble protein antigens for which it is obligatory. The nonlectin T cell mitogen, sodium periodate, also acts directly on the lymphocyte by oxidizing surface glycoproteins. Therefore, as with the lectins, it seems that the only macrophage help required for T cell activation by periodate is supplied by LAF. However, just as with the lectins, there is an alternate pathway of activation, and periodate-treated macrophages will activate nontreated T lymphocytes. For all these T cell mitogens, it is not clear whether there are distinct T cell subpopulations that respond via each pathway, or if one pathway *in vitro* is utilized in preference to the other.

The macrophage requirement for B cell activation is more complex and depends on whether or not the stimulants are thymus-dependent or -independent. B cell activation by soluble protein antigens that are generally thymus-dependent requires the interaction of T helper cells and consequently macrophages. In this response, macrophages must first function to produce T cell activation by the mechanisms that have already been discussed. T cell activation in turn, results in the release of the soluble T cell factor, TRF, which acts as one signal for the B cell. How macrophages are acting on the B cell in this response is less clear, but presumably they may function to convert the antigen into the polymeric configuration necessary for activation. Whether soluble factors from macrophages such as LAF, or synthetic analogs, such as 2-ME, also act on B cells, or whether they act only on T cells is not yet known.

On the other hand, many nonprotein antigens and even some, but not all, protein antigens that are thymus-independent activate B cells directly without requiring macrophage or T cell help. To some extent it is possible to reconcile these differences within the framework of the two signal hypothesis of B cell activation.

Thymus-independent antigens and B cell mitogens, which are generally related, are usually macromolecular compounds with multiple repeating epitopes. Therefore, they are already in an appropriate configuration to satisfy the first requirement for B cell activation—cross-linking of multiple receptors. The means by which they supply the second signal is still controversial. Nevertheless, with a few notable exceptions, most available data demonstrate that these compounds will activate B cells directly without the need for T cells or macrophages to supply this second signal.

B cell activation by sheep erythrocytes (SRBC) is also macrophage-dependent, but here macrophages seem to be required only for their soluble factors. There is an alternative pathway of B cell activation by SRBC that is also dependent on a soluble factor released from macrophages. This factor "solubilizes" SRBC and the resulting fragments possess the necessary polymeric configuration to trigger B cells in a manner similar to thymus-independent antigens. If this is an important mechanism in this response, T cells must also be involved, presumably by causing macrophage activation and enhanced release of the "solubilizing" factor.

The macrophage requirements for lymphokine synthesis by both B and T cells appear to parallel those for proliferation. Therefore, it is likely that macrophages play a role in the actual interaction of lymphocyte activation and not merely in the prolongation or enhancement of phenomena that occur later.

While it is now possible to outline roughly the mechanism of action of macrophages in B and T lymphocyte activation by a variety of stimulants, there remain a host of unanswered questions about macrophage function in these systems. For one, it is still not known whether the phenomenon of macrophage "presentation" represents merely the ordering of a stimulant in the polymeric array that is appropriate for lymphocyte activation, or whether the cell surface itself possesses unique properties that are important for triggering of cells. Second, the nature and mode of action of macrophage soluble factors remain unexplained. It is not clear whether there is only one factor or several. It is not known whether the factor(s) acts as a "second signal" that completes the inductive stimulus for lymphocyte activation or whether it also acts at later stages by promoting viability or cell differentiation. Finally, there are no data at all on how such factors work at a subcellular molecular level—do they act via the cyclic nucleotide pathway or through some other mechanism? Related to this last point is the question of whether synthetic compounds, such as 2-ME, are acting in fashions similar to the macrophage factors. Appropriate technology and expertise are now available to answer many of these questions. Research efforts within the next few years should produce a much more precise understanding of the mechanism of action of macrophages.

ACKNOWLEDGMENTS

We would like to thank our technicians Lynda Weedon and Sue Dougherty who performed many of the experiments reported here; Drs. Sharon Wahl, Mark Wilton, and Michael Glode for generously furnishing appropriate data; Mrs. Dorothy Earman for her always excellent secretarial assistance; and our wives for their patience, cooperation, and encouragement in this and many other projects.

REFERENCES

Alter, B. J., and Bach, F. H. (1970). *Cell. Immunol.* **1**, 207–218.

Bach, F. H., Alter, B. J., Solliday, S., Zoschke, D. C., and Janis, M. (1970). *Cell Immunol.* **1**, 219–227.

Baumgarten, A., and Geczy, A. F. (1970). *Immunology* **19**, 205–217.

Biniaminov, M., Ramot, B., and Novogrodsky, A. (1974). *Clin. Exp. Immunol.* **16**, 235–241.

Blaese, R. M., Oppenheim, J. J., Seeger, R. C., and Waldman, T. A. (1972). *Cell. Immunol.* **4**, 228–242.

Bona, C., Robineaux, R., Anteunis, A., Heuclin, C., and Astesano, A. (1973). *Immunology* **24**, 831–840.

Broome, J. D., and Jeng, M W. (1973). *J. Exp. Med.* **138**, 574–592.

Calkins, C. E., and Golub, E. S. (1972). *Cell. Immunol.* **5**, 579–586.

Campbell, P. A., Cooper, H. R., Heinzerling, R. H., and Tengerdy, R. P. (1974). *Proc. Soc. Exp. Biol. Med.* **146**, 465–469.

Chen, C., and Hirsch, J. G. (1972a). *J. Exp. Med.* **136**, 604–617.

Chen, C., and Hirsch, J. G. (1972b). *Science* **176**, 60–61.

Click, R. E., Benck, L., and Alter, B. J. (1972). *Cell. Immunol.* **3**, 264–276.

Cline, M. J., and Swett, V. C. (1968). *J. Exp. Med.* **128**, 1309–1325.

Cohen, B. E., Rosenthal, A. S., and Paul, W. E. (1973). *J. Immunol.* **111**, 820–828.

Cosenza, H., and Leserman, L. D. (1972). *J. Immunol.* **108**, 418–424.

Coutinho, A., and Möller, G. (1973). *Nature (London), New Biol.* **245**, 12–14.

Elfenbein, G. J., Harrison, M. R., and Green, I. (1973). *J. Immunol.* **110**, 1334–1339.

Engers, H. D., and Unanue, E. R. (1974). *J. Immunol.* **112**, 293–304.

Epstein, L. B., Kreth, H. W., and Herzenberg, L. A. (1974). *Cell. Immunol.* **12**, 407–421.

Fanger, M. W., Hart, D. A., Wells, J. V., and Nisonoff, A. (1970). *J. Immunol.* **105**, 1043–1048.

Feldmann, M. (1972). *J. Exp. Med.* **135**, 1049–1058.

Feldmann, M. (1975). *Contemp. Top. Mol. Immunol.* **3**, 57–84.

Feldmann, M., and Palmer, J. (1971). *Immunology* **21**, 685–699.

Geha, R. S., Schneeberger, E., Rosen, F. S., and Merler, E. (1973). *J. Exp. Med.* **138**, 1230–1247.

Geiger, B., Gallily, R., and Gery, I. (1973). *Cell. Immunol.* **7**, 1–9.

Gery, I., and Handschumacher, R. E. (1974). *Cell. Immunol.* **11**, 162–169.

Gery, I., and Waksman, B. H. (1972). *J. Exp. Med.* **136**, 143–155.

Golstein, P., Svedmyr, E. A. J., and Wigzell, H. (1971). *J. Exp. Med.* **134**, 1385–1402.

Granger, G. A., Moore, G. E., White, J. G., Matzinger, P., Sundsous, J. S., Shupe, S., Kolb, W. P., Kramer, J., and Glade, P. R. (1970). *J. Immunol.* **104**, 1476–1485.

Hamaoka, T., Takatsu, K., and Kitagawa, M. (1971). *Immunology* **21**, 259.

Hämmerling, G. J., and McDevitt, H. D. (1974). *J. Immunol.* **112**, 1734–1740.

Harris, G. (1965). *Immunology* **9**, 529–541.

Havemann, K., and Schmidt, W. (1974). *Proc. Leucocyte Cult. Conf., 8th, 1973* pp. 181–185.

Heber-Katz, E., and Click, R. E. (1972). *Cell. Immunol.* **5**, 410–418.

Hersh, E. M., and Harris, J. E. (1968). *J. Immunol.* **100,** 1184–1194.
Hoffmann, M., and Dutton, R. W. (1971). *Science* **172,** 1047–1048.
Horton, J. E., Oppenheim, J. J., Mergenhagen, S. E., and Raisz, L. G. (1974). *J. Immunol.* **113,** 1278–1287.
Julius, M. H., Simpson, E., and Herzenberg, L. A. (1973). *Eur. J. Immunol.* **3,** 645–649.
Kagnoff, M. F., Billings, P., and Cohn, M. (1974). *J. Exp. Med.* **139,** 407–413.
Katz, D. H., and Unanue, E. R. (1973). *J. Exp. Med.* **137,** 967–990.
Levis, W. R., and Robbins, J. H. (1970a). *Transplantation* **9,** 515–518.
Levis, W. R., and Robbins, J. H. (1970b). *Exp. Cell Res.* **61,** 153–158.
Levis, W. R., and Robbins, J. H. (1970c). *J. Immunol.* **104,** 1295–1299.
Levis, W. R., Whalen, J. J., and Miller, A. E. (1973). *Lancet* **2,** 389–390.
Lohrmann, H., Novikovs, L., and Graw, R. G., Jr. (1974). *J. Exp. Med.* **139,** 1553–1567.
Mackler, B. F., Altman, L., Rosenstreich, D. L., and Oppenheim, J. J. (1974). *Nature (London)* **249,** 834–837.
Mosier, D. E. (1967). *Science* **158,** 1573–1575.
Mosier, D. E. (1969). *J. Exp. Med.* **129,** 351–362.
Munakata, N., and Strauss, B. (1972). *Cell. Immunol.* **4,** 243–255.
Munder, P. G., and Madolell, M. (1973). *Int. Arch. Allergy Appl. Immunol.* **45,** 133–135.
Munder, P. G., Madolell, M., Ferber, E., and Fischer, H. (1970). *In* "Mononuclear Phagocytes" (R. van Furth, ed.), Vol. I, pp. 445–460. Blackwell, Oxford.
Mundy, G. R., Luben, R. A., Raisz, L. G., Oppenheim, J. J., and Buell, D. N. (1974). *N. Engl. J. Med.* **290,** 867–871.
Namba, Y., and Hanaoka, M. (1972). *J. Immunol.* **109,** 1193–1200.
Novogrodsky, A., and Gery, I. (1972). *J. Immunol.* **109,** 1278–1281.
Novogrodsky, A., and Katchalski, E. (1971). *FEBS (Fed. Eur. Biochem. Soc.) Lett.* **12,** 297–300.
Oppenheim, J. J., Hersh, E. M., and Block, J. B. (1966). *In* "The Biological Effects of Phytohemagglutinin," pp. 183–189. The Robert Jones and Agnes Hunt Orthopaedic Hospital, Oswestry, England.
Oppenheim, J. J., Leventhal, B. G., and Hersh, E. M. (1968). *J. Immunol.* **101,** 262–270.
Oppenheim, J. J., Elfenbein, G. J., and Rosenstreich, D. L. (1975). *In* "Mononuclear Phagocytes" (R. van Furth, ed.). Blackwell, Oxford.
Papageorgiou, P. S., Henley, W. L., and Glade, P. R. (1972). *J. Immunol.* **108,** 494–504.
Pierce, C. W., and Benacerraf, B. (1969). *Science* **166,** 1002–1004.
Ramseier, H. (1974). *J. Exp. Med.* **140,** 603–618.
Rode, H. N., and Gordon, J. (1974). *Cell. Immunol.* **13,** 87–94.
Rosenstreich, D. L. (1975). In preparation.
Rosenstreich, D. L., and Rosenthal, A. S. (1973). *J. Immunol.* **110,** 934–942.
Rosenstreich, D. L., and Rosenthal, A. S. (1974). *J. Immunol.* **112,** 1085–1093.
Rosenstreich, D. L., and Wilton, J. M. (1975). *In* "Immune Recognition" (A. S. Rosenthal, ed.), pp. 113–132. Academic Press, New York.
Rosenstreich, D. L., Blake, J. T., and Rosenthal, A. S. (1971). *J. Exp. Med.* **134,** 1170–1186.
Rosenstreich, D. L., Nowotny, A., Chused, T., and Mergenhagen, S. E. (1973). *Infec. Immunity* **8,** 406–411.

Rosenstreich, D. L., Asselineau, J., Mergenhagen, S. E., and Nowotny, A. (1974). *J. Exp. Med.* **140,** 1404–1409.
Rosenthal, A. S., and Shevach, E. M. (1973). *J. Exp. Med.* **138,** 1194–1212.
Rosenthal, A. S., Rosenstreich, D. L., Davie, J., and Blake, J. J. (1972a). *Proc. Leucocyte Cult. Conf., 6th, 1972* pp. 433–454.
Rosenthal, A. S., Davie, J. M., Rosenstreich, D. L., and Blake, J. T. (1972b). *J. Immunol.* **108,** 279–281.
Seeger, R. C., and Oppenheim, J. J. (1970). *J. Exp. Med.* **132,** 44–65.
Seeger, R. C., and Oppenheim, J. J. (1972). *J. Immunol.* **109,** 244–254.
Shortman, K., and Palmer, J. (1971). *Cell. Immunol.* **2,** 399–410.
Shortman, K., Diener, E., Russell, P., and Armstrong, W. D. (1970). *J. Exp. Med.* **131,** 461–482.
Spengler, H., deWeck, A. L., and Geczy, A. (1974). *Proc. Leucocyte Cult. Conf., 8th, 1973* pp. 501–507.
Theis, G. A., and Thorbecke, G. J. (1970). *J. Exp. Med.* **131,** 970–980.
Thurman, G. B., Giovanella, B., and Goldstein, A. L. (1974). *J. Immunol.* **113,** 810–812.
Twomey, J. J., Sharkey, O., Jr., Brown, J. A., Laughter, A. H., and Jordon, P. H., Jr. (1970). *J. Immunol.* **104,** 845–853.
Van Boxel, J. A., and Rosenstreich, D. L. (1974). *J. Exp. Med.* **139,** 1002–1012.
Wahl, L. M., Wahl, S. M., Mergenhagen, S. E., and Martin, G. R. (1975). *Science* **187,** 261–263.
Wahl, S. M., Altman, L. C., Oppenheim, J. J., and Mergenhagen, S. E. (1974a). *Int. Arch. Allergy Appl. Immunol.* **46,** 768–784.
Wahl, S. M., Iverson, G. M., and Oppenheim, J. J. (1974b). *J. Exp. Med.* **140,** 1631–1645.
Wahl, S. M., Wilton, J. M., Rosenstreich, D. L., and Oppenheim, J. J. (1975). *J. Immunol.* **114,** 296–301.
Waldron, J. A., Jr., Horn, R. G., and Rosenthal, A. S. (1973). *J. Immunol.* **111,** 58–64.
Wallen, W. C., Dean, H. J., and Lucas, D. O. (1973). *Cell. Immunol.* **6,** 110–122.
Watson, J. (1973). *J. Immunol.* **111,** 1301–1313.
Watson, J., Trenkner, E., and Cohn, M. (1973). *J. Exp. Med.* **138,** 699–714.
Wilson, A. B., and Coombs, R. R. A. (1973). *Int. Arch. Allergy Appl. Immunol.* **44,** 544–552.
Wilton, J. M., Rosenstreich, D. L., and Oppenheim, J. J. (1975). *J. Immunol.* **114,** 388–393.
Wood, D. D., and Gaul, S. L. (1974). *J. Immunol.* **113,** 925–933.
Yam, L. T., Li, C. Y., and Crosby, W. H. (1971). *Amer. J. Clin. Pathol.* **55,** 283–290.
Yoshida, T., Sonozaki, H., and Cohen, S. (1973). *J. Exp. Med.* **138,** 784–797.
Yoshinaga, M., and Waksman, B. H. (1973). *Ann. Immunol. Inst. Pasteur* **124C,** 97–120.
Yoshinaga, M., Yoshinaga, A., and Waksman, B. H. (1972). *J. Exp. Med.* **136,** 956–961.

8

The Ability of Macrophages to Augment *in Vitro* Mitogen- and Antigen-Stimulated Production of Interferon and Other Mediators of Cellular Immunity by Lymphocytes

Lois B. Epstein

I. Introduction 202
II. The Ability of Macrophages to Augment Mitogen-Stimulated Production of Interferon by Lymphocytes 203
A. Experimental Conditions 204
B. Extent of Response 206
C. Evidence That Lymphocytes Are Source of Mitogen Stimulated Interferon and Not Macrophages 207
D. T and B Lymphocyte Origin of Mitogen-Stimulated Interferon 208
E. Studies with Agents That Affect the Mitogen-Stimulated Interferon Response 209
F. Effect of Monocytes versus Effect of Macrophages in the Mitogen-Stimulated Interferon System ... 211
G. Observations as to the Functional Integrity of Patients' Macrophages Judged by Their Ability to Augment Lymphocyte Interferon 212
III. The Ability of Macrophages to Augment Bacterial and Viral Antigen-Stimulated Production of Interferon by Lymphocytes 214
IV. Macrophages and Their Relationship to the Production of Other Mediaters of Cellular Immunity by Lymphocytes 219
A. Migration Inhibitory Factor 220
B. Lymphotoxin 221
C. Monocyte Chemotactic Factor 221
D. Macrophage Activating Factor 223

E. Osteoclast Activating Factor.................. 224
F. General Comments........................... 224
V. Macrophages and Their Role in Affecting the Production of Viral-Induced Interferon by Leukocytes.. 225
Leukocyte Origin of Interferon Induced by Certain Viruses................................ 225
VI. Summary.................................... 229
References.. 231

I. INTRODUCTION

Interferon is an antiviral protein, well known for its role in host defense. It is produced *in vitro* as well as *in vivo* by numerous cell types in response not only to viruses, but to many nonviral agents as well, such as synthetic polynucleotides and bacterial, fungal, and mitogenic plant extracts. Interferon is effective against a wide range of viruses, both *in vivo* and *in vitro*. Ever since its discovery in 1957 (Isaacs and Lindemann, 1957; Isaacs *et al.*, 1957), a vast body of literature on the subject has appeared. Recent excellent reviews include those by Grossberg (1972), Kleinschmidt (1972), and Finter (1973). Although the exact mechanism of induction and mechanism of action of interferon have not been clearly elucidated, the following concepts are generally accepted at the present time. Most interferon inducers act by derepression of the cell genome: they stimulate the formation of new cellular messenger RNA and new cellular proteins. Correspondingly, induction of interferon can be blocked by treatment of the cells to be challenged by an interferon inducer with actinomycin D (Wagner, 1964) or puromycin (Wagner and Huang, 1965).

With regard to mechanism of action of interferon, it is known that interferon exerts no direct effect on viruses, as preincubation of viruses with interferon has no antiviral effect. On the other hand, pretreatment with interferon of cells to be challenged with virus does protect those cells against the virus. The interferon acts to inhibit the translation of viral, and not cellular, messenger RNA, presumably through its ability to stimulate the formation of another antiviral protein within cells. This is supported by the observations that exposure of cells to inhibitors of RNA or protein synthesis prior to their treatment with interferon prevents the expression of interferon's antiviral action.

The purpose of this chapter is to discuss what is known about certain cellular interactions, specifically between macrophages and lymphocytes in the production of interferon and other mediators of cellular immunity. It will become apparent that considerably more is known about the interaction of macrophages and lymphocytes in the production of a type of interferon induced by nonviral agents, such as nonspecific mitogens and specific antigens, than is known about the interaction of these two cell types in the production of interferon induced by viruses.

In 1965 the presence of an interferon-like substance in the supernatants of human leukocyte cultures stimulated with the nonspecific mitogen, phytohemagglutinin (PHA), was described (Wheelock, 1965). The interferon produced in such cultures in response to mitogen had many physical, chemical, and biological properties in common with interferon produced *in vitro* by human leukocytes in response to virus (i.e., sensitivity to trypsin, lack of response to DNase, RNase, or centrifugation at 105,000 *g*, and stability to pH 3–9 and 56°C for 1 hour). However, differences between the two types of interferon were also noted (Wheelock, 1965). Mitogen-stimulated human leukocyte interferon had less stability to a prolonged exposure to extremes of pH (i.e., $\leq$ pH 2 and $\geq$ pH 10 for 24 hours) and to a brief exposure to heat (i.e., 56° or 70°C for 1 hour) than did virus-stimulated human leukocyte interferon.

The precise cell of origin of the mitogen-stimulated interferon was not determined at that time. However, since the lymphocyte was known by then to be affected in many ways by phytohemagglutinin, e.g., with enhanced RNA synthesis (McIntyre and Ebaugh, 1962; Epstein and Stohlman, 1964), new protein synthesis (Epstein, 1966), and DNA synthesis (MacKinney *et al.*, 1962), the inference was that the lymphocyte was also the cell responsible for interferon production in response to the PHA.

Subsequently, interferon was found in supernatant culture fluids of human leukocytes or mouse splenic leukocytes stimulated with other mitogens, such as pokeweed (Friedman and Cooper, 1967; Wallen *et al.*, 1973), concanavalin A (Con A) (Wallen *et al.*, 1973; Stobo *et al.*, 1974), and in some instances with streptolysin O (Friedman and Cooper, 1967).

II. THE ABILITY OF MACROPHAGES TO AUGMENT MITOGEN-STIMULATED PRODUCTION OF INTERFERON BY LYMPHOCYTES

Extensive studies have been performed over the past several years to characterize the optimal conditions for the *in vitro* production of interferon by human leukocytes in response to mitogens, and to define the precise leukocyte cell type or types involved. For these studies techniques for the preparation of pure populations of human lymphocytes and macrophages were developed and employed. Because these techniques have already been described in great detail in the literature (Epstein *et al.*, 1970, 1971a, 1974a,b; Epstein and Cline, 1974; Epstein, 1975), these and other methods employed in our studies will be summarized only briefly below.

A. Experimental Conditions

1. Preparation of Macrophage Monolayers

Macrophage monolayers are prepared by the growth and differentiation of human peripheral blood monocytes on cover slips in Leighton tubes in McCoy's medium enriched with 30% pooled AB plasma. The resulting cultures are 99–100% pure as determined by morphological studies and functional phagocytic studies. Representative cultures can be counted by removal of the macrophages with concentrated EDTA, and each culture can be assessed for extent of differentiation by microscopic criteria.

2. Preparation of Purified Lymphocytes

a. Nylon Fiber Column Technique. Leukocyte-rich plasma diluted with 30% AB serum-enriched McCoy's medium is passed slowly through a nylon fiber column maintained at 37°C by means of a waterjacket. The eluates from such columns contain more than 99% lymphocytes. They are highly enriched for thymus-derived (T) lymphocytes, as only 4–9% of them are bone marrow-derived or B lymphocytes which bear surface immunoglobulin, as determined by immunofluorescence studies.

b. Fluorescence Activated Cell Sorter Technique. The fluorescence activated cell sorter (FACS) sorts and physically separates populations of cells on the basis of their size and fluorescence (Bonner *et al.*, 1972; Hulett *et al.*, 1973; Kreth and Herzenberg, 1974; Epstein *et al.*, 1974a,b). Thus, by virtue of the fact that human B lymphocytes bear detectable quantities of immunoglobulin on their surface and that T lymphocytes do not, the two populations of cells can be separated by the FACS after their treatment with fluoresceinated anti-immunoglobulin reagents. Such reagents will label the B lymphocytes and not the T.

Lymphocytes from nylon fiber column effluents from which the erythrocytes have been removed by NH_4Cl lysis or lymphocytes from Ficoll gradients from which the monocytes have been removed by adsorbtion to glass are then labeled with a fluoresceinated anti-Cohn fraction II, washed, and passed through the FACS. The cells are forced under pressure through a micronozzle into the center of a stream of fluid that is illuminated by two lasers. One, a helium-neon laser, produces a signal that is proportional to the volume of the cell being illuminated, while the other, an argon ion unit, produces a signal by the activation of the fluorescent label on the labeled cells. The cell stream is vibrated to break it into 40,000 droplets per second, and those droplets containing labeled cells of the proper size are given a positive electric charge and deflected into a collection vessel. Those droplets containing no labeled cells are given a negative charge and deflected into another collection vessel. Empty droplets or those containing cells not of the proper size remain uncharged and pass into a center container. Thus, the instrument can be adjusted so that those cells which contain $>10^5$ immunoglobulin molecules, or B lymphocytes, are collected in one container and those containing $<5 \times 10^3$ immunoglobulin molecules per cell, or T lymphocytes, are collected in another. Evidence has been established that the immunoglobulin-bearing cells separated by the instrument were B cells (Kreth and Herzenberg, 1974), as such cells develop into mature plasmacytes with demonstrable intracytoplasmic immunoglobulin after prolonged culture with pokeweed mitogen (PWM). Also, such immunoglobulin-bearing cells are unaffected by anti-human T lymphocyte serum in the presence of complement (Bobrove *et al.*, 1974). By contrast, those cells containing $<5 \times 10^3$ immunoglobulin are killed by the anti-human T lymphocyte serum in the presence of complement (Bobrove *et al.*, 1974), thus confirming their identity as T lymphocytes. The purity of the T cell preparations obtained in this manner is always greater than 99.9% and that of B cells 70–95%, with a mean of 83%.

3. Preparation of Cultures with Mitogens

Cultures are prepared with either macrophages, lymphocytes, or the two cells combined, and mitogens or other stimulating agents are added at the initiation of cultures. Cultures usually contain 0.9×10^6 to 1.0×10^6 lymphocytes and 2×10^4 to 5×10^4 macrophages per milliliter, and duplicate or triplicate cultures are prepared for each concentration of mitogen used. The cultures are maintained at 37°C in CO_2 incubator for the desired length of time.

4. Harvesting the Cultures

One hour prior to termination of the cultures 1 μCi of [^{3}H]thymidine (specific activity 2.1 Ci/mmole) is added and the cultures incubated at 37°C for the final hour. Using sterile technique, the culture supernatants are collected by their passage through a Hoefer multiport filtration apparatus and refrigerated at 4°C for subsequent interferon assay. The cells are collected on glass filter paper circles, washed, and the cold TCA-precipitable material extracted, washed, and rinsed with cold absolute methanol. The filters are then transferred to scintillation vials where the precipitate is dissolved by Nuclear Chicago Solubilizer, combined with a toluene base scintillator, and counted on a Packard Tri-Carb Liquid Scintillator.

5. *Interferon Assay*

Confluent monolayers of human foreskin fibroblasts are exposed at 37°C in a 5% Co_2 atmosphere for 18–24 hours to various dilutions of the supernatant culture fluids to be tested. The supernatants are then removed, the monolayers washed, and exposed to bovine vesicular stomatitis virus for 45 minutes at 37°C. The monolayers are then overlayed with 0.9% agar in Eagle's medium with 5% bovine serum for 48 hours to allow for plaque development and stained with neutral red. Interferon titer is defined as the dilution of sample that in a 4 ml volume results in 50% reduction of viral plaques. Two to six dilutions for each culture supernatant are made for testing along with the controls for the interferon assay, i.e., fibroblast monolayers with virus and no interferon samples to be tested, and fibroblast monolayers with virus and a known interferon standard. This method is adapted from that originally described by Merigan *et al.* (1966).

B. Extent of Response

Using the techniques described above the following was observed (Epstein *et al.*, 1970, 1971a). No interferon was found in cultures containing 96–100% pure macrophages either in the presence or absence of PHA. In cultures containing only lymphocytes, low levels of interferon were detected in the presence, but not in the absence, of PHA. An average fivefold increase in interferon titers occurred when pure lymphocytes were combined with the macrophages in culture with PHA. In the absence of PHA, no interferon was detected in combined lymphocyte–macrophage cultures. The peak response of interferon occurred 3 days after initiation of the PHA-stimulated combined cultures, and for maximum response PHA was required for the duration of the culture, as was intimate contact between the lymphocytes and macrophages. Separation of the two cell types by a Millipore filter did not allow for maximum interferon production, and medium from either unstimulated or PHA-stimulated macrophages or lymphocytes could not substitute for the corresponding cell type. An increase in lymphocyte concentration to 1.8×10^6/ml or an increase in macrophage concentration to 2.1×10^5/ml resulted in an increase in the amount of interferon produced.

The ability to augment interferon production was a property unique to the macrophage, as syngeneic fibroblasts, HeLa cells, or mouse macrophages were ineffective in augmenting PHA-stimulated interferon production. Although all cultures that produced interferon showed a proliferative response to the PHA, no direct correlation was observed between the degree of PHA-induced interferon and the degree of lymphocyte transformation. Physical and chemical characterization of the interferon found in the PHA-stimulated lymphocyte–macrophage cultures paralleled the observations made originally by Wheelock (1965). The interferon was sensitive to trypsin, unaffected by DNase and RNase, and not sedimentable at 100,000 *g* for 1 hour. It had no direct effect on vesicular stomatitis virus (VSV), but considerable activity was lost after exposure of the interferon to pH 2 for 18 hours and exposure to 56°C for 1 hour.

C. Evidence That Lymphocytes Are Source of Mitogen-Stimulated Interferon and Not Macrophages

Several observations pointed to the lymphocyte origin of interferon in PHA-stimulated combined lymphocyte–macrophage cultures (Epstein *et al.*, 1970, 1971a). First, a small amount of interferon was detected in the supernatants of PHA-stimulated pure lymphocyte cultures, but never in PHA-stimulated pure macrophage cultures. Second, repeated freeze thawing of lymphocytes (which resulted in cell death and fragmentation) obliterated the PHA-induced interferon response in combined cultures, whereas repeated freeze-thawing of macrophages did not. Preparations of frozen-thawed macrophages added to PHA-stimulated lymphocytes were still capable of augmenting interferon production, although to a lesser degree than intact cells.

Final proof of the lymphocyte origin of the PHA-induced interferon came from studies in which mouse macrophages were combined with human lymphocytes in the presence of PHA. The supernatants of these cultures were tested for interferon activity on mouse monolayers as well as on the customary human foreskin monolayers against the same challenge virus, VSV. The interferon produced in the combined human lymphocyte–mouse macrophage cultures with PHA was species specific; it had no protective effect on the mouse monolayers, but did have protective effect on the human monolayers, thus attesting to the human lymphocyte origin of the interferon.

Human lymphocytes from sources other than peripheral blood can produce interferon in response to mitogens. Lymphocytes from human tonsil produce interferon in response to PHA (Sugiyama *et al.*, 1972), and discontinuous density gradient centrifugation of such tonsillar lymphocyte preparations indicated that the small lymphocytes of highest density were the cell source of the interferon (Sugiyama *et al.*, 1974).

D. T and B Lymphocyte Origin of Mitogen-Stimulated Interferon

Studies using the fluorescence activated cell sorter (FACS) with which human T and B lymphocytes can be separated, further characterized the human lymphocyte populations capable of producing interferon in response to both PHA and PWM (Epstein *et al.*, 1974a,b; Epstein, 1975). Both human T and B lymphocytes can produce interferon *in vitro* in the presence of macrophages in response to both PHA and PWM. However, the B cell response is delayed as compared with the T cell response. At 3 days after initiation of cultures, only those macrophage-enriched cultures containing T lymphocytes and mitogen had detectable interferon; those with B lymphocytes did not. The lack of response of B cells after 3 days of culture was not a function of the cell concentration in culture or of the presence of fluoresceinated anti-immunoglobulin complexes on the surface of the B lymphocytes. Increasing the concentration of B cells in culture or removing the fluoresceinated complex still did not result in the production of interferon by B lymphocytes at 3 days of culture. Similarly, the addition of varying amounts of T lymphocytes or T cell products to cultures of macrophage-enriched B lymphocytes also did not result in production of interferon by the B lymphocytes. It was not until the mitogen-stimulated B lymphocyte–macrophage cultures were incubated for 5 and 7 days that interferon was detected from the B lymphocytes. The mechanism underlying the delayed response of mitogen-stimulated B lymphocytes is yet to be elucidated.

Both the proliferative and interferon responses of T and B human lymphocytes to PHA and PWM were macrophage-dependent. In every instance addition of macrophages to purified mitogen-stimulated T or B cell preparations resulted in augmentation of the interferon response. In most instances the proliferative response was enhanced also.

Ancillary evidence that human B as well as T lymphocytes can produce interferon was provided by studies on supernatants of bone marrow cultures prepared from patients with multiple myeloma (Epstein and Salmon, 1974). Such cultures contain large numbers of plasma cells, the end stage in the differentiation of B lymphocytes. Interferon was detected in the supernatant culture fluids of 10 of 12 patients with myeloma. The plasma cell origin of the interferon was attested to by the observation that enrichment of the myeloma cells by gradient techniques resulted in increased interferon production, and no interferon was detected in cultures in which there were low or no plasma cells, i.e., in those obtained from the peripheral blood leukocytes of the patients with myeloma or from bone marrow of normal individuals.

The nature of the stimulus for the production of interferon by the malignant plasma cells was not clear. Normal human B lymphocytes, progenitors of plasma cells, never produce interferon when cultured alone or with macrophages for up to 7 days in culture unless stimulated with PHA or PWM. The malignant plasma cells produced the interferon within 24 hours, and without apparent stimulus. Possibly, the production of interferon by the malignant plasma cells may be a concomitance of the malignant state itself, with its attendant proliferation and differentiation of the cells for protein synthesis and secretion.

Additional evidence that cells of the B lymphocyte series have the ability to produce interferon come from the observations that interferon has been detected in long-term cultures of immunoglobulin-secreting lymphoblastoid lines derived from patients with Burkitt's lymphoma (Henle and Henle, 1965) and infectious mononucleosis (Kasel *et al.*, 1968; McCombs and Benyesh-Melnick, 1967).

Thus, there is evidence in the human that both T and B lymphocytes have the ability to produce interferon. In studies on the mouse, Wallen *et al.* (1973) demonstrated that the interferon production which occurred after stimulating mouse splenic lymphocytes with PHA, Con A, and purified protein derivative of tuberculin (PPD) could be eliminated by treatment of the cells with complement and anti-θ serum, but that the interferon production that occurred after stimulation with PWM could not. Those studies suggested that in the mouse, T cells produce interferon in response to PHA, Con A, and PPD, but B cells produce interferon only in response to PWM. In other studies on the mouse, Stobo *et al.* (1974) confirmed the T cell origin of PHA-induced interferon. Treatment of mixed B and T splenic lymphocyte populations with anti-θ antibody and complement to kill the T cells ablated the PHA-induced interferon response, whereas treatment with anti-κ chain serum and complement to kill the B cells had no effect. They also demonstrated that peripheralized T cells were required for PHA-induced interferon, since cultures of immunologically immature thymus cells and somewhat more mature cortisone-resistant thymus cells failed to produce interferon in response to PHA. In contrast with the human system, in the mouse system, peak interferon production occurred at 24 hours, some 24 hours before the time of peak proliferative response.

E. Studies with Agents That Affect the Mitogen-Stimulated Interferon Response

Several agents that increase cellular cyclic AMP (cAMP) content or mimic the action of the endogenous nucleotide also inhibit the production of interferon by human lymphocytes (Epstein and Bourne, 1975). When

Dibutyrl cAMP (10^{-3} *M*), prostaglandin E, (10^{-5} *M*), or cholera toxin (30 ng/ml) are added to combined lymphocyte–macrophage cultures 10 minutes prior to PHA, marked reduction in the amount of interferon produced is noted. Cell viability was not affected by any of the agents tested. The cyclic AMP content of the lymphocytes so treated with one of these agents—the cholera toxin—increased approximately threefold. Despite the fact that the cholera toxin also caused a threefold rise in cyclic AMP in the human foreskin fibroblasts used in the assay of interferon, it did not interfere with the progress of the assay, as it had no effect on the ability of the challenge virus to cause plaque formation in the fibroblasts.

The inhibition of PHA-stimulated interferon production observed with these cyclic AMP-active agents could have resulted either from a direct effect on the ability of the lymphocytes to produce interferon, or on the ability of macrophages to augment lymphocyte interferon production. The unique pharmacological feature of one of these agents, i.e., cholera toxin, permitted the analysis of this situation.

The toxin produces a delayed increase in cyclic AMP content with a lag period of 30 minutes. Removal of the toxin from the extracellular medium at 10 minutes (by washing or by addition of specific anti-toxin antibody) fails to abrogate the toxin's subsequent effects on cyclic AMP levels. In contrast, antitoxin added to cells before the toxin completely prevents the toxin's effects. Consequently, when macrophages are exposed to the toxin for 10 minutes, followed by sequential addition of anti-toxin, lymphocytes, and PHA, the toxin had no significant inhibitory effect on interferon production. In contrast, when the toxin was added to lymphocytes for 10 minutes, followed by sequential addition of anti-toxin, macrophages, and PHA, the toxin did inhibit interferon production. These experiments thus indicated that the toxin prevented PHA-induced interferon production by an action on lymphocytes, rather than macrophages.

There is suggestive evidence that in the mouse, the population of lymphocytes which proliferates in response to mitogens might be separate from that which produces interferon (Wallen *et al.*, 1973). When mouse spleen cells were separated by albumin discontinuous density gradient centrifugation, the fraction of cells producing interferon were found to belong to a different population of cells than those undergoing a proliferative response. These results might also be explained by the fact that sufficient macrophages were present to augment lymphocyte interferon production in only some of the fractions tested, and not in others.

In the human, irradiation of lymphocytes (at 1000, 2000, or 5000 rads) prior to their combination in culture with macrophages and PHA or PWM will prevent $>90\%$ of the DNA synthesis or proliferative response usually seen after 3 days of culture. In contrast, interferon production is not affected (L. B. Epstein, unpublished). In these same cultures RNA synthesis is markedly depressed, but protein synthesis proportionally is less depressed. This suggests one of two possibilities. The first of these is that the proliferative response per se is not a requisite for the production of interferon by lymphocytes or its augmentation by macrophages, and that the proliferative response is just more radiosensitive than the interferon response. The second possible interpretation is that a separate population of lymphocytes proliferates in response to mitogens than produces interferon. This question is still unresolved for the human situation, but hopefully studies using density gradient separation of human lymphocyte populations, with careful monitoring of the number of macrophages present, should allow a satisfactory resolution of the problem.

F. Effect of Monocytes versus Effect of Macrophages in the Mitogen-Stimulated Interferon System

To employ the standard lymphocyte–macrophage culture system described by Epstein *et al.* (1970, 1971a) two donations of blood, 1 week apart, are required. The first is used to prepare the macrophage monolayers (from the growth and differentiation of peripheral blood monocytes), and the second is used to prepare the purified lymphocytes. From 30–150 ml of blood are required on each occasion, and frequently, especially when studying donors in the pediatric population, such a double donation schedule is not feasible. Therefore in attempts to shortcut the double donation procedure, attempts have been made to study mitogen stimulated interferon in Ficoll gradient preparations of lymphocytes and monocytes obtained from only one donation of blood. But although this technique allows for only one donation of blood, certain problems have arisen with the technique that give some insight as to monocyte versus macrophage effects in the mitogen-stimulated interferon system (L. B. Epstein, unpublished).

First of all, interferon production is never observed in combined lymphocyte—macrophage cultures from which mitogens have been omitted. In contrast, low levels of interferon are routinely observed in cultures prepared from the lymphocyte—monocyte layer of Ficoll gradients, in the absence of mitogenic stimulation. One possible interpretation of this phenomenon is that the Ficoll gradients are perturbing the cellular membranes of one or both cell types to induce interferon on a nonspecific basis. Associated with this nonspecific production of interferon in the lymphocyte—monocyte cultures is an antagonist to interferon. This manifests itself in the interferon assay where, for example, human foreskin fibroblast monolayers exposed to a $\frac{1}{3}$, $\frac{1}{10}$, or $\frac{1}{30}$ dilution of the lymphocyte—monocyte culture supernatant will show no reduction, or even a slight increase in the number of virus-induced plaques, whereas when the monolayers are exposed to a $\frac{1}{100}$ or greater dilution of supernatant the number of plaques will be greatly reduced. This suggests that the interferon antagonist is diluted out, and by the $\frac{1}{100}$ dilution allows expression of the interferon present.

Such an interferon antagonist is never seen in either mitogen-stimulated or unstimulated lymphocyte macrophage cultures, however. Monocytes were proved to be the source of such an antagonist in the following manner. Purified monocytes were obtained from the lymphocyte–monocyte layer of Ficoll gradients and allowed to adhere to glass cover slips in Leighton tubes in the presence of 30% AB positive human serum in McCoy's medium. They were then combined with nylon fiber column separated lymphocytes and stimulated with PHA. The interferon produced in these cultures was compared with that produced in Ficoll gradient isolated, fluorescence activated cell sorter separated, purified T or B lymphocyte-mature macrophage cultures stimulated with PHA. The antagonist to interferon appeared only in those cultures that contained the Ficoll gradient separated monocytes, and not in those which contained Ficoll gradient separated lymphocytes.

Therefore, either monocytes as they differentiate to macrophages lose their ability to produce an interferon antagonist or there is something unusual about a Ficoll gradient treated monocyte which allows for the production of an interferon antagonist. The former possibility is supported by the observation by numerous investigators that cultures of unstimulated leukocytes obtained from buffy coats often show this same antagonist effect in the concentrated culture supernatants and then show some interferon in the diluted supernatants. This, therefore, suggests that some leukocyte cell type, presumeably the monocyte, even when not exposed to Ficoll, can produce this antagonist.

In view of the complexities of the Ficoll gradient lymphocyte–monocyte culture technique with its attendant spontaneous nonspecific production of interferon and the production of an antagonist to interferon, the lymphocyte–macrophage culture system seems infinitely more practicable for the study of patients, despite its requirement for two samples of blood. And, in fact, this is the technique employed in the clinical studies to be described below.

G. Observations as to the Functional Integrity of Patients' Macrophages Judged by Their Ability to Augment Lymphocyte Interferon

In studies with the fluorescence activated cell sorter (Epstein *et al.*, 1974a,b), it was demonstrated that the interferon detected in combined lymphocyte–macrophage cultures stimulated with either PHA or PWM at 3 days was produced exclusively by the human T lymphocytes. Thus, measurement of mitogen-stimulated interferon after 3 days can be used as an effective new tool to monitor the effector competence of human T lymphocyte populations in various disease states.

Consequently, 11 patients with immunodeficiency diseases along with another group of 10 normal donors were studied in this manner (Epstein and Ammann, 1974). The competence of T cell effector function was evaluated by measuring the amount of interferon in supernatants of macrophage-enriched, nylon fiber column purified T lymphocyte cultures after 3 days of stimulation with PHA and PWM. Normal *in vitro* T cell interferon production was found in one patient with congenital sex-linked hypogammaglobulinemia, 3 with acquired hypogammaglobulinemia, and 2 patients who had received successful thymus transplants—one of whom had a pretransplant diagnosis of thymic hypoplasia, and the other, severe, sex-linked combined immunodeficiency. A depressed T cell interferon response was observed in 3 of 4 patients with selective IgA deficiency and in another patient with selective IgA deficiency and underlying thymic hypoplasia who had shown no clinical response to a thymus transplant. The marked depression in PHA- and PWM-stimulated T lymphocyte interferon production in these patients with selective IgA deficiency was of considerable interest. Presumably, such a depressed response could occur either because of a defect in T lymphocyte productive capacity, a dilution of T lymphocytes with abundant numbers of B lymphocytes (analogous to that which occurs in chronic lymphocytic leukemia), or because of some abnormality in the ability of the patients' macrophages to augment mitogen-stimulated interferon production. The latter of two possibilities seem very unlikely, as marked increases in the proportion of circulating B cells have never been reported in these patients, and microscopic examination of their macrophages revealed them to be well differentiated and abundant.

In subsequent studies (Epstein and Ammann, 1975), a macrophage defect in these patients was ruled out. PHA-stimulated allogeneic combinations of patients' macrophages with normal lymphocytes or normal macrophages with patients' lymphocytes indicated that the patients' macrophages functioned well to augment normal lymphocyte interferon production, but that even normal macrophages could not repair the inability of the patients' T lymphocytes to produce interferon.

A T cell defect has long been suspected in patients with selective IgA deficiency because of the association of IgA deficiency with thymic abnormalities in other disease states, such as ataxia telangiectasia (Peterson *et al.*, 1966). However, heretofore, T cell competence in patients with selective IgA deficiency could be assessed only by the proliferative response of T cells to mitogens, and in this study and those of others (Nell *et al.*, 1972; Hobbs, 1968) this was within normal limits. Thus the finding of a T cell defect in these patients may help in some way to explain the repeated occurrence of upper respiratory infections in some of these patients.

Similar studies were performed on patients with chronic lymphocytic leukemia (Epstein and Cline, 1974). In these studies however, PHA- and PWM-stimulated proliferative and interferon responses were examined not only after 3 days of culture (a measure of T cell response) but also after 6 days (a measure of both T and B cell responses). This was possible because (as compared with normal blood) the blood of patients with chronic lymphocytic leukemia contains a higher proportion of cells with surface immunoglobulin (B cells). Consequently, the nylon fiber column effluent obtained from the patients' blood contained a higher proportion of B cells (22–40%) than that obtained from normals (4–9%).

T cell function as measured by T cell interferon production and proliferative response to PHA and PWM was markedly depressed in all 5 patients studied; B cell function was impaired in 3 of these, as compared with 14 normal donors studied at the same time. At this time the possibility that the depressed T cell response observed with the patients' lymphocytes resulted from an inhibitory effect of the contaminating leukemic B cells cannot be ruled out. However, it has been shown previously that the presence of normal B cells does not inhibit T cell interferon or proliferative response (Epstein *et al.*, 1974a,b), and until procedures become available for the separation of leukemic from normal B cells, this question cannot be resolved.

It is unlikely that a defect in the ability of the patients' macrophages to augment lymphocyte interferon production was responsible for the depressed interferon response, as macrophages from the patients were shown to augment the PHA- and PWM-stimulated production of interferon by normal lymphocytes. On the other hand, normal macrophages could not correct either the T or B cell lymphocyte depressed interferon response, and so the defect appears to be intrinsic to the lymphocyte population.

III. THE ABILITY OF MACROPHAGES TO AUGMENT BACTERIAL AND VIRAL ANTIGEN-STIMULATED PRODUCTION OF INTERFERON BY LYMPHOCYTES

Green *et al.* (1969, 1970) demonstrated that cultures of leukocytes from individuals with positive skin test responses to purified protein derivative (PPD) or recent immunization with tetanus toxoid or diptheria toxoid would respond to those respective antigens with lymphocyte proliferation and the production of interferon. This was the first demonstration that immune-specific induction of interferon could occur *in vitro* in human cells, and in response to nonviral antigens. The exact cell source of the antigen-induced interferon was not determined in those studies, but because of the associated proliferative response of immune lymphocytes in the antigen-stimulated cultures, the lymphocyte was the prime suspect. Subsequently, Milstone and Waksman (1970) demonstrated that tuberculin-sensitized mouse peritoneal cells exposed to PPD *in vitro* release an interferon-like substance and that the release or production of such material required the interaction of sensitized lymphocytes with peritoneal exudate macrophages from either immune or nonimmune animals. In contrast with the human situation, the mouse interferon was produced much earlier, i.e., within the first 24 hours of culture. In another experimental system, mouse lymphocytes immunized *in vivo* to L cells responded to the L cells *in vitro* with the production of interferon, also within the first 24 hours of culture, but macrophages were not required (Borecky *et al.*, 1971). The earlier production of interferon by mouse cells was not just a property of the murine system, but was probably due to other factors in the experimental design of those studies, the antigen employed, or the immune status of the animals. In another mouse system, i.e., when mouse lymphocytes are challenged with allogeneic lymphocytes in a mixed lymphocyte cell culture system, interferon is produced, but considerably later, at 72 to 96 hours after initiation of the cultures and at the time of peak proliferative response (Gifford *et al.*, 1971).

That human lymphocytes were the source of *in vitro* antigen-stimulated interferon and that such lymphocyte interferon production was augmented by macrophages was demonstrated by Epstein *et al.* (1971b, 1972a). Nylon column purified lymphocytes from the peripheral blood of normal donors with positive skin test to the bacterial antigen, PPD, produced small amounts of interferon *in vitro* after challenge with the antigen. The addition of macrophages to such PPD stimulated cultures resulted in a greater than threefold increase in the production of interferon by the lymphocytes. Maximum interferon levels occurred at 7–8 days after the initiation of the cultures, and usually 1–2 days after the peak proliferative response of the sensitized lymphocytes to PPD. Thus, with human lymphocytes, antigen-stimulated interferon peaks later in culture than mitogen-stimulated interferon, as does the proliferative response as well. Also, less interferon is produced and less lymphocyte proliferative response is observed in antigen-stimulated cultures than in mitogen-stimulated cultures.

No interferon was produced, even in the presence of macrophages and PPD, however, if the lymphocytes were obtained from donors whose response to intradermal PPD was negative, thus indirectly demonstrating the immune-specific basis of antigen-stimulated interferon production by sensitized lymphocytes. The ability to augment antigen-stimulated lymphocyte interferon was specific for macrophages: autochthonous polymorphonuclear leukocytes were ineffective in substituting for the macrophages.

In addition to reacting to bacterial antigens with the production of interferon, sensitized human lymphocytes can also produce interferon *in vitro* if challenged with viral antigens in the presence of macrophages (Epstein *et al.*, 1972b; Merigan *et al.*, 1973). Using a heat-killed vaccinia virus as antigen, Epstein *et al.* (1972b) demonstrated that lymphocytes from donors vaccinated with vaccinia virus 2–30 years previously responded to the viral antigen *in vitro* by proliferating in the presence of macrophages. However, no interferon was detected in the *in vitro* test system unless the same donors were reimmunized with live vaccinia virus and their lymphocytes studied 4–7 weeks later. No increase in the already significant degree of lymphocyte proliferation after recent reimmunization was noted, suggesting that a separate population of lymphocytes proliferated from that which produced interferon. The presence of macrophages augmented the production of interferon by the lymphocytes of recently immunized donors, but no correlation was observed between the amount of interferon produced and the extent of lymphocyte transformation at the time of peak response of each parameter of *in vitro* cellular immunity.

In the cultures prepared from recently reimmunized donors, peak interferon production always occurred at least 2 days after peak lymphocyte transformation. Here again, the interferon was produced on an immune-specific basis, as donors who had never been vaccinated showed no *in vitro* lymphocyte transformation or interferon response to the vaccinia antigen.

The macrophage dependence of the production of interferon by sensitized human lymphocytes in response to viral antigens was confirmed by Rasmussen *et al.* (1974) and Valle *et al.* (1975). Using the same lymphocyte macrophage culture system as employed in the studies by Epstein *et al.* (1972b) but with heat-inactivated herpesvirus hominis (herpes simplex) as viral antigen, they studied *in vitro* lymphocyte transformation and interferon production by adults during and after infection with herpes simplex. Although lymphocyte transformation and serum antibody levels were constant throughout a 12-week period after active disease in the donors, many of them demonstrated a selective increase in *in vitro* lymphocyte interferon production 2–6 weeks after active disease, and macrophages were required for optimum interferon production in response to the viral antigen.

T lymphocytes were demonstrated to be the source of the interferon. Elimination of the T lymphocytes by treatment with an anti-T cell serum plus complement diminished the amount of interferon produced. Also by using the macrophages of one donor in combination with the lymphocytes of another, Valle *et al.* (1975) were able to demonstrate that the amount of interferon produced in response to the herpes simplex antigen was a function of the immune status of the lymphocyte donor and not that of the macrophage donor. Thus, the memory for the immune-specific production of interferon in response to the particular viral antigen was carried by T lymphocytes and not by macrophages.

Not only herpes simplex viral antigen preparations, but also herpes simplex virus–antibody complexes are capable of stimulating immune lymphocytes to undergo proliferation and to produce interferon (Hooks *et al.*, 1975). Thus antibody-neutralized virus, which presumably has certain viral antigen sites masked, can still induce sensitized lymphocytes to produce interferon.

In contrast to the observations with herpes simplex, stimulation of human macrophage–lymphocyte cultures obtained from adult donors after an attack of herpes zoster with antigens of varicella-zoster virus (V-Z) resulted in no detectable interferon production (Jordan and Merigan, 1974). Although no interferon was detected, lymphocyte transformation from the same donors did occur in lymphocyte–macrophage cultures in response to the V-Z antigen preparation, but it was unrelated to the activity of the disease state. Interferon was observed in response to this viral antigen, but only if cultures were prepared from the lymphocyte–monocyte layer of a Ficoll gradient. But interestingly enough, such interferon was not produced on an immune-specific basis, i.e., it was observed with lymphocytes from both immune adult and nonimmune seronegative childhood donors. Thus in that situation, the production of interferon was related to the method of preparation of the lymphocytes, but not to immune status, and was probably induced by nonantigenic products of the V-Z virus-infected cells used in the preparation of viral antigen. The authors suggested that the negative interferon responses observed in the lymphocyte–macrophage culture system may have been due to technical factors, such as the low titer of the V-Z antigen preparation or to blocking substances in the AB human serum that was employed in the preparation of the cultures.

Thus, a considerable body of knowledge has accumulated on the macrophage-dependent *in vitro* production of interferon by lymphocytes in response to mitogens and bacterial and viral antigens. Such *in vitro* studies have proved of value in understanding the cellular interactions in the production of mitogen- and antigen-induced interferon, but they also are of considerable relevance as a model for studying events that are known to occur *in vivo* as well. For example, L. B. Epstein and T. C. Merigan (unpublished, 1968) observed low levels of interferon in the serum of mice for several days after the intravenous injection of PHA. The kinetics of response roughly paralleled the transformation of lymphocytes noted in the lymph nodes of these animals (Epstein and Smith, 1968).

Antigen- as well as mitogen-induced interferon can occur *in vivo* and on an immune-specific basis. Mice infected with *Mycobacterium tuberculosis,* strain BCG, produced interferon that reached a peak 6 hours after intravenous challenge with tuberculin (Stinebring and Absher, 1970). Subsequent studies (Youngner and Salvin, 1973; Salvin *et al.*, 1973, 1974, 1975) have confirmed and extended the earlier observations. Not only interferon was found in the serum of mice infected with *Mycobacterium tuberculosis* strain BCG and challenged with old tuberculin (OT) or living BCG cells but also migration inhibitory factor (MIF) as well. The intravenous route of sensitization was associated with maximum production of mediators, and both protein and certain lipid components of the BCG are necessary for sensitization. The interferon and MIF were produced on an immune-specific basis, as uninfected animals challenged for the first time with large doses of OT or living BCG did not produce either mediator of cellular immunity. The interferon produced on an immune-specific basis in this *in vivo* system was found to have physical and chemical properties similar to that described previously for *in vitro* mitogen- and antigen-induced interferon, which distinguish it from Newcastle disease virus- (NDV) induced interferon produced either *in vivo* or *in vitro.* The immune-specific interferon was labile to pH 2 and heating at 56°C. Youngner and Salvin (1973) named this type of interferon Type II, and the interferon induced *in vivo* in BCG infected or control mice by either bacterial lipopolysaccharide (LPS) or NDV, Type I interferon. Type I interferon was considerably more stable to pH 2 and to heating at 56°C and was neutralized by antibodies prepared against highly purified L cell interferon induced by NDV. In contrast, Type II interferon was not affected by high concentrations of antibody raised to the NDV-induced interferon, implying a difference in antigen determinants in the Type II and Type I interferon molecules. However, at present it is not known what significance the difference in heat and pH sensitivity between mitogen- *or* antigen-induced interferon and viral-induced interferon means, either in terms of molecular structure or range of antiviral activity. It is hoped that future purification and biochemical characterization of Type I and Type II interferons will clarify these issues.

The question also remains as to the significance in host defense of interferon produced as a mediator of cellular immunity, especially in situations where nonviral antigens are involved as the inducers. The answer probably lies in the fact that Type II interferon probably has many effects on cell proliferation and immune response other than its antiviral properties, as has been so thoroughly documented for Type I interferon. For example, preparations of viral- or polynucleotide-induced interferon have been shown to inhibit the growth of hematopoietic colonies (McNeill and Fleming, 1971; McNeill and Gresser, 1973), normal and malignant cells *in vitro* (Lindahl-Magnusson *et al.*, 1971; Fontaine-Brouty-Boye *et al.*, 1969; Gresser *et al.*, 1970a), and tumor cells *in vivo* (Gresser *et al.*, 1969, 1970b; Gresser and Bourali, 1969, 1970). Such interferon also has effects on the immune response and specific functions of macrophages and lymphocytes. It inhibits the proliferation of mouse lymphocytes in response to PHA and allogeneic cells (Lindahl-Magnusson *et al.*, 1972) or human lymphocytes in response to PHA, Con A, PPD, and allogeneic cells (Blomgren *et al.*, 1974); enhances cytotoxicity by sensitized lymphocytes (Lindahl *et al.*, 1972); and enhances phagocytosis by macrophages (Huang *et al.*, 1971). In addition, it suppresses antibody-producing spleen cells in mice (Chester *et al.*, 1973; Brodeur and Merigan, 1974) and enhances the expression of surface antigens on murine leukemia cells (Lindahl *et al.*, 1973).

However, until Type II interferon can be purified and separated from the other mediators of cellular immunity induced by and found in supernatants of mitogen- and antigen-stimulated lymphocyte–macrophage cultures or purified from the serum of sensitized, antigen-challenged animals, similar studies to those described above for Type I interferon cannot be performed as yet.

IV. MACROPHAGES AND THEIR RELATIONSHIP TO THE PRODUCTION OF OTHER MEDIATORS OF CELLULAR IMMUNITY BY LYMPHOCYTES

Interferon is only one of a group of substances known as "mediators of cellular immunity," all of which have been detected *in vitro* in supernatant culture fluids of lymphocytes that have been activated by mitogens or antigens. These mediators of cellular immunity are also called lymphokines (Dumonde *et al.*, 1969) or lymphocyte activation products (LAP) (Kelly *et al.*, 1972) and they have been recently reviewed thoroughly (Lawrence and Landy, 1969; Bloom and Glade, 1971; Bloom, 1971; David, 1972; World Health Organization, 1973). Well known among such mediators are migration inhibitory factor (MIF) (David,

1972), lymphotoxin (LT) (Granger and Williams, 1971); chemotactic (CTX) factors for monocytes, granulocytes, eosinophils, and lymphocytes (Ward *et al.*, 1970); macrophage activating factor (MAF) (Hammond and Dvorak, 1972); mitogenic factor (MF) (Dumonde *et al.*, 1969); skin reactive factor (SRF) (Dumonde *et al.*, 1969); osteoclast activating factor (OAF) (Horton *et al.*, 1972); and proliferation inhibitory factor (PIF) (Cooperband and Green, 1971).

The assays for each of these factors have been described in detail (Bloom and Glade, 1971), and recent advances in studies to determine their cellular origin and biological significance have been summarized (Greaves *et al.*, 1973). The *in vitro* effects of these substances presumably reflect their role *in vivo*. Intracutaneous injection of supernatants from activated lymphocytes can produce delayed cutaneous reactivity (Bennett and Bloom, 1968), and intralymphatic injection of lymphokines can produce germinal center hyperplasia of the draining lymph node (Kelly and Wolstencroft, 1974). Mediators of cellular immunity have been detected *in vivo* in the serum of sensitized animals (Salvin *et al.*, 1973) and in the efferent lymphatic drainage of antigen- or mitogen-stimulated lymph nodes (Hay *et al.*, 1973; Hay, 1973).

There has been considerable discussion in the literature as to whether these mediators represent separate, distinct substances or whether several of these factors are, in fact, identical but have multiple functions, depending on the nature of the assay. It is important to note that although interferon is found in some of the same mitogen- and antigen-stimulated culture supernatants as these other factors, it has always been distinguished from them by its molecular weight of 18,000 and its property of general species-specificity. In addition, for the human, *in vitro* mitogen- and antigen-stimulated interferon occurs much later in cultures than do most of the other mediators.

Table I summarizes the results of numerous studies in which attempts were made to determine if the production of various mediators by lymphocytes in response to mitogen or antigen is macrophage-dependent, as it is with interferon.

A. Migration Inhibitory Factor

Migration inhibitory factor (MIF) activity is measured by its ability to inhibit the migration of normal macrophages from capillary tubes. When highly purified preparations of guinea pig lymphocytes [obtained by the passage over glass bead columns of lymph node cells from animals previously immunized with bovine γ-globulin (BGG)] are challenged *in vitro* with BGG, no MIF is produced (Nelson and Leu, 1975). However, when such purified lymphocyte preparations are enriched by as little as 5% additional peritoneal exudate macrophage cells obtained either from BGG immune or nonimmune guinea pigs, BGG-stimulated MIF production by the lymphocytes is restored. Thus, a macrophage–lymphocyte interaction in the antigen-induced production of MIF by lymphocytes has been demonstrated. How the macrophage serves to augment lymphocyte MIF production in this system has not yet been elucidated, however. The production of the mediator occurs early in culture prior to the peak lymphocyte transformation response to antigen, thus implicating a role for the macrophage early in the activation of the lymphocyte.

B. Lymphotoxin

Yoshinaga and Waksman (1973) demonstrated that the production of lymphotoxin (LT) by glass bead purified rat lymph node lymphocytes in response to PHA and ovalbumin was macrophage-dependent. Furthermore, they demonstrated that in that system, supernatants from activated macrophages could replace intact macrophages in their ability to reconstitute the production of lymphotoxin by the rat lymphocytes. Macrophages were also implicated in the triggering of the proliferative response of normal rat lymph node cells to low doses of PHA or Con A, but were not required in the proliferative response of rat lymphocytes to PWM. Of interest was the observation that only with PHA and not with specific antigens, that the higher the number of macrophages, the more the degree of activation, and the higher the dose of PHA, the greater an inhibitory effect of the macrophages on lymphocyte transformation was manifested.

C. Monocyte Chemotactic Factor

In studies on the guinea pig (Wahl *et al.*, 1975), purified (>96% pure), sensitized T lymphocytes obtained by the passage of spleen cells through a nylon fiber column and challenged either with dinitrophenylated ovalbumin (DNP-OA) or PPD produced monocyte chemotactic factor (MNL-CTX) only when the cultures were supplemented by peritoneal exudate macrophages. When similar purified T cell populations were stimulated with Con A or PHA, some MNL-CTX was produced, but considerably more was produced by the lymphocytes in the presence of peritoneal exudate macrophages. Macrophages pulsed with DNP-OA, PPD, or PHA and then washed to remove excess stimulant were also effective in augmenting lymphocyte production of MNL-CTX to these agents. However, viable macrophages were essential; freeze-thawed, nonviable cells were not effective.

TABLE I

Macrophage Dependence of the Production of Mitogen or Antigen Stimulated Mediators of Cellular Immunity by Lymphocytes

Mediator	Species examined	Source of lymphocytes	Class of lymphocytes	Stimulant	Macrophage dependence	Reference
Interferon	Human	Peripheral blood	T	PHA or PWM	+	Epstein *et al.*, 1974a, b
Interferon	Human	Peripheral blood	B	PHA or PWM	+	Epstein *et al.*, 1974a,b
Interferon	Human	Peripheral blood	Sensitized T	PPD	+	Epstein *et al.*, 1971b, 1972a
Interferon	Human	Peripheral blood	Sensitized T	Vaccinia antigen	+	Epstein *et al.*, 1972b
Interferon	Human	Peripheral blood	Sensitized T	Herpesvirus hominis antigen	+	Rasmussen *et al.*, 1974; Valle *et al.*, 1975
Migration inhibitory factor	Guinea pig	Lymph nodes	Sensitized T	Bovine γ-globulin	+	Nelson and Leu, 1975
Lymphotoxin	Rat	Lymph nodes	Sensitized T	PHA or oval-bumin	+	Yoshinaga and Waks-man, 1973
Monocyte chemotactic factor	Guinea pig	Spleen	Sensitized T	DNP-OA, PPD, Con A, or PHA	+	Wahl *et al.*, 1975
Monocyte chemotactic factor	Guinea pig	Spleen	B	LPS	–	Wahl *et al.*, 1975
Macrophage activating factor	Guinea pig	Spleen	Sensitized T	DNP-OA or PPD	+	Wahl *et al.*, 1975
Osteoclast activating factor	Human	Peripheral blood	T	PHA	+	Horton *et al.*, 1974

In these same studies (Wahl *et al.*, 1975), B lymphocytes, isolated from E rosette-forming T lymphocyte-depleted spleen cell preparations (Wilson and Coombs, 1973; Wahl *et al.*, 1974) responded to a B cell mitogen, a lipopolysaccharide (LPS) prepared from *Salmonella typhimurium* with the production of MNL-CTX. The addition of macrophages to the LPS-stimulated B cell cultures, however, had no enhancing effect on MNL-CTX production. Thus in this system, B cells do not require the presence of macrophages for maximum production of mediator in response to LPS.

No MNL-CTX was produced by purified B cell cultures in response to a T cell stimulant, DNP-OA, and even the presence of macrophages did not enable the B cells to respond. Likewise, purified T cell cultures did not produce any MNL-CTX in response to the B cell stimulant, LPS, either with or without the presence of macrophages.

Those situations in which macrophage dependence was demonstrated for MNL-CTX production paralleled the requirement for macrophages in the proliferative response. For example, the proliferative response of guinea pig purified T cells to DNP-OA, PPD, or PHA was found to be macrophage-dependent.

Macrophages were thus implicated as helpers in the T lymphocyte proliferative reaction and production of guinea pig MNL-CTX in response to mitogens and antigens, but were not essential for the production of the mediator by B lymphocytes. Here again, because mediator production occurred early in culture, within the first 4 hours, the importance of an early action of macrophages was noted.

According to Altman *et al.* (1973), the molecular weight of human mononuclear chemotactic factor distinguishes it from the guinea pig material described above and by Ward *et al.* (1969). In studies on the origin of this factor, *glass* bead purified human T lymphocytes were shown to produce MNL-CTX in response to PHA, without the presence of macrophages (Altman *et al.*, 1973). However, in these studies no experiments were performed to determine if addition of human macrophages could augment production of the mediator.

D. Macrophage Activating Factor

Using the same experimental system as they did with their studies on MNL-CTX, Wahl *et al.* (1975) found the same requirements for macrophages in the maximum T lymphocyte production of guinea pig MAF in response to specific antigens. Similarly, macrophages were not required for maximum B lymphocyte production of MAF in response to LPS. MAF activity was quantitated by the incorporation of ^{14}C-labeled glucosamine by macrophage monolayers.

E. Osteoclast Activating Factor

Supernatant fluids from cultures of human leukocytes stimulated with PHA or antigenic material prepared from dental plaques, contain a mediator of cellular immunity—osteoclast activating factor (OAF)—which induces osteoclasts to resorb fetal rat bone in organ cultures (Horton *et al.*, 1972). Purified preparations of human lymphocytes obtained from glass bead columns (and thus presumably T lymphocytes) did not produce OAF in response to PHA (Horton *et al.*, 1974). Similarly, purified preparations of X-irradiated, glass-adherent macrophages produced no OAF in response to PHA. However, when the two cell types were combined in culture with PHA, OAF production occurred, and to as great an extent as that observed with unfractionated mononuclear cell cultures. PHA-stimulated OAF production by mononuclear cells is sensitive to X irradiation, suggesting a lymphocyte origin of the mediator. Thus, it was concluded that OAF is produced by lymphocytes, but that its production is dependent on a macrophage–lymphocyte interaction. Supernatants of nonstimulated or PHA-stimulated macrophages could not replace the intact cell in enhancing lymphocyte OAF production. OAF production is maximal 12 hours after initiation of cultures with PHA and thus, like most mediators, but in contrast with interferon, precedes the time of peak lymphocyte proliferation.

F. General Comments

In reviewing the studies concerned with macrophage dependence of lymphocyte mediator production, it is apparent that macrophages from numerous sources are competent in this regard. For lymphotoxin production (Yoshinaga and Waksman, 1973) rat macrophages from either spleen or peritoneum were effective; for interferon and osteoclast activating factor production, macrophages derived from the growth and differentiation of human peripheral blood monocytes were effective; and for guinea pig monocyte chemotactic factor and macrophage activating factor production, guinea pig peritoneal macrophages sufficed.

Although macrophages from several sources are competent to augment lymphocyte mediator production, the requirement for intact, viable macrophages varies depending on the mediator under examination. For example, frozen and thawed macrophages will augment, although to a lesser degree than intact cells, lymphocyte interferon production in response to PHA (Epstein *et al.*, 1971a). However, frozen and thawed guinea pig macrophages are totally ineffective in augmenting guinea pig lymphocyte MNL-CTX (Wahl *et al.*, 1975).

There is also a mediator-dependent difference in the capability of macrophage supernatants to replace intact macrophages in their ability to augment lymphocyte mediator production. Unstimulated or PHA-stimulated macrophage supernatants do not augment human lymphocyte interferon production. In contrast, lymphotoxin production by rat lymphocytes in response to specific antigen is augmented by macrophage supernatants. In this system, macrophage supernatants were far more effective in the presence of autochthonous (rat) serum than they were in the presence of xenogeneic serum (fetal calf serum) (Yoshinaga and Waksman, 1973). Although the source of the serum in which the action of the macrophage supernatants were tested therefore assumes some importance, species-specific serum does not always allow for demonstration of a supernatant effect. In the human interferon studies (Epstein *et al.*, 1971a) human serum was used throughout, but still no effect of the macrophage supernatants was demonstrated.

To date, the mechanism by which macrophages augment lymphocyte mediator production is not clearly understood. The most widely accepted theory is that the macrophage presents antigen or mitogen to the lymphocyte in a form that allows for enhanced triggering of lymphocyte mediator formation, but further extensive study in this area is needed.

V. MACROPHAGES AND THEIR ROLE IN AFFECTING THE PRODUCTION OF VIRAL-INDUCED INTERFERON BY LEUKOCYTES

Leukocyte Origin of Interferon Induced by Certain Viruses

Two questions are relevant at this point. First, can lymphocytes serve as a source of virus induced interferon, and, second, is there a macrophage–lymphocyte interaction in the production of interferon in response to virus similar to that seen in responses to mitogens and antigens?

The situation with regard to virus-induced interferon is somewhat more complex to study than with mitogens or antigens. Although many viruses are capable of inducing interferon in many different types of cells *in vivo* and *in vitro,* not all viruses are capable of inducing interferon in leukocytes. Furthermore, as will be seen below, not all viruses that are capable of inducing interferon in leukocytes induce it in the same leukocyte cell type, i.e., some viruses induce interferon in lymphocytes, and others, possibly, in macrophages.

That leukocytes from several animal species and anatomic locations could, in fact, produce interferon in response to certain viruses was shown in several early reports. Human peripheral blood leukocytes challenged with Sendai or measles virus (Gresser, 1961), Balb C or CD-1 mouse peritoneal leukocytes challenged with vaccinia virus (Glasgow and Habel, 1963; Glasgow, 1965), rabbit splenic as well as peripheral blood leukocytes challenged with Sindbis virus (Kono and Ho, 1965), and glycogen-stimulated rabbit peritoneal exudate leukocytes challenged with NDV (Smith and Wagner, 1967) were all shown to produce interferon. For human peripheral blood leukocytes, NDV (either live or UV irradiated) and Sendai virus were found to be better inducers of interferon than vaccinia, vesicular stomatitis virus, or several of the influenza viruses (Strander and Cantell, 1966). The suggestion that in the human mononuclear leukocytes were the predominant cell source of Sendai virus-induced interferon was made by Lee and Ozere (1965). They succeeded in preparing for virus challenge >97% pure mononuclear cell suspensions (containing lymphocytes and monocytes) by magnetic elimination of polymorphonuclear cells which, by virtue of their phagocytic properties, had ingested freely particulate iron particles. Because more interferon was observed in 24 hour virus-stimulated cultures that contained both polymorphonuclear and mononuclear cells than was observed with cultures that contained only mononuclear cells, these authors also concluded that under appropriate conditions, polymorphonuclear leukocytes could also produce interferon. However, subsequent, more definitive studies by Wheelock (1966), in which highly purified preparations of human polymorphonuclear leukocytes were obtained by EDTA elution from siliconized glass bead columns (Rabinowitz, 1964), indicated that such cells could not produce interferon in response to another virus, i.e., NDV.

In these same studies (Wheelock, 1966) definitive evidence implicating the human lymphocyte as the only leukocyte and mononuclear cell responsible for NDV-induced interferon was set forth. Pure cultures (99%) of human peripheral blood lymphocytes obtained by their passage through a siliconized glass bead column were an excellent source of NDV-induced interferon. Subsequently, human lymphocytes from sources other than peripheral blood have been shown to produce interferon in response to viruses. Ficoll gradient separated lymphocytes from human colostrum and human breast milk produce interferon upon *in vitro* challenge with NDV (Emodi and Just, 1974). Also, human cord blood leukocytes (97.5–100% lymphocytes) and peripheral blood lymphocytes from 8- to 17-week-old fetuses, premature infants, newborns, and children, as well as from adults, produced interferon upon *in vitro* challenge with Sendai virus (Cantell *et al.*, 1968). Both in this study and in that of Ray (1970), consistent differences in the quantitative production of lymphocyte interferon with advancing age were not found. The calculated average interferon yield per lymphocyte did not show any clear correlation with the age of the individual. From the third month of gestation on, lymphocytes could respond to Sendai virus with the production of interferon (Cantell *et al.*, 1968).

It should be noted, however, that there is a wide range of variation from donor to donor of interferon titers observed in virus-stimulated human lymphocyte cultures (Rassiga-Pidot *et al.*, 1972) and that the interferon produced occurs usually within the first 24 hours of culture (Tovell and Cantell, 1971), much earlier than that seen with mitogen- and antigen-stimulated interferon.

The titers of human interferon observed in the supernatant culture fluids of NDV-stimulated human adult leukocytes were related to the absolute number of lymphocytes as well as to the number of glass-adherent cells (presumably monocytes or macrophages) in the cultures (Rassiga-Pidot and McIntyre, 1974). In comparing the interferon titers observed in NDV-stimulated lymphocyte cultures with that of similar cultures prepared with both lymphocytes and glass-adherent cells, these authors found that more interferon was produced in the latter situation. They suggested that a lymphocyte–glass-adherent cell interaction occurs in the production of virus-induced lymphocyte interferon similar to that seen with mitogen- and antigen-induced interferon.

In retrospect, there was a suggestion that a lymphocyte–macrophage interaction might be occurring in the NDV induction of interferon in bovine leukocyte cultures in an early report by Kono (1967). In those studies bovine leukocytes were cultured for up to 12 days. After the first day in culture 95% of the cells were mononuclear leukocytes, presumably because of the early death of the polymorphonuclear cells. The mononuclear cells were lymphocytes and monocytes, the latter of which differentiated into macrophages as the culture period was extended. Many of the cells in the cultures were phagocytic, attesting to their monocyte–macrophage nature. Kono observed that as the culture period increased from 1 to 12 days the number of cells required to produce 1 unit of interferon declined from 4.9×10^4 to $<2.5 \times 10^3$, suggesting an increased sensitivity of cells to the virus as an inducer. Alternatively, one could interpret these results as indicating a lymphocyte–macrophage interaction, wherein monocytes as they differentiate to macrophages increasingly augment the production of virus-induced interferon by lymphocytes.

There is considerable evidence to implicate the lymphocyte as the source of viral-induced interferon in the mouse, as well as in the human. Mice treated with anti-lymphocyte serum and then challenged with NDV *in vivo* show a depressed interferon response (Barth *et al.*, 1969). Further implication of the involvement of cells of the immune system in virus-induced interferon comes from the studies of Glasgow (1966) in which it was demonstrated that cultures of leukocytes from animals immune to Chikungunya virus (CV) produced twofold to tenfold greater amounts of interferon when challenged with CV than those cultures with similar cell content, but from nonimmune control animals.

In a series of elegant studies which employed X irradiation, xenogeneic bone marrow transplantation, and anti-lymphocyte serum treatment, the lymphocyte was confirmed as the cell source of *in vivo* circulating interferon in the mouse after intravenous NDV challenge (De Maeyer *et al.*, 1967, 1969; De Maeyer-Guignard *et al.*, 1969; De Maeyer-Guignard and De Maeyer, 1971; Jullien *et al.*, 1974). These authors demonstrated that production of circulating interferon after *in vivo* NDV challenge was markedly depressed in mice following a course of 1000 R total body X irradiation, or even after only 125 R. They ascribed the depressed interferon response to radiation-induced depression of hematopoietic function, which could be corrected by either syngeneic or xenogeneic bone marrow transplants to lethally irradiated recipients. The species specificity of interferon allowed for the determination that in xenogeneic radiation chimeras the circulating interferon induced by NDV was of donor origin, and hence from some line of hemopoietic cells. Since both lymphocytes and granulocytes are radiosensitive, these authors employed anti-lymphocyte serum to identify the actual cells producing interferon in the radiation chimeras, and it was at this point that the lymphocyte was implicated.

However, the studies of De Maeyer, De Maeyer-Guignard and colleagues with other viruses suggested that the lymphocyte may not be the only leukocyte or other cell type in the mouse that can respond to certain viruses with the production of interferon. For example, whereas induction of interferon by NDV, a myxovirus, is a very radiosensitive process, induction by encephalomyocarditis virus (EMC), vaccinia virus, or a nonviral inducer, poly(I·C), is relatively insensitive to radiation or anti-lymphocyte serum. In fact, EMC virus-induced interferon remained of recipient type in xenogeneic chimeras up to 3 months after lethal irradiation and xenogeneic bone marrow transplantation, indicating that the interferon observed after EMC challenge had originated from a cell population not derived from the hemopoietic system at all. In contrast, interferon induced by poly(I·C) became donor type within 3 months after xenogeneic bone marrow grafting, suggesting that it was made by cells from the hemopoietic system. When xenogeneic chimeras were subjected to radiation 1 month after the initial bone marrow transplant, interferon production by donor cells in response to poly(I·C) was not affected, thus implicating a hemopoietic cell more radioresistant than a lymphocyte, i.e., the macrophage, as the cell source of this type of interferon (Jullien *et al.*, 1974).

Also, these authors have shown that interferon induction by arboviruses or by vesicular stomatitis virus (VSV) shows intermediate sensitivity to X irradiation and anti-lymphocyte serum, and it has yet to be proved in comparable experiments to those described above whether the lymphocyte, macrophage, or both cells can produce interferon in response to these agents.

Thus, the lymphocyte is well established as a cell source of interferon in response to certain viruses. However, with the exception of the studies with NDV and human lymphocytes by Rassiga-Pidot and McIntyre (1974), information is lacking as to whether lymphocyte interferon production in response to numerous viruses is macrophage-dependent or not.

All the studies described in this chapter which demonstrate a macrophage–lymphocyte interaction (either in the production of mitogen-, antigen-, or virus-induced interferon, or in the production of other mediators of cellular immunity in response to mitogen and antigen) have been performed *in vitro*. To date, no studies have been performed which actually indicate that such macrophage–lymphocyte interactions in the production of mediators do occur *in vivo*. But it is not too unrealistic to imagine that such macrophage–lymphocyte interactions do exist. In view of the close anatomic relationship of the two cell types *in vivo* and the intimate relationship of macrophages with both T and B lymphocytes in the proliferative and antibody responses to antigenic stimuli (Unanue, 1972), it is quite probable that in the very near future confirmation of the *in vivo* interaction of macrophages and lymphocytes in the immune-specific induction of mediators of cellular immunity will also occur.

VI. SUMMARY

Lymphocytes can respond *in vitro* to numerous mitogens with the production of the antiviral protein interferon. Either syngeneic or allogeneic macrophages can augment *in vitro* mitogen-stimulated lymphocyte interferon production. Intimate macrophage–lymphocyte contact is required for the interaction of these two cell types for maximum interferon production. In studies on human cells, both T and B lymphocytes can produce interferon *in vitro* in response to PHA and PWM, but the B cell response is delayed. The amount of interferon produced after 3 days of culture of lymphocytes (in the presence of macrophages) with mitogen is a measure of the effector competence of T lymphocytes.

Macrophages augment both T and B lymphocyte interferon production.

Monocytes support lymphocyte interferon production also, but they appear to elaborate an antagonist to the expression of the antiviral effect of interferon.

Agents that increase the intracellular level of cyclic AMP depress mitogen-stimulated interferon production by T lymphocytes, and one of them, i.e., cholera toxin, does not affect the ability of macrophages to augment lymphocyte interferon production.

Whereas X irradiation depresses the lymphocyte proliferative response to mitogens, it does not affect the mitogen-stimulated production of interferon.

The study of 3 day T lymphocyte interferon production in response to mitogens proved to be an effective tool with which to assess T lymphocyte effector competence in patients with various diseases. A defect in T cell effector function was noted in patients with selective IgA deficiency and chronic lymphocytic leukemia. Macrophages prepared from such patients were functionally competent to augment lymphocyte interferon production by lymphocytes from normal donors.

Previously sensitized lymphocytes can respond *in vitro* to bacterial and viral antigens with the production of interferon, as well as with proliferation. Both the production of interferon and the proliferative response are augmented by the presence of macrophages, but often, the macrophages are just as effective whether they be from immune or nonimmune donors. Often there is a dissociation in time between peak interferon production and the maximum proliferative response, with the latter occurring first in human culture systems. Recent reexposure to live virus is necessary for demonstration of *in vitro* viral antigen-stimulated interferon, whereas the lymphocyte proliferative response appears to reflect more the prior immune status of the lymphocyte donor rather than the active state of the viral infection.

Interferon is also produced *in vivo* on an immune-specific basis, and its possible role in host defense, especially against nonviral antigens, is discussed. It is not yet known whether a macrophage–lymphocyte interaction similar to that observed *in vitro* actually occurs in the *in vivo* production of immune interferon.

Macrophages also augment the *in vitro* mitogen- or antigen-stimulated production of other mediators of cellular immunity by lymphocytes, i.e., MIF, LT, MNL CTX, MAF, and OAF. The exact mechanism by which the macrophage augments lymphocyte mediator production is not known.

The dependence of *in vitro* virus-stimulated lymphocyte interferon on the presence of macrophages has been demonstrated with Newcastle disease virus. However differences in stability to heat and low pH distinguish viral-induced interferon from mitogen- or antigen-stimulated interferon. Further study is needed to define the relationship between the two types of interferon. Macrophages appear to augment production of both types of interferon by lymphocytes, but it is not known whether they do so via the same mechanism.

ACKNOWLEDGMENTS

The experimental results from the author's laboratory and the work on this chapter were supported by grants from the National Institutes of Health (CA 11067, 14508, and AI 12481), from the Damon Runyon Memorial Fund (DRG 1205), and from the California Division, American Cancer Society. The author wishes to thank Carol Stadum, Dorothy Metcalf, and Cathy Ploetz for typing the manuscript.

REFERENCES

Altman, L. C., Snyderman, R., Oppenheim, J. J., and Mergenhagen, S. E. (1973). *J. Immunol.* **110,** 801–810.

Barth, R. F., Friedman, R. M., and Malmgren, R. A. (1969). *Lancet* **2,** 723–724.

Bennett, B., and Bloom, B. R. (1968). *Proc. Nat. Acad. Sci. U.S.* **59,** 756–762.

Blomgren, H., Strander, H., and Cantell, K. (1974). *Scand. J. Immunol.* **3,** 655–664.

Bloom, B. R. (1971). *Advan. Immunol.* **13,** 102–208.

Bloom, B. R., and Glade, P. R., eds. (1971). "*In Vitro* Methods of Cell-Mediated Immunity." Academic Press, New York.

Bobrove, A., Strober, S., Herzenberg, L. A., and DePamphilis, J. D. (1974). *J. Immunol.* **112,** 520–527.

Bonner, W. A., Hulett, H. R., Swett, R. G., and Herzenberg, L. A. (1972). *Rev. Sci. Instrum.* **43,** 404–409.

Borecky, L., Fuchsberger, N., Zemla, J., and Lackovic, V. (1971). *Eur. J. Immunol.* **2,** 213–218.

Brodeur, B. R., and Merigan, T. C. (1974). *J. Immunol.* **113,** 1319–1325.

Cantell, K., Strander, H., Saxén, L., and Meyer, B. (1968). *J. Immunol.* **100,** 1304–1309.

Chester, T. J., Paucker, K., and Merigan, T. C. (1973). *Nature (London)* **246,** 92–94.

Cooperband, S. R., and Green, J. A. (1971). *In* "*In Vitro* Methods in Cell-Mediated Immunity" (B. R. Bloom and P. R. Glade, eds.), pp. 381–400. Academic Press, New York.

David, J. R. (1972). *Progr. Allergy* **16,** 300–449.

DeMaeyer, E., Jullien, P., and DeMaeyer-Guignard, J. (1967). *Int. J. Radiat. Biol.* **13,** 417–431.

DeMaeyer, E., DeMaeyer-Guignard, J., and Jullien, P. (1969). *Proc. Soc. Exp. Biol. Med.* **131,** 36–41.

DeMaeyer-Guignard, J., and DeMaeyer, E. (1971). *Nature (London), New Biol.* **229,** 212–214.

DeMaeyer-Guignard, J., DeMaeyer, E., and Jullien, P. (1969). *Proc. Nat. Acad. Sci. U.S.* **63,** 732–739.

Dumonde, D. C., Wolstencroft, R. A., Panayi, G. S., Matthew, M., Morley, J., and Howson, W. T. (1969). *Nature (London)* **244,** 38–42 (1969).

Emodi, G., and Just, M. (1974). *Scand. J. Immunol.* **3,** 157–160.

Epstein, L. B. (1966). *Fed. Proc., Fed. Amer. Soc. Exp. Biol.* **25,** 439.
Epstein, L. B. (1975). *In* "Effects of Interferon on Cells, Viruses and the Immune System" (A. Geraldes, ed.), pp. 393–408. Academic Press, New York.
Epstein, L. B., and Ammann, A. J. (1974). *J. Immunol.* **112,** 617–626.
Epstein, L. B., and Ammann, A. J. (1975). Submitted for publication.
Epstein, L. B., and Bourne, H. R. (1975). *In* "Mitogens in Immunobiology" (D. L. Rosenstreich and J. J. Oppenheim, eds.) (in press).
Epstein, L. B., and Cline, M. J. (1974). *Clin. Exp. Immunol.* **16,** 553–563.
Epstein, L. B., and Salmon, S. E. (1974). *J. Immunol.* **112,** 1131–1138.
Epstein, L. B., and Smith, C. W. (1968). *J. Immunol.* **100,** 421–435.
Epstein, L. B., and Stohlman, F., Jr. (1964). *Blood* **24,** 69–75.
Epstein, L. B., Cline, M. J., and Merigan, T. C. (1970). *In* "Proceedings of the Fifth Leukocyte Culture Conference" (J. E. Harris, ed.), pp. 501–513. Academic Press, New York.
Epstein, L. B., Cline, M. J., and Merigan, T. C. (1971a). *J. Clin. Invest.* **50,** 744–753.
Epstein, L. B., Cline, M. J., and Merigan, T. C. (1971b). *Cell. Immunol.* **2,** 602–613.
Epstein ,L. B., Cline, M. J., and Merigan, T. C. (1972a). *In* "Proceedings of the Sixth Leukocyte Culture Conference" (R. Schwarz, ed.), pp. 265–282. Academic Press, New York.
Epstein, L. B., Stevens, D. A., and Merigan, T. C. (1972b). *Proc. Nat. Acad. Sci. U.S.* **69,** 2632–2636.
Epstein, L. B., Kreth, H. W., and Herzenberg, L. A. (1974a). *In* "Lymphocyte Recognition and Effector Mechanisms" (K. Lindahl-Kiessling and D. Osoba, eds.), pp. 169–174. Academic Press, New York.
Epstein, L. B. Kreth, H. W., and Herzenberg, L. A. (1974b). *Cell. Immunol.* **12,** 407–421.
Finter, N. B., ed. (1973). "Interferons and Interferon Inducers." North-Holland Publ., Amsterdam.
Fontaine-Brouty-Boye, E., Gresser, I., Macieira-Coelho, A., Rosenfeld, C., and Thomas, M. T. (1969). *C. R. Acad. Sci.* **269,** 406–408.
Friedman, R. M., and Cooper, H. L. (1967). *Proc. Soc. Exp. Biol. Med.* **125,** 901–905.
Gifford, G. E., Tibor, A., and Peavy, D. L. (1971). *Infec. Immunity* **3,** 164–166.
Glasgow, L. A. (1965). *J. Exp. Med.* **121,** 1001–1017.
Glasgow, L. A. (1966). *J. Bacteriol.* **91,** 2185–2191.
Glasgow, L. A., and Habel, K. (1963). *J. Exp. Med.* **117,** 149–160.
Granger, G. A., and Williams, T. W. (1971). *In* "Progress in Immunology" (B. Amos, ed.), pp. 437–445. Academic Press, New York.
Greaves, M. F., Owen, J. J. T., and Raff, M. C. (1973). "T and B Lymphocytes—Origins, Properties and Roles in Immune Responses," pp. 105–111. Amer. Elsevier, New York.
Green, J. A., Cooperband, S. R., and Kibrick, S. (1969). *Science* **164,** 1415–1417.
Green, J. A., Cooperband, S. R., Kleinman, L. F., and Kibrick, S. (1970). *Ann. N.Y. Acad. Sci.* **173,** 736–741.
Gresser, I. (1961). *Proc. Soc. Exp. Biol. Med.* **108,** 799–805.
Gresser, I., and Bourali, C. (1969). *Nature (London)* **223,** 844–845.
Gresser, I., and Bourali, C. (1970). *J. Nat. Cancer Inst.* **45,** 365–376.
Gresser, I., Brouty-Boye, D., Thomas, M. T., and Macieira-Coelho, A. (1969). *Proc. Nat. Acad. Sci. U.S.* **63,** 51–57.
Gresser, I., Brouty-Boye, D., Thomas, M. T., and Macieira-Coelho, A. (1970a). *Proc. Nat. Acad. Sci. U.S.* **66,** 1052–1058.
Gresser, I., Bourali, C., Chouroulinkov, I., Fontaine-Brouty-Boye, D., and Thomas,

M. T. (1970b). *Proc. New York Acad. Sci.* **173,** 694–707.
Grossberg, S. E. (1972). *N. Engl. J. Med.* **287,** 13–19, 79–85, and 122.
Hammond, E. M., and Dvorak, H. F. (1972). *J. Exp. Med.* **136,** 1518–1532.
Hay, J. B. (1973). *Int. Arch. Allergy Appl. Immunol.* **44,** 569–584.
Hay, J. B., Lachman, P. J., and Trenka, Z. (1973). *Eur. J. Immunol.* **3,** 127–131,
Henle, G., and Henle, W. (1965). *J. Bacteriol.* **89,** 252–258.
Hobbs, J. R. (1968). *Lancet* **1,** 110–114.
Hooks, J., Fujibashi, T., and Notkins, A. L. (1975). *Fed. Proc., Fed. Amer. Soc. Exp. Biol.* **34,** 869.
Horton, J. E., Raisz, L. G., Simmons, H. A., Oppenheim, J. J., and Mergenhagen, S. E. (1972). *Science* **177,** 793–795.
Horton, J. E., Oppenheim, J. J., Mergenhagen, S. E., and Raisz, L. G. (1974). *J. Immunol.* **113,** 1278–1287.
Huang, K. Y., Donahoe, R. M., Gordon, R. B., and Dressler, H. (1971). *Infec. Immunity* **4,** 581–588.
Hulett, H. R., Bonner, W. A., Sweet, R. G., and Herzenberg, L. A. (1973). *Clin. Chem.* **19,** 813–816.
Isaacs, A., and Lindemann, J. (1957). *Proc. Roy. Soc., Ser. B* **147,** 258–267.
Isaacs, A., Lindemann, J., and Valentine, R. C. (1957). *Proc. Roy. Soc., Ser. B* **147,** 268–273.
Jordan, G. W., and Merigan, T. C. (1974). *J. Infec. Dis.* **130,** 495–501.
Jullien, P., DeMaeyer-Guignard, J., and DeMaeyer, E. (1974). *Infec. Immunity* **10,** 1023–1028.
Kasel, J. A., Haase, A. T., Glade, P. R., and Chessin, L. N. (1968). *Proc. Soc. Exp. Biol. Med.* **128,** 351–353.
Kelly, R. H., and Wolstencroft, R. A. (1974). *Clin. Exp. Immunol.* **18,** 321–336.
Kelly, R. H., Wolstencroft, R. A., Dumonde, D. C., and Balfour, B. M. (1972). *Clin. Exp. Immunol.* **10,** 49–65.
Kleinschmidt, W. J. (1972). *Annu. Rev. Biochem.* **41,** 517–542.
Kono, Y. (1967). *Proc. Soc. Exp. Biol. Med.* **124,** 155–160.
Kono, Y., and Ho, M. (1965). *Virology* **25,** 162–166.
Kreth, H. W., and Herzenberg, L. A. (1974). *Cell. Immunol.* **12,** 396–406.
Lawrence, H. S., and Landy, M., eds. (1969). "Mediators of Cellular Immunity." Academic Press, New York.
Lee, S. H. S., and Ozere, R. L. (1965). *Proc. Soc. Exp. Biol. Med.* **118,** 190–195.
Lindahl, P., Leary, P., and Gresser, I. (1972). *Proc. Nat. Acad. Sci. U.S.* **69,** 721–725.
Lindahl, P., Leary, P., and Gresser, I. (1973). *Proc. Nat. Acad. Sci. U.S.* **70,** 2785–2788.
Lindahl-Magnusson, P., Leary, P., and Gresser, I. (1971). *Proc. Soc. Exp. Biol. Med.* **138,** 1044–1050.
Lindahl-Magnusson, P., Leary, P., and Gresser, I. (1972). *Nature (London), New Biol.* **237,** 120–121.
McCombs, R. M., and Benyesh-Melnick, M. (1967). *J. Nat. Cancer Inst.* **39,** 1187–1196.
McIntyre, O. R., and Ebaugh, F. G. J. (1962). *Blood* **19,** 443–453.
MacKinney, A. S., Jr., Stohlman, F., Jr., and Brecher, G. (1962). *Blood* **19,** 349–358.
McNeill, T. A., and Fleming, W. A. (1971). *Immunology* **21,** 761–766.
McNeill, T. A., and Gresser, I. (1973). *Nature (London), New Biol.* **244,** 173–174.
Merigan, T. C., Gregory, D. F., and Petralli, J. K. (1966). *Virology* **29,** 515–522.
Merigan, T. C., Stevens, D. A., Rasmussen, L. E., and Epstein, L. B. (1973). *In* "Non-Specific Factors Influencing Host Resistance" (W. Braun and J. Ungar, eds.), pp. 430–437. Karger, Basel.

Milstone, L. M., and Waksman, B. H. (1970). *J. Immunol.* **105,** 1068–1071.
Nell, P. A., Ammann, A. J., Hong, R., and Stiehm, R. (1972). *Pediatrics* **49,** 71–79.
Nelson, R. D., and Leu, R. W. (1975). *J. Immunol.* **114,** 606–609.
Peterson, R. D. A., Cooper, M. D., and Good, R. A. (1966). *Amer. J. Med.* **41,** 342–359.
Rabinowitz, Y. (1964). *Blood* **23,** 811–828.
Rasmussen, L. E., Jordan, G. W., Stevens, D. A., and Merigan, T. C. (1974). *J. Immunol.* **112,** 728–736.
Rassiga-Pidot, A. L., and McIntyre, O. R. (1974). *Cancer Res.* **34,** 2995–3002.
Rassiga-Pidot, A. L., O'Keefe, G., III, McManus, N., and McIntyre, O. R. (1972). *Proc. Soc. Exp. Biol. Med.* **140,** 1263–1269.
Ray, C. G. (1970). *J. Pediat.* **76,** 94–98.
Salvin, S. B., Youngner, J. S., and Lederer, W. H. (1973). *Infec. Immunity* **7,** 68–75.
Salvin, S. B., Nishio, J., and Shonnard, J. T. (1974). *Infec. Immunity* **9,** 631–635.
Salvin, S. B., Ribi, E., Granger, D. L., and Youngner, J. S. (1975). *J. Immunol.* **114,** 354–359.
Smith, T. J., and Wagner, R. R. (1967). *J. Exp. Med.* **125,** 559–577.
Stinebring, W. R., and Absher, M. (1970). *Ann. N.Y. Acad. Sci.* **173,** 714–718.
Stobo, J., Green, I., Jackson, L., and Baron, S. (1974). *J. Immunol.* **112,** 1589–1593.
Strander, H., and Cantell, K. (1966). *Ann. Med. Exp. Biol. Fenn.* **44,** 265–273.
Sugiyama, M., Yamamoto, K., Kinoshita, Y., Kimura, S., Shibata, T., and Watanabe, M. (1972). *Jap. J. Tonsil.* **11,** 106–112.
Sugiyama, M., Yamamoto, K., Kinoshita, Y., Kimura, S., Shibata, T., and Watanabe, M. (1974). *Jap. J. Tonsil.* **13,** 104–113 (1974).
Tovell, D., and Cantell, K. (1971). *J. Gen. Virol.* **13,** 485–489.
Unanue, E. R. (1972). *Advan. Immunol.* **15,** 95–165.
Valle, M. J., Bobrove, A. M., Strober, S., and Merigan, T. C. (1975). *J. Immunol.* **114,** 435–441.
Wagner, R. R. (1964). *Nature (London)* **204,** 49–51.
Wagner, R. R., and Huang, A. S. (1965). *Proc. Nat. Acad. Sci. U.S.* **54,** 1112–1117.
Wahl, S. M., Iverson, G. M., and Oppenheim, J. J. (1974). *J. Exp. Med.* **140,** 1631–1645.
Wahl, S. M., Wilton, J. M., Rosenstreich, D. L., and Oppenheim, J. J. (1975). *J. Immunol.* **114,** 1296–1301.
Wallen, W. C., Dean, J. H., and Lucas, D. O. (1973). *Cell. Immunol.* **6,** 110–122.
Ward, P. A., Remold, H. G., and David, J. R. (1969). *Science* **163,** 1079–1081.
Ward, P. A., Remold, H. G., and David, J. R. (1970). *Cell. Immunol.* **1,** 162–174.
Wheelock, E. F. (1965). *Science* **149,** 310–311.
Wheelock, E. F. (1966). *J. Bacteriol.* **92,** 1415–1421.
Wilson, A., and Coombs, R. R. A. (1973). *Int. Arch. Allergy Appl. Immunol.* **44,** 544–552.
World Health Organization. (1973). *World Health Organ., Tech. Rep. Ser.* **519.**
Yoshinaga, M., and Waksman, B. H. (1973). *Ann. Immunol. Inst. Pasteur* **124C,** 97–120.
Youngner, J. S., and Salvin, S. B. (1973). *J. Immunol.* **111,** 1914–1922.

9

Nonspecific Immunoregulation by Macrophages and Their Products

D. S. Nelson

I. Introduction 235
II. Potentiation of Lymphoid Cell Responses 236
III. Inhibition of Lymphoid Cell Responses 239
IV. Mode of Action of Macrophages in Depressing Lymphocyte Responses 243
V. Significance of Lymphoid Cell Stimulation and Inhibition by Macrophages and Their Products 250
References 253

I. INTRODUCTION

It may be some time before there is a full elucidation of the multiple roles of macrophages in specific immune responses. Their vital roles in many responses have been discussed by other contributors to this volume, as have their roles in lymphocyte activation and lymphokine production. My aims in this chapter are to examine situations in which macrophages may exert a nonspecific regulatory effect, particularly in depressing lymphocyte responses; ways in which such effects may be produced; and some experimental, biological, and clinical phenomena that may be explicable in terms of macrophage-dependent inhibition. A consideration of nonspecific inhibitory effects must, however, be put into the perspective of other effects of macrophages and their products. Personal experience in this field, especially in the study of soluble factors produced by macrophages, has been chastening and has led to a realization of the need for the most careful control and scrutiny of the technical conditions in which experiments have been carried out. Despite these reservations, it seems reasonable to draw some conclusions and to offer some speculations about the significance of macrophage activity in this area of immunology.

II. POTENTIATION OF LYMPHOID CELL RESPONSES

The ways in which macrophages may promote or play an essential role in the production of antibodies by B cells and their progeny have been discussed by Pierce and Kapp (Chapter 1), Mosier (Chapter 2), and Basten and Mitchell (Chapter 3). As studied *in vitro,* these may involve (1) handling of a specific antigen so that it is presented in an appropriate fashion or in appropriate amounts to responding B cells, (2) production of factors that can provide a second signal for the stimulation of B cells, (3) promotion of viability, or (4) production of soluble factors that can amplify B cell responses. Of special relevance in the present context are (3) and (4).

The presence of macrophages increases the viability of lymphoid cells in culture; in this function it seems that macrophages can be replaced by 2-mercaptoethanol (2-ME) (Chen and Hirsch, 1972; Gisler *et al.*, 1973; Pierce *et al.*, 1974; Watson *et al.*, 1974). Supernatant fluids from cultured macrophages have been reported to serve this function, if only partially (Shortman and Palmer, 1971; Hoffmann and Dutton, 1971), but this appears not to be easily reproducible, possibly because the supernatant factor(s) is unstable (Cosenza *et al.*, 1971; D. D. Wood, unpublished observations, 1974, cited by Pierce *et al.*, 1974).

The response of cultured B cells to thymus-dependent antigens may be rendered wholly or partially independent of the presence of live T cells by soluble factors (see Basten and Mitchell, Chapter 3). By and large, these factors are produced in lymphocyte cultures stimulated by allogeneic cells (mimicking the allogeneic effect) or by T cell mitogens (Dutton *et al.*, 1971; for further discussion and references see Sjöberg *et al.*, 1972, 1973; Armerding and Katz, 1974; Britton, 1974; Rubin *et al.*, 1974). Such factors may either increase the incidence of potentially responsive B cells or improve the performance of individual cells (Hunter and Kettmann, 1974). Both physicochemically and, in all likelihood, functionally "T cell replacing factors" are heterogeneous (Watson, 1973).

Because T cell replacing factors have generally been found in supernatants from cultures containing stimulated T cells, it has been assumed that they were produced by T cells. Macrophages can, however, produce factors with similar effects (Schrader, 1973; Wood and Gaul, 1974). On the basis of his own experiments and those of others, Britton (1974) has suggested that activated T cells trigger (or "alarm") macrophages to produce factors supporting B cell maturation. The heterogeneity of factors, the finding that some are inhibitory, and the somewhat shadowy distinction between an immunological second signal and an immunological amplifier all militate against a final pronouncement on this subject.

It has been known for some time that macrophages are essential for, or markedly promote, lymphocyte transformation induced by antigens, allogeneic cells, and, to an apparently lesser extent, nonspecific T cell mitogens, such as phytohemagglutinin (PHA), concanavalin A (Con A), or periodate (Oppenheim *et al.*, 1968; Hersh and Harris, 1968; Gordon, 1968; Alter and Bach, 1970; Levis and Robbins, 1970; Biniaminov *et al.*, 1974). Similarly, macrophages play a part in the production by lymphocytes of interferon and other lymphokines (Epstein *et al.*, 1971; Epstein, Chapter 8). One role for macrophages appeared to be the presentation of antigen to reacting lymphocytes (Cline and Swett, 1968; Hanifin and Cline, 1970). Another role, in mixed lymphocyte reactions (MLR's), appeared to be the provision of soluble factors enhancing transformation (Bach *et al.*, 1970). The latter role could, it was suggested, be filled by 2-ME both for the proliferative response (Herber-Katz and Click, 1972) and for the generation of alloimmune cytotoxic cells (Bevan *et al.*, 1974).

Much clarification of the roles of macrophages in lymphocyte transformation has been achieved as a result of the studies reviewed in detail by Rosenthal *et al.* (Chapter 6), Rosenstreich and Wilton (1975), and Rosenstreich and Oppenheim (Chapter 7). Their work was carried out for the most part with guinea pigs, but their conclusions are likely to be applicable to other species in which, indeed, important related and supporting data have been obtained.

The key technical feature of Rosentreich's work is the exhaustive depletion of macrophages from the cell populations studied. When this was done, macrophages were found to be required for optimum stimulation of T cells by nonspecific mitogens, such as PHA, Con A, or periodate. Supernatants from macrophage cultures contained a factor(s) capable of restoring the responsiveness of macrophage-depleted lymphocyte cultures. It is suggested that this factor might be identical with the lymphocyte activating factor (LAF) previously described by Gery *et al.* (1971) (discussed below) and might act as a vital second signal for the transformation of T cells. The first signal could come from mitogens reacting directly with T cells, as is the case with PHA, Con A, and periodate, or from mitogenic stimuli presented by macrophages, as is the case with specific antigens and, in some experimental circumstances, nonspecific mitogens such as PHA. In MLR's, macrophages constitute a far more potent stimulus than do T cells to allogeneic T cells and thus function as the antigen. 2-ME could not replace macrophages or macrophage supernatants in their helper or second signal functions, although it could act synergistically with them. Essentially similar findings were reported by Rode and Gordon (1974) for human MLR's. Suggestions, cited above, that 2-ME or macrophage supernatants could *entirely* replace macrophages in MLR's probably stem from a failure to deplete macrophages adequately from the cell suspensions being tested. The beneficial effect of 2-ME appears to be a general phenomenon in lymphocyte cultures (Fanger *et al.*, 1970; Chen and Hirsch, 1972; Click *et al.*, 1972; Broome and Jeng, 1973).

Macrophages are not required for and, in general, markedly depress the response of B cells to mitogens. They appear not to inhibit the responses of B cells from immunized animals to specific antigens, at least in the presence of T cells (Yoshinaga *et al.*, 1972; Rosenstreich and Oppenheim, Chapter 7). It is of interest that a murine myeloma synthesizing IgM requires macrophages, or products thereof, for replication (Namba and Hanaoka, 1972).

In the light of these current interpretations, the lymphocyte activating factor (LAF) described by Gery and his colleagues attracts great interest (Gery *et al.*, 1971, 1972; Gery and Waksman, 1972; Novogrodsky and Gery, 1972; Gery and Handschumacher, 1974). LAF is produced by adherent cells, presumably macrophages, from a variety of species and sources, e.g., mouse peritoneal cavity and spleen, human peripheral blood, especially if the cells have been stimulated directly (e.g., by endotoxin) or are present in cultures stimulated with, for example, PHA. The most notable features of LAF are its capacities to potentiate the response of mouse thymocytes to T cell mitogens (PHA, Con A, periodate), to potentiate the response of macrophage-depleted human peripheral blood lymphocytes to PHA, and, to a lesser extent, to cause direct stimulation of mouse thymocytes. LAF (from human or mouse cells) has been partially characterized as a nondialyzable protein with a molecular weight of about 15,000, stable to modest changes in pH (5.5–10.5), partially destroyed at 60° to 80°C, and totally destroyed at 80°C in the presence of normal serum. It is tempting to attribute many of the helper effects of macrophages to LAF, but only further chemical characterization of the factors responsible for these effects will show whether this simplification is as justifiable as it seems desirable.

One additional intriguing property of macrophages deserves mention. Blomgren (1974) has adduced evidence that human monocytes (or macrophages) produce a factor that protects PHA or pokeweed mitogen-stimulated human lymphocytes from the inhibitory effects of a corticosteroid (prednisolone).

III. INHIBITION OF LYMPHOID CELL RESPONSES

Evidence that macrophages can inhibit lymphoid cell responses falls into two broad classes: that derived from experiments in which cells from animals with modified (usually stimulated) macrophages fail to respond in a normal fashion *in vitro* or *in vivo,* and that derived from experiments in which the direct addition of macrophages or their products results in inhibition of the response of lymphoid cells cultured *in vitro.*

The inhibitory effect of graft versus host reactions on active immune responses in affected animals has been known for some time (Howard and Woodruff, 1961; Blaese *et al.*, 1964; see Sjöberg, 1972, for more extensive references). Generally, a phase during which responsiveness is increased precedes a phase of profound depression of cell-mediated and humoral responses, both thymus-dependent and thymus-independent, e.g., to bacterial lipopolysaccharide (LPS) and Type III pneumococcal polysaccharide (S III) (Sjöberg, 1972; Byfield *et al.,* 1973). There is also a decreased responsiveness to PHA *in vitro* (Sjöberg, 1972). Mice with graft versus host reaction possess activated macrophages (Blanden, 1969). Removal of macrophages from the spleens of such mice partially restored their *in vitro* responsiveness to antigen and to PHA (Sjöberg, 1972), whereas removal of T cells did not. In the experiments of Byfield *et al.* removal of T cells and macrophages was required to give partial restoration of responsiveness to the spleen cells, as tested by transfer to irradiated hosts. Despite a lack of complete correlation, both sets of experiments are consistent with the development of the concept of "suppressor macrophages."

Corynebacterium parvum is one of the most powerful stimulants of the mononuclear phagocytic system *in vivo* (Halpern *et al.*, 1964, 1973). It is of particular interest because its administration is accompanied by marked suppression of tumor growth (Halpern *et al.*, 1964, 1973; Woodruff and Dunbar, 1973; Woodruff, *et al.*, 1973). Scott (1972a,b) found that certain T cell functions, responsiveness to PHA or allogeneic lymphocytes *in vitro* and graft versus host reactivity, were depressed in the spleens of *C. parvum*-injected mice, whereas responsiveness to a predominantly B cell mitogen, pokeweed mitogen (PWM), was scarcely affected. Reviewing these and other results, Howard *et al.* (1973) also noted that responsiveness to LPS, another B cell mitogen, was unaffected. The production of antibodies to thymus-dependent antigens (sheep and rat erythrocytes) and a thymus- independent antigen (S III) was decreased. Warr and Šljivić (1974) also found decreased antibody responses to sheep erythrocytes and to S III in *C. parvum*-injected mice. They found that increased responses could also occur, depending on the dose of antigen and the timing of its administration in relation to *C. parvum*. Kirchner *et al.* (1975a) have also investigated the effect of *C. parvum* injections on lymphocyte responses and have found that both T cell responses (to PHA and Con A) and B cell responses (to LPS) were depressed. There is substantial evidence that the depressive effect can be attributed to macrophages. Scott (1972b) removed adherent cells by passage over glass beads and restored the responsiveness of spleen cells to PHA. As discussed further below, not all glass-adherent cells are macrophages. The experiments of Kirchner *et al.* (1975a) implicate macrophages much more directly as suppressor cells in this system. Responsiveness to PHA was largely restored by removal of cells which (a) could adhere to rayon, (b) could take up iron, allowing their removal by means of a magnet, and (c) were susceptible to carrageenan. They further showed that the addition to normal spleen cells of living spleen cells from *C. parvum*-injected mice depressed the responses of the normal cells; this makes it unlikely that a change in the distribution of cell types, leading to a dilution of T cells by macrophages, could cause the depression.

BCG is a long established stimulant of the phagocytic system, its antitumor activity and safety qualifying it as the most popular agent for "nonspecific" immunotherapy of human malignant disease (Yashphe *et al.*, 1971; Baker and Taub, 1973). The spleen cells of mice injected with BCG were found to contain increased numbers of macrophages and to respond less well than normal spleen cells to T cell mitogens (PHA and Con A) but equally well to a B cell mitogen (LPS) (Mitchell *et al.*, 1973). They also showed higher resting or baseline DNA synthesis. Removal of adherent cells restored their responsiveness to PHA to levels equal to those of normal nonadherent spleen cells and partially restored responsiveness to Con A. Baseline levels of DNA synthesis were still high. These observations are again consistent with the suppressor macrophage concept. In an apparent paradox, however, cultured cells, either unfractionated or adherent, from the spleens of BCG-treated mice produced more LAF *in vitro* than did cells from normal mice. This raises the question, to be discussed below, of the relationship between LAF and lymphocyte depressive factors.

LPS produces, *in vivo,* a short-lived stimulation of macrophages (Rowley, 1955; Shilo, 1959). Although LPS can act as an adjuvant to antibody production, inappropriate timing of the injection of antigen in relation to LPS can lead to depressed antibody production in rabbits (Franzl and McMaster, 1968). Exposure of the appendix of irradiated rabbits to endotoxin is followed by marked local stimulation of macrophages, accompanied by a failure of normal regeneration of the lymphoid cells (Blythman and Waksman, 1973).

The development or carriage of tumors, in experimental animals and in man, can lead to a considerable degree of stimulation of macrophages (Nelson, 1974) as well as to nonspecific depression of immunological reactivity (Smith, 1972). Interpretation of analyses of immunodepression in tumor-bearing experimental animals is a task fraught with difficulties because of the great variety in number, type, and biological behavior of model systems. Even tumors that are generally similar to one another, such as methylcholanthrene-induced fibrosarcomas in mice, can vary widely in their specific immunogenicity, the nature of the effector cells capable of inducing their destruction, and the functional and histological changes in lymphoid tissues that accompany their growth (Kearney and Nelson, 1973; Kearney *et al.*, 1975; Simes *et al.*, 1975; D. S. Nelson and R. Kearney, unpublished observations).

The clearest examples of macrophages contributing to depression of lymphocyte responses come from the studies of Kirchner *et al.* (1974a,b, 1975a,b) on mice bearing Moloney sarcoma virus-induced tumors. Spleen cells from such mice had grossly decreased responses to PHA and Con A, significantly decreased responses to PWM, but only slightly decreased responses to LPS. Passage through rayon columns restored the responsiveness and removed 75% of the cells. The depressed response could thus be due to the operation of suppressor cells or to dilution of responsive cells. Responsiveness was restored by treatment with iron and a magnet or with carrageenan, but not by irradiation. Addition of cells from the spleens or peritoneal cavities of tumor-bearing animals inhibited the responses of normal spleen cells. Thus, whether or not a dilution effect was occurring, there was clear evidence for the existence of suppressor cells with the properties of macrophages. Suppressor cells were also detected in the spleens of Moloney sarcoma-bearing mice by Gorczynski (1974) who found that they were susceptible to treatment with anti-immunoglobulin sera and complement; this suggested that they were B cells, but the possibility that they were macrophages bearing large amounts of cytophilic immunoglobulin cannot be excluded. The suppressor cells in both sets of experiments were wholly resistant to treatment with anti-θ serum and complement, clearly eliminating the possibility that suppressor T cells (Gershon, 1974) made any direct contribution.

In somewhat more extensive experiments, Kirchner *et al.* (1974a) found that the spleens of mice bearing primary methylcholanthrene-induced sarcomas had depressed responses to PHA. Although cells actively depressing PHA responses of normal lymphocytes were not identified, the spleen cells inhibited the growth of a lymphoma (Kirchner *et al.*, 1975a; see Section V). Konda *et al.* (1973) and Smith and Konda (1973) made extensive studies with transplanted methylcholanthrene-induced sarcomas, particularly one each in CBA and C57Bl mice. The PHA responses of the spleens of the tumor-bearing mice were decreased on a "per cell" basis, whereas the responses of B cells to LPS were normal, on the same basis. There was, in fact, only a relative decrease in T cell numbers, with an absolute increase in T cell numbers outweighed by a greater absolute increase in B cell numbers. Here a dilution effect could be operating, but a role for suppressor cells clearly cannot be excluded.

The direct addition of normal macrophages in excessive numbers has long been known to inhibit primary antibody production by cultured mouse lymphoid cells (Perkins and Makinodan, 1965; Parkhouse and Dutton, 1966; Diener *et al.*, 1970). Likewise, the *in vitro* induction of a cell-mediated immune reaction of mouse spleen cells to xenogeneic target cells is inhibited by excess macrophages, although their presence in moderate numbers is required for induction (Lonai and Feldman, 1971). The response of rat splenic B cells to LPS was noted above not to require macrophages; peritoneal macrophages in excessive numbers (5% of the number of lymphocytes) can profoundly depress the response (Yoshinaga *et al.*, 1972). DNA synthesis by unstimulated cultured rat spleen cells was found to be inhibited by excess macrophages (Waldman and Gottlieb, 1973). The rat lymph node cell response to PHA is also suppressed, at high PHA doses, by excess macrophages (again 5%) (Yoshinaga and Waksman, 1973; Folch *et al.*, 1973). With spleen cells, however, the response to PHA was increased by removal of adherent cells on glass wool columns, and the addition of peritoneal macrophages (2%) had no depressive effect; this was also true when high doses of PHA were used. Folch *et al.* postulated the presence in rat spleen of a population of adherent cells, differing from peritoneal macrophages, which exerted a suppressive effect on T cells at high PHA doses. A similar effect was exerted on mixed lymphocyte reactions (Folch and Waksman, 1974b). More extensive studies (Folch and Waksman, 1974a) revealed that suppressor cell activity of this type was readily demonstrable in spleens of young rats, but that the behavior of spleen cells changed as the rats aged. Unfractionated, the spleen cells of older rats responded more vigorously than did those of young rats. The response was lowered after removal of adherent cells but could then be restored by the addition of peritoneal macrophages.

Keller (1974; Chapter 19) has found that proliferation of rat lymphocytes in response to Con A, LPS, or allogeneic cells was depressed or abolished by excessive numbers of *activated* peritoneal macrophages, but scarcely or not affected by normal macrophages. ("Activation" was induced by intraperitoneal injection of proteose–peptone broth). In his experiments and those of Yoshinaga, Folch, and Waksman, the macrophages were substantially free of other cells. For reasons that are unclear, but which may be technical, Keller's results differ in detail from those of Yoshinaga, Folch, and Waksman, but again in principle strongly support the concept of suppressor macrophages.

There is thus evidence from studies in both rats and mice that a variety of lymphoid cell responses to specific and nonspecific stimuli can be inhibited by macrophages that either are present in excess numbers or have been activated. The same sets of experiments have yielded evidence that macrophages can promote or stimulate responses (see Section II) and that cells other than macrophages can also exert a nonspecific inhibitory effect. This last point highlights the importance of precise definitions and/or characterization of inhibitory or stimulatory cells, in this case the fallacy of equating "adherent cells" with "macrophages." Passage of cells from spleens, or other lymphoid organs, through columns of fibers or beads of glass, rayon, nylon, etc., certainly removes *most* macrophages. It also removes many other cells—30–50% of the total nucleated cell population of rat or mouse spleens or lymph nodes, in our hands and those of others (Folch *et al.*, 1973; Nelson and Shneider, 1974)—and selectively enriches for T cells (Julius *et al.*, 1973). Conversely, the peritoneal cavities, stimulated or unstimulated, of mice, rats, and guinea pigs contain cells other than macrophages; some potential pitfalls of equating "peritoneal cells" or "peritoneal exudate cells" with "macrophages" are illustrated in Section IV.

IV. MODE OF ACTION OF MACROPHAGES IN DEPRESSING LYMPHOCYTE RESPONSES

The two principal questions which now arise are the following. Do macrophages depress lymphocyte responses by a mechanism predominantly cytotoxic, or by one predominantly cytostatic? Does the mechanism of depression mainly involve cell contact, or does it mainly involve the production of a soluble mediator? Attempts to answer these questions involve a preliminary consideration of the target cell specificity of the depressive effect of macrophages, discussed again in Section V, and a consideration of the relation of soluble depressive factors produced by macrophages to other depressive factors.

Much of the current interest in macrophages has been stimulated by the compelling evidence that macrophages, acting in a variety of ways, can exert a cytolytic, cytotoxic, or cytostatic* effect on many target cells (see Chapters 18 to 21). The *nonspecific* effects of macrophages, activated or otherwise, can be of any of these sorts (Lohmann-Matthes, Chapter 18; Keller, Chapter 19; Alexander and Evans, Chapter 21; Hibbs, 1974). Very little evidence is available concerning the mode of action of macrophages (activated or otherwise) on normal lymphoid cells. Waldman and Gottlieb (1973) found that inhibition by peritoneal cells of lymphocyte DNA synthesis was not accompanied by ^{51}Cr release, indicating an absence of cytolytic activity. The evidence summarized by Keller (Chapter 19) suggests that the effect of activated rat macrophages on mitogen-stimulated cells is cytostatic and reversible. Lymphomas have been used as targets for macrophages. The extent to which the susceptibilities of murine lymphomas reflect those of replicating normal lymphoid cells is, of course, debatable. There are, however, suggestions from a variety of experimental approaches that specifically immune T cells rapidly exert a predominantly cytolytic effect, whereas the nonspecific effect of activated macrophages is cytostatic, or, if prolonged, cytotoxic (Grant and Alexander, 1974; Olivotto and Bomford, 1974; Kirchner *et al.,* 1975a,b).

The roles of contact and soluble medators are still not clearly defined. In a negative way, the failure of culture supernatants to inhibit normal lymphocyte responses suggested that cell contact might be very important (Perkins and Makinodan, 1965; Diener *et al.,* 1970; Scott, 1972b; Sjöberg, 1972). When nonlymphoid cells are used as targets of activated macrophages, nonspecific cytotoxicity depends on cell contact (Hibbs, 1974). Several investigators have found that macrophage culture supernatants could inhibit lymphoid cell proliferation, though generally to a lesser extent than could live macrophages added in numbers equivalent to those producing the supernatants. This has been reported for mouse spleen cells producing antibody in culture (Hoffmann and Dutton, 1971) (their supernatants promoted antibody production in smaller quantities), for mitogen-stimulated mouse lymphocytes (Nelson, 1973) and rat lymphocytes (Keller, Chapter 19), for unstimulated rat lymphocytes (Waldman and Gottlieb, 1973), and for a leukemia (Olivotto and Bomford, 1974). If the effect of such supernatant factors is truly cytostatic, it is likely that they differ from the cytolytic factor released from macro-

* The words are used in the following senses. Cytolytic, causing overt lysis of cells revealed by release of an intracellular marker, e.g., ^{51}Cr. Cytostatic, inhibiting the proliferation of cells as reflected in uptake of DNA precursors. Cytotoxic, a term for the gray area in which cell survival is diminished but there is no demonstration of cytolysis or cytostasis.

phages in the experiments of Sintek and Pincus (1970), McIvor and Weiser (1971), and Melsom *et al.* (1974).

Does a macrophage-produced soluble factor account entirely for the inhibitory effects of excess numbers or excessively active macrophages? In some of the experiments cited, soluble factors simply were not detected, although they were sought, and in others the soluble factors were less inhibitory than the parent macrophages. The detection of soluble inhibitors produced by macrophages is beset with technical problems, some of which are discussed below. It is conceivable or even probable that the factor(s) produced is unstable. The physically close association so often prevailing between macrophages and lymphocytes (Rosenthal *et al.*, Chapter 6) would enhance the effectiveness of molecules, especially unstable ones, just leaving the macrophages. The question is, however, unresolved.

Our own experiments on the production by stimulated macrophages of factor(s) depressing lymphocyte transformation suggest some insights into the immunoregulatory role of macrophages and provide some cautionary tales.

Our interest began with work on the nonspecific inhibitory effect on PHA-induced human lymphocyte transformation of serum from patients with leprosy (Nelson *et al.*, 1971). Serum factors depressing lymphocyte transformation are present in a wide variety of human conditions, particularly those in which there is some depression of cell-mediated immunity (reviewed by Nelson, 1975; Nelson and Gatti, 1976). Many of these conditions are also characterized by heavy macrophage involvement and/or granuloma formation, notably infections such as leprosy, histoplasmosis, and syphilis. In an attempt to set up an experimental model, we began by examining the effect of mouse serum on mouse spleen cell responses to mitogens. We found that normal mouse serum had an inhibitory effect on the responses to T and B cell mitogens and to allogeneic lymphocytes (Nelson and Shneider, 1974). Others had found a similar effect of normal mouse serum on primary antibody production to thymus-dependent antigens (Mishell and Dutton, 1967; Veit and Michael, 1972; Britton, 1972; Bullock and Möller, 1972). Mice with deficiencies in T cells following the administration of anti-thymocyte globulin after adult thymectomy alone or combined with X irradiation and bone marrow reconstitution or nude mice all had normal inhibitory activity in their serum. Mice subjected to procedures that resulted in macrophage stimulation had increased depressive activity in their serum. These included the induction of a graft versus host reaction, infection with BCG, infection with *Salmonella enteritidis* 11RX, and the injection of levamisole. Table I shows typical results and illustrates the lack of correlation of macro-

TABLE I

Effect of Abnormal Mouse Sera on Mouse Spleen Lymphocyte Responses to PHA

Procedure[a]	Extent[b] and time[c] of maximum depressive effect of serum	Extent[d] and time[c] of maximum stimulation of macrophage DNA synthesis
1. Injection of live BCG (second)	59%, 14 days	not done
2. Infection with *Salmonella enteritidis* 11RX	32%, 11 days	3.6%, 11 days
3. Injection of levamisole (25 μg, intravenously)	68%, 4 days	no change
4. Induction of graft versus host reaction	43%, 11 days	13.5%, 8 days

[a] 1, SW mice; 2 and 3, Balb/c mice; 4, 5×10^7 A/J spleen cells → (C57Bl/6J × A/J) F_1 mice.

[b] PHA-induced incorporation of tritiated thymidine in the presence of 5% test mouse serum, as a percentage of incorporation in the presence of 5% control mouse serum (see Nelson and Shneider, 1974).

[c] Time after procedure.

[d] Percentage of resident peritoneal macrophages synthesizing DNA (normal, 1–2%). Increases are frequently an expression of cell-mediated immunity (More *et al.*, 1973).

phage proliferation with the production of increased serum depressive activity.

The possibility that stimulated mouse macrophages produced a depressive factor(s) was investigated directly (Nelson, 1973). Mouse peritoneal cells were cultured in petri dishes, nonadherent cells being removed by vigorous washing after 3 hours of incubation. The washing procedure used left a population of adherent cells that was 95–99% macrophages as judged by morphology, phagocytosis of colloidal gold, and the possession of cytophilic antibody receptors (More *et al.*, 1973; Simes, 1973). Stimulated macrophages were obtained, for most experiments, from mice injected with LPS, and normal macrophages were obtained from uninjected mice. Table II summarizes typical results, showing that the supernatants from cultured macrophages taken from LPS-treated mice inhibited PHA-induced DNA synthesis by spleen cells. Table II also illustrates differences between two strains of mice in the extent and time course of the macrophage response. Normal macrophages have very rarely, in our hands, yielded inhibitory supernatants; generally the supernatants produce a mildly stimulatory effect, which is sometimes statistically sig-

TABLE II

Production of Lymphocyte Depressive Factor by Macrophages from Mice Injected with Endotoxin[a]

Strain	Time of harvest of macrophages[b] (days)	Transformation as percent of transformation in control supernatants[c] (mean ± SE)
CBA/J	1	45 ± 9
	2	33 ± 9
	3	114 ± 10
	4	122 ± 30
C57Bl/6J	1	59 ± 8
	2	49 ± 1
	3	66 ± 11
	4	51 ± 3

[a] Lipopolysaccharide (Boivin) of *Salmonella typhimurium* 400 μg subcutaneously.

[b] After endotoxin injection.

[c] PHA-induced transformation of mouse spleen lymphocytes in presence of stimulated macrophage supernatants. For details of methods, see Nelson (1973). Macrophages were cultured for 24 hours in medium RPMI 1640 containing $6\frac{1}{4}\%$ human serum. 4.5×10^6 spleen cells in 0.6 ml RPMI 1640 were mixed with 0.4 ml of supernatant and 0.1 ml PHA. Tritiated thymidine incorporation was measured after 48 hours.

nificant. Inhibitory supernatants have also been obtained from macrophages of mice with graft versus host reaction (Nelson, 1973) or injected with sheep red cells (D. S. Nelson and J. M. Penrose, unpublished results). Other basic experiments with macrophages from LPS-treated mice showed that the supernatants (a) depressed T cell responses (to PHA, Con A, and allogeneic spleen cells) but not B cell responses (to another LPS), (b) had a variably depressive effect on base line DNA synthesis, (c) were most depressive if present throughout the full period of culture with PHA and least depressive if present only late in the culture period, and (d) had their depressive effect overridden by a large dose of PHA. Experiments on the effect of mouse serum suggest that the activity of the *serum* factor is not directly related to macrophage proliferation (Table I). Experiments in which macrophages from normal or LPS-treated mice were cultured at varying densities similarly showed that the production of the inhibitory factor by macrophages depended on stimulation of the cells rather than on an increase in their number.

At one stage in our investigation of lymphocyte depressive factors produced by macrophages, we were disturbed by the lack of consistent results with cells from LPS-injected mice. A number of factors probably contributed to this, among them the differences in the responsiveness of different strains of mice (cf. Table I), the stress to the mice, associated with temporary accommodation in noisy quarters, and differences among human sera, routinely used in all the cultures, from different donors. An inhibitory effect of stress was noted by Folch and Waksman (1974a) in their studies of splenic suppressor cells, stressed rats (exposed to building construction noise!) losing their suppressor cells. Likewise, LAF produced by macrophages, or the detection of its activity, varies widely according to the source of xenogeneic serum (B. H. Waksman, personal communication). Perhaps most striking were the combined influences of the concentration of human serum in the test *lymphocyte* cultures and of the concentration of macrophage supernatants. Table III shows an illustrative experiment, the key findings in which are (1) that the same *amount* of supernatant in the presence of 4% normal human serum caused much more inhibition than it did in the presence of 2% serum; (2) that a distinct *potentiation* of the response by diluted supernatant from normal macrophages occurred, again only in the presence of the higher concentrations of serum; and (3) that the inhibitory effect of the supernatants from macrophages from treated mice was lost quite rapidly on dilution. That the experimental system is so susceptible to quite small variations in culture conditions indicates the need for very precise definition of conditions and suggests possible explanations for the failure of others to demonstrate activity in culture supernatants. Well-defined and technically adequate or appropriate conditions will allow answers to be obtained to important questions, for example, whether the inhibitory factor is related to LAF, perhaps representing a gross excess of LAF; whether it is preformed and released, or actively synthesized; and what its chemical nature may be.

Another technical point of very considerable importance is the necessity to avoid confusion between the population of macrophages and the total population of the peritoneal cavity, stimulated or unstimulated, of an experimental animal. We have found that supernatants from cultures from nonadherent peritoneal cells, or the total peritoneal cavity population, from normal mice have a profoundly inhibitory effect on PHA-induced transformation. This effect is lost after dialysis. Calderon *et al.* (1974) described an inhibitor of the proliferation of lymphoma cells found in supernatants of mouse peritoneal exudates. This factor(s) was dialyzable and was present in supernatants from peritoneal exudates from mice whose peritoneal macrophages were otherwise normal, or whose macrophages were activated following *Listeria monocytogenes* infection.

TABLE III

Effect of Xenogeneic Serum Concentration on the Effect of Mouse Macrophage Supernatants on PHA-Induced Lymphocyte Transformation[a]

Human serum in culture	Dilution of supernatant	DNA synthesis in supernatants		Inhibition (%)
		Normal[b]	Endotoxin[b]	
4%	4:5	63,321 ± 2,456	27,241 ± 3,721	57
	2:5	89,247 ± 4,415	43,593 ± 804	51
	1:5	58,721 ± 2,599	50,533 ± 1,768	14
	No supernatant	44,730 ± 2,305		
2%	2:5	75,292 ± 922	60,702 ± 1,562	17
	1:5	75,795 ± 1,881	70,078 ± 1,634	8
	No supernatant	66,695 ± 828		

[a] Cultures were set up of macrophages from CBA/J mice injected 72 hours previously with 300 μg of *Salmonella enteritidis* LPS (Boivin) and from normal CBA/J mice. After 3 hours in 35 mm plastic petri dishes, each containing peritoneal washings from 3 mice, the cultures were washed vigorously then incubated for a further 24 hours in medium RPMI 1640 with 5% heated (56°C, 30 minutes) human serum. The supernatants were added in 0.8 ml volumes undiluted, diluted 1:2, or diluted 1:4 to 0.2 ml of mouse spleen cells suspension containing 22×10^6 cells per ml of RPMI 1640. The diluents were RPMI 1640 containing heated normal human serum to maintain the concentration (now at 4%) or to halve it (to 2%). Controls received diluent only, containing normal human serum at the proper concentration. The cultures were stimulated with PHA, and tritiated thymidine incorporation was measured in the last 24 hours of a 48 hour culture period (Nelson, 1973; Nelson and Shneider, 1974).

[b] Normal, supernatants from macrophages of normal mice; endotoxin, supernatants from macrophages of mice injected with endotoxin.

Quite conceivably the factor(s) in these experiments was produced by contaminating nonadherent cells and not by macrophages. A dialyzable factor, inhibiting primary antibody production *in vitro,* was also found by Watson (1973) in supernatants from cultures of cells from the spleens of T cell-reconstituted irradiated mice. This activity, too, could have been derived from the T cells rather than from the residual radioresistant macrophages in the spleens.

The inhibitory effect of *activated* rat macrophages on rat lymphocyte responses to mitogens has been studied by Keller (Chapter 19) (see Section III above). He has found the effect to be attributable, at least in part, to a soluble factor. In his hands, normal macrophages did not either inhibit directly or produce a soluble inhibitor, but some of the experiments of Waldman and Gottlieb (1973) implicate a soluble, low molecular weight product in the depressive activity of normal rat macrophages.

Much less information is available about guinea pig macrophages. Rosenstreich and Wilton (1975) found that supernatants from macrophages in oil-induced peritoneal exudates of guinea pigs inhibited guinea pig lymphocyte responses to PHA; after dialysis, the inhibitory activity was lost and stimulatory activity became apparent (see Section II). We have likewise found that supernatants from guinea pig macrophages (normal or in oil-induced exudates) mildly inhibited guinea pig lymphocyte responses to PHA, but we have attempted no further characterization.

Even less is known about the possible production of soluble factors by human macrophages. Human lymphoblastoid cell lines have been reported to contain (Papageorgiou *et al.*, 1974) and release (Smith *et al.*, 1970; Hersh *et al.*, 1974) an inhibitory of lymphoid cell activity. An unusual glass-adherent malignant lymphoma cell line was also found to produce an inhibitory of human lymphocyte blastogenesis (Hersh and Drewinko, 1974). Such activity may be more closely related to the inhibitory activity found in cultures of "nonmacrophages" than to the activity in macrophage supernatants.

The present confused situation about soluble inhibitors from macrophages can receive only the most superficial summary, by reason of the technical difficulties outlined and species variations. It seems clear that macrophages can and do produce soluble inhibitors and that, in the case of mice and rats, stimulation of macrophages either is required for or greatly enhances the production of the inhibitors. It is not clear whether soluble factors account entirely for the inhibitory effects of macrophages. Nonadherent cells can produce potent inhibitors of lymphoid cell responses to antigens or mitogens. Macrophages can also produce factors essential for potentiating the responses of lymphoid cells to antigens or mitogens (Section II). The net effect of mixed populations of cells may be inhibitory or stimulatory, depending on culture conditions (see Armerding and Katz, 1974), the proportion of different cell types (Rich and Pierce, 1974; Kishimoto and Ishizaka, 1974), the degree of stimulation of macrophages (as described here), and the degree and nature of stimulation of other cells (Watson, 1973; Armerding and Katz, 1974; Rich and Pierce, 1974).

V. SIGNIFICANCE OF LYMPHOID CELL STIMULATION AND INHIBITION BY MACROPHAGES AND THEIR PRODUCTS

The most basic question one can ask is whether macrophages play an important or critical role in regulating, nonspecifically, the intensity of lymphoid cell responses to antigens. That they *can* do so is clearly apparent, especially in well-defined experimental situations, such as those described above involving *C. parvum,* graft versus host reactions, or Moloney virus-induced tumors. A particularly attractive hypothesis is that macrophages may play an important part in the homeostasis of cell-mediated immune reactions. This they could do in the following way. The interaction of effector T cells with antigen results in the production of lymphokines with a variety of effects, including chemotaxis, immobilization, and activation of macrophages (see Blanden *et al.*, Chapter 15). Once cells, especially activated macrophages, have accumulated in adequate numbers at a site of infection (or antigen concentration) it is in the interest of the host to halt the process, lest excessive tissue damage occur (see Allison and Davies, Chapter 17). The production by activated macrophages, in increasing amounts as they accumulate, of inhibitors of T cell activity would constitute an elegant mechanism for switching off cell-mediated immune reactions. A similar mechanism could operate in lymphoid tissues during the inductive phase of a cell-mediated immune response or possibly of a thymus-dependent humoral antibody response.

Although this hypothesis has attractions, its acceptance is hindered by two sets of arguments. First, the inhibitory effect of stimulated macrophages and their soluble products lacks target cell specificity. Not only are lymphocyte responses inhibited (Keller, Chapter 19) (Nelson, 1973), but stimulated rat macrophages exert a cytostatic effect on rapidly replicating cells of almost any sort regardless of tissue or species origin (Keller, Chapter 19). Arguing teleologically, the nonspecific cytostatic effects of macrophages may be a primitive defense mechanism that is utilized in the control of immunological processes, rather than one evolved specifically for such control. Nevertheless, as Keller points out, rapidly replicating lymphoid cells are among those most susceptible to inhibition by activated macrophages. Second, lymphoid cells, especially as blasts, themselves produce potent inhibitors, as noted above; they may therefore provide for their own homeostasis. The inhibitors produced by lymphoblastoid cell lines may have species and target cells specificity (Hersh and Drewinko, 1974), though an inhibitor produced by stimulated human and mouse normal lymphoid cells ("proliferation inhibiting factor") lacks such specificity (Badger *et al.*, 1973, 1974).

Regardless of its overall biological significance, the immunoregulatory effect exerted by macrophages may involve cell contact or it may involve soluble mediators. There is no doubt that soluble mediators exist and can be demonstrated. It is possible that they are unstable and that this instability affects the ease with which they can be demonstrated. Quite possibly a soluble mediator of considerable instability could nevertheless exert a drastic effect on cells in the immediate neighborhood; the microanatomical relations between macrophages and other cells in lymphoid tissues would then markedly influence the overall effects of the mediators (Basten and Mitchell, Chapter 3).

Whether soluble factors are involved or not, the pathways by which macrophages are induced to exert regulatory roles deserve further investigation. Although macrophage activation in microbial infections (Blanden *et al.*, Chapter 15) and graft versus host reactions (Sjöberg, 1972) requires the participation of effector T cells, macrophages can be stimulated to increased anticellular activity, adjuvant activity, or release of soluble inhibitors either in the absence of T cells (Woodruff *et al.*, 1973) or by LPS, which does not affect T cells and may affect macrophages directly (Alexander and Evans, 1971; Nelson, 1973) or by way of B cells (Wilton *et al.*, 1975). The mechanisms whereby the growth of Moloney virus-induced tumors, and possibly other tumors, stimulates macrophages seem particularly to deserve attention (see Section III).

The relationship between macrophage-produced soluble depressive factors and serum factors with similar effects has not been clarified. Normal human serum contains a factor referred to as immunoregulatory α-globulin (Cooperband *et al.*, 1972) or normal immunosuppressive protein (Nelken, 1975). The relationship between these proteins and the substances responsible for serum lymphocyte depressive activity in a variety of diseases remains to be clarified. Even further from clarification is the question of the origin of such factors from macrophages. With mice likewise, normal serum inhibits mitogen transformation of T and B cells, and serum from mice with stimulated macrophages is more inhibitory (Table I), but evidence of the identity of factors in normal and abnormal sera and those produced by macrophages is totally lacking.

Despite the scarcity of hard data, some brief speculations on the possible inhibitory role of macrophages in some experimental and clinical situations seem justified. The best evidence exists for such a role in the immunosuppression induced experimentally in graft versus host reactions and tumor carriage (Section III). The protection by macrophages of certain tumor cells from lymphocyte cytotoxicity may be an example of such an effect *in vitro* (Hersey and MacLennan, 1973). Where target cells are killed solely or primarily by cytolytic effector T cells, the presence of excess macrophages and/or activated macrophages can inhibit cytolysis (Kiessling *et al.*, 1974; Vasudevan *et al.*, 1974).

Antigenic competition, at least that of the "sequential" type (Taussig, 1973) could involve a nonspecific soluble inhibitor, perhaps produced by macrophages under the stimulating influence of T cells (Pross and Eidinger, 1974). A more general role for macrophages as mediators of effects of suppressor T cells has been suggested (Folch and Waksman, 1973; Gershon, 1974), but such a role would require that macrophages exert their effects over a very short range when *specific* suppression is involved.

Con A has a depressive effect on primary antibody production by mouse spleen cells *in vitro* (Dutton, 1972). This depends on the presence of T cells (Dutton, 1973), and a soluble noncytotoxic inhibitor has been implicated (Rich and Pierce, 1974). Again it is conceivable that macrophages stimulated as a consequence of Con A–T cell interaction are the source of the factor.

Immunodepression in some infections may be associated with macrophage proliferation and stimulation. This is noteworthy in leprosy, being most emphasized with the lepromatous type but also observed with the tuberculoid type (Bullock, 1968; Turk and Waters, 1971). There is no direct evidence that macrophages are directly or indirectly (by way of a soluble depressive factor) responsible for immunodepression in leprosy, but the possibility seems a likely one. Although less well worked out, malaria (Greenwood *et al.*, 1971) and trypanosomiasis (Mansfield and Wallace, 1974) may offer examples of similar phenomena. Immunodepression occurs during and after a wide variety of acute viral infections in man, notably measles (von Pirquet, 1908; Mellman and Wetton, 1963), but also including rubella (Kauffman *et al.*, 1974), influenza (Kantzler *et al.*, 1974), and infectious mononucleosis (Mangi *et al.*, 1974). Although some viruses may exert a direct effect on lymphocyte function, an indirect effect by way of macrophages may contribute to the depression in other cases.

In conclusion, it is apparent that macrophages can exert nonspecific immunoregulatory effects, but that there is a need for much further work at the technical, biological and clinical level before the nature and significance of these effects are understood.

ACKNOWLEDGMENTS

The work of the author's laboratory is supported by grants from the National Health and Medical Research Council, the New South Wales State Cancer Council, the Postgraduate Medical Foundation of the University of Sydney, and the Australian Kidney Foundation. The experiments described here were carried out with the assistance of Cynthia N. Shneider and Jean M. Penrose.

REFERENCES

Alexander, P., and Evans, R. (1971). *Nature (London), New Biol.* **232,** 76–78.
Alter, B. J., and Bach, F. H. (1970). *Cell. Immunol.* **1,** 207–218.
Armerding, D., and Katz, D. H. (1974). *J. Exp. Med.* **140,** 19–37.

Bach, F. H., Alter, B. J., Solliday, S., Zoschke, D. C., and Janis, M. (1970). *Cell. Immunol.* **1**, 219–227.
Badger, A. M., Cooperband, S. R., Merluzzi, V. J., and Green, J: A. (1973). *Clin. Exp. Immunol.* **15**, 435–443.
Badger, A. M., Cooperband, S. R., and Merluzzi, V. (1974). *J. Immunol.* **112**, 1435–1443.
Baker, M. A., and Taub, R. N. (1973). *Progr. Allergy* **17**, 227–299.
Bevan, M. J., Epstein, R., and Cohn, M. (1974). *J. Exp. Med.* **139**, 1025–1030.
Biniaminov, M., Ramot, B., and Novogrodsky, A. (1974). *Clin. Exp. Immunol.* **16**, 235–242.
Blaese, R. M., Martinez, C., and Good, R. A. (1964). *J. Exp. Med.* **119**, 211–224.
Blanden, R. V. (1969). *Transplantation* **7**, 484–497.
Blomgren, H. (1974). *Scand. J. Immunol.* **3**, 655–664.
Blythman, H. E., and Waksman, B. H. (1973). *J. Immunol.* **111**, 1081–1085.
Britton, S. (1972). *Scand. J. Immunol.* **1**, 361–370.
Britton, S. (1974). *Scand. J. Immunol.* **3**, 433–444.
Broome, J. D., and Jeng, M. W. (1973). *J. Exp. Med.* **138**, 574–592.
Bullock, W. E. (1968). *N. Engl. J. Med.* **278**, 298–304.
Bullock, W. W., and Möller, E. (1972). *Eur. J. Immunol.* **2**, 514–517.
Byfield, P., Christie, G. H., and Howard, J. G. (1973). *J. Immunol.* **111**, 72–81.
Calderon, J., Williams, R. T., and Unanue, E. R. (1974). *Proc. Nat. Acad. Sci. U.S.* **71**, 4273–4277.
Chen, C., and Hirsch, J. G. (1972). *J. Exp. Med.* **136**, 604–617.
Click, R. E., Benck, L., and Alter, B. J. (1972). *Cell. Immunol.* **3**, 156–160.
Cline, M. J., and Swett, V. C. (1968). *J. Exp. Med.* **128**, 1309–1325.
Cooperband, S. R., Badger, A. M., Davis, R. C., Schmid, K., and Mannick, J. A. (1972). *J. Immunol.* **109**, 154–163.
Cosenza, H., Leserman, L. D., and Rowley, D. A. (1971). *J. Immunol.* **107**, 414–421.
Diener, E., Shortman, K., and Russell, P. (1970). *Nature (London)* **225**, 731–732.
Dutton, R. W. (1972). *J. Exp. Med.* **136**, 1445–1460.
Dutton, R. W. (1973). *J. Exp. Med.* **138**, 1496–1505.
Dutton, R. W., Falkoff, R., Hirst, J. A., Hoffmann, M., Kappler, J. W., Kettman, J. R., Lesley, J. F., and Vann, D. (1971). *In* "Progress in Immunology" (B. Amos, ed.), Vol. 1, pp. 355–368. Academic Press, New York.
Epstein, L. B., Cline, M. J., and Merigan, T. C. (1971). *J. Clin. Invest.* **50**, 744–753.
Fanger, M. W., Hart, D. A., Wells, J. V., and Nisonoff, A. (1970). *J. Immunol.* **105**, 1043–1051.
Folch, H., and Waksman, B. H. (1973). *Cell. Immunol.* **9**, 12–24.
Folch, H., and Waksman, B. H. (1974a). *J. Immunol.* **113**, 127–139.
Folch, H., and Waksman, B. H. (1974b). *J. Immunol.* **113**, 140–144.
Folch, H., Yoshinaga, M., and Waksman, B. H. (1973). *J. Immunol.* **110**, 835–839.
Franzl, R. E., and McMaster, P. D. (1968). *J. Exp. Med.* **127**, 1087–1107.
Gershon, R. K. (1974). *Contemp. Top. Immunobiol.* **3**, 1–40.
Gery, I., and Waksman, B. H. (1972). *J. Exp. Med.* **136**, 143–155.
Gery, I., and Handschumacher, R. E. (1974). *Cell. Immunol.* **11**, 162–169.
Gery, I., Gershon, R. K., and Waksman, B. H. (1971). *J. Immunol.* **107**, 1778–1780.
Gery, I., Gershon, R. K., and Waksman, B. H. (1972). *J. Exp. Med.* **136**, 128–142.
Gisler, R. H., Staber, F., Rüde, E., and Dukor, P. (1973). *Eur. J. Immunol.* **3**, 650–652.
Gorczynski, R. M. (1974). *J. Immunol.* **112**, 1826–1838.

Gordon, J. (1968). *Proc. Soc. Exp. Biol. Med.* **127,** 30–33.

Grant, C. K., and Alexander, P. (1974). *Cell. Immunol.* **14,** 46–51.

Greenwood, B. M., Playfair, J. H. L., and Torrigiani, G. (1971). *Clin. Exp. Immunol.* **8,** 467–478.

Halpern, B. N., Prévot, A. R., Biozzi, G., Stiffel, C., Mouton, D., Morard, J. C., Bouthillier, Y., and Decreusefond, C. (1964). *J. Reticuloendothel. Soc.* **1,** 77–96.

Halpern, B., Fray, A., Crepin, Y., Platica, O., Corinet, A. M. Rabourdin, A., Sparros, L., and Isac, R. (1973). *In* "Immunopotentiation," Ciba Found. Symp. No. 18, New Ser., pp. 217–234. Associated Scientific Publishers, Amsterdam.

Hanifin, J. M., and Cline, M. J. (1970). *J. Cell Biol.* **46,** 97–105.

Heber-Katz, E., and Click, R. E. (1972). *Cell. Immunol.* **5,** 410–418.

Hersey, P., and MacLennan, I. C. M. (1973). *Immunology* **24,** 385–393.

Hersh, E. M., and Drewinko, B. (1974). *Cancer Res.* **34,** 215–220.

Hersh, E. M., and Harris, J. E. (1968). *J. Immunol.* **100,** 1184–1194.

Hersh, E. M., McCredie, K. B., and Freireich, E. J. (1974). *Clin. Exp. Immunol.* **17,** 463–473.

Hibbs, J. B., Jr. (1974). *Science* **184,** 468–471.

Hoffmann, M., and Dutton, R. W. (1971). *Science* **172,** 1047–1048.

Howard, J. G., and Woodruff, M. F. A. (1961). *Proc. Roy. Soc., Ser. B* **154,** 532–539.

Howard, J. G., Scott, M. T., and Christie, G. H. (1973). *In* "Immunopotentiation," Ciba Found. Symp. No. 18, New Ser., pp. 101–116. Associated Scientific Publishers, Amsterdam.

Hunter, P., and Kettman, J. R. (1974). *Proc. Nat. Acad. Sci. U.S.* **71,** 512–516.

Julius, M. H., Simpson, E., and Herzenberg, L. A. (1973). *Eur. J. Immunol.* **3,** 645–649.

Kantzler, G. B., Lauteria, S. F., Cusumano, C. L., Lee, J. D., Ganguly, R., and Waldman, R. H. (1974). *Infec. Immunity* **10,** 996–1002.

Kauffman, C. A., Phair, J. P., Linnemann, C. C., and Schiff, G. M. (1974). *Infec. Immunity* **10,** 212–215.

Kearney, R., and Nelson, D. S. (1973). *Aust. J. Exp. Biol. Med. Sci.* **51,** 723–735.

Kearney, R., Basten, A., and Nelson, D. S. (1975). *Int. J. Cancer* **15,** 438–450.

Keller, R. (1974). *Immunology* **27,** 285–298.

Kiessling, R., Bataillon, G., Lamon, E. W., and Klein, E. (1974). *Int. J. Cancer* **14,** 642–648.

Kirchner, H., Herberman, R. B., Glaser, M., and Lavrin, D. H. (1974a). *Cell. Immunol.* **13,** 32–40.

Kirchner, H., Chused, T. M., Herberman, R., Holden, H. T., and Lavrin, D. H. (1974b). *J. Exp. Med.* **139,** 1473–1487.

Kirchner, H., Holden, H. T., and Herberman, R. B. (1975a). *J. Immunol.* in press

Kirchner, H., Muchmore, A. V., Chused, T. M., Holden, H. T., and Heberman, R. B. (1975b). *J. Immunol.* **114,** 206–210.

Kishimoto, T., and Ishizaka, K. (1974). *J. Immunol.* **112,** 1685–1697.

Konda, S., Nakao, Y., and Smith, R. J. (1973). *Cancer Res.* **33,** 2247–2256.

Levis, W. R., and Robbins, J. H. (1970). *J. Immunol.* **104,** 1295–1299.

Lonai, P., and Feldman, M. (1971). *Immunology* **21,** 861–867.

McIvor, K. L., and Weiser, R. S. (1971). *Immunology* **20,** 307–313.

Mangi, R. J., Niederman, J. C., Kelleher, J. E., Dwyer, J. M., Evans, A. S., and Kantor, F. S. (1974). *N. Engl. J. Med.* **291,** 1149–1153.

Mansfield, J. M., and Wallace, J. H. (1974). *Infec. Immunity* **10,** 335–339.

Mellman, W. J., and Wetton, R. (1963). *J. Lab. Clin. Med.* **61,** 453–458.

Melsom, H., Kearny, G., Gruca, S., and Seljelid, R. (1974). *J. Exp. Med.* **140,** 1085–1096.
Mishell, R. I., and Dutton, R. W. (1967). *J. Exp. Med.* **126,** 423–442.
Mitchell, M. S., Kirkpatrick, D., Mokyr, M. B., and Gery, I. (1973). *Nature (London), New Biol.* **243,** 216–218.
More, D. G., Penrose, J. M., Kearney, R., and Nelson, D. S. (1973). *Int. Arch. Allergy Appl. Immunol.* **44,** 611–630.
Namba, Y., and Hanaoka, M. (1972). *J. Immunol.* **109,** 1193–1200.
Nelken, D. (1973). *J. Immunol.* **110,** 1161–1162.
Nelson, D. S. (1973). *Nature (London)* **246,** 306–307.
Nelson, D. S. (1974). *Transplant. Rev.* **19,** 226–254.
Nelson, D. S. (1975). *In* "Nuclear Techniques in Helminthology Research," Proc. Panel, Nairobi, 1973, pp. 19–40. IAEA, Vienna.
Nelson, D. S., and Gatti, R. A. (1976). *Progr. Allergy* (to be published).
Nelson, D. S., and Schneider, D. N. (1974). *Eur. J. Immunol.* **4,** 79–86.
Nelson, D. S., Nelson, M., Thurston, J. M., Waters, M. F. R., and Pearson, J. M. H. (1971). *Clin. Exp. Immunol.* **9,** 33–41.
Novogrodsky, A., and Gery, I. (1972). *J. Immunol.* **109,** 1278–1281.
Olivotto, M., and Bomford, R. (1974). *Int. J. Cancer* **13,** 478–488.
Oppenheim, J. J., Leventhal, B. G., and Hersh, E. M. (1968). *J. Immunol.* **101,** 262–270.
Papageorgiou, P. S., Tibbetts, L., Sorkin, C. F., and Glade, P. R. (1974). *Cell. Immunol.* **11,** 354–366.
Parkhouse, R. M. E., and Dutton, R. W. (1966). *J. Immunol.* **97,** 663–669.
Perkins, E., and Makinodan, T. (1965). *J. Immunol.* **94,** 765–777.
Pierce, C. W., Kapp, J. A., Wood, D. D., and Benacerraf, B. (1974). *J. Immunol.* **112,** 1181–1189.
Pross, H. F., and Eidinger, D. (1974). *Advan. Immunol.* **18,** 133–168.
Rich, R. R., and Pierce, C. W. (1974). *J. Immunol.* **112,** 1360–1368.
Rode, H. N., and Gordon, J. (1974). *Cell. Immunol.* **13,** 87–94.
Rosenstreich, D. L., and Wilton, J. M. (1975). *In* "Immune Recognition" (A. S. Rosenthal, ed.), pp. 113–132. Academic Press, New York.
Rowley, D. (1955). *Lancet* **1,** 232–234.
Rubin, A. S., MacDonald, A. B., and Coons, A. H. (1974). *J. Exp. Med.* **139,** 439–444.
Schrader, J. W. (1973). *J. Exp. Med.* **138,** 1466–1480.
Scott, M. T. (1972a). *Cell. Immunol.* **5,** 459–468.
Scott, M. T. (1972b). *Cell Immunol.* **5,** 469–479.
Shilo, M. (1959). *Annu. Rev. Microbiol.* **13,** 255–278.
Shortman, K., and Palmer, J. (1971). *Cell. Immunol.* **2,** 399–410.
Simes, R. J. (1973). Thesis, Department of Bacteriology, University of Sydney, Sydney, Australia.
Simes, R. J., Kearney, R., and Nelson, D. S. (1975). *Immunology* **29,** 343–352.
Sintek, D. E., and Pincus, W. B. (1970). *J. Reticuloendothel. Soc.* **8,** 508–521.
Sjöberg, O. (1972). *Clin. Exp. Immunol.* **12,** 365–375.
Sjöberg, O., Andersson, J., and Möller, G. (1972). *J. Immunol.* **109,** 1379–1385.
Sjöberg, O., Möller, G., and Andersson, J. (1973). *Clin. Exp. Immunol.* **13,** 213–223.
Smith, R. T. (1972). *N. Engl. J. Med.* **287,** 439–450.
Smith, R. T., and Konda, S. (1973). *Int. J. Cancer* **12,** 577–588.
Smith, R. T., Bausher, J. A. C., and Adler, W. H. (1970). *Amer. J. Pathol.* **60,** 495–504.
Taussig, M. J. (1973). *Curr. Top. Microbiol. Immunol.* **60,** 125–174.

Turk, J. L., and Waters, M. F. R. (1971). *Clin. Exp. Immunol.* **8,** 363–376.

Vasudevan, D. M., Brunner, K. T., and Cerottini, J.-C. (1974). *Int. J. Cancer* **14,** 301–313.

Veit, B. C., and Michael, J. G. (1972). *Nature (London), New Biol.* **235,** 238–240.

von Pirquet, C. (1908). *Deut. Med. Wochenschr.* **34,** 1297–1300.

Waldman, S. R., and Gottlieb, A. A. (1973). *Cell. Immunol.* **9,** 142–156.

Warr, G. W., and Šljivić, V. S. (1974). *Clin. Exp. Immunol.* **17,** 519–532.

Watson, J. (1973). *J. Immunol.* **111,** 1301–1313.

Watson, J., Thoman, M., Ralph, P., and Trenkner, E. (1974). *J. Immunol.* **112,** 1873–1883.

Wilton, J. M., Rosenstreich, D. L., and Oppenheim, J. J. (1975). *J. Immunol.* **114,** 388–393.

Wood, D. D., and Gaul, S. L. (1974). *J. Immunol.* **113,** 925–933.

Woodruff, M. F. A., and Dunbar, N. (1973). *In* "Immunopotentiation," Ciba Found. Symp. No. 18, New Ser., pp. 287–300. Associated Scientific Publishers, Amsterdam.

Woodruff, M., Dunbar, N., and Ghaffar, A. (1973). *Proc. Roy. Soc., Ser. B* **184,** 97–102.

Yashphe, D. J. (1971). *In* "Immunological Parameters of Host-Tumor Relationships (D. W. Weiss, ed.), pp. 90–107. Academic Press, New York.

Yoshinaga, M., and Waksman, B. H. (1973). *Ann. Immunol. Inst. Pasteur* **124C,** 97–120.

Yoshinaga, M., Yoshinaga, A., and Waksman, B. H. (1972). *J. Exp. Med.* **136,** 956–961.

10

Macrophage Membranes

Janet M. Oliver and Richard D. Berlin

I. Introduction 259
II. Probes of Macrophage Surface Organization 261
III. Random Mobility of Macrophage Surface Proteins 262
IV. Organized Movement of Macrophage Surface Elements 264
V. Control of Translational Movement of Receptors and Transport Proteins within the Plane of the Membrane 266
VI. Summary 271
References 272

I. INTRODUCTION

The macrophage participates in biological phenomena primarily through its surface. Phagocytosis, pinocytosis, cell recognition, antigen binding, etc., are essentially surface phenomena. Much is known in a descriptive sense about the presence of surface receptors, for example, but on the whole observations on macrophage surfaces have not been put in the perspective of modern theories of membrane physiology nor correlated with observations on other cell types not generally in the purview of immunologists. On the other hand, it is often not appreciated that the macrophage has several unique advantages in the study of membrane phenomena which are applicable to all cells. In this chapter we shall indicate the general status of information on macrophage surfaces and interpret it in the light of current membranology. At the same time we shall point out some important insights gained through macrophage studies.

The membrane of an animal cell can best be viewed in terms of Singer's (1974) "fluid mosaic membrane" model. According to this now familiar scheme, the cell surface consists of a bilayer of phospholipid in which proteins are embedded, their hydrophobic regions inserting into the lipid and hydrophilic regions extending into the aqueous phase. Proteins may be associated with one or other leaflet of the bilayer or may extend through the bilayer forming a bridge between the cytoplasm and the extracellular milieu. The model predicts that there are no long-range forces within the membrane restraining the free diffusion of the proteins so that they tend to assume a random or homogeneous topographical distribution. However, recent studies suggest that the distribution is not always random. At least under some circumstances subcellular structures act to constrain or even to direct the movement of membrane proteins (Berlin *et al.*, 1974).

The macrophage provides an ideal model system to study membrane organization and function and to test the fluid mosaic model. Sufficient numbers of cells can be obtained from peritoneal exudates and alveolar wash fluid for compositional analyses of isolated membranes, and the cells can be maintained in long-term tissue culture so that studies of membrane turnover by radioactive tracer techniques are possible. Furthermore, macrophages express several distinct types of surface receptor proteins that bind particulates by either immunological or nonimmunological mechanisms, thus providing specific markers for studies of surface topography. Other functional markers, such as activities of surface enzymes and membrane transport carriers, are available to complement and extend receptor studies. Importantly, macrophages are also capable of removing a large proportion of the plasma membrane during pinocytosis and phagocytosis. The membrane is thus sampled for the distribution of surface markers during a physiologically significant cell activity.

We will review and sometimes reinterpret current information about the mobility (random and nonrandom) of macrophage surface elements under various conditions. We will also discuss the role of two classes of subcellular structures, microtubules (MT) and microfilaments (MF), in regulating macrophage surface topography and function. We have been highly selective in the choice of material, taking the opportunity to present in a concise manner a new framework in which to study the role of the macrophage surface in biological events. We apologize in advance for the omission of a great deal of significant data, for example, on the composition and turnover of macrophage membranes and on the nature of membrane receptors, which have been discussed in other published reviews (e.g., Unanue, 1972; Gordon and Cohn, 1973) and are presented elsewhere in this book.

II. PROBES OF MACROPHAGE SURFACE ORGANIZATION

As noted above, macrophages express many different surface receptors, and these can all be regarded as potential probes of surface topography. Most have not been identified biochemically with any degree of precision, but all of them can be recognized by specific binding reactions. We will simply list properties that facilitate studies of membrane organization.

The best characterized group of receptors are the Fc receptors that bind γ-globulins (IgG), either free or in the form of antigen–antibody complexes, through the Fc segments of the globulin molecules (Berken and Benacerraf, 1966). The Fc receptor is a particularly useful marker, since it is found on all macrophages and is stable during long-term culture (Rabinovitch and De Stefano, 1972). Its chemical nature is unclear. It is reported to be stable to trypsin and other proteolytic enzymes (LoBuglio and Reinehard, 1970) and to neuraminidase but can be destroyed by crude phospholipases (Allen and Cook, 1970) (which may also cause extensive cell damage and so represent a nonspecific destruction of the receptor). Receptor activity is demonstrated by exposing macrophages to antibody-coated particles, such as red blood cells (RBC), or by using antigen–antibody complexes in a soluble or aggregated form (Arend and Mannik, 1972; Steinman and Cohn, 1972). Antibody-coated RBC attach in characteristic rosette forms and are subsequently ingested by the cell.

Macrophages can also bind erythrocyte–antibody–complement complexes via a receptor for the C3 factor of complement (Lay and Nussenzweig, 1969). Trypsinization abolishes binding. It is not yet clear whether the C3 binding is to a specific membrane receptor or to cell-bound immunoglobulin, since macrophages lose reactivity in long-term culture (Rabinovitch and De Stefano, 1972).

Other macrophage receptors that are less well characterized include a class of nonspecific receptors (Steinman and Cohn, 1972) that binds particles, such as latex beads, protein aggregates, aldehyde-treated RBC, and hemocyanin. Binding, movement, and internalization of hemocyanin can be visualized directly by electron microscopy (Unanue and Calderon, 1975). In addition, mouse macrophages express specific H-2 antigens that bind antibody-coated RBC (Gordon and Cohn, 1973).

All macrophages bind an array of plant lectins. These agglutinins bind with specific carbohydrate residues of surface glycoproteins or glycolipids. Competing hapten sugars inhibit binding and can displace bound lectins from their receptors. Lectins provide particularly convenient tools for mapping surface topography, since they are readily purified, can be labeled with radioactive and fluorescent markers (Fig. 1) and can be visualized under the electron microscope by several techniques involving their conjugation to hemocyanin, ferritin, and horseradish peroxidase (Oliver, 1975).

The binding of migration inhibition factor (MIF) to macrophages is analogous to lectin binding (Remold, 1973). Macrophages treated with trypsin or α-fucosidase are no longer influenced by MIF, suggesting that the MIF receptor is a specific glycoprotein. In addition, the MIF effect is specifically inhibited by α-fucose.

Thus, receptors for IgG (Fc), complement, phagocytic particles, lectins, and even MIF, as well as specific membrane antigens, all represent potential markers for the study of the distribution and mobility of macrophage surface components. As noted above, still other probes of surface topography are available. Transport carriers for essential nutrients, and membrane-associated enzymes, such as ATPase and 5′-nucleotidase, have been used to study the topography of macrophage membranes.

III. RANDOM MOBILITY OF MACROPHAGE SURFACE PROTEINS

The elegant cell fusion studies of Gordon and Cohn (1970, 1971, 1973) establish that at least under some conditions macrophage surface proteins can diffuse at random in the lipid membrane, as predicted by the fluid mosaic membrane model. They fused mouse macrophages and mouse melanoma cells with Sendai virus and followed the fate of two macrophage membrane markers, the Fc receptor and membrane ATPase, neither of which is present on the melanoma cell. The heterokaryons expressed Fc receptor activity (measured by uptake of antibody-coated RBC) shortly after fusion but activity was lost over the next 12 hours. Treatment of these 12-hour heterokaryons with trypsin appeared to unmask the receptor, which was lost again on further cultivation. However, both inhibition of heterokaryon protein synthesis by cycloheximide and inhibition of melanoma cell RNA synthesis by drugs or UV irradiation before fusion blocked the "masking" of the Fc receptor in heterokaryons. Thus, the loss of Fc binding activity was due to proteins coded by melanoma RNA in the hybrid and not to a simple loss of a macrophage membrane component.

The interpretation of these experiments can be enriched by concepts derived from recent studies on the surfaces of fibroblasts. It has long been known that viral transformed cells are more agglutinable by plant lectins, such as concanavalin A (Con A), than normal parental cells. This increased agglutinability is correlated with the distribution of surface-bound Con A into clusters on the malignant cell (Nicolson, 1973). The clustering of Con A presumably increases the density of cell–cell Con A bridges at sites of contact between cells, thereby favoring their agglutination. Recently it has become clear that the clusters of Con A are induced by addition of the multivalent Con A (Rosenblith *et al.*, 1973). That is, Con A receptors are inherently disperse over all surfaces, but in transformed cells they can be cross-linked by the multivalent ligand (Con A) and drawn into patches. Light trypsinization enables Con A to induce clusters even in normal cells (Berlin, 1975).

By analogy, it is probable that the binding of antibody-coated RBC by Fc receptors requires movement of these receptors from a random distribution into aggregates or clusters on the macrophage surface to form multiple bridges at points of contact between the macrophage and RBC. The functional assay for Fc receptor activity, therefore, is not simply a measure of existence of receptors, but also of their ability to move within the surface. Consequently, the apparent loss of Fc receptors after heterokaryon formation could be due to their effective immobilization. Conversely the "unmasking" of Fc receptors by trypsinization could be the result of movement of Fc receptors into clusters. According to this interpretation, Fc receptors do not disappear with heterokaryon formation or reappear after trypsinization, rather their capacity to move within the membrane is altered. This hypothesis makes the study of macrophage heterokaryons of potentially even greater importance, since the forces that control the movement of surface proteins and receptors are key to the understanding of a broad range of biological phenomena, including the nature of the transformed or malignant state.

The distribution of surface ATPase in the hybrids was also observed by cytochemical techniques. The unfused macrophages showed a randomly distributed label, while little reaction product was formed on the surface of unfused melanoma cells. Immediately after fusions the reaction product was distributed in isolated patches on the heterokaryon membrane. However, within a short time the enzyme became evenly distributed on the surface of the heterokaryon. This shift in distribution indicates translation movement of the ATPase in the plane of the membrane.

These data provide some of the most compelling evidence now available for the ability of proteins to diffuse in the membrane and achieve a homogeneous surface distribution. They are in some respects more satisfactory than the more widely quoted experiments of Frye and Edidin (1970), who reported a similar random mixing of antigen–antibody complexes in mouse–human fibroblast hybrids. In Frye and Edidin's study, the possibility that cross-linking of multivalent antibodies with surface antigens induced redistribution of antigens cannot be excluded. Gordon and Cohn, on the other hand, studied the distribution of an enzyme cytochemically, where the added markers (enzyme substrates) are highly unlikely to change the topographical distribution of the enzyme.

IV. ORGANIZED MOVEMENT OF MACROPHAGE SURFACE ELEMENTS

In addition to random diffusion of macrophage membrane elements, which has been demonstrated in a restricted number of situations, there is very good evidence that macrophage surface proteins and lipids can move in a *directed* manner during the physiologically important process of phagocytosis.

The first evidence for this came from studies in our laboratory on the fate of membrane transport carriers for amino acids and purine bases and nucleosides after removal of membrane by extensive phagocytosis of latex beads (Tsan and Berlin, 1971). Between 30 and 50% of the surface membrane of alveolar macrophages in monolayer culture was internalized during phagocytosis. The cell monolayers were then tested for their ability to transport nutrients using a technique that permitted measurement of the initial rate of influx. The experimental results established that membrane transport was completely unchanged after phagocytic internalization of a large proportion of the total membrane. Other studies showed that no new compensatory transport sites were inserted into the membrane during phagocytosis. This clearly indicates that transport carriers are excluded from phagocytic areas of the membrane and are selectively preserved on the cell surface. Further study showed that rabbit peritoneal polymorphonuclear leukocytes (PMN), like macrophages, also exclude transport carriers from the membrane that engulfs phagocytic particles.

In contrast to transport carriers, macrophages and PMN selectively include surface glycoprotein receptors for plant lectins in phagocytic vesicles. Lutton (1973) showed that binding of [^{125}I]Con A to monolayers of macrophages is reduced by 25–30% immediately after phagocytosis of latex beads. Binding activity rose progressively toward the original levels during the first 8 hours after phagocytosis, and cycloheximide prevented this recovery of binding. Similarly we have titrated receptors for Con A and another plant lectin, *Ricinus communis* agglutinin (RCA), on isolated membranes of PMN before and after phagocytic ingestion of bovine serum albumin-coated paraffin oil droplets. These cells show a 40 to 50% decrease in the surface density of lectin binding sites that develops in parallel with the degree of phagocytes (Oliver *et al.*, 1974).

A further example of nonrandom movement of surface proteins during phagocytosis in macrophages was described by Schmidt and Douglas (1972). Cells were allowed to engulf polystyrene particles or formaldehyde-pretreated sheep erythrocytes for 45 minutes, then the phagocytic particles were removed and the cells maintained in culture. Binding and/or phagocytosis of antibody-coated sheep or human red cells was used to detect the IgG receptor at various times after phagocytosis. Before phagocytosis greater than 90% of macrophages showed IgG receptor activity. However, in the first 10 minutes after removing the latex particles or formaldehyde-treated RBC, IgG receptors were detected in only 9% of macrophages. Receptor activity increased with time until at 6 hours after phagocytosis 78% of macrophages again showed binding and uptake of antibody-coated RBC. Cycloheximide prevented the reappearance of the receptor. We interpret these data, like Lutton's data with Con A receptors, as evidence for selective internalization of IgG receptors during phagocytosis followed by synthesis and replacement of new receptors.

In addition to partitioning of membrane proteins into or out of phagocytic vesicles, there may also be segregation of membrane phospholipids during phagocytosis. Mason and co-workers (1972) compared the lipid composition of rabbit alveolar macrophages and of phagocytic vesicles isolated from these cells. They observed higher cholesterol to phospholipid ratios in the vesicles than in whole cells or in cell pellet fractions. In addition, there were significant differences in phospholipid composition between these fractions, and, in general, the phospholipids of the vesicle fraction contained more saturated and less polyunsaturated fatty acids than whole cells or cell pellets. A higher degree of saturation in fatty acids from phagocytic vesicle membranes than from surface membranes has also been demonstrated in PMN by Mason *et al.* and by Smolen and Shohet (1974). These differences could result from metabolic events occurring during phagocytosis which alter fatty acids, as suggested by Shohet. Alternatively during phagocytosis the fatty acids could be partitioned so that phosphatides containing more saturated fatty acids are interiorized.

Thus, the ability to show nonrandom or directed movement of certain surface elements (transport carriers, IgG and lectin receptors, and phospholipids) would seem to be a general property of leukocytes. The potential significance of the partitioning of surface proteins and lipids during phagocytosis is that certain functions are preserved at the surface, while, on the other hand, in the absence of certain receptors, the phagocyte becomes refractory to specific stimuli. Moreover the unique composition of the phagocytic vesicle that results from partitioning of membrane components may determine the fate of endocytized materials.

These data have been obtained in phagocyte systems and are of course relevant to the processing of particulate antigens. However, there is some reason to suppose that similar segregative movements occur with the binding and interiorization of macromolecules. For example, binding of Con A or RCA leads to the selective depletion of their receptors from the PMN surface (Oliver *et al.*, 1974). Similarly, binding of hemocyanin with macrophage receptors is followed by rapid interiorization of most of the hemocyanin–receptor complexes, leaving a small amount (1 to 10%) of the bound hemocyanin either isolated or in small clusters on the surface. The persistent molecules may indicate a heterogeneity in functional membrane receptor sites (Unanue and Calderon, 1975). In general, it is likely that interiorization of membrane always leads to the selective loss of specific surface components and the preservation of others, thereby affecting all subsequent surface events as well as the fate of internalized substances.

V. CONTROL OF TRANSLATIONAL MOVEMENTS OF RECEPTORS AND TRANSPORT PROTEINS WITHIN THE PLANE OF THE MEMBRANE

The selective translational movement of surface receptors has now been documented. For example, it is clear that Con A receptors that are initially dispersed over the surface are drawn into the membrane that envelopes phagocytized particles. Conversely, transport proteins are excluded from internalization. But how do these movements come about? As noted, Singer's fluid mosaic membrane model provides for no long-range forces that could direct the movement of surface constituents. Several lines of evidence indicate that the interaction of microtubules (MT) with membranes is an essential requirement for directed movement of certain membrane components. These studies have been done mainly in PMN, but their extension to the macrophage is strongly suggested. When PMN phagocytize after pretreatment with colchicine (which prevents MT assembly) transport systems are no longer preserved on the surface (Ukena and Berlin, 1972). The selective movement of lectin receptors into the endocytized membrane also no longer occurs (Oliver *et al.*, 1974).

In some cells, for example, lymphocytes, (Edelman *et al.*, 1973) the movement of fluorescein-labeled Con A bound to the surface results in its aggregation at one pole of the cell into a so-called cap. This appears to result from the formation of a lattice composed of the multivalent

Con A and surface receptors. Free mobility of Con A receptors is essential for cap formation. In other cells, for example, PMN (Oliver *et al.*, 1975) and SV40 virus-transformed 3T3 fibroblasts (Rosenblith *et al.*, 1973), cap formation will not occur unless they are incubated in the cold or pretreated with colchicine, both of which tend to disassemble MT. Rabbit alveolar macrophages fall into this latter category (J. M. Oliver and R. D. Berlin, unpublished observations). Cells exposed briefly to fluorescein-conjugated Con A in the absence of serum show a random distribution of fluorescence (Fig. 1a). Pretreatment of the cells with colchicine permits movement of Con A into a surface cap (Fig. 1b). Cells pretreated with serum show rapid internalization of surface-bound Con A (Fig. 1c). This does not require prior cap formation, but very likely involves a local aggregation of Con A–receptor complexes into patches that can be removed from the surface by endocytosis. These results all suggest that a microtubular system is essential for the directed movement or stabilization of the distribution of Con A receptors.

This interaction of colchicine-sensitive structures (presumably MT) with membranes is apparently a dynamic one. Reaven and Axline (1973) have shown that in mouse peritoneal macrophages, microfilaments (MF) and MT are assembled only at the adherent surface. During phagocytosis, however, MF and MT are assembled in membrane regions near the particle. In PMN it appears that complement factors, particularly C5a, induce the proliferation of polymerized MT (Goldstein *et al.*, 1973). Thus, the emerging picture is that elements adsorbed to the surface bring about MT polymerization that in turn "feeds back" to influence the behavior of membrane constituents.

What is the nature of the signal by which surface events induce MT polymerization? Recent studies in our laboratory suggest that cyclic GMP may serve as such a signal. These observations arose in conjunction with studies on the Chediak–Higashi (CH) syndrome. The syndrome occurs in man (Wolff *et al.*, 1972) and in several other species including the so-called beige mouse (C576J bg/bg) (Gallin *et al.*, 1974). The syndrome is familiar to immunopathologists, since it is characterized in part by defective bacterial killing in phagocytes. We have observed that CH mouse and human PMN and CH mouse peritoneal macrophages behave like colchicine-treated normals and show extensive surface cap formation by Con A (on about 50% of PMN and 20% of macrophages during a 10 minutes incubation at 37°C). By contrast, untreated normal cells show very little Con A capping. This suggests that MT assembly is impaired in CH cells. Most importantly this surface abnormality is corrected by cyclic GMP or agents that increase cyclic GMP level, namely, carbamylcholine (carbachol) and PMA (phorbol myristate acetate) (Oliver, 1975;

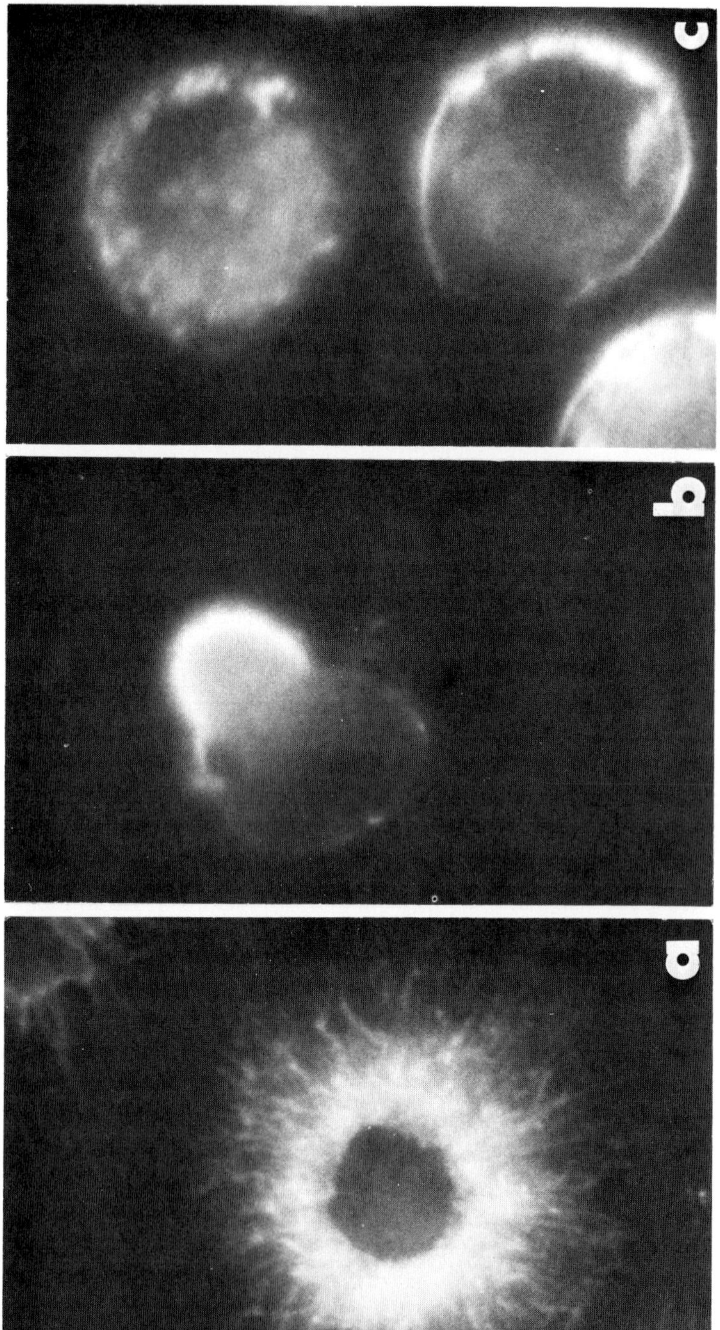
c
b
a

Oliver *et al.*, 1975; J. M. Oliver and R. D. Berlin, unpublished results). Thus cyclic GMP may stimulate MT assembly and control MT-dependent cell surface properties in leukocytes.

Further studies with CH macrophages suggest a direct relationship between plasma membrane properties and intracellular membrane organization. We have observed that CH mouse peritoneal macrophages develop the giant lysosomal granules that are pathognomonic of the disease during maturation *in vitro* (Fig. 2A). Previous investigators have proposed that this aberrant morphology may result from compositional changes in the lysosomal membrane (White, 1966; Wolff *et al.*, 1972). However, when carbachol, which promotes MT–plasma membrane interactions is included in the medium, the cells develop normal lysosomes *in vitro* (Fig. 2B). It is possible that carbachol normalizes these two characteristics of CH cells (defective MT assembly and generation of giant lysosomes) by separate mechanisms that depend on cyclic GMP. It seems more likely, however, that abnormal lysosome formation is a consequence of the MT–membrane defect. Membranes of secondary lysosomes are derived in part from endocytized plasma membrane, which may in fact provide the stimulus for generation of lysosomal granules (Cohn, 1970; Gordon and Cohn, 1973). Furthermore, our studies (reviewed above) establish that the composition of endocytic vesicles is different from that of the bulk membrane and is regulated by MT–membrane interactions. We propose therefore that inadequate MT assembly in CH macrophages may result in an abnormality in endocytic vesicle composition that leads to abnormal composition and morphology of lysosomes (for example, a

---

Fig. 1. Distribution of Con A on rabbit alveolar macrophages. Cell monolayers on coverslips were preincubated for 60 minutes, (a) with serum-free modified Hanks' medium, (b) with serum-free medium containing colchicine (10^{-5} *M*), and (c) with medium containing 10% fetal calf serum. The coverslips were rinsed and incubated for 5 minutes at 37°C with serum-free medium containing fluorescein-conjugated Con A (5 μg/ml). The cells were then fixed with 2% (w/v) paraformaldehyde for 10 minutes and examined with a Zeiss fluorescence microscope. In the absence of colchicine or serum the macrophages spread, exposing a large ruffled surface that binds Con A uniformly. Colchicine prevents the spreading of all cells and promotes movement of surface-bound Con A into caps on about 20% of cells. Lower doses of colchicine (10^{-6} *M*) will promote extensive (greater than 50%) Con A capping on rabbit PMN (Oliver, 1975; Oliver *et al.*, 1975). This suggests that microtubule polymerization in macrophages is less sensitive to colchicine than microtubule polymerization in PMN. Macrophages preincubated with serum show a very rapid internalization of Con A into intracellular vesicles. This probably reflects movement of Con A–receptor complexes into patches that are removed by endocytosis. These endocytic vesicles fuse together upon further incubation (15 minutes and longer) to form a small number of large, intensely fluorescent vesicles (Edelson and Cohn, 1974a,b; J. M. Oliver and R. D. Berlin, unpublished observations).

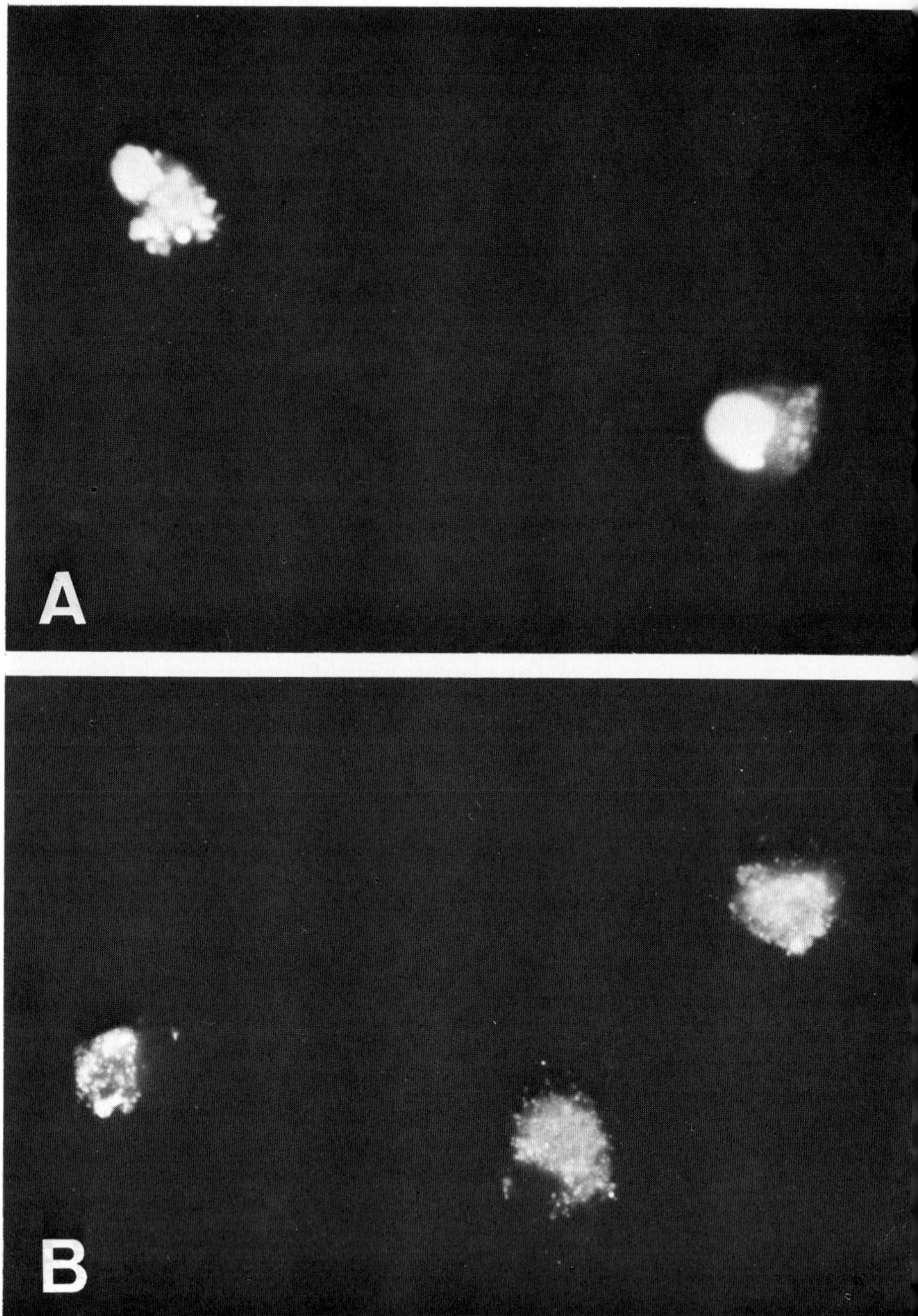
A
B

surface-derived recognition signal that regulates fusion of lysosomes with lysosomes may be absent). Cyclic GMP, by promoting MT assembly, may restore the normal segregation of surface components and so normalize the composition and function of CH lysosomes.

VI. SUMMARY

The macrophage surface has been reexamined from the viewpoint of modern theories of membrane organization. Membrane proteins that correspond to various receptors for Fc, complement, lectins, and enzymes, etc., are freely or randomly mobile in the plane of the membrane under certain conditions. This is clearly shown, for example, for ATPase in heterokaryons of macrophages and melanocytes. We also postulate that the binding of antibody-coated RBC to macrophage surfaces requires the free mobility of Fc receptors and that internalization of surface-bound Con A by macrophages depends on the ability of lectin–receptor complexes to move and form surface patches that can be pinocytized. Under other conditions, particularly phagocytosis, membrane components, such as lectin receptors and transport proteins, show a mobility that is highly directed in orientation with respect to the endocytized membrane. There is a specific partitioning of membrane constituents between residual surface membrane and that which is internalized. This partitioning appears to depend on microtubules that are extrinsic to the membrane proper. The interaction of microtubules (and probably microfilaments) with the membrane is dynamic and appears to be induced by events at the external aspect of the surface, such as the binding of lectins or phagocytic particles. Recent studies with PMN and macrophages from normal mice and from the mouse homolog of Chediak–Higashi disease suggest that binding

---

Fig. 2. Prevention of giant granule formation in Chediak–Higashi mouse macrophages by carbachol. Resting (essentially agranular) peritoneal macrophages were collected from beige (Chediak–Higashi) mice by peritoneal lavage and cultured *in vitro* in Dulbecco's modified Eagle's medium supplemented with 20% fetal calf serum with and without carbachol (10^{-5} M). After 6 days in culture the lysosomal granules were observed by staining with acridine orange ($1{:}10^6$) for 3 minutes and observing the cells by fluorescence microscopy. Lysosomes develop an intense fluorescence that can be recorded by black and white photography. In the absence of drugs (A) Chediak–Higashi macrophages contain a small number of very large lysosomal granules. These are pathognomonic of the disease. By contrast, when these macrophages mature *in vitro* in the presence of carbachol (B) granule morphology is indistinguishable from that of normal macrophages (J. M. Oliver, J. A. Krawiec, and R. D. Berlin, unpublished results).

promotes microtubule polymerization and its interaction with the membrane by turning on cyclic GMP production.

The consequences of MT-dependent segregation of membrane constituents during endocytosis are far-reaching and only partially understood at present. Normally, the selective partitioning preserves certain surface functions, such as transport, which are presumably essential for recovery, repair, etc. At the same time the cell may become refractory to certain stimuli due to the selective removal of specific surface receptors. This may allow the macrophage to exempt itself from certain immunologic events and free it to process antigens or interact with lymphocytes. The fate of antigens may also be indirectly determined by this segregation of membrane components, since the fusion of endocytic vesicles with lysosomes and hence the degradation of antigens may be dependent on the composition of the vesicle and lysosomal membranes.

Thus we consider that the organization and function of macrophage cell surfaces is controlled by a balance between extracellular events (such as the movement of randomly distributed receptors into clusters during the binding of antigens and phagocytic particles) and intracellular events (such as the assembly of microtubules and microfilaments that act on the membrane to promote specific changes in surface topography). Furthermore, we propose that tight control of surface organization permits the cell to preserve essential functions during endocytosis, determines how antigens are presented by lymphocytes, regulates the intracellular fate of endocytized material, etc. This dynamic view of the macrophage membrane provides a new framework for future studies of macrophage functions that involve surface interactions.

REFERENCES

Allen, J. M., and Cook, G. M. W. (1970). *Exp. Cell Res.* **59,** 105–116.

Arend, W. P., and Mannik, M. (1972). *J. Exp. Med.* **136,** 514–529.

Berlin, R. D. (1975). *Ann. N.Y. Acad. Sci.* **256,** 445–454.

Berken, A., and Benacerraf, B. (1966). *J. Exp. Med.* **123,** 119–144.

Berlin, R. D., Oliver, J. M., Ukena, T. G., and Yin, H. H. (1974). *Nature (London)* **247,** 45–46.

Cohn, Z. A. (1970). *In* "Mononuclear Phagocytes" (R. van Furth, ed.), pp. 50–61. Blackwell, Oxford.

Edelman, G. M., Yahara, I., and Wang, J. L. (1973). *Proc. Nat. Acad. Sci. U.S.* **70,** 1442–1446.

Edelson, P. J., and Cohn, Z. A. (1974a). *J. Exp. Med.* **140,** 1364–1386.

Edelson, P. J., and Cohn, Z. A. (1974b). *J. Exp. Med.* **140,** 1387–1403.

Frye, L. D., and Edidin, M. (1970). *J. Cell Sci.* **7,** 319–335.

Gallin, J. I., Bujak, J. S., Patten, E., and Wolff, S. M. (1974). *Blood* **43,** 201–206.

Goldstein, I. M., Hoffstein, S., Gallin, J., and Weissmann, G. (1973). *Proc. Nat. Acad. Sci. U.S.* **70,** 2916–2920.

Gordon, S., and Cohn, Z. A. (1970). *J. Exp. Med.* **131,** 981–1003.
Gordon, S., and Cohn, Z. A. (1971). *J. Exp. Med.* **134,** 947–962.
Gordon, S., and Cohn, Z. A. (1973). *Int. Rev. Cytol.* **36,** 171–214.
Lay, W. H., and Nussenzweig, V. (1969). *J. Exp. Med.* **128,** 991–1007.
LoBuglio, H. F., and Reinehard, J. (1970). *Clin. Res.* **18,** 409.
Lutton, J. D. (1973). *J. Cell Biol.* **56,** 611–617.
Mason, R. J., Stossell, T. P., and Vaughan, M. (1972). *J. Clin. Invest.* **51,** 2399–2407.
Nicolson, G. L. (1973). *Nature (London), New Biol.* **243,** 218–220.
Oliver, J. M. (1975). *In* "Immune Recognition" (A. S. Rosenstreich, ed.), pp. 445–471. Academic Press, New York.
Oliver, J. M., Ukena, T. E., and Berlin, R. D. (1974). *Proc. Nat. Acad. Sci. U.S.* **71,** 394–398.
Oliver, J. M., Zurier, R. D., and Berlin, R. D. (1975). *Nature (London)* **253,** 471–473.
Rabinovitch, M., and De Stefano, M. J. (1972). *J. Immunol.* **110,** 695–701.
Reaven, E. P., and Axline, S. G. (1973). *J. Cell Biol.* **59,** 12–27.
Remold, H. G. (1973). *J. Exp. Med.* **138,** 1065–1076.
Rosenblith, J. Z., Ukena, T. E., Yin, H. H., Berlin, R. D., and Karnovsky, M. J. (1973). *Proc. Nat. Acad. Sci. U.S.* **70,** 1625–1629.
Schmidt, M. E., and Douglas, S. D. (1972). *J. Immunol.* **109,** 914–917.
Singer, S. J. (1974). *Annu. Rev. Biochem.* **43,** 805–833.
Smolen, J. E., and Shohet, S. B. (1974). *J. Clin. Invest.* **53,** 726–734.
Steinman, R. M., and Cohn, Z. A. (1972). *J. Cell Biol.* **55,** 616–634.
Tsan, M. F., and Berlin, R. D. (1971). *J. Exp. Med.* **134,** 1016–1035.
Ukena, T. E., and Berlin, R. D. (1972). *J. Exp. Med.* **136,** 1–7.
Unanue, E. R. (1972). *Advan. Immunol.* **15,** 95–165.
Unanue, E. R., and Calderon, J. (1975). *Fed. Proc., Fed. Amer. Soc. Exp. Biol.* **34,** 1737–1742.
White, J. G. (1966). *Blood* **28,** 143–156.
Wolff, S. M., Dale, D. C., Clark, R. A., Root, R. K., and Kimball, H. R. (1972). *Ann. Intern. Med.* **76,** 293–306.

11

Macrophage Cell Lines and Their Uses in Immunobiology

Vittorio Defendi

I. Introduction.................................... 275
II. Growth of Primary Macrophages *in Vitro*.......... 276
A. Assay for Growth of Macrophages............. 277
B. Macrophage Growth Factor, Properties and Sources.. 280
C. Conditions for the Production of Macrophage Growth Factor.............................. 281
D. Macrophage Growth Factor Purification......... 282
III. Permanent Lines with Properties of Macrophages... 283
A. Macrophage Lines Transformed by SV40....... 284
B. Tumor Lines with Macrophage Properties....... 287
IV. Conclusion.. 288
References.. 289

I. INTRODUCTION

In recent years it has become evident that macrophages play a role in a variety of immunological reactions far more complex than the function that gave them their name. (1) They are necessary intermediary for the immunological processing of particulate antigens. (2) They act as effector cells in processes of cell-mediated immunity. (3) They are themselves the target of products originated from interacting lymphoid cells. Yet, because of the lack of refined morphological and functional criteria of identification, it is not clear whether all these properties are characteristic of a single cell population, which modulates its functions in different environments and at different stages of maturation, or different populations, which although superficially similar, actually have different lineages with fixed and unchangeable functional profiles. It has been difficult to resolve these questions because of two interrelated problems: (1) the inability to obtain a population of macrophages, as defined by whichever criteria one chooses, that is completely devoid of other cell types and (2) the lack of replication *in vitro* by macrophages, a phenomenon that would allow experimental approaches that have been extremely useful in the analysis of other heterogeneous cell systems. Recent developments, however, suggest that a more critical and satisfactory analysis of this problem will be possible in the near future. Thus it has been reported that mouse peritoneal macrophages, under certain conditions, can be stimulated to grow *in vitro* for several cell generations (Virolainen and Defendi, 1967; Lin and Stewart, 1973), and some permanent lines have been established that maintain several of the properties of primary macrophages (Mauel and Defendi, 1971c; Stone and Takemoto, 1970). This chapter deals with these two aspects of macrophage biology.

II. GROWTH OF PRIMARY MACROPHAGES *IN VITRO*

Mouse peritoneal macrophages can be maintained *in vitro* for several weeks, but do not proliferate under culture conditions in which most other primary or established cell lines do replicate. Macrophages derived from other tissues or organs divide *in vitro,* but the rate of proliferation is lower and of short duration (Bennett, 1966). In 1967, however, Virolainen and Defendi demonstrated that peritoneal macrophages could be induced to replicate if medium conditioned (CM) by other cells were added to the normal culture medium.* This observation has been confirmed in other laboratories for macrophages derived from the peritoneal cavity (Lin and Stewart, 1973) as well as from other sources (Soderland and Naum, 1973). In the process of these studies not only has a method to obtain proliferating cultures of macrophages been developed, but also it has been shown that macrophages are a distinct biological system in the sense that their capacity to proliferate appears to be totally dependent upon other cell populations.

The macrophage system *in vitro* has been studied to a certain extent, and some of the conditions required for the proliferation to occur have been defined. Macrophage replication *in vitro* appears to depend upon

* Activity of conditioned medium (CM) and macrophage growth factor (MGF) are used interchangeably, since it has been shown that the DNA stimulating activity resides in a discrete component of the CM.

three elements: (1) a factor (MGF) that is produced by other cells, (2) dialyzable factor(s) present in the serum; and (3) "activation" of the macrophages, for example, by injection of irritants, such as starch or thioglycollate, in the peritoneal cavity. Ascitic fluid, however, from Freund's adjuvant inoculated mice can reduce or abolish all these requirements and represents a complete growth medium even for nonactivated macrophages (Cifone *et al.*, 1975).

A. Assay for Growth of Macrophages

In routine assay for macrophage proliferation, peritoneal fluid is collected from mice that have been injected intraperitoneally 3 or 4 days before with starch (2%) (Virolaninen and Defendi, 1967) or thioglycolate (Lin and Stewart, 1973). After centrifugation, the cells are suspended in complete medium and seeded at a concentration of 5×10^4 nucleated cells per cm^2. Thirty minutes later the medium with nonattached cells, mostly lymphocytes and fibroblasts, is suctioned off, and fresh medium is added to the cultures. If necessary, 2 or 3 days later the culture can be incubated with trypsin for a short period of time, a treatment that removes residual fibroblasts but leaves the macrophages attached on the plastic or glass surface. Conditioned medium or purified factor at different concentrations is then added to the medium.

The growth response can be assayed either by pulse labeling with tritiated thymidine ([^{3}H]TdR) or by continuous labeling and harvest 5 days later [a time at which more than 90% of the cells capable to be stimulated to DNA synthesis have incorporated [^{3}H]TdR (Virolainen and Defendi, 1967)] or by colony formation in agar (Lin and Stewart, 1973) or in liquid medium (Stewart *et al.*, 1975).

If there are no fibroblasts, the percentage of labeled macrophages is less than 1% over a 5 to 10 day period. A typical response is illustrated in Fig. 1. From this figure several facts are immediately apparent. There is considerable delay before the macrophages are induced into DNA synthesis, at least 24–36 hours before the first macrophages show [^{3}H]TdR incorporation; the response itself of the cell population is protracted over a long period of 4 to 5 days. The proportion of cells capable of being labeled by [^{3}H]TdR decreases thereafter. Occasionally, a second wave of cell labeling can be observed at optimal CM concentration. The lag of response in the DNA synthesis induction immediately differentiates the macrophage system from many other systems in which cells are stimulated to grow; for example, stimulation of proerythroblasts by erythropoietin (Chui *et al.*, 1971) or stimulation of confluent fibroblasts with fresh medium or with serum after serum starvation (Holley and Kiernan,

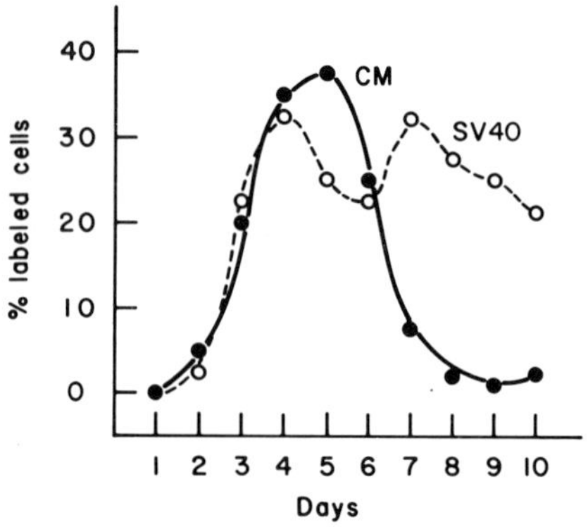

Fig. 1. Induction of DNA synthesis in mouse peritoneal macrophages measured at various times after SV40 infection or addition of CM by pulse labeling with [^{3}H]TdR.

1968). The lag period cannot be modified by maintaining macrophages for several days prior to the addition of CM or by several other manipulations. Thus, macrophages appear to be a more orthodox model of a cell population that is in a genuine G_0 state of the cell cycle.

Only with Ehrlich ascites fluid can the peak of DNA synthesis be shortened by about 2 days (Cifone *et al.*, 1975); the reason for this difference in the kinetics of response to CM from two different sources is not known at present.

Also not known, are the macromolecular events that precede the DNA synthesis in this system. The only changes preceding the initiation of DNA synthesis which have been reported are a flattening of the cells on the substrate, an increase in the number of pseudopods, and an increase in membrane activity (Virolainen and Defendi, 1967).

The proportion of macrophages initially induced into DNA synthesis is grossly proportional to the concentration of CM up to a certain level; with most of the preparation, a concentration higher than 40% (Mauel and Defendi, 1971b) begins to be inhibitory. Even under optimal concentration of CM, not all macrophages can be induced into DNA synthesis; actually, the maximum percentage varies considerably from preparation to preparation of macrophages, ranging from 40 to 90%. This clearly indicates a considerable heterogeneity in the macrophage population in terms of its capacity to initiate DNA synthesis. The basis for this heterogeneity is not known; an attractive hypothesis is the possibility that macrophages, at different levels of their differentiation, vary in their distribution or quantity of receptors for macrophage growth factor (MGF) if the activity of this factor is mediated through such a mechanism.

Mitosis and increase in cell number follows the incorporation of [^{3}H]TdR; the number in mitosis, however, is less than could be expected from the proportion in cell DNA synthesis. This, combined to the fact that several of the stimulated cells become binucleated (Virolainen and Defendi, 1967; Stewart *et al.*, 1975), indicates that only a fraction of the stimulated macrophages have the potentiality to resume successive cycles of proliferation. By the labeled mitosis method, it has been established that mouse peritoneal macrophages under these conditions have an S period of 15–16 hours (Virolainen and Defendi, 1967).

Several factors influence the proportion of stimulated macrophages. Serum is essential for the macrophage response; this appears not only to be due to the complex serum components that are needed for most cell proliferation *in vitro* but also to dialyzable factor(s) present in the serum. Thus, dialyzed serum does not allow the [^{3}H]TdR incorporation to take place even in the presence of CM. A normal response can be restored with a nondialyzed serum (Mauel and Defendi, 1971b). Such low molecular weight components of the serum could be similar to the nucleotides deemed to be necessary by Landau and Sachs (1971) for the formation of bone marrow colonies in agar.

The density of macrophages in the initial preparation also determines the proportion of macrophages which can be stimulated; thus, the denser the culture, the earlier the initial rise of proliferation and the greater its extent within a range of cell densities (3×10^3 to 5×10^4 per cm^2). From recombination experiments in which low and high density cultures are incubated in the same medium, it appears that macrophages per se produce some conditioning factor (Virolainen and Defendi, 1967), although mouse macrophages do not produce a detectable amount of MGF.

Another condition that appears essential for the response to MGF is that "activated" macrophages have to be used. Macrophages obtained from the peritoneal cavity of untreated mice give only very low response or no response at all. The precise nature of the "activated state" is not clear; it has been shown that phagocytosis stimulates specific enzyme formation (Axline and Cohn, 1970) and, in particular, an increased production of plasminogen activators (Gordon *et al.*, 1974). Since ascitic fluid, in contrast to conditioned medium, can also stimulate nonactivated macrophages (Cifone *et al.*, 1975), it is probable that macrophages *in vitro* in order to respond to MGF by DNA synthesis need to be preconditioned *in vivo*. It would be of great interest if the soluble factor produced by antigenically stimulated lymphocytes (Nathan *et al.*, 1971) was able to precondition *in vitro* nonactivated macrophages; if this were the case, the phenomenon of growth stimulation of macrophages would have a clear physiological linkage to the life cycle and the function of this cell population.

As indicated above, to sustain proliferation of macrophages *in vitro* it is necessary to renew the supply of CM; actually, changes at any time to fresh medium without CM, blocks further recruitment of macrophages, although cells that have initiated DNA synthesis appear to be able to complete it. On the basis of this observation and other experimental evidence, it has been suggested that macrophages utilize or inhibit the MGF (Virolainen and Defendi, 1967); this interesting problem cannot be resolved until labeled purified MGF will be available to study its interaction with the target cells.

Although it is possible to induce successive waves of DNA synthesis by continuous supply of fresh CM, the macrophage cultures cannot be carried for more than a few generations. The phenomenon has not been studied in detail; however, it can be explained on the basis that a considerable proportion of the population in each cell generation becomes binucleated (see above) or undergoes a final mitosis. Thus, the ability of macrophages to replicate *in vitro* even in the presence of MGF and the other permissive conditions outlined above is self-limiting. It is attractive to consider that this may be true *in vivo* as well, since it could reflect the pattern of a cell population that is needed for rapid expansion under certain stimuli or factors provided by other cells to fulfill specific functions, but at the same time it is of limited duration.

In cloning experiments under similar conditions Iin and Stewart (1973) have demonstrated that about 4–6% of activated mouse peritoneal macrophages *in vitro* have the capacity to form a colony. This proportion represents the presumed fraction of stem macrophage cells present in the injected peritoneal cavity at the time of harvesting.

B. Macrophage Growth Factor, Properties and Sources

Macrophage growth factor has been found in the medium conditioned by several mouse fibroblastic lines or strains in addition to ascitic fluid. Until recently, no mouse lines with clear epithelial characteristics were available, and it is not known whether other mouse cell lines besides mesenchimal are MGF producers. Although only the MGF obtained from L cells or from ascitic fluid has been studied to any extent (Mauel and Defendi, 1971a; Cifone, 1974), it is presumed that the various MGF's are similar. It has to be remembered, however, that the bone marrow colony stimulating factors (CSF), which appear to be identical to MGF (see below) when obtained from different sources, differ in terms of their physical properties as well as in their range of biological activity (Metcalf, 1974).

The range of activity of MGF appears to be species-specific, at least when mouse peritoneal macrophages are the targets. CM from cells of other species, such as human, monkey, hamster, rabbit, or rat, are not effective over a wide range of concentration (Mauel and Defendi, 1971a), although they can stimulate macrophages of their own species.

What is of some interest, although of unknown biological implications, is that some mouse cell lines do not produce MGF; these cell lines are lymphoid cells (L-5178 Y and AKR-A), histamine releasing cells (P-815 and HC), lines with macrophage properties (IC-21 and P-388), and neuroblastoma lines (MS-20 and Neuro 2-A) (Mauel and Defendi, 1971a; Cifone, 1974). The lack of activity is not due to production of an inhibitor for MGF. The modality of monolayer growth versus suspension does not determine whether a certain cell type is a producer or not. In summary, within the range of the source tested, the capability of producing MGF seems to reside in fibroblastic cells.

The restriction of MGF production to certain cell types is in favor of MGF being a regulatory substance with physiological activity, i.e., conveying a message specific for macrophages. This would assure a better control over the size of the macrophage population than if the MGF were a general metabolite excreted by all cells. In support of this interpretation, it has been recently found that MGF is produced *in vivo* as well and found in ascitic fluid induced with Freund's adjuvant (Cifone *et al.*, 1975). Presumably MGF is released wherever an inflammatory reaction occurs with fibroblast proliferation.

C. Conditions for the Production of Macrophage Growth Factor

The appearance of MGF in the medium is related to the degree of proliferation of the culture during the time of exposure to the medium; thus, the production of MGF is maximal under conditions that increase the rate of cell division, for example, optimal pH and high serum concentration (Cifone, 1974). If cells are adapted to grow in medium without serum, such as a subclone of L cells (MCTC-2071), then MGF can be obtained even in the absence of serum, a condition that has facilitated the attempt to purify this material.

The dependence upon cell division rather than on the absolute number of cells for the appearance of MGF in the supernatant has been clarified in a series of experiments. It was found that MGF could be released from the cells' monolayer by mild trypsinization (4 minutes with 0.05% purified trypsin), but not by EDTA treatment (Cifone and Defendi, 1974).

The cells' viability and morphology were not affected by these conditions. When cells were synchronized, it was observed that MGF activity could be trypsin-released only during the S phase, with almost no activity being recoverable during the periods between S′. Spontaneously released MGF appeared in the medium as the activity disappeared from the cell surface. By a variety of experimental treatments, it was finally demonstrated that MGF activity is present in the cell lysate at all times during the cell cycle, but it appears in trypsin releasable form at the cell surface only during the S period. It remains there all through mitosis, and then begins to be spontaneously released into the medium.

These initial findings remain to be verified at the single cell level (Cifone and Defendi, 1974), possibly by the use of immunofluorescence or immunoradiolabeled probes. However, it can be reasonably concluded that the expression of MGF on the cell surface is cycle-dependent.

It is not yet clear whether the spontaneously released MGF from cells in G_1 is transferred to the cell surface during the preceeding S phase or synthesized after mitosis. An elucidation of this point could have bearing on the interpretation of the physiological role that MGF may play *in vivo*. It is conceivable that there is a chronological restriction (cell cycle and replication) in addition to cell-type restriction (fibroblasts) on the regulation of macrophage multiplication by other cells.

D. Macrophage Growth Factor Purification

In initial studies, it was shown that MGF from L cells conditioned medium was stable to a variety of enzyme treatments, including proteolytic enzymes, but was destroyed by periodate and heating to 100°C for 10 minutes (Virolainen and Defendi, 1967). These findings indicated that the active moiety contains carbohydrates, a suggestion that is compatible with the fact that trypsin releases glycopeptides from the surface of plasma membranes (Kraemer, 1971), and the presumed synthesis and transfer of this factor is in accord with the model of synthesis of glycoproteins (Schachter and Rodin, 1971).

In studies of partially purified MGF from the medium of L cells grown in absence of serum, it was apparent that it is an acidic material of large and heterogeneous molecular weight (Mauel and Defendi, 1971a). Similar findings were obtained with the trypsin-released MGF, except that MGF from CM eluded from QAE-Sephadex column in two peaks at different salt concentrations, while MGF from trypsin eluded in a single peak (Cifone *et al.*, 1975). It is possible, therefore, that trypsin removes MGF from cells in a form that is different from MGF spontaneously released in the medium. MGF can also be separated by affinity column of concanavalin A–Sepharose, from which it can be specifically eluded by α-methyl-D-mannoside, although not all MGF activity is absorbed to concanavalin A (Con A) (Cifone, 1974).

Complete purification of MGF has not yet been achieved; four different factors have been separated on the basis of their size (Sephadex G-200 gel filtration) and ability to bind Con A with a molecular weight from 40,000 to 70,000 and higher. The small molecular fraction represents only a minor portion of the total recovered activity (Stanley *et al.*, 1975).

At present, the definition of MGF in terms of its physical and chemical properties seems premature. What is significant is that with the method indicated above MGF copurifies with CSF, which stimulates precursor cells from the bone marrow to proliferate and differentiate to form colonies of granulocytes and macrophages (Bradley and Metcalf, 1966; Ichikawa *et al.*, 1966). Actually, the two factors appear identical by several biological and physicochemical criteria, including heterogeneity in size and charge and antigenic properties. Thus, neutralization curves of MGF and CSF with an antiserum produced against L cells CSF are the same (Stanley *et al.*, 1975). It is also important to note that antibodies neutralize not only MGF from the same source, yet with different molecular weights and carbohydrate content, but also MGF from a variety of other sources, such as ascitic fluid and trypsin digest of plasma membranes (Cifone, 1974). It is highly probable, therefore, that CSF and MGF belong to the same, if not identical, family of growth regulatory factors whose heterogeneity depends more on the source than on the active groups, which affect cells of the myelocyte–monocyte series at different levels of differentiation. Thus, the different response obtained in the test systems for MGF and for CSF may reflect differences in the target cells of the same lineage rather than different factors.

III. PERMANENT LINES WITH PROPERTIES OF MACROPHAGES

Macrophages stimulated to grow with CM have only a limited life span *in vitro*, and only colonies with a small number of cells can be obtained (Carleton *et al.*, 1975). These colonies, whether in agar or in liquid medium, cannot be subcultured. Because of this limitation, their use to resolve several of the problems inherent to the functions of macrophages is somewhat restricted. As indicated above, however, permanent lines have been obtained after SV40 infection which have morphological and functional properties of macrophages. Furthermore, very recently, some tumor mouse lines carried *in vivo* or *in vitro*, whose origin was not known as to the specific cell type, have now been found to be macrophage-like.

A. Macrophage Lines Transformed by SV40

In two separate studies Stone and Takemoto (1970) and Mauel and Defendi (1971c) infected SV40 mouse peritoneal macrophages, respectively, from Balb-c and C57 B1 strains. As in several other mammalian cell systems, it was observed that SV40 infection at a multiplicity of 100 PFU/cells induced DNA synthesis and the appearance of the virus-specific intranuclear T antigen. In both studies the proportion of cells incorporating [^{3}H]TdR reached 100% by 5–10 days after infection; concomitantly all the cells became T antigen positive as tested by immunofluorescence. Since mouse cells are not permissive for SV40 replication, and indeed no replicating SV40 DNA molecules could be demonstrated (Mauel and Defendi, 1971c), [^{3}H]TdR incorporation represents cell DNA replication. There are two unique features to DNA synthesis induction by SV40 in these cells: (1) After CM treatment the proportion of induced cells declines after 4–5 days, while after SV40 infection the proportion of labeled cells is maintained at a steady state, at least as long as it had been tested (Fig. 1). Many infected macrophages become tetraploid within the first cell generation (Lehman *et al.*, 1971). (2) While in other systems of cells which are in a resting phase (G_1), the induction of cell DNA synthesis begins at 12–18 hours postinfection, in the macrophages the viral-induced DNA synthesis is delayed to 48–60 hours. Thus, the kinetics of DNA synthesis induction by virus or by CM are essentially identical. Furthermore, induction of T antigen in this system clearly precedes that of DNA synthesis by several hours, giving support to the hypothesis that identifies this new antigen as a regulatory protein for DNA synthesis (Defendi *et al.*, 1966).

Morphological alterations follow the SV40 infection, which are somewhat similar to those observed after CM treatment but are of an ill-defined nature. The populations appear rather pleomorphic, with some cells of clear macrophage morphology and others fibroblastic-like. Capacity to phagocytize carbon particles and acid phosphatase activity also varies.

Only after several weeks, in experiments from both laboratories, a rapid proliferating population emerged which in one case (Mauel and Defendi, 1971c; Moçarelli *et al.*, 1973) has been fully characterized.

It appears, therefore, that while permanent lines can be obtained from macrophages after SV40 infection, their occurrence is a rare event, rarer than has been observed with other cell populations. The reason for this is unknown, although possibly related to the terminal proliferation state of these cells. From a practical point of view, it is clear, however, that permanent lines from macrophages or monocytes should be obtainable from any species that is susceptible to SV40 infection.

1. The Phenotype of IC-21

From the infected culture a colony has been isolated, identified as IC-21, and has been propagated *in vitro* for over 6 years. The line is not strictly, but probably, of clonal origin. Morphologically, the cells maintain the characteristic of primary macrophages, with the exception of having a larger nuclear size. They have a high mobility on the substrate, with very active endocytosis and membrane ruffling. Like primary macrophages, the cells grow as discrete units and rarely form confluent monolayers, probably resulting from the rapid shift in migrating direction wherever the leading edge of the cells touch other cell membranes (S. Dienstman, personal communication). Contrary to primary macrophages, they can be easily removed from the surface by trypsin. They maintain high acid phosphatase activity that varies, however, from cell to cell. Their growth requirements are not unusual, although the line is infected by mycoplasma. Some fetal calf sera are toxic, and an optimal serum needs to be selected, a requirement that appears to be common to the growth *in vitro* of cells of the lymphocytic–monocytic lineage.

A distinct difference from primary macrophages is that the IC-21 line does not require CM for growth nor does its addition accelerate the rate of cell division. The IC-21 does not produce CM or CSF (Cifone, 1974; Stanley *et al.*, 1975).

SV40-transformed cells, in general, have a reduced requirement for serum and can grow at a much higher cell density than the parental population (Holley and Kiernan, 1968; Dulbecco, 1970); but the IC-21 share these characteristics only to some extent with other SV40-transformed cells. What is unique to this cell line is that transformation results in a loss of growth control as exercised by another cell population. It is possible, however, that SV40 may have selected a rare stem macrophage that may be initially independent from extrinsic growth factors.

In respect to other characteristics of the transformed phenotype, the IC-21 does not grow in soft agar, has an increased amount of surface receptor for concanavalin A, and lacks density-dependent regulation of growth when cultured in low serum concentration. All the cells remain T antigen positive, and their karyotype is heteroploid with a high percentage (35–45%) of near tetraploid cells (G. Garotta and V. Defendi, unpublished observation). Despite these changes, the IC-21 failed to induce tumors when injected in syngeneic C57 B1 newborns or irradiated adults (G. Garotta and V. Defendi, unpublished observation) or in nude mice (B. Giovanella and V. Defendi, unpublished observation), even at inocula as high as 10^7 cells.

It appears, therefore, that while several properties of IC-21 are those of a transformed cell population, many others are not. It is interesting that in this case, in which no procedures were applied to select for the transformed phenotype after SV40 infection, a cell line was obtained with intermediate properties between "normal" and transformed cells. It is probably for this reason that so many of the functional properties of the parental differentiated population have remained after SV40 transformation.

2. *Functional Properties of IC-21*

The interest in this particular line lies in the fact that many macrophages properties do persist after several hundred generations *in vitro*. The IC-21 cells phagocytize carbon particles and red blood cells at a high rate; the rate of phagocytosis appears to be quite different among various cells, with a proportion of them showing little activity at any one time. Actually, in quantitative assay (Mauel and Defendi, 1971c), it was found that the distribution of cells with engulfed RBC is quite similar in primary peritoneal macrophages and IC-21. Red cells coated with antibodies are rapidly phagocytized, with 100% of the cell becoming loaded with numerous RBC. Of particular interest is that the IC-21 cells are capable of substituting for primary macrophages in the induction *in vitro* of plaque-forming cells in a purified lymphocytic population exposed to red cells (Mocarelli *et al.*, 1973). The dose–response curves for the primary peritoneal macrophages and IC-21 were essentially similar, indicating also that only one cell in either of the two populations of macrophages is interacting with the nonprimed lymphocyte. Also high concentration of IC-21 ($>2.5 \times 10^5$ per 10^7 lymphocytes) inhibited the immune response.

The IC-21 cells appear to respond to macrophage inhibitory factor, but they are much less sensitive than mouse peritoneal macrophages (G. Garotta and V. Defendi, unpublished observation).

Presence of Fc receptors, distinct for IgG2a and IgG2b myeloma proteins, phospholipase sensitive but trypsin resistant, have been shown by Walker and Demus (1975). These authors have demonstrated that IC-21 have the capacity to lyse chicken red cells in the presence of target-specific antibodies and that such effector activity is independent of phagocytosis. The possibility that IC-21 may act as effector cells against tumor cells (Hibb *et al.*, 1972) has not yet been critically tested. Walker and Demus (1975) also indicate that the IC-21 can be separated into

TABLE I

Lines with Macrophages Properties

Lines	IC-21 (C57 Bl)	P388/D_1 (DBA/2)	J.774 Balb/c/NIH
Macrophage morphology	+++	+	++
Acid phosphatase	+	+	
Phagocytosis			
Carbon	+	+	+
SRBC	+		+
Fc receptor	+	+	+
C_3 receptor	+	+	
Production of lysozyme	+	+	
"Macrophage" antigen	+		
Effector activity	+	+	+
Immunological processing of antigen	+		−

density-dependent subclasses similar to primary macrophages. This is to be expected considering the pleomorphism of the IC-21 population.

The IC-21 have been shown to produce and release lysozyme at a rate comparable to that of primary macrophages (Mauel and Defendi, 1971c). The cells reacted specifically with an antisera against purified macrophages (Mauel and Defendi, 1971c). The properties of IC-21 are summarized in Table I.

B. Tumor Lines with Macrophage Properties

Very recently, two mouse tumor lines that have been carried *in vivo* as transplantable tumors or *in vitro* for several years have been found to have macrophage properties. The J-774 is a Balb/c reticulum cell sarcoma, of type A in the Dunn (1954) classification, which has been carried in ascitic form in syngeneic mice. It metastasizes very rapidly; only recently it has been adapted to grow *in vitro* with moderate success (Ralph *et al.*, 1975). The properties that these tumor cells share with macrophages are adhesiveness to substrate, phagocytosis of carbonyl iron, and capacity to form rosettes with erythrocytes in the presence of the corresponding antiserum. In addition, the cells act as effector cells against erythrocytes by mediating antibody-dependent cellular immunity. The tumor cells also bear receptors for IgG_{2a} and IgG_{2b} immunoglobulin. These cells, however, do not replace the function of adherent cells in the induction of immune response *in vitro*. The general usefulness of this line will depend upon how many other macrophages-like properties the cells have and their susceptibility to grow *in vitro* without functional changes. It is of interest that probably many of the tumors induced in a similar manner and with similar morphological properties could have some, if not all, of the macrophage properties. One can visualize a library of different lines, each one expressing different patterns of the macrophage phenotype. Actually another transplantable myelomonocytic leukemia in Balb/c was reported by Warner *et al.* (1969). These cells were characterized by a large production of lysozyme.

Of unusual interest, because it could not have been expected, is the finding of another line with macrophage properties (Koren *et al.,* 1975). This is the P-388D1 line that was isolated from a methycholantrene-induced lymphoma in a DBA/2 mouse 20 years ago (Dawe and Potter, 1957). The lymphoma tumor was adapted to grow *in vitro* and carried in such a way ever since; during the initial adaptation *in vitro* the emergence of a population with ameboid character was observed. This line has been widely used for a variety of experimental purposes, such as for growth of polyomavirus (Rabson and Legallais, 1959), for transfer of genetic markers (Roosa and Bailey, 1970), and in studies of intercellular metabolic cooperation (Roosa, 1971). Yet, except for the observed capacity to phagocytize carbon particles, a property that is not uncommon in several cell lines *in vitro,* there was little to suggest macrophage properties. Thus, the cells, in general, grow in small clumps that are poorly attached to the substrate and which continuously shed cells into the supernatant, although occasional adherence and spreading have been observed. But in these cells, Koren *et al.* (1975) have demonstrated high esterase activity and receptor for the Fc fragments of immunoglobulin and for C3; furthermore, the cells have effector activity against red cells coated with specific antibodies. The advantage of this line is that it has already been used in a variety of tissue culture techniques and, therefore, should be easily adaptable to a variety of experimental purposes.

IV. CONCLUSION

In this brief survey, it has been shown that proliferating population of cells with macrophage characteristics can be obtained, from primary cultures or as permanent lines. While this has been accomplished so far only with murine cells, it should be possible to use the same methodology to obtain similar results with macrophages from other species. This would be particularly interesting, since surface and functional properties of monocyte–macrophages appear to differ in different species. It is also conceivable that, even within the same species, macrophages isolated from different organs may vary in different ways. By growing these populations *in vitro* a systematic comparison could be performed.

The population of macrophages *in vitro,* now available, appear to differ in terms of the extent of macrophage properties they manifest; this probably reflects the stage of maturation along differentiating pathways at which the proliferating stimulus has acted. Thus, replicating cells with the whole spectrum of characteristics can be obtained *in vitro* from the fully differentiated macrophages of the peritoneal cavity to the monocytic tumor. Since by technical variations it should be possible to obtain clonal populations with a fixed phenotype from each of them, functional lineage could be firmly established. Most important, as pure populations, whose growth cycle can be controlled are becoming available, it will be possible to study the factors that modulate expression of the macrophage phenotype and to determine how the various parameters are genetically or phenotypically coordinated.

It is conceivable that availability of these cell populations may have the same impact on the solution of problems of an immunological nature, in particular, and of cell cooperation, in general, as the availability of differentiated nerve cells *in vitro* is having on the approaches and methodology to understand the function of the neural tissues.

REFERENCES

Axline, S. G., and Cohn, Z. (1970). *J. Exp. Med.* **131,** 1239–1260.

Bennett, B. (1966). *Amer. J. Pathol.* **48,** 165–182.

Bradley, T. R., and Metcalf, D. (1966). *Aust. J. Exp. Biol. Med.* **44,** 287–300.

Chui, D., Djaldetti, M., Marks, P. A., and Rifkind, R. A. (1971). *J. Cell Biol.* **51,** 585–595.

Cifone, M. (1974). Ph.D. Thesis, University of Pennsylvania, Philadelphia.

Cifone, M., and Defendi, V. (1974). *Nature (London)* **252,** 151–153.

Cifone, M., Mocarelli, P., and Defendi, V. (1975). *Exp. Cell Res.* (in press).

Dawe, C. J., and Potter, M. (1957). *Amer. J. Pathol.* **33,** 603.

Defendi, V., Carp, R. I., and Gilden, R. V. (1966). *In* "Viruses Inducing Cancer" (W. J. Burdette, ed.), pp. 269–287. Univ. of Utah Press, Salt Lake City.

Dulbecco, R. (1970). *Nature (London)* **227,** 802–806.

Dunn, T. (1954). *J. Nat. Cancer Inst.* **14,** 1281–1433.

Gordon, S., Unkeless, J. C., and Cohn, Z. (1974). *J. Exp. Med.* **140,** 995–1010.

Hibb, J. B., Lambert, L. H., and Remington, J. S. (1972). *Science* **177,** 998–1000.

Holley, R., and Kiernan, J. (1968). *Proc. Nat. Acad. Sci. U.S.* **60,** 300–304.

Ichikawa, Y., Pluznik, D. H., and Sachs, L. (1966). *Proc. Nat. Acad. Sci. U.S.* **56,** 488–495.

Koren, H. S., Handwerger, B. S., and Wunderlich, J. R. (1975). *J. Immunol.* **114,** 894–897.

Kraemer, P. M. (1971). *Biomembranes* **1,** 67–190.

Landau, T., and Sachs, L. (1971). *FEBS (Fed. Eur. Biochem. Soc.) Lett.* **17,** 339.

Lehman, J. M., Mauel, J., and Defendi, V. (1971). *Exp. Cell Res.* **67,** 230–233.

Lin, H., and Stewart, C. C. (1973). *Nature (London), New Biol.* **243,** 176–177.
Mauel, J., and Defendi, V. (1971a). *Exp. Cell Res.* **65,** 33–42.
Mauel, J., and Defendi, V. (1971b). *Exp. Cell Res.* **65,** 377–385.
Mauel, J., and Defendi, V. (1971c). *J. Exp. Med.* **134,** 335–350.
Metcalf, D. (1974). *In* "Control of Proliferation in Animal Cells" (B. Clarkson and R. Baserga, eds.), pp. 887–905. Cold Spring Harbor Lab., Cold Spring Harbor, New York.
Mocarelli, P., Palmer, J., and Defendi, V. (1973). *Immunol. Commun.* **2,** 441–447.
Nathan, C. F., Karnovsky, M. L., and David, J. R. (1971). *J. Exp. Med.* **133,** 1356–1376.
Rabson, A. S., and Legallais, F. Y. (1959). *Proc. Soc. Exp. Biol. Med.* **100,** 229–233.
Ralph, P., Prichard, J., and Cohn, M. (1975). *J. Immunol.* **114,** 898–905.
Roosa, R. A. (1971). *In* "Informational Molecules in Biological Systems" (L. Ledoux, ed.), pp. 67–79. North-Holland Publ., Amsterdam.
Roosa, R. A., and Bailey, E. (1970). *J. Cell. Physiol.* **75,** 137–150.
Schachter, H., and Rodén, L. (1973). *In* "Metabolic Conjugation and Metabolic Hydrolysis" (W. H. Fishman, ed.), Vol. 3, pp. 2–149. Academic Press, New York.
Soderland, S. C., and Naum, Y. (1973). *Nature (London)* **245,** 150–152.
Stanley, R., Cifone, M., and Defendi, V. (1975). In preparation.
Stewart, C. C., Lin, H. S., and Adles, C. (1975). *J. Exp. Med.* **141,** 1114–1132.
Stone, L. B., and Takemoto, K. K. (1970). *J. Virol.* **6,** 621–627.
Virolainen, M., and Defendi, V. (1967). *Wistar Inst. Symp. Monogr.* **7,** 67–86.
Walker, W. S., and Demus, A. (1975). *J. Immunol.* **114,** 765–769.
Warner, N. L., Moore, M. A. S., and Metcalf, D. (1969). *J. Nat. Cancer Inst.* **43,** 963–982.

12

Monocyte Kinetics and Their Changes in Infection

Alvin Volkman

I. Introduction 291
II. Theoretical and Methodological Background 293
III. Cell Kinetics of the Monocytes 295
A. The Proliferative Compartment 295
B. The Monocyte in the Blood 302
C. Fate of the Monocyte: Relationships to Other Mononuclear Cell Populations 308
IV. Cell Kinetics of Monocytes in Infection 311
V. Concluding Remarks 319
References 320

I. INTRODUCTION

A great deal of attention within the past decade has been focused on the functional activities of macrophages in immunological processes and in nonspecific host defense mechanisms mounted against infection and malignant growth. In many instances the macrophages under study are predominantly the immigrant cells in inflammatory exudates. These cells are known to be more highly differentiated or developed monocytes (Ebert and Florey, 1939; Volkman and Gowans, 1965a; Spector *et al.*, 1965). Looked at in another way, the monocytes in the blood constitute a mobile pool from which the macrophages of inflammation may be drawn. Interestingly, the monocytes in most mammalian species are a minority population, generally constituting of between 3 and 8% of the nucleated cells in the blood. Inflammatory lesions of several kinds, whether due to nonliving antigens, infectious agents, or certain tumors, can effect the accumulation of vast numbers of hematogenous macrophages in relatively short intervals. Since the capacity of monocytes and macrophages to proliferate appears to be limited, it follows that the provision of adequate numbers of macrophages for participation in host defenses is highly dependent upon the mechanisms assuring the sustained supply and delivery of blood monocytes. The purpose of this chapter is to present and discuss pertinent data relating to the cell kinetics of this supply and delivery system and their responses in infection, a realistic situation of challenge to host defenses.

The earliest kinetic assessments of monocytes in the blood (Fliedner *et al.*, 1962; Volkman and Gowans, 1965a) were made possible by the development of the powerful investigative tools of labeling dividing cells with tritiated thymidine (^{3}HT) combined with high resolution autoradiography (Fitzgerald *et al.*, 1951; Hughes *et al.*, 1958). These methods provided an objective means for the study of the proliferative behavior and migration of visually identifiable cells. When applied to the study of monocytes in the rat, it became evident that the cytokinetic behavior of these cells distinguished them from other classes of mononuclear leukocytes (Volkman and Gowans, 1965a) and served in addition to identify them as the exclusive antecedents of immigrant macrophages in inflammation (Volkman and Gowans, 1965a; Spector *et al.*, 1965). By further employing ^{3}HT as an indelible marker, it was possible to demonstrate the origin of monocytes from a rapidly proliferating precursor pool in the bone marrow (Volkman and Gowans, 1965b). In brief, these studies in the rat clearly defined the monocytes as a discrete class of cells with dividing precursors in the bone marrow and a mobile pool in the blood with the capacity to emigrate and develop into highly functional macrophages of inflammatory exudates following appropriate stimulation. Later investigations demonstrated comparably lineal relationships of monocytes in the mouse (Van Furth and Cohn, 1968; Virolainen, 1968) and in man (Wulff and Sparrevohn, 1966; Leder, 1967a,b). Additional observations on monocyte progenitors in the bone marrow of the guinea pig (Nichols *et al.*, 1971) and the rabbit (Nichols *et al.*, 1971) are also supportive, as are the ^{3}HT labeling studies of macrophages in tubercles experimentally induced with BCG in the rabbit (Dannenberg *et al.*, 1972).

Many of the structural details of the respective compartments of the monocyte series are becoming known, and some will be discussed in this chapter. However, the full extent of the monocyte system is still a matter of controversy and has not been wholly defined as yet. To help achieve such definition, evidence bearing on certain putative relationships that the author regards as doubtful or incompletely resolved will be reviewed.

The major focus of this chapter, however, will be predominantly on the monocyte and its immediate precursors.

II. THEORETICAL AND METHODOLOGICAL BACKGROUND

A brief review will be adequate to set the stage for the bulk of the discussion to follow. Several detailed accounts dealing at length with theories of cell kinetics and their methods of study are available for consultation (Athens *et al.*, 1959; Cronkite *et al.*, 1959; Bond *et al.*, 1965; Cleaver, 1967; Killmann, 1968).

With regard to the cell cycle, a postmitotic diploid cell is said to be in a phase called G_1. When such a cell begins to synthesize DNA, it enters a phase termed S, during which the DNA content of the nucleus is doubled. The cessation of DNA synthesis is followed by a generally brief period, G_2, or premitotic rest phase before entering mitosis (M). The time from one mitosis to the next is the generation or cell cycle time (T_C).

An actively cycling cell will incorporate thymidine, a specific precursor of DNA, during the period of DNA synthesis. When tritium (^3H) is substituted for one of the hydrogens on the thymidine molecule the incorporation of tritiated thymidine (^3HT) rapidly results in the labeling of newly formed DNA. The labeled DNA is metabolically stable and is decreased only by cell division. The activity of the contained label is expressed in an autoradiograph as the number of grains in the photographic emulsion overlying the nucleus of a labeled cell after a given period of exposure. High resolution of the localized isotope is made possible by the low energy of the β particle emitted by the slowly decaying ^3H. Following division, each daughter cell should have statistically half of the activity and hence half the grain count of the parent cell. In a defined proliferating population, the fraction of cells in DNA synthesis that becomes labeled with ^3HT is the immediate labeling index (LI). The LI is in turn equal to the fraction of the cell cycle time which a cell spends in DNA synthesis. It follows that if the LI and either the duration of S (T_S) or T_C are known, the other can be calculated.

$$\text{Fraction of cells in DNA synthesis (LI)} = \frac{T_S}{T_C} \qquad (1)$$

from which

$$\text{Average cell production rate} = \frac{\text{LI}}{T_S} \qquad (2)$$

Several assumptions underlie the use of these equations. One is that all the labeled cells under consideration divide. A second is that all the cells of the observed population are in cycle. The third is that DNA synthesis is continuous, without gaps that may coincide with the period of ^{3}HT availability (Alpen and Johnston, 1967).

With respect to computations based on reductions in grain counts, errors may be imposed by the cessation of regular division of labeled cells after one or more cycles, although proliferating and nonproliferating cells may be morphologically indistinguishable. Depending on their proportion, the persistance of such noncycling cells in a dividing population could reduce the rate of decline of the average grain count and lead to overestimations of T_C.

As will be seen later, the disappearance of monocytes from the blood is exponential, therefore random, and not due to senescence. Half-times for the loss of these cells can be calculated from the equation:

$$T_{1/2} = \frac{\ln 2}{\lambda} \tag{3}$$

where λ is the fractional loss constant. Semilogarithmic plots of the decline of unlabeled cells or 100 — LI, during the influx of labeled monocytes provide rapid estimates of $T_{1/2}$. From Eq. (3) the average transit or sojourn time for monocytes in the blood is then $1/\lambda$ or $T_{1/2}/\ln 2$.

After a pulse of ^{3}HT the percentage of labeled cells that enter the blood reaches a peak and then declines. If no appreciable division takes place in the blood, $T_{1/2}$ of a labeled population can be estimated from the rate of this decline of the LI by selecting cells relatively homogeneous with respect to their time of birth, i.e., the cohort of daughter cells with the highest mean grain counts. The greater the homogeneity of the cohort, the greater the accuracy of the estimate. Inaccuracies in this method may also be due to undetected proliferation, the reentry of labeled cells into the blood, and the reutilization of label. Overestimates of half-time can result from all three.

The half-time of cells in the blood may be estimated by the steepest rate of increase of labeled cells first entering this compartment after pulse labeling. If unlabeled cells enter concurrently, the apparent entry rate of labeled cells will be reduced. Transit times can therefore also be overestimated by this method.

In another approach, a sustained excess of isotopic label can be provided by either repeated administration at intervals shorter than a generation time or by the continuous infusion of this agent (Osgood *et al.*, 1962). From the decline of the unlabeled cells, the $T_{1/2}$ and life-span in the blood can be estimated. Reutilization of labeled thymidine liberated as a consequence of the death of labeled cells obviously cannot influence the results obtained by this method. Sources of error could, as in other methods, arise from failure to identify a proportion of members of a particular cell population morphologically. Conversely, it is possible that morphologically identical cells may have differing kinetic behavior that could influence labeling data.

Still another approach to the study of the kinetics of a cell population in the blood is by the infusion of a known number of labeled histocompatible cells. Such a technique has proved to be highly effective for the investigation of the population dynamics of human granulocytes (Athens *et al.*, 1959). An advantage of this method is that it permits better assessment of the distribution of the injected cells without the confusion imposed by any additional influx of labeled cells. For the same reason, measurements of the loss of the labeled population are, in theory, highly accurate. Computations in this method are obviously based on the principle of dilutions of isotopic label. Several other considerations merit comment. It is crucial that the extra-corporeal handling of the cells should not inflict damage resulting in an altered life expectancy or in any way alter the capacity of a cell to emigrate from the blood. The label should have a high degree of stability, and ideally no element of the procedure should influence the mechanisms regulating the dynamics of the cell population under study in the subject. In this connection, either the removal or infusion of excessive numbers of blood cells would be undesirable.

III. CELL KINETICS OF THE MONOCYTES

A. The Proliferative Compartment

1. Recognizable Precursors

The existence of a monocyte progenitor pool with distinctive proliferative behavior, localized in the bone marrow and to a lesser extent in the spleen, was established in experiments employing isotopic labeling by Volkman and Gowans (1965a,b). It is interesting, in retrospect, that bone marrow was considered as a source for circulating monocytes in normal mammals in morphological studies (Sabin *et al.*, 1936). In a still earlier study, noting the abundant presence of apparently immature monocytes in foci of cellular hyperplasia brought about by the administration of

Listeria monocytogenes, Witts and Webb (1927) concluded that bone marrow and spleen were major sites of monocyte production in the rabbit.

Leder (1967a,b) was able to identify dividing and nondividing cells as precursors of monocytes by employing selective cytochemical reactions for the activities of α-naphthylacetate esterase, naphthol-AS-acetate esterase and peroxidase. He termed these cells promonocytes. Similar esterase activities are also manifested by granulocyte precursors, which are said to be distinguishable from promonocytes by the more apparent azurophilic granules in the cytoplasm of the former. Supportive observations on partially differentiated bone marrow cells that share cytochemical and ultrastructural characteristics with monocytes have been made by others (Van Furth and Cohn, 1968; Schmalzl and Braunsteiner, 1969; Nichols *et al.*, 1971). These then are the recognizable precursors of monocytes. The term promonocyte, employed in the literature for many years, is for the present an adequate designation for these cells, although future investigations may prove it to be too general.

2. *Stem Cells*

a. In Vivo. It has been impossible to identify by morphological means progenitors of monocytes more poorly differentiated than promonocytes. Leder (1967a,b) contends, on the basis of cytochemical examinations, that monocytes are derived from promyelocytes. Additional links between granulocytes and monocytes are provided by studies of stem cell proliferation and differentiation *in vivo* and *in vitro.*

When bone marrow cells are injected into heavily irradiated mice, nodular hemopoietic colonies appear in the spleen (Till and McCulloch, 1961). Although most other major cell lines have been identified in discrete or mixed colonies, no monocytogenic colonies have ever been described. In view of the known origin of monocytes from precursors in bone marrow, this is somewhat surprising. Virolainen and Defendi (1968) have shown, however, that mononuclear phagocytes that originated in donor bone marrow could be isolated principally from granulocytic nodules. Such evidence allies the monocytic and granulocytic lines but does not explain why monocytopoiesis cannot be more readily demonstrated in these splenic nodules. Two explanations can be proposed to explain these observations. One is that monocytopoiesis apparently involves fewer divisions than granulocytopoiesis, at least so far as the recognizable precursors are concerned. Thus, the yield of monocytes would be lower than the yield of granulocytes, which would, in turn, render the monocytes inconspicuous. The second is that monocytes do not tarry in hemopoietic tissue following their last precursor division but

TABLE I Kinetics of Monocytopoiesis[a]

Species	T_S (hours)	T_C (hours)	Marrow transit time (hours)	Total pro-monocyte pool (cells/kg body wt)	DNA synthesizing fraction (%)	Output (cells/kg/hour)	Minimum emergence time (hours)	Reference
Man	34[b]	40–82[b]	—	—	—	5.6×10^5 [j]	13–26	Whitelaw (1972)
Man	9.5–11.0[b]	29[b]	54	5.8×10^8	12 (observed) 35 (expected)	6.8×10^6 [k]	5–7	Meuret (1974)
Man	—	—	—	—	—	—	12–24	Fliedner *et al.* (1969)
Rat	12.5[b]	21[b]	—	—	—	—	8	Whitelaw *et al.* (1968)
Rat	—	—	—	—	—	—	6	Volkman (1967, 1970)
Rat	12[b]	18[b]	—	—	66.7 (expected)	—	6	Volkman (Fig. 1)
Rat	—	34[c]	—	—	—	—	—	Volkman and Collins (1974)
Mouse	—	—	—	—	—	—	1	Van Furth and Cohn (1968)
Mouse	13.6[d]	19.5[e]	—	1.3×10^7 [f]	47 (observed)[h] 69.8 (observed)[k]	1.3×10^6 [l]	—	Van Furth and Diesselhoff-Den Dulk (1970)
Mouse	11.8[d]	16.2[e]	—	2.0×10^7 [g]	6.18 (observed)[h] 72.9 (observed)[i]	2.5×10^6 [m]	6	Van Furth *et al.* (1973)

[a] Data relating to monocyte formation in several species are tabulated for comparison. Means are given but standard deviations have been deleted. The original reports should be consulted for these and other details.

[b] Determined from maxima and minima of labeling curves in blood following pulse label of ^{3}HT.

[c] $T_{1/2}$ of decline of median grain count of blood monocytes following pulse label of ^{3}HT.

[d] T_S equals initial LI per hourly increase in LI.

[e] $T_C = T_S$/LI, when LI taken from *in vivo* determination 1 hour after pulse of ^{3}HT.

[f] 3.3×10^5/25 gm mouse.

[g] 5×10^5/25 gm mouse.

[h] *In vitro.*

[i] *In vivo.*

[j] Calculation based on assumed mean weight of 70 kg; original figure is 9.4×10^8/24 hours given as output.

[k] Monocyte birth rate.

[l] 3.3×10^4/25 gm mouse; marrow release rate.

[m] 6.3×10^4/25 gm mouse; monocyte production rate.

rapidly gain entry into the blood as indicated by a relatively short emergence time (Table I). Similar behavior may also occur within the hemopoietic spleen colonies. If so, monocytes would never accumulate to form aggregates of proportions large enough to permit detection.

b. In Vitro. Additional observations relating stem cells of the granulocytic and monocytic series comes from the studies of cells which form hemopoietic colonies when grown *in vitro* (Bradley and Metcalf, 1966; Pluznik and Sachs, 1966). Such colony-forming cells (CFC) are believed to be stem cells and are said to display clonal growth (Paran and Sachs, 1969; Bradley and Metcalf, 1966) in enriched soft agar or methyl cellulose gels. The most common result is the outgrowth of discrete colonies of differentiating granulocytes which later give way to macrophages (Metcalf *et al.*, 1967). One explanation is that each cell type takes origin from its own stem cell (Paran and Sachs, 1969). Metcalf (1971) however, on the basis of single-cell isolation and subculture believes that ring-nucleus myelocytes can actually transform into macrophages. There are clearly conceptual difficulties that prevent the full acceptance of the compelling results of this painstaking experiment. Although Metcalf's experiment appears to be closely controlled, our imperfect knowledge of the morphology of the formative cells of the monocytic series limits the conclusions that can be drawn from these observations. Possibly a cell resembling a ring-nucleus myelocyte is derived from a still more primitive progenitor already committed to form monocytes but not granulocytes. Thus, it may be that differently committed cells, possibly arising from a common stem cell, are morphologically poorly distinguishable.

3. *Kinetics of Monocytopoiesis*

The average duration of some phases of the cell cycle of monocyte precursors can be estimated indirectly from ^{3}HT labeling data of monocytes in the blood. If samples of blood are drawn at closely spaced periods after a pulse of ^{3}HT, the resulting labeling pattern in the rat (Whitelaw *et al.*, 1968) and man (Meuret, 1974) resembles a series of overlapping waves. Some of the author's data to illustrate this point are shown in Fig. 1. The time between the intravenous injection of ^{3}HT and the appearance of labeled cells in the blood, the minimum emergence or "flushing" time (Fliedner *et al.*, 1969), is seen to be about 6 hours. From this point, the first rise in the labeling index in Fig. 1 represents the entry of labeled monocytes. It is terminated at about 18 hours by the dilution of label, presumably imposed by a wave of unlabeled monocytes whose precursors were not yet in S during the hour or less in which ^{3}HT was available

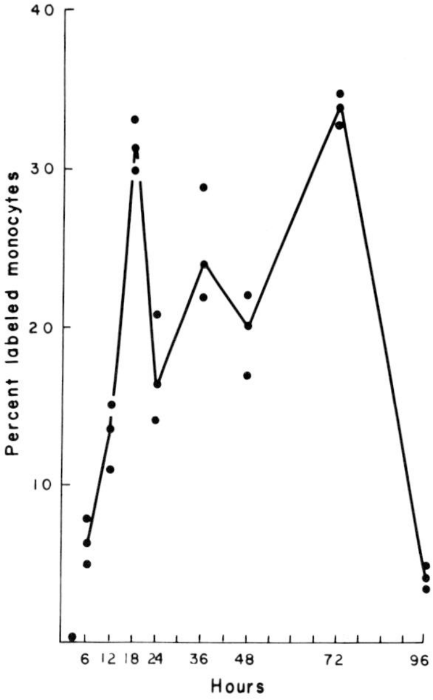

Fig. 1. Percentage of labeled monocytes entering the blood of normal rats after a single intravenous injection of ^{3}HT. The lines connect the median percentages for three rats. Three hours after the administration of ^{3}HT the percentage of labeled blood monocytes was less than 1% in all instances.

for incorporation into newly forming DNA (Rubini *et al.*, 1960). Since G_2 and M are generally very brief, the 6–18 hour interval approximates the average duration of S for monocyte precursors. It follows that the interval between adjacent pairs of maxima or minima in Fig. 1, should provide a crude approximation of the average cell cycle time, which can be estimated from these data to be about 18 to 24 hours. Greater accuracy is probably obtained by employing the earliest waves, since the accumulation of labeled cells in the blood tends to blur this phasic phenomenon. Moreover, in Fig. 1, the later determinations are too widely spaced to be used for quantitative data. A DNA synthesis time of 12 hours and a cell cycle time of 18 to 24 hours determined from Fig. 1 agree with most of the published measurements for these phases in rats and other species as summarized in Table I.

With respect to the DNA synthesis time, the close agreement of all but one of the determinations (Whitelaw, 1972) is particularly interesting, since three different species are being compared. Excluding the figure of 34 hours, the mean duration of S is approximately 12 ± 1.4 hours (SD). In Whitelaw's study (1972), the period of DNA synthesis was taken to be the interval between the point where the labeling index begins its first rise and the point where it reaches its first peak, as described above. Meuret (1974) also employed this method plus two additional and independent methods to determine the duration of S in man, thereby providing a great deal of power to his data.

Whitelaw (1972) estimated the cell cycle time as roughly between 40 and 80 hours more. Aside from these figures, there is a remarkably small range of cell cycle times from species to species. In Whitelaw's study (1972) a precise calculation of T_C was impossible because the mean grain count per labeled cell remained near the maximum for about 65 hours before declining slowly. All other calculations of T_C in Table I vary about a mean of 23 hours.

The only available measurement of the marrow transit time for monocyte precursors was recorded by Meuret (1974). By employing [^{3}H]DFP as an *in vivo* label, it was possible to follow the course of labeled monocytes as they disappeared from the blood. The measurement is based on the principle that virtually all promonocytes and monocytes become labeled in this procedure. It should be noted that this study was carried out in a 68-year-old patient suffering from severe cardiac insufficiency. Influences of possible concomitant disturbances, such as alterations in blood volume, blood chemistry, or bone marrow function, must be taken into account in interpreting these results; nevertheless, the data are of considerable interest. Maximum labeling occurred rapidly after the injection of [^{3}H]DFP, after which the proportion of labeled blood monocytes fell to about 30%. This plateau was maintained until 54 hours postinjection, when the labeling indices abruptly began to decline exponentially with a half-time of about 45 hours. Meuret's (1974) interpretation was that the extent of the initial phase of the curve to the end of the plateau roughly corresponded to the transit time of monocyte precursors through the bone marrow from the stem cell through the last promonocyte division. A bone marrow transit time of 54 hours would permit two consecutive promonocyte cell cycles based on the cell cycle time of 29 hours calculated by Meuret (1974).

The DNA synthesizing fraction of promonocytes (Table I) has been determined in man and mouse and represented by an extrapolated value in the rat. The percentage "observed" refers to the labeling index of promonocytes incubated either *in vitro* or "flash" labeled *in vivo*. The "expected" percentages refer to labeling indices determined from the ratio of the DNA synthesis time to the cell cycle time. In man, the expected value exceeds the observed, suggesting that a proportion of promonocytes is out of cycle, perhaps in a state of G_0. Alternatively, a proportion of the promonocytes may have protracted cell cycle times, possibly signifying an extended G_1. It is also worth considering that there may be morphological difficulties involved in the identification of promonocytes. If true, unlabeled cells belonging to other classes, if incorrectly classed as promonocytes, could lead to an underestimation of the DNA synthesizing fraction.

If the last possibility is discounted, the ratio, observed LI/expected LI may be taken as the growth fraction of the dividing compartment, about 35% in man. No estimate can be made from the available data in the mouse, since the calculation of T_C is dependent on the observed LI (Table I).

The monocyte birthrate in man (Table I) cannot be compared with the figures for monocyte production rates or output estimated in the mouse and rat, since the output (K_{out}) from a multiplicative compartment is equal to the input (K_{in}) plus the birthrate (K_B), provided there is no cell death within the compartment (Quastler, 1959). Assuming for the moment that there is no cell death in the promonocyte compartment, then K_B is an underestimate of the monocyte production rate. The degree of inaccuracy could be substantial, since amplification during monocytopoiesis appears to be low, one stem cell yielding four monocytes (Meuret, 1974). Human granulocytopoiesis, for sake of comparison, may involve a 16-fold amplification (Cronkite and Vincent, 1969). For purposes of illustration we will take the liberty of employing Meuret's data (1974) to estimate the influx (K_{in}) from the stem cell pool. From Quastler (1959),

$$K_B = K_{out} - K_{in} \quad (4)$$

and

$$K_{out} = 2^n K_{in} \quad (5)$$

where n is the number of mitotic divisions in the proliferative compartment. According to Meuret (1974), $n = 2$, $K_B = 7 \times 10^6$/kg/hour, and $K_{out} = 4K_{in}$ [Eq. (5)]. Substituting these values in Eq. (4), K_{in} is equal to about 2.3×10^6 cells/kg/hour. By comparison, the influx from the stem cell compartment into the proliferative compartment in human granulocytopoiesis has been estimated at about 4.2×10^6 cells/kg/hour (Cronkite and Vincent, 1969). When the approximate values of K_{in} and K_B for promonocytes are summed, K_{out} is roughly 9.3×10^6 cells/kg/hour, the theoretical monocyte production rate. As will be shown elsewhere (Section III,B,2), this figure exceeds the monocyte turnover rate in the blood to which it should, in theory, be equal under steady-state conditions. Taken further, the calculations suggest that promonocyte formation may be excessive and that the surplus cells may normally die in the marrow. Further speculation along these lines is prompted by the ability of an acute infectious stimulus to evoke the release into the blood of immature monocytes whose proliferative cycles had been apparently aborted or suspended (Volkman and Collins, 1974; see also Section IV). These observations prompt a comparison with the studies of Patt and Moloney (1964) of granulocytopoiesis in the dog, which indicated that myelocyte production exceeds the influx into the metamyelocyte compartments and that the excess myelocytes die in the marrow.

B. The Monocyte in the Blood

In most instances, the kinetics of monocytes in the blood have been measured by the use of ^{3}HT as described in Section II. Meuret and Hoffmann (1973) and Meuret (1974) have, in addition, employed the autologous transfusion of white blood cells previously withdrawn into plastic bags and labeled with [^{3}H]DFP. An earlier study by Kurth *et al.* (1961) indicated that [^{3}H]DFP was not a wholly stable marker for leukocytes. Meuret (1974; Meuret and Hoffmann, 1973), however, employed [^{3}H]DFP of a much higher specific activity than Kurth *et al.* (1961) and found that although some reduction of labeling intensity was encountered, the proportion of cells labeled did not fall except as a function of loss from circulation. In humans virtually all monocytes and their recognizable precursors can be labeled *in vivo* or *in vitro* (Meuret, 1974). Seeking to adapt this useful technique to studies in rats, the author was unfortunately unable to achieve a useful degree of labeling of monocytes despite the use of high specific activity [^{3}H]DFP and prolonged exposure of autoradiographs.

1. Life-Span in the Blood

It is clear from the data summarized in Table II that substantial disagreement exists with respect to the half-time of the monocyte circulation. The discrepancies do not seem to find explanation in species differences. Intravascular division of the blood monocyte (Table II) clearly does not contribute to the problem. The reason for these wide-ranging values must surely be methodological; alternatively they could be explained by kinetic heterogeneity among the monocytes, one portion of the population having a much shorter life-span in circulation than the other. Still another explanation is that morphological criteria are inadequate for the identification of a proportion of monocytes (Zucker-Franklin, 1974). This is a distinct possibility but is not a wholly satisfactory explanation, since widely differing values have been obtained within the same laboratory (Table II) depending upon methodology and mode

TABLE II

Kinetic Characteristics of Monocytes in the Blood of Normal Subjects

Species	$T_{1/2}$ (hours)	Average life-span in blood (hours)	Blood monocytes in DNA synthesis (%)	Reference
Man	24	35	0	Fliedner *et al.* (1969)
Man	71	102	0	Whitelaw (1972)
Man	8	12	0.05–3.28	Meuret (1974)
Rat	75	108	—	Whitelaw (1966)
Rat	42	61	0.1	Volkman (1967, 1970)
Rat	35, 61	51, 88	0.1	Volkman and Collins (1974)
Rat	13	19	—	Whitelaw *et al.* (1968)
Rat	14	20	—	Whitelaw and Batho (1972)
Mouse	22	32	0	Van Furth and Cohn (1968)
Mouse	—	—	2.3	Van Furth *et al.* (1973)

of calculation. In such instances, one would expect that morphologic identification should have been a constant factor. The lowest values for the half-time of monocytes in the blood were recorded following the infusion of labeled cells into autologous or isologous recipients (Meuret and Hoffmann, 1973; Whitelaw and Batho, 1972). Low values were also obtained, although not invariably, when calculated from the initial rise of the labeling index following a pulse of ^{3}HT. In Whitelaw's laboratory the application of this procedure (Whitelaw *et al.*, 1968) yielded shorter half-times in rats than other methods (Whitelaw, 1966), but this was not the case in man (Whitelaw, 1972). In searching for an explanation, one could suggest that calculations performed on the first rise of the labeling index deal with relatively small proportions of labeled cells in a numerically small population. Minor, even transient, fluctuations, therefore, could conceivably exert a great influence on the results. The same comment pertains to procedures involving the transfusion of labeled cells. Here again, the percentage of labeled monocytes appearing in the blood of recipients must necessarily be low in face of the large dilutions involved. It is also conceivable that, despite all care during the procedure of labeling the cells outside the body or in concentrating them *in vitro*, either stimulation or injury of the monocytes could have occurred, thereby shortening their life expectancy in the blood. It can be argued, however, that isotopic labeling if carefully performed outside the body does not appear to adversely affect the life span of granulocytes (Athens *et al.*,

1959). On the other hand, in contrast with results in monocytes, good agreement among several mammalian species is found between data from autotransfusion (Mauer *et al.*, 1960, Raab *et al.*, 1964) and other methods (Gerecke *et al.*, 1973) in studies of granulocyte kinetics, suggesting that these cells may not be as sensitive to handling as monocytes.

The determinations of $T_{1/2}$ by Van Furth and Cohn (1968), Fliedner *et al.* (1969), and Volkman and Collins (1974) were based on measuring the slope of the decline of the most highly labeled cohorts of monocytes in the blood as explained in Section II,B. The value of 61 hours reported by Volkman and Collins (1974) may be excessive, and their alternative calculations yielded a lower figure that is also shown in Table II. Whitelaw's (1966) estimate of 75 hours was determined by repeatedly administering doses of ^{3}HT at intervals presumed to be shorter than a generation time. Assuming the samples to be representative and a kinetically homogeneous population, the results should be highly accurate. A variant of this approach was employed by Volkman (1967, 1970) who continuously infused ^{3}HT into rats by means of femoral vein cannulas. Results taken from those experiments are shown in Fig. 2. Although the mean $T_{1/2}$ for the six animals infused for 4 and 5 days is approximately 40 hours, this calculation was influenced by a somewhat longer $T_{1/2}$, observed in one of the rats (Fig. 2). Taken without this value, $T_{1/2}$ calculated from the data of the remaining five rats is about 35 hours. The theoretically sound methodology of the experiments based on the repeated or continuous infusion of ^{3}HT, makes it exceedingly difficult to reconcile some of the extreme values of $T_{1/2}$ in Table II.

Meuret (1974) found that the incidence of DNA synthesis by blood monocytes *in vitro* was inversely related to their maturity. The presence of incompletely matured monocytes in the blood is not surprising in view of their relatively short sojourn in bone marrow. It is quite conceivable that many such cells escape identification as monocytes in routine observations (Zucker-Franklin, 1974). Not all observers were able to find evidence for proliferation of monocytes (Table II); however, immigrant macrophages derived from monocytes retain the capacity to divide upon appropriate stimulation (Volkman, 1966). The mature blood monocyte apparently is not in a regular proliferative cycle and may be in G_0, or in a protracted G_1. In either case, the monocyte is clearly not an end cell.

2. *Distribution and Turnover*

Studies carried out in man (Mauer *et al.*, 1960; Athens *et al.*, 1961) employing autotransfused DF^{32}P-labeled granulocytes showed that at the

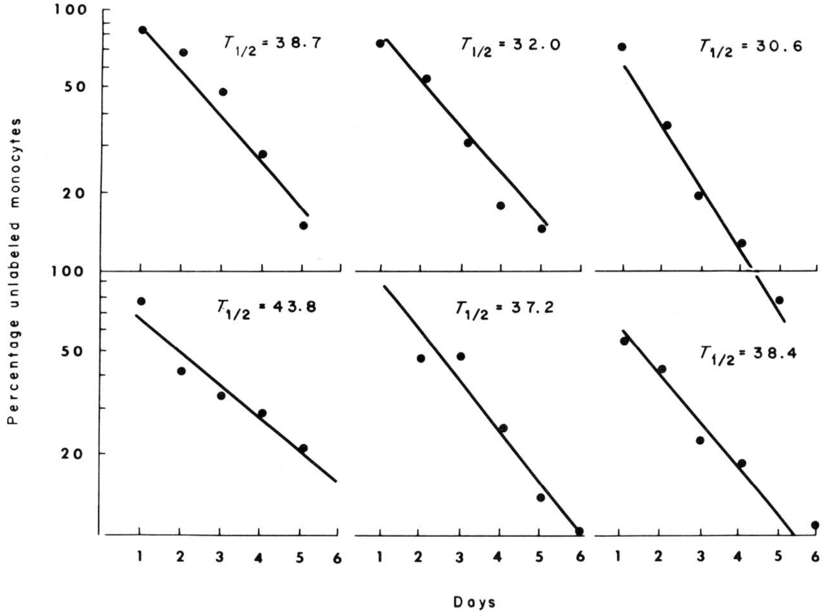

Fig. 2. The loss of unlabeled monocytes from the blood of normal rats continuously infused with ^{3}HT via femoral canulas. Infusion was maintained for 4 days (top half of figure) and 5 days (bottom half of figure); sampling was continued for 1 additional day. Each point = 100 — percent monocytes labeled. Regression lines were fitted by the method of least squares. The half-time in hours is shown next to each regression. Data based on observations reported by Volkman (1967, 1970).

completion of infusion only about 50% of the labeled cells could be accounted for in circulation. To explain this occurrence, it was proposed that a proportion of the infused cells had become distributed in the blood between a circulating granulocyte pool (CGP) and a marginal granulocyte pool (MGP) in equilibrium with each other. The two pools together make up the total blood granulocyte pool (TBGP). The absolute granulocyte count per milliliter multiplied by the blood volume provides the estimate of the CGP; the TBGP is the CGP divided by the fraction of labeled cells remaining in the CGP at the completion of the infusion of The MGP therefore is the difference between TBGP and CGP. It follows that the turnover rate cannot be accurately determined without knowing the total pool size. In concept, the marginal pool results from a slowing of blood flow through certain vascular beds, which permits nucleated cells to leave the axial flow and come into contact with the endothelium (Vejlens, 1938). The marginal pool is additionally important, since it is presumably from this pool that cells can emigrate into tissues.

Whitelaw and Batho (1972) and Meuret and Hoffmann (1973) have demonstrated the presence of a marginal monocyte pool (MMP) in the rat and in man, analogous to the marginal granulocyte pool. It can be seen in Table III that the estimates of the MMP differ widely. The size of the MMP calculated by Whitelaw and Batho (1972) may be an overestimate, since this group infused a number of labeled monocytes into each recipient which by calculation was roughly between 46–69% of the size of the circulating monocyte pool (CMP). It is thus conceivable that this procedure evoked compensatory activity on the part of regulatory mechanisms to displace the excess cells rapidly from the blood. Unpublished experiments in the author's laboratory, based on the exchange transfusion of whole blood between heavily labeled donors and syngeneic recipient rats, have led to calculations of MMP approximately 3.5 times the circulating monocyte pool. This figure lies near the ratios determined in man by Meuret and Hoffmann (1973) as shown in Table III.

Figures for monocyte turnover rates are quoted directly from the sources but are expressed on a per kilogram basis in Table III to provide easy comparison with corresponding measurements in man. The author's approximations are from composite data rather than from one experiment and are used merely to illustrate what the turnover of monocytes may be in the rat.

3. *Reserve Capacity*

There appears to be virtually no evidence for a reserve pool of monocytes anywhere near the magnitude of the reserves of the granulocyte series. It was shown, for example, by Volkman and Collins (1968) that when precursor proliferation was impaired by whole body ionizing radiation, the blood levels of monocytes dropped precipitously. There is also no evidence to indicate that monocytes recirculate to any extent in the manner of long-lived small lymphocytes. From these considerations, it is clear that the maintenance of normal blood levels of monocytes is dependent upon unimpaired precursor cell proliferation and the sustained release of effective numbers of cells from the bone marrow.

4. *Oscillation of Blood Monocyte Levels*

A low amplitude oscillation of the absolute blood monocyte count was described by Meuret (1974) in young male students. When sampled at

TABLE III

The Distribution and Turnover of Monocytes in the Blood of Normal Subjects

	Circulating monocyte pool		Total blood monocyte pool				
Species	Total cells	Cells/kg body weight	Total cells	Cells/kg body weight	CMP/MMP	Monocyte turnover rate (cells/kg/hour)	Reference
Man	1.4×10^9	18×10^6	6.4×10^9	81×10^6	0.3	7.5×10^6	Meuret (1974)
Rat	—		—		0.04	—	Whitelaw and Batho (1972)
Rat[a]	17.7×10^6	89×10^6	79.6×10^6	400×10^6	0.29	6.9×10^6	A. Volkman (unpublished)

[a] These calculations are based on composite data from several experiments with male and female rats weighing about 200 gm with a mean blood volume of 6.8% body weight CMP, circulating monocyte pool; MMP, marginal monocyte pool.

the same time each day, fluctuations in the monocyte count resulted in a series of maxima and minima with a modal periodicity of 5 days (range 3–6 days). This behavior corresponds in type to oscillations in the blood counts reported for neutrophils and thrombocytes in man (Morley, 1966, 1969) and reticulocytes in dogs (Morley and Stohlman, 1969), although the oscillatory period is shorter among monocytes. The phenomenon has been attributed to the presence of a regulatory mechanism of a negative feedback loop linking the peripheral blood cell compartment and the stem cell differentiation rate. A time delay largely due to the bone marrow transit time from stem cell to egress into the blood would be inherent in such a system and could account for the oscillatory nature of the blood monocyte level (Morley *et al.*, 1970).

C. Fate of the Monocyte: Relationships to Other Mononuclear Cell Populations

Steady-state conditions demand that as many monocytes leave as enter the blood each day. Since the duration of the sojourn of monocytes in the blood is not age-dependent, it is logical to look for a functionally significant extravascular role for the emigrant cells. The ability of the monocyte to emigrate into a focus of inflammation and develop into a larger, more active and effective cell, the macrophage, is now a fact established by a substantial quantity of evidence (reviewed by Volkman, 1970).

Whether the monocyte in leaving the blood plays any role in the renewal, under physiological conditions, of resident ("fixed") populations of macrophages located predominantly in the liver, the pulmonary alveolar spaces, the areolar tissues, and body cavities is still a moot point. There is evidence that resident macrophage populations, for example, the Kupffer cells in the liver (Edwards and Klein, 1961; Kelly *et al.*, 1962) and peritoneal macrophages (Volkman, 1966) divide and turn over at a slow rate and are therefore capable of self-renewal. In addition, there have been no objective demonstrations that monocytes contribute to the renewal of any of these resident populations under anything approaching physiological conditions. Physiological conditions may be defined readily for the purpose of making the point, as the conventional ambience conducive to sustained good health and opposed to those conditions that occur during or after lethal whole body irradiation, a systemic graft versus host reaction, subtotal hepatectomy, systemic administration of a potent granuloma-forming or immunostimulating agent, and estrogenic or other hormonal stimulation. These, in fact, are the conditions under which the ostensible development of circulating cells into "fixed" or resident-type macrophages has been demonstrated (see review by Volkman, 1970). The objections to conclusions reached under such experimental conditions are obvious, but some qualifications are in order.

Balner (1963) and Goodman (1964) employed specifically cytotoxic antisera to demonstrate that peritoneal macrophages could be derived from donor-type bone marrow cells administered to lethally irradiated rats and mice. Even under these conditions, the derivation of resident macrophages from bone marrow would be of considerable interest. It is plausible, however, that the milieu of the peritoneal cavity becomes inflammatory following lethal irradiation due to the presence of products liberated from damaged and dead cells. If true, then the newly appearing peritoneal macrophages could merely represent a monocytic response to inflammation; if not true, the interpretation of these experiments is still limited in the present context. The conditions attending the establishment of radiation chimeras are drastic and may evoke stem cell activities not normally expressed in adult animals. The same arguments apply to the carefully executed experiment of Pinkett *et al.* (1966), who employed the T_6 chromosome marker in CBA mice to determine the origins of pulmonary alveolar macrophages in bone marrow-restored radiation chimeras. Two-thirds to four-fifths of the dividing alveolar macrophages under these conditions proved to be of donor type. An additional consideration in this connection is that the alveolar spaces are open to the external environment, and it would not be unexpected to find a consistent hematogenous contribution to the alveolar macrophage population in ostensibly normal animals. Taken further, these are physiological conditions for alveolar spaces, and the "resident" population of mononuclear phagocytes may always be of dual origin starting from several hours after birth.

Van Furth and Cohn (1968), who employed ^{3}HT labeling in mice, concluded on the basis of the labeling patterns of the respective populations that resident peritoneal macrophages were normally derived from monocytes. Their data in that paper are wholly consistent with this interpretation, but alternative explanations were by no means eliminated by any experimental data in that study. When the experimental protocols of Van Furth and Cohn (1968) were replicated and extended by others (Takahashi *et al.*, 1973), it was found that following a pulse ^{3}HT, the grain counts in the labeled peritoneal macrophages were consistently higher than in labeled blood monocytes. This evidence weighs strongly against the possibility that the labeled resident macrophages had been derived from immigrant monocytes. In another study, Whitelaw and Batho (1972) could find no emigration of labeled monocytes into the unstimulated peritoneal cavities of rats intravenously infused with large numbers of heavily labeled syngeneic white blood cells. The emigration of autotransfused labeled monocytes into foci of inflammation was, on the other hand, demonstrable (Meuret *et al.*, 1971).

Another question that arises at this point is whether the so-called resident macrophages might not originate by the accumulation of monocytes from successive responses to repeated inflammatory stimuli. Distinct ultrastructural and cytochemical differences, however, distinguish resident-type macrophages from monocyte-derived macrophages (Daems and Brederoo, 1973; Wisse, 1974), adding further evidence against the possibility that a lineal relationship exists between the blood monocytes and resident populations of macrophages. The observations of Daems *et al.* (1973; Daems and Brederoo, 1973) indicate in addition that exudate macrophages and resident peritoneal macrophages maintain the distinguishing characteristics of their respective classes within an exudate. It seems a logical corollary, therefore, that the protracted sojourn of "free" macrophages in tissue or a serous cavity would not be grounds for contending that such cells had become identical with the resident macrophage population.

From the foregoing discussion it is clear that there is no objective support for the view proposed by Van Furth *et al.* (1972) that the monocyte system includes the resident macrophages of tissues, sinusoidal linings, and serosal cavities. Indeed, there is some strong evidence to the contrary as cited above. In short, it appears that by virtue of their emigratory properties monocytes may serve to reinforce local macrophage populations, but it is highly doubtful that the monocytes serve as a physiological renewal mechanism for resident cells.

What then is the fate of monocytes? Since their sojourn via the blood is not terminated by senescence and there is no evidence for reentry, the existence of a one-way portal for vigorous cells appears logical. One can propose routes of exit dependent on the notion that low-grade multifocal "trivial" inflammation may be occurring constantly and "normally." This may be the result of physical trauma, minute microbial invasions, and the intestinal absorption and pulmonary inhalation of nonspecific irritants and antigenic materials. A "background" drainage of relatively constant magnitude may thus account for the steady removal of monocytes from the blood. There is some evidence that granulocytes may leave the blood for reasons of this sort. Thus, blood and sputum granulocytes label synchronously after a single injection (Fliedner *et al.*, 1964) or during the continuous infusion of ^{3}HT (Gerecke *et al.*, 1973). A substantial efflux of labeled macrophages into the oropharynx was observed in rats following the intravenous administration of ^{3}HT (Spritzer *et al.*, 1968). Presumably these cells migrated from the blood into pulmonary alveoli and then into the oropharynx. An objection to this conclusion is that the indwelling polyethylene catheter necessary for the collection of the cells could have provoked local inflammation.

As a final consideration, the life span of monocytes may be determined by an intrinsic control mechanism responsive to, but independent of, peripheral demands. The normal levels would then be in excess of peripheral demands, and the daily surplus discharged in some unknown way. Teleologically, this may seem uneconomical. On the other hand, the blood monocyte pool in such a system would represent a highly mobile reserve. It seems plausible that small demands could be met without any resulting perturbation of the regulatory mechanism if the normal daily loss were not exceeded, the only change involved being the portal of exit.

IV. CELL KINETICS OF MONOCYTES IN INFECTION

Infection is a realistic context in which to explore the cytokinetic adjustments of monocytes as a component of the defenses of the host. Quantitative information on this subject, however, is meager. Data discussed earlier indicate that the monocytes are a closely regulated system. It would be anticipated, therefore, that significant increases in the emigration of monocytes from the blood in response to infection could initiate or augment signals for an increased output in order to maintain normal levels of monocytes in the blood. Quite conceivably, small changes in the production of monocytes might not be reflected in the absolute blood monocyte count but could be revealed by cytokinetic studies.

Some data of altered monocyte kinetics in infection have recently been obtained in humans (Meuret and Hoffmann, 1973) and in rats (Volkman and Collins, 1974). In man, each sample represented one patient at a point during an ongoing infection; alterations in variety of infections were observed. A sequential study of altered kinetic mechanisms was possible, however, during systemic infection with *Salmonella enteritidis* in experimental rats (Volkman and Collins, 1974). This study extended from a point 2 days before infection to a point 8 days after infection. Data emerging from the respective studies are summarized in Table IV.

Taking the absolute blood monocyte count as a guide, data relating to clinical infection (Meuret and Hoffmann, 1973) were arbitrarily divided into two groups in Table IV. In one group, the monocyte count was almost doubled and classed in Table IV as a moderate response. Included in the group were one case of acute pyelonephritis, one of subacute tonsillitis, one of chronic cholangitis, and three of tuberculosis. High monocyte responses with counts five to seven times normal were found in two patients with septicemia (agent not given) and one with sporotricho-

TABLE IV

***Distribution and Turnover of Monocytes in Infection*[a]**

Species	Status	Absolute monocyte count (cells/mm³)	CMP (cells × 10^9)	MMP (cells × 10^9)	CMP/MMP	TBMP (cells × 10^9)	$T_{1/2}$ (hours)	Monocyte turnover rate (cells × 10^9/hour)	Reference
Man	Normal	260 ± 105	1.4 ± 0.5	5 ± 2.8	0.3 ± 0.2	6.4 ± 3.1	8.4 ± 1.9	0.6 ± 0.4	Meuret and Hoffmann (1973)
	Infection moderate response	489 ± 178	2.1 ± 1.2	12.8 ± 11	0.28 ± 1.2	14.9 ± 9.9	7.7 ± 2.6	1.3 ± 1.1	
	Infection high response	1455 ± 237	9.2 ± 2.9	29.7 ± 4.8	0.29 ± 0.1	38.9 ± 4.4	11.1 ± 4.6	2.9 ± 1.6	
	Boeck's sarcoid	7840	39.6	131.9	0.3	170.3			

Species	Status	Absolute monocyte count (cells/mm³)	CMP (cells × 10^7)	MMP (cells × 10^7)	CMP/MMP	TBMP (cells × 10^7)	$T_{1/2}$ (hours)	Monocyte turnover rate (cells × 10^6/hour)	Reference
Rat	Normal	1200	(1.4)	(4.9)	(0.29)	(6.3)	35, 61	(1.2, 0.72)	Volkman and Collins (1974)
	Infection	4100	(4.8)	(16.8)	(0.29)[b]	(21.6)	15, 25	(10, 6)	

[a] The figures in the table are means and (where available) standard deviations. Data in parentheses did not appear in the reference but were calculated retrospectively on the basis of later observations. CMP, circulating monocyte pool; MMP, marginal monocyte pool; TBMP, total blood monocyte pool; $T_{1/2}$, half-time of loss of monocytes from the blood.

[b] This ratio is assumed, only for purposes of discussion, to be unchanged from normal on the basis of the observations of Meuret and Hoffmann (1973) shown in the table and is included with derivative data merely to illustrate possible results.

sis who, in fact, also displayed the highest monocyte counts among the three patients. Data from a case of Boeck's sarcoid are included in Table IV, as a matter of interest in view of the extremely high elevations of the blood monocyte count and other parameters. It is curious that in most instances there was very little change observed in the half-time of monocytes in the blood and virtually no alteration in the ratio of the marginal monocyte pool to the circulating monocyte pool. By contrast, Fliedner *et al.* (1969) observed a small (25%) reduction of half-time in a patient with bacterial infection.

Since the data in the rat demonstrate something of the development of monocytosis in relation to a defined systemic infection, this model will be discussed in greater detail. In this study employing isotopic labeling and autoradiography, a single intravenous injection of ^{3}HT was given at varying intervals with respect to the time of the intravenous injection of 10^6 living *Salmonella enteritidis*. This organism is a facultative intracellular parasite to which rats generally display a high degree of resistance. The rapid inactivation or organisms by the host is associated with widespread formation of granulomas, the emergence of high levels of specific delayed-type hypersensitivity, and a high incidence of a destructive polyarthritis (Volkman and Collins, 1973). Within 3 weeks after inoculation the organism cannot be recovered from most organs and tissues; however, small numbers of salmonellae continue to grow in the kidneys and some lymph nodes, indicating the presence of a stable carrier state (Volkman and Collins, 1973).

In Fig. 3 the absolute monocyte and white blood cell counts are shown in relation to the rapid decline in the growth of *S. enteritidis* in the liver and spleen. It is interesting to note the initial fall in blood monocytes, which may represent acute depletion, is followed by an apparently linear increase that finally stabilizes at a plateau over three times the normal level on day 5. This plateau probably represents the imposition of a new steady state.

The $T_{1/2}$ of monocytes in the blood was estimated from the decline in the percentage of labeled monocytes in a highly labeled cohort. Regression lines computed from these data (Fig. 4) clearly demonstrate that the $T_{1/2}$ of monocytes in the blood was reduced in Fig. 4A–4C of infected rats to less than 50% of the value calculated in the control (uninfected) rats. Since the $T_{1/2}$ in the controls exceeded the figures previously obtained in this laboratory, a second calculation was made after raising the grain count threshold to define the most highly labeled cohort (Volkman and Collins, 1974). This recalculation yielded a $T_{1/2}$ of 35 hours in the uninfected and 15 hours in the infected rats. These values remain in approximately the same ratio as the initially calculated 61 and 25 hours;

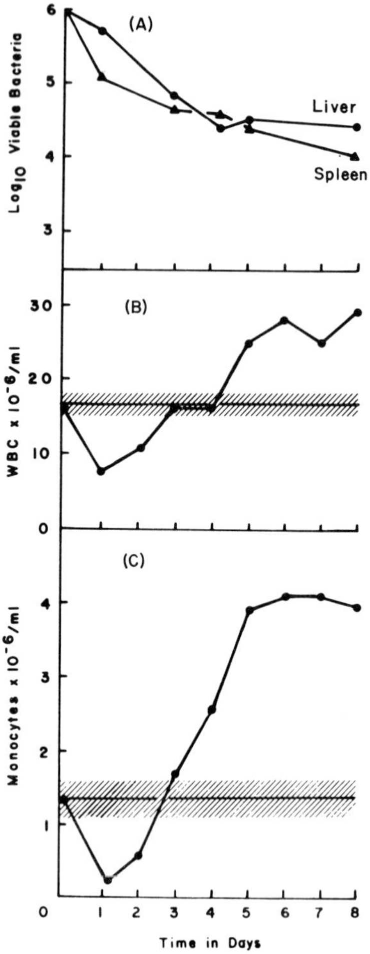

Fig. 3. The development of monocytosis during acute systemic infection with *S. enteritidis* in (Lewis × BN) F_1 hybrid rats. (A) The decline in numbers of viable *S. enteritidis* in the liver and spleen is shown at increasing intervals after the intravenous injection of 10^6 living salmonellae on day 0. (B) White blood cell counts. The mean and 95% confidence intervals for 18 uninfected rats are indicated by the shaded band. (C) Absolute monocyte counts/milliliter. The mean and 95% confidence intervals for 18 uninfected rats are indicated by the shaded band. Data taken from Volkman and Collins (1974).

moreover, the figure of 35 hours is in close agreement with the earlier determination based on the continuous infusion of ^{3}HT (Section III,B,1).

The average generation or cell cycle time (T_G) for dividing monocyte precursors in bone marrow was estimated by fitting a regression line to

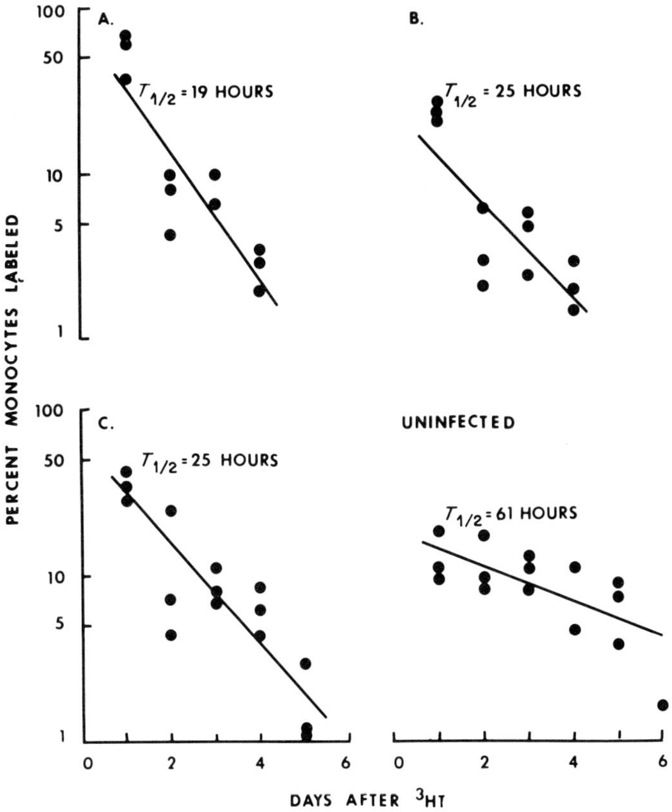

Fig. 4. Estimation of the half-time ($T_{1/2}$) of monocytes in the blood of rats during progressive phases of primary infection with *S. enteritidis*. Regression lines were fitted by the method of least squares (Volkman and Collins, 1974). Reproduced by courtesy of the publishers of *J. Exp. Med.*, The Rockefeller University Press.

the decline in median grain counts; the halving time of the regression was taken as the approximation of T_G. Data in Fig. 5 shows that T_G was reduced to about 15 hours from days 1–3 (Fig. 5A and 5B) of infection but on days 4–8 (Fig. 5C) the computed cell cycle time was 35 hours, a value close to 32 hours determined in the interval before infection (A′) and 31 hours in the uninfected controls. The slopes thus actually fall into two families mathematically. This reduction in the cell cycle time undoubtedly contributed substantially to the increased output of monocytes into the blood. Comparable behavior within the monocyte proliferative pool was also observed to occur in human infections (Meuret, 1974) (Table IV). An apparently stable absolute monocytosis was maintained from days 5–8 in the presence of a normal T_G, a reduced $T_{1/2}$ of monocytes

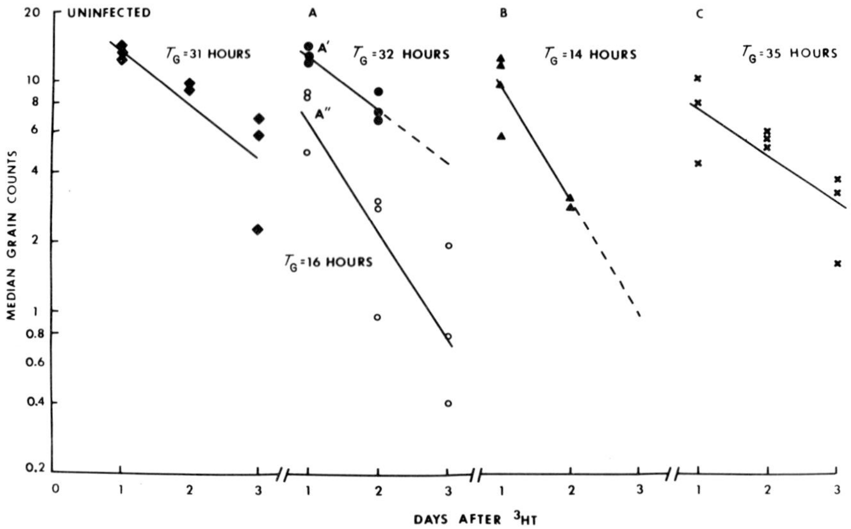

Fig. 5. Estimation of the average generation time (T_G) of proliferating monocyte precursors in rats during progressive phases of acute primary infection with *S. enteritidis*. The T_G is taken to be equal to the halving time of the median grain count. The regression lines were fitted by the method of least squares. The dashed lines indicate extrapolations (Volkman and Collins, 1974). Reproduced by courtesy of the publishers of *J. Exp. Med.*, The Rockefeller University Press.

in the blood, and an increased monocyte turnover rate. In addition, monocyte reserves proved to be inconsequential, and intravascular division trivial (Volkman and Collins, 1974). Under these conditions it seems fair to conclude that the sustained increase in monocyte output must have been due to an enlarged precursor pool in the bone marrow. The data provide no indication of the mechanisms by which this inferred enlargement was brought about. One possibility is that more monocyte precursors were induced into active cycle; another is that increased numbers of undifferentiated stem cells were diverted into monocyte formation.

One additional feature of this study merits comment. The rises in labeling indices in uninfected rats (Fig. 6D) were comparable until 48 hours after administration of ^{3}HT at which time one (Fig. 6A) was injected with live *S. enteritidis*. The increase in labeling index was sustained for another day in Fig. 6A in contrast with the decline observed starting at 48 hours in the uninfected controls and in Fig. 6C. The decline in the labeling index occurred still earlier in Fig. 6B. The increase in the labeling index occurring soon after infection in Fig. 6A was correlated with the appearance in the blood of monocytes (promonocytes?) with grain counts in excess of the early median grain counts. These cells consti-

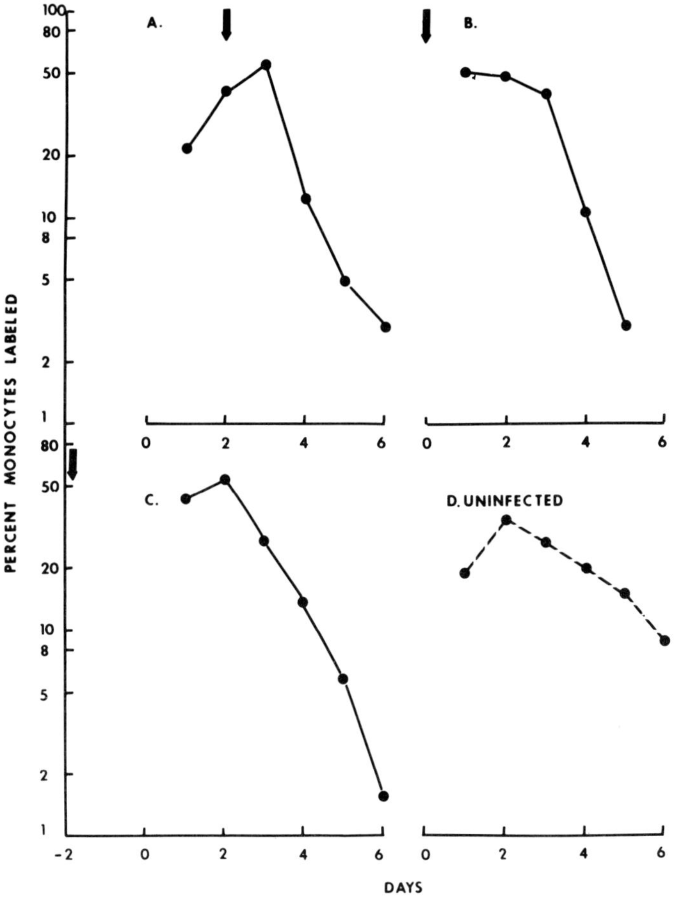

Fig. 6. The median percentages of labeled monocytes in panels of infected (A)–(C) and uninfected (D) rats on successive days after single intravenous injection of ^{3}HT. The time of intravenous infection with 10^6 viable *S. enteritidis* is indicated by the arrows (Volkman and Collins, 1974). Reproduced by courtesy of the publishers of *J. Exp. Med.*, The Rockefeller University Press.

tuted about 22% of the labeled monocyte population in Fig. 6A on the third day after the administration of ^{3}HT. This unique occurrence probably represented an immediate response of the monocyte system to infection or to endotoxic stimulation. The observation suggests, in addition, that some proportion of the monocyte precursors had not completed the usual number of divisions before their release into the blood. In short, the proliferative cycle of these highly labeled cells had either been interrupted or was more protracted in relation to the bulk of the population. Since labeling of rats (Fig. 6A) was performed before infection, one can also infer that the observed behavior occurs normally. One is tempted to speculate that these cells with an altered cycle could account for the discrepancy between the theoretical and actual K_{out} discussed in Section III,A,3. In a strict sense these highly labeled cells constituted a reserve population; however, their numbers were obviously too few to compensate for the depression in the peripheral monocyte count that occurred after infection (Fig. 3); absolute monocyte counts did not return to the normal range for approximately 48 hours.

In summary, three mechanisms were observed in the response of monocytes to infection. One was the release of premature monocytes that are apparently normally retained in the bone marrow, whose cycle is as possibly in suspended cycle. A second was the temporary shortening of the cell cycle time to about 50% of normal, thereby potentially doubling the output of monocytes. The third mechanism was the apparent sustained enlargement of the monocyte precursor pool, possibly achieved by increasing the proportion of promonocytes actively cycling and/or the recruitment of stem cells into monocytopoiesis.

Since the marginal monocyte pool was not actually measured in these studies the size of the total blood monocyte pool can only be approximated by assuming, on the basis of the observations of Meuret and Hoffmann (1973), that the ratio of the circulating to the marginal monocyte pool in infection did not deviate appreciably from normal. The monocyte turnover rate thus estimated (Table IV) was found to be substantially increased in the *Salmonella*-infected rats.

The stability of the $T_{1/2}$ in man during infection compared with the distinct reduction of $T_{1/2}$ in the infected rats is interesting but unexplained. Seeking analogies in granulocyte kinetics provides little help, since the $T_{1/2}$ of granulocytes in infection is either unchanged or increased (Cronkite and Vincent, 1969). This is surprising, since one would predict a reduced $T_{1/2}$ to the increased drainage of cells from the blood into foci of infection. Cronkite and Vincent (1969) interpret the increase in the $T_{1/2}$ of granulocytes in infection to signify an alteration of the usual random loss pattern in order to increase the number of blood granulocytes available for emigration to the site of infection without a generalized and pronounced increase in the granulocyte turnover rate. The monocyte data permit no conclusions of this sort, since in man increased half-times were associated with some of the highest turnover rates (Meuret and Hoffmann, 1973), and in *Salmonella*-infected rats, the half-times were consistently shortened. One can only speculate that alterations in the length of the sojourn of the monocyte in the blood during infection may be determined in part by the extent of the pathology and in part by the nature of the infectious agent.

V. CONCLUDING REMARKS

The kinetics of the proliferating and circulating compartments of the monocyte system and their alterations in infection have been presented in profile. Despite the fact that the monocytes constitute a minority of the nucleated blood cells, their proliferative pool appears to be capable of great expansion in face of demand. Since there is no large reserve of monocytes in bone marrow and the emergence time is brief, it is probable that great increases in monocytopoiesis can take place without intramedullary "crowding." A large number of gaps in our knowledge concerning this important cell system still exist. One such gap concerns the nature of the unrecognized monocyte precursors in bone marrow and their relationship to the stem cells assessed in *in vitro* studies of hemopoiesis. In turn, further information is needed concerning the relationship of these formative cells to other cell systems, particularly the granulocytic series. The fine structure of the monocyte precursor pool still needs further clarification. Variations in cell cycle, the proportion of precursors in active cycle (growth fractions), and the factors that influence them are virtually unknown. The life span of monocytes in the blood, as described in the literature, varies so extensively that further investigation is required to resolve this problem. More attention must be given to the distribution of monocytes into circulating and marginal pools and to the factors that may influence this distribution. The relationship of the marginal pool to cellular emigration also merits additional investigation. The demonstration of oscillatory behavior of the blood monocyte count suggests the constant operation of a feedback system; however, our knowledge concerning regulatory mechanisms of monocyte production is at present rudimentary.

Since the time when the participation of mononuclear phagocytes in host defense mechanisms was first appreciated, numerous attempts have been made to increase the number and activity of these cells in favor of the host. Indeed, this approach still constitutes a very active area of immunobiological research. All too often, the term "reticuloendothelial stimulation" has been used to characterize the effect being sought. It is doubtful, according to the evidence reviewed in this chapter, that a lineal relationship exists between the monocyte system and the so-called reticuloendothelial cells ("fixed" or resident macrophages).

It is clearly desirable to define the mononuclear phagocytes and their properties with as much precision as is demanded in dealing with lymphocytic populations. Hopefully, the further clarification of the compartments of the monocyte system, their kinetic responses, and their regulatory mechanisms will help to provide an objective basis for achieving this goal.

ACKNOWLEDGMENTS

Some of the author's work described in this chapter was supported by the United States Public Health Service grants CA 17756 and AM 17159 from the National Institute of Arthritis, Metabolism and Digestive Diseases. The author thanks Mrs. Anne L. Jones for her help in preparing the manuscript.

REFERENCES

Alpen, E. L., and Johnston, M. E. (1967). *Exp. Cell Res.* **47,** 177–192.

Athens, J. W., Raab, S. O., Haab, O. P., Mauer, A. M., Ashenbrucker, H., Cartwright, G. E., and Wintrobe, M. M. (1961). *J. Clin. Invest.* **40,** 159–164.

Athens, J. W., Mauer, A. M., Ashenbrucker, H., Cartwright, G. E., and Wintrobe, M. M. (1959). *Blood* **4,** 303–333.

Balner, H. (1963). *Transplantation* **1,** 217–223.

Bond, V. P., Fliedner, T. M., and Archambeau, J. O. (1965). "Mammalian Radiation Lethality: A Disturbance in Cellular Kinetics." Academic Press, New York.

Bradley, T. R., and Metcalf, D. (1966). *Aust. J. Exp. Biol. Med. Sci.* **44,** 287–300.

Cleaver, J. E. (1967). "Thymidine Metabolism and Cell Kinetics." Wiley, New York.

Cronkite, E. P., and Vincent, P. C. (1969). *Ser. Haematol.* [N.S.] **2,** 3–43.

Cronkite, E. P., Fliedner, T. M., Bond, V. P., and Rubini, J. R. (1959). *Ann. N.Y. Acad. Sci.* **77,** 803–820.

Daems, W. T., and Brederoo, P. (1973). *Z. Zellforsch. Mikrosk. Anat.* **144,** 247–297.

Daems, W. T., Poelmann, R. E., and Brederoo, P. (1973). *J. Histochem. Cytochem.* **21,** 93–95.

Dannenberg, A. M., Ando, M., and Shima, K. (1972). *J. Immunol.* **109,** 1109–1121.

Ebert, R. H., and Florey, H. W. (1939). *Brit. J. Exp. Pathol.* **20,** 342–356.

Edwards, J. L., and Klein, R. E. (1961). *Amer. J. Pathol.* **38,** 937–951.

Fitzgerald, P. J., Eidinoff, M. L., Knoll, J. E., and Simmel, E. B. (1951). *Science* **114,** 494–498.

Fliedner, T. M., Cronkite, E. P., and Bond, V. P. (1962). *Proc. Congr. Eur. Soc. Haematol., 8th, 1961* Paper No. 62.

Fliedner, T. M., Cronkite, E. P., and Robertson, J. S. (1964). *Blood* **24,** 402–414.

Fliedner, T. M., Laeger, F., and Cronkite, E. P. (1969). *In* "Der Monozyt" (H. Brucher, ed.), pp. 39–51. Lehmanns, Munich.

Gerecke, D., Scultze, B., and Maurer, W. (1973). *Cell Tissue Kinet.* **6,** 369–378.

Goodman, J. W. (1964). *Blood* **23,** 18–26.

Hughes, W. L., Bond, V. P., Brecher, G., Cronkite, E. P., Painter, R. B., Quastler, H., and Sherman, F. G. (1958). *Proc. Nat. Acad. Sci. U.S.* **44,** 476–483.

Kelly, L. S., Brown, B. A., and Dobson, E. L. (1962). *Proc. Soc. Exp. Biol. Med.* **110,** 555–559.

Killmann, S.-A. (1968). *Ser. Haematol.* [N.S.] **1,** 38–102.

Kurth, D., Athens, J. W., Cronkite, E. P., Cartwright, G. E., and Wintrobe, M. M. (1961). *Proc. Soc. Exp. Biol. Med.* **107,** 1422–1426.

Leder, L.-D. (1967a). *Blut* **16,** 86–97.

Leder, L.-D. (1967b). "Der Blutmonocyt." Springer-Verlag, Berlin and New York.

Mauer, A. M., Athens, J. W., Ashenbrucker, H., Cartwright, G. E., and Wintrobe, M. M. (1960). *J. Clin. Invest.* **39,** 1481–1486.
Metcalf, D. (1971). *J. Cell. Physiol.* **77,** 277–280.
Metcalf, D., Bradley, T. R., and Robinson, W. (1967). *J. Cell. Physiol.* **69,** 93–107.
Meuret, G. (1974). *Exp. Hematol.* **2,** 238–249.
Meuret, G., and Hoffmann, G. (1973). *Brit. J. Exp. Haematol.* **24,** 275–285.
Meuret, G. M., Djawari, D., Berlet, R., and Hoffmann, G. (1971). *In* "The Reticuloendothelial System and Immune Phenomena" (N. R. DiLuzio and K. Flemming, eds.), pp. 33–46. Plenum, New York.
Morley, A. A. (1966). *Lancet* **2,** 1220–1222.
Morley, A. A. (1969). *Australas. Ann. Med.* **18,** 127–129.
Morley, A. A., and Stohlman, F., Jr. (1969). *Science* **165,** 1025–1027.
Morley, A. A., King-Smith, E. A., and Stohlman, F., Jr. (1970). *In* "Hemopoietic Cellular Proliferation" (F. Stohlman, Jr., ed.), pp. 3–14. Grune & Stratton, New York.
Nichols, B. A., Bainton, D. F., and Farquhar, M. G. (1971). *J. Cell Biol.* **50,** 498–515.
Osgood, E. E., Tivey, H., Davison, K. B., Seaman, A. J., and Li, J. G. (1962). *Cancer (Philadelphia)* **5,** 331–335.
Paran, M., and Sachs, L. (1969). *J. Cell. Physiol.* **73,** 91–92.
Patt, H. M., and Moloney, M. A. (1964). *Ann. N.Y. Acad. Sci.* **113,** 515–522.
Pinkett, M. O., Cowdrey, D. R., and Nowell, P. C. (1966). *Amer. J. Pathol.* **48,** 859–867.
Pluznik, D. H., and Sachs, L. (1966). *Exp. Cell Res.* **43,** 553–563.
Quastler, H. (1959). *In* "Kinetics of Cellular Proliferation" (F. Stohlman, ed.), pp. 431–433. Grune & Stratton, New York.
Raab, S. O., Athens, J. W., Haab, O. P., Boggs, D. R., Ashenbrucker, H., Cartwright, G. E., and Wintrobe, M. M. (1964). *Amer. J. Physiol.* **206,** 83–88.
Rubini, J. R., Cronkite, E. P., Bond, V. P., and Fliedner, T. M. (1960). *J. Clin. Invest.* **39,** 909–918.
Sabin, F. R., Miller, F. R., Smithburn, K. C., Thomas, R. M., and Hummel, L. E. (1936). *J. Exp. Med.* **64,** 97–120.
Schmalzl, F., and Braunsteiner, H. (1969). *Klin. Wochenschr.* **47,** 887–888.
Spector, W. G., Walters, M. N.-I., and Willoughby, D. A. (1965). *J. Pathol. Bacteriol.* **90,** 181–192.
Spritzer, A. A., Watson, J. A., Auld, J. A., and Guettnoff, M. A. (1968). *Arch. Environ. Health* **17,** 726–730
Takahashi, H., Enzan, H., and Ohkita, T. (1973). *Recent Advan. RES Research (Tokyo)* **11,** 85–109.
Till, J. E., and McCulloch, E. A. (1961). *Radiat. Res.* **14,** 213–222.
Van Furth, R., and Cohn, Z. A. (1968). *J. Exp. Med.* **128,** 415–433.
Van Furth, R., and Diesselhoff-Den Dulk, M. M. C. (1970). *J. Exp. Med.* **132,** 813–828.
Van Furth, R., Cohn, Z. A., Hirsch, J. G., Humphrey, J. H., Spector, W. G., and Langevoort, H. L. (1972). *Bull. W.H.O.* **46,** 845–852.
Van Furth, R., Diesselhoff-Den Dulk, M. M. C., and Mattie, H. (1973). *J. Exp. Med.* **138,** 1314–1330.
Vejlens, G. (1938). *Acta Microbiol. Scand., Suppl.* **33.**
Virolainen, M. (1968). *J. Exp. Med.* **127,** 943–952.
Virolainen, M., and Defendi, V. (1968). *Nature (London)* **217,** 1069–1070.
Volkman, A. (1966). *J. Exp. Med.* **124,** 241–254.

Volkman, A. (1967). *Haematol. Lat.* **10**, 61–63.
Volkman, A. (1970). *Ser. Haematol.* [N.S.] **3**, 62–90.
Volkman, A., and Collins, F. M. (1968). *J. Immunol.* **101**, 846–859.
Volkman, A., and Collins, F. M. (1973). *Infect. Immunity* **8**, 814–818.
Volkman, A., and Collins, F. M. (1974). *J. Exp. Med.* **139**, 264–277.
Volkman, A., and Gowans, J. L. (1965a). *Brit. J. Exp. Pathol.* **46**, 50–61.
Volkman, A., and Gowans, J. L. (1965b). *Brit. J. Exp. Pathol.* **46**, 62–70.
Whitelaw, D. M. (1966). *Blood* **28**, 455–464.
Whitelaw, D. M. (1972). *Cell Tissue Kinet.* **5**, 311–317.
Whitelaw, D. M., and Batho, H. F. (1972). *Cell Tissue Kinet.* **5**, 215–225.
Whitelaw, D. M., Bell, M. F., and Batho, H. F. (1968). *J. Cell. Physiol.* **72**, 65–71.
Wisse, E. (1974). *J. Ultrastruct. Res.* **46**, 499–520.
Witts, L. J., and Webb, R. A. (1927). *J. Pathol. Bacteriol.* **30**, 687–712.
Wulff, H. R., and Sparrevohn, S. (1966). *Acta Pathol. Microbiol. Scand.* **68**, 401–407.
Zucker-Franklin, D. (1974). *J. Immunol.* **112**, 234–240.

13

Chemotaxis of Macrophages

Ralph Snyderman and Stephan E. Mergenhagen

I. Introduction 323
II. Methods for Quantifying Macrophage Chemotaxis 324
A. Chemotaxis of Peritoneal Macrophages 326
B. Chemotaxis of Peripheral Blood Macrophages 328
C. Measurement of Chemotaxis *in Vivo* 328
III. Humoral Factors Chemotactic for Macrophages 329
A. Chemotactic Factors Derived from Complement 329
B. Chemotactic Activity in Serum and Plasma 331
IV. Lymphocyte-Derived Chemotactic Factors 333
A. Chemotactic Activity Produced *in Vitro* 333
B. Chemotactic Activity Produced *in Vivo* 336
V. Chemotactic Factors from Bacteria 337
VI. Factors Which Alter Monocyte Chemotactic Function 337
VII. Abnormalities of Monocyte Chemotaxis in Human Diseases 340
VIII. Summary and Conclusions 345
References 346

I. INTRODUCTION

The importance of macrophage function in inflammation and wound healing has been recognized for nearly a century, but the mechanism by which these cells accumulate at local tissue sites is still poorly defined. Macrophages are phagocytic, wandering cells with intracellular digestive properties and promote wound healing by eliminating tissue debris and fibrin deposits. In immunologically mediated inflammation, macrophages function to degrade antigens as well as to phagocytize neutrophil debris.

These processes are essential to host defense and depend upon the rapid accumulation of an adequate number of cells at local tissue sites where antigen or tissue breakdown products are concentrated.

One mechanism that could account for the local accumulation of wandering cells such as macrophages is chemotaxis, the unidirectional migration of cells along a concentration gradient of a chemoattractant. Boyden (1962) developed a quantitative assay for the measurement of leukocyte chemotaxis *in vitro*. In subsequent years, this methodology has been modified to allow the quantitative analysis of locomotion of macrophages and monocytes derived from a number of species. From studies of macrophage migration *in vitro* and *in vivo* a number of points have become clearer. Macrophages migrate toward chemotactic factors produced as a consequence of immunological reactions or tissue breakdown (Snyderman and Stahl, 1974). Furthermore, dysfunctions of human monocyte chemotaxis may have pathophysiological significance in a number of human diseases marked by increased susceptibility to infections and neoplasms (Snyderman *et al.*, 1974b; Snyderman and Stahl, 1975). In the following discussion, we will review methodology for the quantification of macrophage and monocyte chemotaxis *in vitro* and *in vivo,* define factors that are chemotactic for macrophages, and discuss recent findings of depressed monocyte chemotaxis in human disease states.

II. METHODS FOR QUANTIFYING MACROPHAGE CHEMOTAXIS

It has been recognized since the latter part of the nineteenth century that leukocytes have the ability to migrate unidirectionally along a concentration gradient of an attractant substance. A dramatic demonstration of leukocyte chemotaxis *in vivo* was first described by Leber in 1888, who injected inflammatory agents into rabbit corneas and observed the migration of cells towards the site of injection. Since these early experiments, present concepts of leukocyte chemotaxis have evolved from the use of various techniques for studying cell migration. A number of techniques are available which allow direct visualization and measurement of cellular movement. One such method is time lapse cinematography of cell migration on glass slides. Techniques such as these are laborious, only semiquantitative, and allow sampling of only very few cells at a given time. The development by Boyden (1962) of an *in vitro* method for quantifying polymorphonuclear leukocyte migration has allowed major advances in our understanding of the mechanisms of cell accumulation in inflammatory states. Moreover, by modifying Boyden's original technique, the study of macrophage chemotaxis *in vitro* has also become possible. Detailed descriptions of the methodology for studying leukocyte chemotaxis can be found in a number of recent articles or reviews (Ward *et al.*, 1965; Keller, 1966; Snyderman *et al.*, 1968, 1970, 1971b, 1972a; Stroud *et al.*, 1973; Wilkinson, 1974). The following outline is meant to serve as a general description of the more commonly employed techniques for quantifying macrophage or monocyte chemotaxis *in vitro*.

The Boyden technique essentially involves the measurement of leukocyte migration through porous filters. The filter employed separates a chemotaxis chamber into an upper and lower compartment. Leukocytes are placed on the upper surface of the filter and a solution containing material to be tested for chemotactic activity is placed on the lower side of the filter. The chemotaxis chamber itself can be made of plastic or stainless steel. An example of a chemotaxis chamber now in use in the authors' laboratories is seen in Fig. 1. The chambers containing leuko-

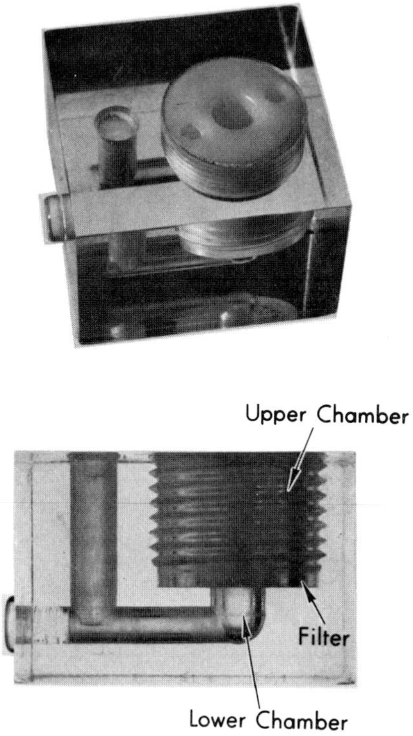

Fig. 1. Chemotaxis chamber. A standardized cell suspension (0.4 ml) is placed in the upper compartment of the chamber and is separated from the chemotactic stimulant (0.85 ml) or medium alone in the lower compartment by a polycarbonate or nitrocellulose filter.

cytes and chemotactic factor or control medium are incubated at 37°C for varying times depending upon the cell type being studied and the filter being used. Following a suitable incubation period, the chambers are emptied, the filters are removed and stained, and the number of cells that migrated through the filter are counted. Two general types of filters have been successfully used in this system. The most widely used are nitrocellulose filters of ~150 μm thickness, which have convoluted pores and are available in pore sizes ranging from 0.4 to 8 μm in diameter. Most investigators choose an 8.0 μm pore filter for macrophage studies. Using this type of filter, one can score chemotaxis by measuring the total number of cells per microscopic field which have migrated completely through the filter during the chosen incubation time. An alternative method of quantifying chemotaxis is to measure the depth into the filter to which the leading front of cells has migrated in a given period of time (Zigmond and Hirsch, 1973). This method may be slightly more reproducible than counting the cells that have migrated entirely through the filter, but is valuable only when one is dealing with a homogeneous cell population because it is difficult to delineate the morphology of cells within the filter. Error in measurement can also occur because cells within the filter itself elongate as they migrate and may extend to 30 μm or more in length. Determining the leading front of any given cell then becomes quite difficult. The other type of filter that has been successfully used in the Boyden chamber is the polycarbonate filter (Nuclepore) (Horwitz and Garrett, 1971; Snyderman *et al.*, 1972a). This type of filter is approximately 15 μm in thickness and has linear pores that are produced by neutron beams penetrating the filter. Filters are available with pore sizes ranging from 1 to 10 μm in diameter, but most investigators use 5 μm pore filters for the study of macrophage migration. The polycarbonate filter allows measurement only by counting the cells on the lower surface of the filter (Fig. 2). The advantage of the polycarbonate filter is that the time necessary for the chemotaxis assay is far less than the time necessary for studies using the nitrocellulose filter.

A. Chemotaxis of Peritoneal Macrophages

Macrophages derived from the peritoneal cavities of guinea pigs, rabbits, and mice have been effectively used in the Boyden chemotaxis assay (Ward, 1968; Snyderman *et al.*, 1971b, 1975b; Hausman *et al.*, 1972; Wahl *et al.*, 1974a). In general, animals are injected intraperitoneally with inflammatory agents, such as glycogen, starch, mineral oil, or proteose–peptone, and 3–4 days later the peritoneal cavities are lavaged with saline or tissue culture medium. The cells harvested in this manner usu-

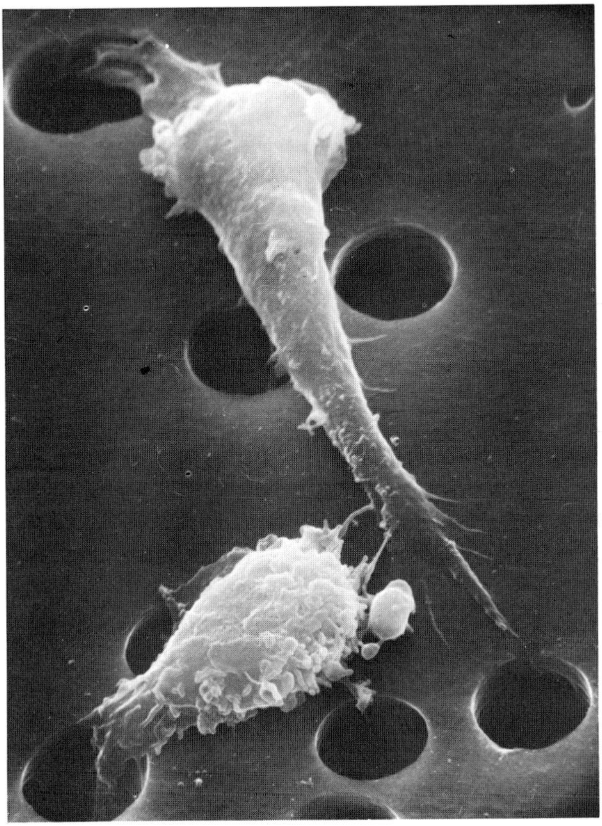

Fig. 2. Scanning electron micrograph of two normal human monocytes which have migrated in response to lymphocyte-derived chemotactic factor (LDCF) to the bottom surface of a polycarbonate filter (×3120). The cell at the top has completely emerged from a 5.0 μm pore and has advanced diagonally across the filter's surface On the lower left, another cell has migrated onto the bottom surface of the membrane.

ally contain at least 70% macrophages. We have found glycogen and mineral oil to be most suitable for studies in guinea pigs and rabbits and proteose-peptone (10%) most suitable for obtaining mouse macrophages (Snyderman *et al.*, 1971b, 1975b; Hausman *et al.*, 1972; Wahl *et al.*, 1974a). One can also obtain peritoneal macrophages by lavage of unstimulated animals, but these cells are, in general, less chemotactically responsive than macrophages obtained from inflammatory exudates. The peritoneal cells are washed, counted, and standardized to contain approximately 1.5×10^6 macrophages/ml of the tissue culture medium to be used in the chemotaxis assay. The use of peritoneal macrophages in this assay is convenient, since it does not involve separation techniques once the cells are obtained. It must be realized, however, that peritoneal cells have already migrated from the blood into the peritoneal cavity and may be in varying states of "activation," depending upon the stimulant used to obtain them.

B. Chemotaxis of Peripheral Blood Monocytes

In order to study the chemotaxis of cells that have not already migrated out of the circulation to a local tissue site, it is necessary to use peripheral blood cells. Mononuclear leukocytes suitable for use in the chemotaxis assay have been obtained from human and avian blood (Altman and Kirchner, 1972; Snyderman *et al.*, 1972a). The isolation of these cells involves the use of Ficoll-Hypaque gradients onto which whole blood is layered (Böyum, 1968). Mononuclear leukocytes (MNL's) containing approximately 20–30% monocytes and 70–80% lymphocytes can be clearly separated from erythrocytes and granulocytes by this method. The MNL's are then washed and standardized to contain 1.5×10^6 monocytes per ml of tissue culture medium and placed in the upper compartment of the chemotaxis chamber with a 5.0 μm polycarbonate filter used to separate the cells from the lower compartment of the chamber. Only the monocytes stick to the lower surface of the filter and thus are the only cells evaluated in this assay system.

C. Measurement of Chemotaxis *in Vivo*

Understanding the mechanisms of leukocyte accumulation has been greatly hindered by the lack of quantitative, reproducible methods that clearly measure chemotaxis *in vivo*. The accumulation of leukocytes at local tissue sites could be a manifestation of chemotaxis but could also be a result of randomly migrating cells remaining in a local site. Most available methods for the study of leukocyte accumulation *in vivo* cannot distinguish between these two mechanisms for cellular localization. Direct visualization of leukocyte movement *in vivo* can be studied by observing translucent vascular tissues, such as the mesentery or the rabbit ear. These methods, however, are difficult to perform, are not quantitative, and may introduce artifacts during the manipulation necessary to prepare the tissues for study. Methods that allow the quantification of leukocyte accumulation *in vivo* are available, but they do not differentiate chemotaxis from other means of cell localization. However, they do provide useful information concerning the nature of factors that influence the inflammatory response. We have studied the kinetics of leukocyte accumulation and the production of mediators of inflammation *in vivo* by introducing inflammatory agents into the peritoneal cavities of a number of animal species (Snyderman *et al.*, 1971a; Postlethwaite and Snyderman, 1975). The cavities are lavaged at various time intervals after the introduction of antigen or other agents, and the leukocyte content and nature of putative mediators of inflammation in the exudates determined. Other investigators have measured leukocyte accumulation into an enclave created by injection of air subcutaneously (air enclave method) (Larson, 1969; Tempel *et al.*, 1970). Another method recently employed to study inflammatory cell accumulation *in vivo* involves the radiolabeling of circulating leukocytes and measuring the influx of radiolabel into local sites of inflammation (Perper *et al.*, 1974). Skin window techniques and variants have also been used in humans. These techniques involve the denuding of surface epithelial cells, placing cover slips or other material on the skin, and measuring the number of cells that adhere to the cover slip during varying time periods. It is obvious that these methods are at best qualitative.

III. HUMORAL FACTORS CHEMOTACTIC FOR MACROPHAGES

A. Chemotactic Factors Derived from Complement

Activation of the complement (C) system by inflammatory agents, such as endotoxins or immune complexes, results in the cleavage of a number of C components and release of low MW peptides (Nelson, 1974). In previous investigations, we studied the role of the complement system as a mediator of polymorphonuclear leukocyte (PMN) chemotaxis and found that a fragmentation product of the fifth component of complement, C5a, was an important chemotactic factor *in vitro* and *in vivo* (Shin *et al.*, 1968; Snyderman *et al.*, 1970, 1971b). During the course of these studies, purified C5a was injected intradermally in rabbits (Jensen *et al.*, 1969) and guinea pigs (Snyderman and Shin, unpublished observation) and histological sections of the injected skin were prepared at various times. In addition to the massive accumulation of PMN's at the site of C5a injection, we observed large numbers of macrophages. This finding initiated subsequent investigations to determine if C5a mediated the chemotaxis of macrophages as well as that of PMN's.

Highly purified guinea pig C5 was cleaved with either the earlier acting components of complement (EAC $\overline{1423}$) or with trypsin. Cleavage of C5 by either of these means resulted in the production of potent chemotactic activity for guinea pig peritoneal macrophages (Snyderman *et al.*, 1971b). In these experiments, solutions containing C5a in as little as 5×10^{-9} *M* concentrations were strongly chemotactic for macrophages. In order to determine if identical C5 fragments were responsible for chemotactic activity for guinea pig macrophages and PMN's, reaction mixtures of activated C5 were fractionated by polyacrylamide gel electrophoresis and molecular sieve chromatography. Chemotactic activity for the two cell types could not be separated by these methods, indicating that the activity for both resides in a similar or the same fragment of C5 (about 15,000 daltons) (Snyderman *et al.*, 1971b). A purified acid-acting proteinase derived from homogenates of macrophages was also shown to cleave purified C5 and produce chemotactic activity for macrophages and PMN's (Snyderman *et al.*, 1972b). This proteinase, however, cleaved C5 into a number of chemotactically active fragments as shown by gel filtration on Sephadex G-75. These studies suggest that the release of this proteinase by macrophages during phagocytosis could result in cleavage of C5 into a number of chemotactically active fragments that could thus amplify the inflammatory response.

We also sought to determine if complement activated in the more physiologic milieu of whole serum would result in generation of chemotactic activity for macrophages. Antigen–antibody complexes, endotoxin, or cobra venom factor were used to activate serum complement. Each of these factors is known to produce C5a (Snyderman *et al.*, 1970; Snyderman and Mergenhagen, 1972) and to generate chemotactic activity for macrophages when incubated with whole serum (Hausman *et al.*, 1972). The amount of chemotactic activity produced was proportional to the amount of hemolytic complement activity consumed in the treated serum. Fractionation by gel filtration of serum treated with endotoxin, antigen–antibody complexes, or cobra venom factor demonstrated the presence of two peaks of chemotactic activity. One was a low molecular weight (about 15,000 daltons), heat-stable (56°C for 30 minutes) factor found only in activated serum. This activity had an elution profile similar to C5a and was inhibited by incubation with monospecific antibody to C5 or C5a. This established the identity of the chemotactic factor produced in whole serum by complement activation as C5a (Hausman *et al.*, 1972). The other peak of chemotactic activity was of higher molecular weight (about 90,000 daltons) and was present in both activated and untreated serum (see below).

Similar experiments were performed to determine if activated human serum produced chemotactic activity for human peripheral blood monocytes (Snyderman *et al.*, 1972a). Human serum treated with antigen–antibody complexes, endotoxin, or cobra venom factor contained chemotactic activity for human monocytes *in vitro*. The active material had a low molecular weight (about 15,000 daltons), was heat-stable (56°C for 30 minutes), and was inhibited by antibody to human C5. Human C5a derived from activated serum was chemotactic for human monocytes at concentrations as low as 3.3×10^{-9} (Snyderman *et al.*, 1972a). The contention that C5a is chemotactic factor for macrophages has been challenged by Wissler *et al.* (1972). These workers presented data that suggested that C5a is not chemotactic for macrophages but selectively chemotactic for neutrophils and eosinophils. We have recently shown, however, that C5 is required for the production of chemotactic activity in mouse serum by inflammatory agents that activate complement. Serum from mice congenitally deficient in C5 did not produce chemotactic activity when incubated with endotoxin or aggregated γ-globulin, while normal mouse serum treated in an identical manner produced chemotactic activity attributable to C5a (Snyderman *et al.*, 1975b).

Clearly C5a is chemotactic for mononuclear leukocytes as well as PMN's. Since PMN's are not present in the mononuclear leukocyte preparations tested *in vitro*, it can be assumed that prior accumulation of neutrophils is not required for the chemotaxis of macrophages *in vivo*. This assumption is supported by the observation of Simpson and Ross (1972), who showed that macrophages accumulate normally at wound sites in neutropenic animals. The role that C5a plays *in vivo* as a chemotactic factor for macrophages is still a matter of speculation. C5a may be responsible for macrophage accumulation at sites of immune complex-induced inflammation. Since intracellular proteolytic enzymes released by damaged cells can cleave C5 to produce phlogistic peptides, macrophage accumulation at sites of nonspecific tissue trauma may be mediated by C5 fragmentation products (Ward and Hill, 1970; Snyderman *et al.*, 1972b). Similarly, virus-infected cells release a factor that cleaves C5 to produce chemotactic activity for macrophages (Brier *et al.*, 1970; Snyderman *et al.*, 1972c).

B. Chemotactic Activity in Serum and Plasma

As previously mentioned, fresh untreated serum contains chemotactic activity for guinea pig macrophages. It has been reported that serum, but not plasma, is chemotactic for macrophages (Borel and Sorkin, 1969). We studied fresh serum and plasma to determine if chemotactic activity for guinea pig peritoneal macrophages (Snyderman and Stahl, 1974) and human peripheral blood monocytes is present. Substantial and similar amounts of chemotactic activity for macrophages and human monocytes are found in both serum and plasma. However, excessive amounts of heparin (>20 U/ml blood) inhibit the chemotactic activity of both serum and plasma for guinea pig macrophages (Hausman *et al.*, 1972; Snyderman and Stahl, 1974) and human monocytes. The amount of anticoagulant used could, therefore, account for the low chemotactic activity of plasma reported by others (Borel and Sorkin, 1969). Characterization of the chemotactic factor in untreated guinea pig serum showed it to be heat-labile (56°C for 30 minutes) and to elute on Sephadex G-200 in the molecular weight range of 90,000 daltons (Hausman *et al.*, 1972).

The existence of chemotactic activity in normal serum and plasma suggests that similar activity may be circulating in whole blood. Alternatively, this activity may not be present in whole blood, but may be produced by the conversion of whole blood to serum or plasma. Such a conversion might activate the complement, kinin, and/or clotting systems whose activated components possess a range of biologic activities, among them chemotactic activity (Snyderman *et al.*, 1970; Kaplan *et al.*, 1972; Stecher and Sorkin, 1972). We attempted to inhibit activation of these systems following blood drawing to determine how the chemotactic activity present in plasma might be affected. Guinea pigs were bled directly into plastic tubes containing EDTA, citrate, heparin, or hexadimethrene. Other blood samples were collected at 0°C, and formed elements were removed immediately by centrifugation in the cold. Hexadimethrene, an inhibitor of the activation of Hageman factor (Hausman *et al.*, 1972), was also directly inhibitory to macrophage chemotaxis (R. Snyderman and M. S. Hausman, unpublished data); therefore, experiments to determine if this agent inhibited the formation of chemotactic activity in plasma were inconclusive. In all other cases, the resultant plasma contained the same amount of chemotactic activity normally found in fresh serum (Hausman *et al.*, 1972). Although these experiments suggest that the complement and clotting systems need not be activated to produce the chemotactic activity present in normal serum, partial activation may have occurred despite the use of various inhibitors. Moreover, activation of the kinin-forming system may be responsible for the generation of this activity, since the conversion of prekallikrein to kallikrein does result in the formation of chemotactic activity for neutrophils and human blood monocytes (Kaplan *et al.*, 1972; Gallin and Kaplan, 1974). A clue concerning the nature of the chemotactic activity present in normal serum has come from recent work using serum from mice congenitally devoid of C5 (Snyderman *et al.*, 1975b). While normal unactivated mouse serum contains a high molecular weight chemotactic activity for macrophages, serum from mice lacking C5 does not. This finding suggests that the macrophage chemotactic activity in normal serum requires the presence of the fifth component of C.

In summary, the exact nature of the chemotactic activity in fresh serum and plasma remains undetermined. If this activity is present in whole blood, it could function to inhibit migration of monocytes out of the circulation until chemotactic activity at local inflammatory sites reaches a concentration above that found in whole blood. Thus, chemotactic activity in the circulation could have a modulating effect on the inflammatory response. If, on the other hand, this chemotactic activity is generated upon the conversion of whole blood to serum, it could play an important role in wound healing by attracting macrophages to sites of coagulation at areas of tissue injury.

IV. LYMPHOCYTE-DERIVED CHEMOTACTIC FACTORS

A. Chemotactic Activity Produced *in Vitro*

Cell-mediated immune reactions protect the host against microbial invasion, particularly by viral, fungal, and mycobacterial agents. Depression of a host's cellular immune system results in a higher incidence of infections and also higher susceptibility to carcinogenesis. An important effector cell that mediates the destruction of material recognized as foreign by a cellular immune response is the macrophage. The observation that lymphocytes release biologically active effector molecules (lymphokines) after interaction with antigen has greatly enhanced the understanding of how macrophages may accumulate at sites of cellular immune reactions. An important observation made by Ward *et al.* (1969) was that guinea pig lymphocytes, when stimulated with specific antigen, release a factor that is chemotactic for homologous macrophages. The chemotactic factor was estimated to have a MW slightly less than 43,000 and was reported to be separable from migration inhibition factor (MIF) (Ward *et al.*, 1970).

Our laboratories have focused upon mechanisms of macrophage accumulation in human cellular immune inflammation (Snyderman *et al.*, 1972a; Altman *et al.*, 1973). Human peripheral blood leukocytes were isolated from normal individuals and from individuals with known sensitivities to tuberculoprotein (PPD). The incubation of normal leukocytes with the nonspecific mitogen, phytohemagglutinin (PHA), or of leukocytes from tuberculin-sensitive patients with PPD or with PHA resulted in the production of chemotactic activity for autologous or homologous monocytes (Table I) (Snyderman *et al.*, 1972a). Since cultures of column-purified lymphocytes stimulated by a mitogen produced as much chemotactic activity as stimulated leukocyte cultures containing a similar

TABLE I

Chemotactic Activity for Human Monocytes in Supernatants of Tuberculoprotein- (PPD) Stimulated Leukocyte Cultures[a]

Material tested[c]	Chemotactic activity[b] Experiment I (PPD, 0.25 μg/ml)	Experiment II (PPD, 1 μg/ml)
Supernatants of leukocytes incubated with PPD	120 ± 18.3	273 ± 6.0
Supernatants of leukocytes plus PPD added at harvest	22 ± 6.9	36 ± 2.6
Medium alone	19 ± 3.0	41 ± 6.1

[a] Adapted from Snyderman *et al.*, 1972a. Leukocytes were obtained from individuals with positive delayed skin reactivity to PPD.

[b] Each value represents the mean and standard error of triplicate samples expressed as cells per oil immersion field.

[c] 0.5 ml of the indicated material was brought to 1.0 ml with gelatin veronal buffer (pH 7.3), then to 1.7 ml with Gey's medium.

number of lymphocytes plus macrophages and neutrophils, it was concluded that the chemotactic activity must have been produced by lymphocytes (Altman *et al.*, 1973). Studies of the kinetics of lymphocyte-derived chemotactic factor (LDCF) production demonstrated that the factor is released prior to blastogenesis, and that blastogenesis is not necessary for its production (Altman *et al.*, 1973). Release of chemotactic activity from lymphocytes can be detected within 6 hours after stimulation with PHA or with specific antigen *in vitro*. Human LDCF was characterized by gel filtration and sucrose density gradient ultracentrifugation and found to have a molecular weight of approximately 12,000 daltons. In addition, LDCF was shown to be antigenically distinct from the C5a fragment of the complement system (Snyderman *et al.*, 1972a; Altman *et al.*, 1973).

It had generally been assumed that bone marrow derived (B) lymphocytes were exclusively antibody producing cells, whereas thymus derived (T) lymphocytes performed numerous functions including synthesizing lymphokines, mediating target cell cytotoxicity, and playing a "helper" role in the processing of antigen. However, with the availability of new techniques for the separation of B cells from T cells, it has been shown that stimulated B cells also may produce a chemotactic lymphokine. Mackler *et al.* (1974; Altman *et al.*, 1974a) have shown that human B lymphocytes, isolated after rosetting with sensitized sheep erythrocytes carrying the activated third component of complement (EAC3b), produced a chemotactic lymphokine when cultured *in vitro* with PHA or concanavalin A (Con A). Since this method of B cell purification can allow contamination by up to 5% T cells, a possible contribution of T helper cells in this system has to be considered.

The characterization of lymphokine production by guinea pig lymphocytes *in vitro* has been extensively studied by Wahl *et al.* (1974a). Lymphocytes from guinea pigs sensitized with a well-defined antigen (DNP-ovalbumin) to produce delayed hypersensitivity *in vivo* released a low molecular weight (about 12,500 daltons) chemotactic factor when exposed to the same antigen *in vitro*. Production of the guinea pig chemotactic lymphokine occurred within 8 hours after incubation of lymphocytes with antigen or nonspecific mitogen. Similar to the human lymphokine, the guinea pig factor was distinguishable from C5a and sensitive to digestion by proteolytic enzymes.

Further studies by Wahl *et al.* (1974b) have increased our understanding of the mechanisms involved in activation of B lymphocytes to produce chemotactic lymphokines. Polymeric B cell mitogens, including lipopolysaccharides and polymerized flagellin, can activate lymphocytes to produce chemotactic factors for macrophages. Additionally, interaction of appropriate molecules with other B cell surface receptors stimulates the elaboration of a chemotactic lymphokine. Antigen–antibody complexes or aggregated γ-globulin acting through the Fc receptor, anti-immunoglobulin at the Ig receptor, and antigen–antibody–complement complexes interacting with the C3 receptor all served as adequate stimuli for mediator production but not for B cell proliferation. Moreover, since anti-immunoglobulin but not its Fab fragments activated the B cells, this suggested that activation of B cells to produce mediators of macrophage chemotaxis requires binding and cross-linking of B cell membrane receptors. In addition to activation of the B lymphocytes by immune complex-bound C3b, Sandberg *et al.* (1974) have shown that soluble C3b can induce guinea pig B lymphocytes to produce a chemotactic lymphokine. The response was B cell specific and occurred in the absence of detectable proliferation. These latter experiments suggest the possibility that membrane alterations sufficient for triggering of lymphokine synthesis occurs via C3 binding to its respective receptors in the absence of cross-linking.

Our understanding of the role played by the macrophage in the "presentation" of antigens to lymphocytes is at present incomplete (see Rosenthal *et al.*, Chapter 6; Rosentreich and Oppenheim, Chapter 7; Epstein, Chapter 8). It is, however, well established that the activation of lymphocytes by antigens requires "processing" of the antigens by macrophages. The adjuvant effect of macrophages for lymphokine production by subpopulations of lymphocytes has recently been investigated. Wahl *et al.* (1975) have shown that purified T lymphocytes depleted of macrophages do not produce monocyte chemotactic factor in response to specific antigen. When macrophages are added back to these T cell–antigen cultures, the ability of the lymphocytes to produce a chemotactic factor is restored. B lymphocytes, however, produced chemotactic activity when cultured *in vitro* with a B cell mitogen in the absence of macrophages. These findings indicate that macrophages are required for the production of chemotactic factor(s) by T lymphocytes but not by B lymphocytes.

B. Chemotactic Activity Produced *in Vivo*

In vitro studies have contributed greatly to our conceptual understanding of the mechanisms of leukocyte accumulation in cellular immune reactions; however, the actual role played *in vivo* by putative mediators of inflammation is as yet rudimentary. Cohen *et al.* studied extracts from skin sites of delayed hypersensitivity reactions and detected the presence of a chemotactic factor for monocytes (Cohen *et al.*, 1973). The extractable chemotactic activity for monocytes could be separated by sucrose density gradient ultracentrifugation into two broad peaks. One peak sedimented in the region of an IgG marker, and the other sedimented near an albumin marker.

We have recently devised an animal model to study the kinetics of inflammation in cell-mediated immune reactions *in vivo* (Postlethwaite and Snyderman, 1975). Guinea pigs sensitized to specific antigens, which induce primarily delayed hypersensitivity reactions, had silicon plastic catheters placed intraabdominally. The antigen was introduced into the peritoneal cavity through the catheter, and at various time intervals the peritoneal fluid was sampled for the presence of lymphokines or for the quantity and type of leukocytes that had accumulated. Using this methodology, we found that a macrophage chemotactic factor of approximately 12,000 daltons was produced within 24 hours after the introduction of specific antigen into immunized animals. The majority of chemotactic activity could be attributed to a factor that appeared to be identical to the chemotactic lymphokine produced by stimulated lymphocyte cultures *in vitro*. Concomitant with the appearance of this factor was the influx of macrophages into the peritoneal cavity. These data suggest that lymphokines are indeed produced *in vivo* during cellular immune reactions and that a chemotactic lymphokine is responsible for the influx of macrophages to sites of delayed hypersensitivity reactions.

V. CHEMOTACTIC FACTORS FROM BACTERIA

In addition to the chemotactic factors present or produced in normal serum or released by mammalian cells, compounds elaborated by bacteria have been shown to be strongly chemotactic for leukocytes *in vitro* (Keller and Sorkin, 1967; Ward *et al.*, 1968; Tempel *et al.*, 1970; Schiffman *et al.*, 1974). Some of these substances are small, heterogenous peptides with blocked amino groups. Schiffman *et al.*, (1975) recently found that small formylmethionyl peptides analogous to those derived from the N-terminal regions of newly synthesized bacterial proteins are chemotactic for leukocytes. The investigators speculated that these synthetic peptides may be related to some of the bacterial factors. Doses of purified formylmethionine (f-Met) ranging from 10^{-2} to 10^{-4} M were chemotactic for rabbit PMN's *in vitro*. *N*-acylmethionyl peptides such as f-Met-Trp, f-Met-Phe, f-Met-Leu-Gly, and acyl-Met-Leu were chemotactic for guinea pig and human neutrophils and macrophages at doses as low as 10^{-6} and 10^{-9} M. Neither nonacylated peptides nor free methionine have this chemotactic property, suggesting that formylation is specifically necessary for the chemotaxis initiated by these peptides. Since eukaryotic cells appear for the most part to initiate protein synthesis with nonacylated methionine (Yoshida *et al.*, 1970), the chemotactic response of mammalian leukocytes to formylated amino acids may represent a simple recognition system that detects the presence of microbial agents. In addition to the significance these findings may have for our understanding of primitive mechanisms for the differentiation of self from non-self, they also clearly demonstrate that very simple molecules in presumably nondenatured forms can be chemotactic for mammalian leukocytes.

VI. FACTORS WHICH ALTER MONOCYTE CHEMOTACTIC FUNCTION

The cellular and biochemical mechanisms required to enable leukocytes to migrate to chemotactic stimuli are as yet unknown. It has been demonstrated, however, that leukocyte motility is an energy-requiring process that may in fact depend upon myofilament and myofibril formation as well as actin polymerization (Boxer, 1974; Boxer *et al.*, 1974). The leukocyte membrane may also play an important role in the ability of these cells to migrate. Whether factors that initiate chemotaxis do so via binding to specific cell surface receptors or by altering leukocyte transmembrane potential or membrane permeability has not yet been determined. Attempts are now being made to understand the physiochemistry of chemotaxis by utilizing various pharmacological agents to elucidate precisely which biochemical pathways are required for leukocyte migration.

Various chemical agents can be shown to affect monocyte chemotactic responsiveness *in vitro*. One of these agents is prostaglandin PGE_2 (McClatchey and Snyderman, 1974). It was shown that PGE_2, when incubated with normal human monocytes, enhanced the chemotactic responsiveness of these cells to a chemotactic lymphokine. PGE_2 was the only prostaglandin studied which affected the cells in this manner. Recent work in this laboratory has also directly demonstrated the importance of Ca^{2+} flux for monocyte chemotaxis (M. M. Boucek and R. Snyderman, unpublished observations, 1974). Lanthanum chloride was used to block Ca^{2+} movement across human monocyte membranes *in vitro*. Doses of as little as 5×10^{-4} *M* of lanthanum chloride depressed human monocyte chemotaxis by >80%. The data suggested that passive Ca^{2+} influx and active Ca^{2+} efflux are required for chemotaxis. The data moreover are consistent with the hypothesis that rapid polymerization and depolymerization of actomyosin, a contractile protein, is required for leukocyte migration.

We have recently investigated the possibility that certain infectious organisms might inhibit or enhance monocyte function. Indeed, we have recently shown that infection of human mononuclear leukocytes (MNL's) *in vitro* with certain viruses, such as herpes simplex or influenza, markedly depresses the chemotactic responsiveness of monocytes (Kleinerman *et al.*, 1974) (Table II). Treatment of monocytes with identical doses of UV-inactivated viruses produced no effect on chemotactic responsiveness. Infection of monocytes with other viruses, such as vaccinia, reo, or polio viruses, also had no effect on the chemotactic response of these cells. Herpes simplex and influenza are enveloped viruses, deriving their coats from the infected host's cell membrane, whereas reo and polio viruses are unenveloped, and the outer surface structure components of vaccinia virus does not originate from the host's cell membrane. One could speculate that the ability of certain viruses to alter the membranous surface of cells results in the retardation of monocyte chemotactic responsiveness. It will be important to determine if alteration of leukocyte chemotactic responsiveness by certain viruses can result in the depressed cellular immunity found in some human disease states. Another infectious organism that alters monocyte chemotactic function is bacillus Calmette-Guerin (BCG). Immunization with this agent has been shown to enhance monocyte chemotaxis in some patients with cancer (Snyderman *et al.*, 1974a,c,d; Snyderman and Stahl, 1975) (see below). This fact may in part explain the effectiveness of this type of immunotherapy in promoting regressions of tumors such as malignant melanoma.

TABLE II

Depression of Monocyte Chemotaxis by Infection of Mononuclear Leukocytes (MNL's) with Herpes Simplex and Influenza Virus[a]

MNL's incubated with[b]	Chemotactic response[c]	% Inhibition
Herpes simplex virus		
7.0 PFU/MNL	31.4 ± 6.1	62
0.7 PFU/MNL	45.5 ± 2.3	44
0.07 PFU/MNL	54.5 ± 6.3	33
Medium alone	81.8 ± 14.8	
Influenza virus		
10^3 HAU	13.2 ± 2.8	77
10^2 HAU	30.4 ± 11.0	47
10^1 HAU	44.2 ± 16.2	23
Medium alone	57.4 ± 14.1	

[a] Adapted from Kleinerman *et al.*, 1974.

[b] To a 4.5 ml sample of MNL (1.7×10^6 monocytes/ml) was added to 0.5 ml of medium (control) or 0.5 ml of medium containing influenza virus at 10^3, 10^2, or 10 hemagglutinating units (HAU)/ml or 0.5 ml of medium containing herpes simplex virus (HSV) resulting in a multiplicity of infection of 7.0, 0.7, and 0.07 plaque forming units (PFU) of HSV/MNL. After incubation and centrifugation, the cells were resuspended to 5 ml in Gey's medium and tested for chemotactic responsiveness to a chemotactic lymphokine.

[c] Each value represents the mean and standard error of triplicate samples expressed as cells per oil immersion field.

In addition to factors that can influence monocyte chemotaxis by altering the monocyte itself, factors in serum can interact with chemotactic agents to destroy their chemotactic properties. The first evidence that normal serum contained factors that depressed the activity of chemotactic substances was demonstrated by Wilkinson *et al.* (1969). These authors showed that chemotactic factors in serum could be rendered less active by combination with certain serum fractions. Till and Ward (1973) recently reported that normal human serum contains at least two factors that inhibit the activity of chemotactic agents. These substances are reported to inhibit the chemotactic activity of C3a, C5a, the $C\overline{567}$ complex and bacterial chemotactic factors. Ward and Berenberg (1974) recently suggested that the defect in cellular immunity that occurs in patients with Hodgkin's disease may be due to an increased circulatory level of chemotactic factor inhibitors. Serum from patients with Hodgkin's disease was shown to contain increased inhibitor activity for C5a and bacterial chemotactic factors. However, the inhibitory activity present in the serum of the patients studied was not correlated with skin test reactivity or stage of disease, so one cannot evaluate the biological significance of these findings at this time.

VII. ABNORMALITIES OF MONOCYTE CHEMOTAXIS IN HUMAN DISEASES

The accumulation of macrophages at local sites is particularly important for host defense against viral, fungal, and mycobacterial infections as well as for protection against the development and spread of neoplasms. Since tissue macrophages are derived from peripheral blood monocytes, abnormal chemotactic responsiveness by the latter cells could result in increased susceptibility to infectious and neoplastic diseases. Since the development of the methodology for assaying human monocyte chemotaxis has only recently been described (Snyderman *et al.*, 1972a), our knowledge of monocyte chemotactic dysfunctions in human disease processes is rudimentary at present.

The first observation of a defect in human monocyte chemotaxis was made in a child with recurrent mucocutaneous candidiasis and absence of delayed cutaneous reactivity to *Candida* antigen (Snyderman *et al.*, 1973a,b). The patient, a 9-year-old girl, developed oral moniliasis at the age of 2 months. Involvement of her skin occurred soon thereafter, and the diagnosis of chronic mucocutaneous candidiasis was made. Therapy with oral amphoteracin B, topical nystatin, and two courses of intravenous amphoteracin B resulted in clinical improvement, but the development of nephropathy necessitated interruption of therapy. Treatment with 5-fluorouracil resulted in no clinical improvement. Immunologically, the patient had depressed or absent delayed cutaneous reactivity to monilial as well as other ubiquitous antigens, but her lymphocytes transformed normally *in vitro* and were capable of producing MIF. In contrast to normal lymphocyte transformation and lymphokine production, the patient's monocyte chemotactic responsiveness to C5a and to LDCF ranged from 2 to 11% of normal when compared to age matched controls. Transfer factor therapy was used in an attempt to enhance the patient's immune response. Nine months after initiation of this treatment, the patient's monocyte chemotaxis had improved to approximately 80% of normal. In addition, after transfer factor treatment and concomitant with the improvement of her monocyte chemotaxis, the patient's delayed skin reaction to *Candida* became positive and clinical improvement of her disease ensued. Depressed monocyte chemotactic responsiveness was recently reported by Gallin (1975) and co-workers in another patient with chronic mucocutaneous candidiasis. Treatment with dialyzable transfer factor, however, failed to correct the defect in this patient.

During the past 20 years much data has accumulated which suggest a central role for the immune system in protecting the host against the development and spread of neoplasms (Waldmann *et al.*, 1972). Using experimental animals, a number of investigators have shown that cellular immune reactions can destroy tumors and that the accumulation of macrophages is associated with tumor killing (Zbar *et al.*, 1970). It is, therefore, important to determine if the ability of macrophages to respond to chemotactic stimuli and thus accumulate at sites of delayed hypersensitivity reactions is impaired in individuals with tumors. We have recently studied monocyte chemotactic responsiveness to a chemotactic lymphokine (LDCF) in a large group of patients with cancer (Snyderman *et al.*, 1974,a,c,d; Snyderman and Stahl, 1975). Of 98 patients studied, 45 had recurrent malignant melanoma, and the rest had a variety of common neoplasms including carcinoma of the lung, breast, colon, prostate, and kidney. None of the patients were undergoing chemotherapy at the time of testing. Approximately 60% of the patients with cancer had depressed monocyte chemotactic responsiveness with values below the ninety-fifth percentile of the responses of a large population of age matched normals and hospitalized controls (Fig. 3). The patients with recurrent malignant melanoma in this particular study were to be placed on BCG therapy (Seigler *et al.*, 1973). Of patients with melanoma tested prior to receiving BCG, 45% had chemotactic responses at least 2 standard deviations below the normal mean. The chemotactic responses of these individuals were compared to the responses of these and other patients with malignant melanoma following treatment with BCG. Immunization with BCG and subsequent intralesional injection of BCG enhanced the chemotactic responsiveness of eight of nine individuals who had depressed chemotaxis prior to therapy (Fig. 4). In addition, a group of patients with either renal carcinoma or carcinoma of the breast were tested for monocyte chemotactic responsiveness both before and after surgical excision of the tumor. All 7 patients tested with depressed chemotaxis prior to removal of the tumor had enhancement of monocyte chemotactic responsiveness postoperatively (Table III). These data indicate that the presence of a tumor may directly influence the recognition, activation, or mobilization processes involved in a normal monocyte chemotactic response. This supposition is strengthened by the observation that implantation of tumor cells in mice depresses the ability of these animals to mobilize macrophages to a site of inflammation distant from the tumor.

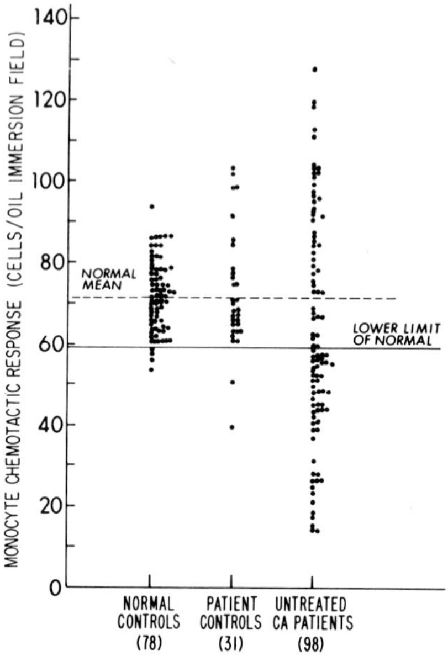

Fig. 3. Monocyte chemotactic responsiveness of normals, hospitalized patients with nonneoplastic disease, and patients with neoplasms. The lower limit of normal indicates the level below which only 5% of the normal responses fall. The responses of approximately 60% of the patients with cancer fall below this level. Taken from Snyderman *et al.*, 1974d.

C3H mice were injected with 5×10^6 syngeneic tumor cells subcutaneously in the thigh. At various times following tumor injection, mice received intraperitoneal injections of either proteose-peptone or phytohemagglutinin (PHA). By 5 days after tumor implantation, the migration of macrophages into the peritoneal cavity in response to these inflammatory agents was reduced by 30 to 70% in tumor-bearing animals. Moreover the chemotactic responsiveness *in vitro* of the peritoneal macrophages recovered from tumor-bearing animals was markedly depressed (Snyderman *et al.*, 1975a).

The hypothesis that neoplasms themselves may produce anti-inflammatory effects has received further recent support (Fauve *et al.*, 1974). These investigators demonstrated that mouse neoplasms growing *in vitro* produce a low molecular weight factor(s) (between 10^3 to 10^4 daltons) that inhibits the accumulation of neutrophils at inflammatory sites *in vivo*. It remains to be determined if tumors release factors that inhibit macrophage chemotactic responsiveness, but if so the characterization of the mechanisms by which neoplasms retard leukocyte function will certainly

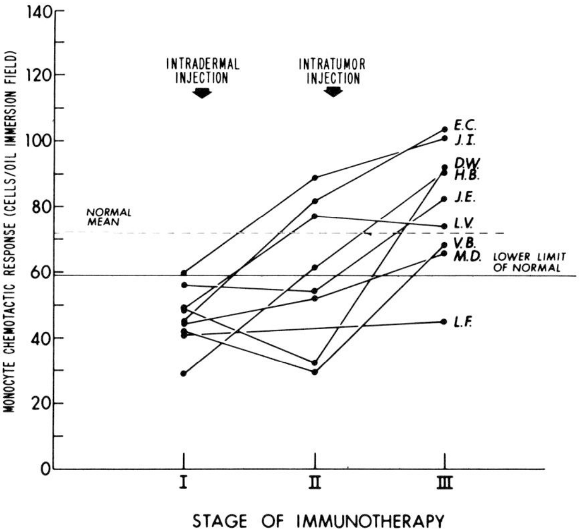

Fig. 4. Effect of BCG immunotherapy on the monocyte chemotactic responsiveness of patients with malignant melanoma whose responses were depressed prior to therapy. Stage I, before BCG administration; stage II, 4 weeks after intradermal injection of BCG; stage III, 4 weeks after inoculation of tumor nodules with BCG. Taken from Snyderman *et al.,* 1974d.

TABLE III

Effect of Tumor Removal on Monocyte Chemotactic Responsiveness[a]

Patient	Neoplasm	Chemotactic Response[b]	
		Preoperative	Postoperative
M.S.	Carcinoma breast	48.3 ± 2.6	69.3 ± 1.9
M.W.	Carcinoma breast	32.9 ± 3.5	40.6 ± 9.4
V.P.	Carcinoma breast	37.5 ± 5.4	52.6 ± 5.0
A.W.	Renal adenocarcinoma	21.3 ± 4.2	83.3 ± 5.6
A.G.	Renal adenocarcinoma	20.9 ± 2.6	86.9 ± 7.6
B.F.	Renal adenocarcinoma	57.6 ± 5.0	91.9 ± 5.2
B.S.	Renal adenocarcinoma	44.6 ± 2.5	68.4 ± 4.6
Mean ± 1 SEM		37.6 ± 4.4	70.4 ± 7.7
		($p < 0.001$)	
H.B.	Benign breast mass	84.9 ± 6.5	70.9 ± 1.3
V.C.	Benign renal mass	115.5 ± 1.2	88.2 ± 1.8

[a] Adapted from Snyderman *et al.,* 1974d.
[b] Each value represents the mean and standard error of triplicate samples expressed as cells per oil immersion field.

enhance one understanding of tumor immunity and perhaps provide prototypes for new forms of immunotherapy.

Boetcher and Leonard (1974) and Hausman *et al.* (1973) have demonstrated a similar depression in monocyte chemotactic responsiveness in patients with cancer. Boetcher and Leonard have shown that of 44 patients with various types of cancer, 24 individuals had depressed monocyte chemotaxis. Hausman *et al.* have shown that 24 patients with renal cell carcinoma have a 34% decrease in chemotactic responsiveness when compared to normal, and 12 patients with transitional cell carcinoma of the bladder had chemotactic responses that were approximately 30% below normal.

Wiskott–Aldrich syndrome is a rare, sex-linked, recessive disorder characterized by thrombocytopenia, eczema, increased susceptibility to infection, arthritis, and a propensity for the development of lymphoreticular neoplasms. Immunologically, these individuals have depressed cellular immunity and defective antibody synthesis, with a striking inability to produce antibody to complex polysaccharide and lipopolysaccharide antigens. Altman *et al.* (1974b) have studied cellular immune effector function in six individuals with Wiskott–Aldrich syndrome. The peripheral blood lymphocytes from these patients produced normal amounts of LDCF when stimulated with nonspecific mitogens or ubiquitous antigens, although the proliferative response of these patients' lymphocytes to the same stimulants was frequently depressed. The chemotactic responsiveness of monocytes from patients with this disease was significantly impaired, and incubation of normal monocytes in the plasma of these patients depressed the chemotactic responsiveness of these cells. An interesting observation made in this study was that peripheral blood lymphocytes from individuals with Wiskott–Aldrich syndrome produced excessive amounts of LDCF when cultured in the absence of antigens or nonspecific mitogens. The authors reasoned that hyperproduction of LDCF by circulating lymphocytes might desensitize peripheral blood monocytes and hinder their chemotactic responsiveness to LDCF produced at local tissue sites. This hypothesis was strengthened by the finding that incubation of normal monocytes with LDCF, followed by washing the cells, diminished the ability of these cells to respond chemotactically. These data indicate that hyperproduction of LDCF by unstimulated peripheral blood lymphocytes from patients with Wiskott–Aldrich syndrome results in the presence of humoral chemotactic inhibitor activity. In other words, elevated plasma levels of LDCF may "deactivate" the circulating monocytes of patients with Wiskott–Aldrich syndrome and thus contribute to the anergy characteristic of this disease. An additional recent observation may further our understanding of the basic immunoglobulin defect in the Wiskott–Aldrich syndrome. Human B lymphocytes, traditionally thought to function primarily as antibody-producing cells, have been shown to produce lymphokines with biological activities similar to those released by stimulated T lymphocytes. Together with the findings that circulating lymphocytes from patients with Wiskott–Aldrich syndrome produce excessive amounts of LDCF, these observations suggest that faulty regulation of B lymphocyte function may be a primary immunological defect in the Wiskott–Aldrich syndrome. This hypothesis might explain why patients with this syndrome have elevated levels of circulating IgE, IgA, and IgG but fail to make a normal antibody response to specific antigens.

VIII. SUMMARY AND CONCLUSIONS

The localization of leukocytes at sites of immune reactions is accomplished by a series of interrelated processes initiated by the recognition of foreign or neoplastic tissues as "non-self." The combination of host recognition factors, such as serum immunoglobulins or lymphocytes with antigens, can result in the production or release of biologically active products that enhance vascular permeability, induce local vascular stasis, and attract circulating leukocytes. A cleavage product of the fifth component of complement, C5a, is highly chemotactic for macrophages. This factor is released when the complement system is activated by immune complexes or endotoxin or when C5 is cleaved directly by the action of proteolytic enzymes derived from lysed or phagocytizing cells. C5a may thus be an important mediator of macrophage accumulation at local sites of humoral immune reactions as well as at sites of nonspecific tissue damage. Chemotactic factors derived from the clotting and kinin-forming systems may similarly be important in attracting macrophages to areas of wounds. Accumulation of macrophages at sites of delayed hypersensitivity appears to be mediated by a chemotactic lymphokine released by stimulated lymphocytes. This factor is released prior to blastogenesis and is distinct from C5a.

The availability of new *in vitro* methods for quantifying human monocyte chemotaxis has allowed evaluation of this important biological function in various disease states. An abnormality in the host's ability to mobilize leukocytes rapidly to sites of immunological reactions could result in the ineffective elimination of foreign substances and render the host more susceptible to infectious and neoplastic diseases. Indeed, most patients with neoplastic disease have depressed monocyte chemotactic responsiveness, and there is some evidence to suggest that neoplasms themselves may directly cause defective macrophage accumulation *in vivo*. It can be expected that within the next few years one will be able to expand the rudimentary knowledge of defects of monocyte chemotaxis provided in this review and offer a clearer insight into the diagnosis and treatment of abnormalities of immune function.

ACKNOWLEDGMENTS

Research reported in this chapter supported in part by grants N01 CP 33313 and 5 R01 DE 03738-02 ALY from the United States Public Health Service.

The authors gratefully acknowledge the excellent assistance of Ms. Marilyn C. Pike in the preparation of this manuscript. We also acknowledge Dr. Charles A. Daniels for the preparation of the scanning electron photomicrograph (Fig. 2) and Dr. Arnold Postlethwaite who designed the modified Boyden chamber (Fig. 2).

REFERENCES

Altman, L. C., and Kirchner, H. (1972). *J. Immunol.* **109,** 1149–1151.

Altman, L. C. Snyderman, R., Oppenheim, J. J., and Mergenhagen, S. E. (1973). *J. Immunol.* **110,** 801–810.

Altman, L. C., Mackler, B. F., and Chassy, B. M. (1974a). *RES, J. Reticuloendothel. Soc.* **16,** Suppl., 15a.

Altman, L. C., Snyderman, R., and Blaese, R. M. (1974b). *J. Clin. Invest.* **54,** 486–493.

Boetcher, D. A., and Leonard, E. J. (1974). *J. Nat. Cancer Inst.* **52,** 1091–1099.

Borel, J. F., and Sorkin, E. (1969). *Experientia* **25,** 1333–1335.

Boxer, L. (1974). *N. Engl. J. Med.* **291,** 1093–1099.

Boxer, L., Hedley-Whyte, T., Glader, B., and Stossel, T. (1974). *Clin. Res.* **22,** 384a.

Boyden, S. (1962). *J. Exp. Med.* **115,** 453–466.

Böyum, A. (1968). *Scand. J. Clin. Lab Invest.* 21, Suppl. 97, 77–89.

Brier, A. M., Snyderman, R., Mergenhagen, S. E., and Notkins, A. L. (1970). *Science* **170,** 1104–1106.

Cohen, S., Ward, P. A., Toshida, T., and Burek, C. L. (1973). *Cell. Immunol.* **9,** 363–376.

Fauve, R. M., Hevin, B., Jacob, H., Gaillard, J. A., and Jacob, F. (1974). *Proc. Nat. Acad. Sci. U.S.* **71,** 4052–4056.

Gallin, J. L. (1975). *In* "The Phagocytic Cell in Host Resistance" (J. A. Bellanti and D. H. Dayton, eds.), pp. 227–248. Raven Press, New York.

Gallin, J. L., and Kaplan, A. P. (1974). *J. Immunol.* **113,** 1928–1934.

Hausman, M. S., Snyderman, R., and Mergenhagen, S. E. (1972). *J. Infec. Dis.* **125,** 595–602.

Hausman, M. S., Brosman, S., Snyderman, R., Mickey, M. R., and Fahey, J. (1973). *Clin. Res.* **21,** 646a.

Horwitz, D. A., and Garrett, N. A. (1971). *J. Immunol.* **106,** 649–655.

Jensen, J., Snyderman, R., and Mergenhagen, S. E. (1969). *Cell. Humoral Mech. Anaphylaxis Allergy Proc. Int. Congr. Allergy Anaphylaxis, 3rd, 1968* pp. 265–278.

Kaplan, A. P., Kay, A. F., and Austen, K. F. (1972). *J. Exp. Med.* **135,** 81–97.

Keller, H. U. (1966). *Immunology* **10,** 225–230.

Keller, H. U., and Sorkin, E. (1967). *Int. Arch. Allergy Appl. Immunol.* **31,** 505–517.

Kleinerman, E. S., Snyderman, R., and Daniels, C. A. (1974). *J. Immunol.* **113,** 1562–1567.

Larson, A. (1969). *J. Bacteriol.* **97,** 445–447.

Leber, T. (1888). *Fortschr. Med.* **4,** 460–480.

McClatchey, W., and Snyderman, R. (1974). *Clin. Res.* **22,** 423a.

Mackler, B. F., Altman, L. C., Rosenstreich, D. L., and Oppenheim, J. J. (1974). *Nature (London)* **249,** 834–837.

Nelson, R. A. (1974). *In* "The Inflammatory Process" (B. W. Zweifach, L. Grant, and R. T. McCluskey, eds.), 2nd ed., Vol. 1, pp. 37–84. Academic Press, New York.

Perper, R. J., Oronsky, A. L., Stecher, V. J., Sanda, M., and Chinea, G. (1974). *Fed Proc., Fed. Amer. Soc. Exp. Biol.* **33,** 631a.

Postlethwaite, A. E., and Snyderman, R. (1975). *J. Immunol.* **114,** 274–278.

Sandberg, A. L., Wahl, S. M., and Mergenhagen, S. E. (1974). *RES, J. Reticuloendothel. Soc.* **16,** Suppl., 16a.

Schiffman, E., Showell, H., Corcoran, B. A., Smith, E., Ward, P. A., and Becker, E. L. (1974). *Fed. Proc., Fed. Amer. Soc. Exp. Biol.* **33,** 631a.

Schiffman, E., Corcoran, B. A., and Wahl, S. M. (1975). *Proc. Nat. Acad. Sci. U.S.* **72,** 1059–1062.

Seigler, H. F., Shingleton, W. W., Metzgar, R. S., Buckley, C. E., and Bergoc, P. M. (1973). *Ann. Surg.* **178,** 352–359.

Shin, H. S., Snyderman, R., Friedman, E., Mellors, A., and Mayer, M. M. (1968). *Science* **162,** 361–363.

Simpson, D. M., and Ross, R. (1972). *J. Clin. Invest.* **51,** 2009–2023.

Snyderman, R., and Mergenhagen, S. E. (1972). *In* "Biological Activities of Complement" (D. G. Ingram, ed.), pp. 117–132. Karger, Basel.

Snyderman, R., and Stahl, C. (1974). *In* "Biology and Biochemistry of Chemotaxis" (E. Sorkin, ed.), pp. 284–295. Karger, Basel.

Snyderman, R., and Stahl, C. (1975). *In* "The Phagocytic Cell in Host Resistance" (J. A. Bellanti and D. H. Dayton, eds.), pp. 267–281. Raven Press, New York.

Snyderman, R., Gewurz, H., and Mergenhagen, S. E. (1968). *J. Exp. Med.* **128,** 259–275.

Snyderman, R., Phillips, J. K., and Mergenhagen, S. E. (1970). *Infec. Immunity* **1,** 521–525.

Snyderman, R., Phillips, J. K., and Mergenhagen, S. E. (1971a). *J. Exp. Med.* **134,** 1131–1143.

Snyderman, R., Shin, H. S., and Hausman, M. S. (1971b). *Proc. Soc. Exp. Biol. Med.* **138,** 387–390.

Snyderman, R., Altman, L. C., Hausman, M. S., and Mergenhagen, S. E. (1972a). *J. Immunol.* **108,** 857–860.

Snyderman, R., Shin, H. S., and Dannenberg, A. M. (1972b). *J. Immunol.* **109,** 869–898.

Snyderman, R., Wohlenberg, C., and Notkins, A. L. (1972c). *J. Infec. Dis.* **126,** 207–209.

Snyderman, R., Altman, L. C., and Mergenhagen, S. E. (1973a). *In* "Nonspecific Factors Influencing Host Resistance" (W. Braun, ed.), pp. 180–189. Karger, Basel.

Snyderman, R., Altman, L. C., Frankel, A., and Blaese, R. M. (1973b). *Ann. Intern. Med.* **78,** 509–513.

Snyderman, R., Dickson, J., Meadows, L., and Pike, M. C. (1974a). *Clin. Res.* **22,** 430a.

Snyderman, R., Altman, L. C., and Pike, M. C. (1974b). *Annu. Rev. Allergy* pp. 325–335.

Snyderman, R., Dickson, J., and Meadows, L. (1974c). Submitted for publication.

Snyderman, R., Pike, M. C., and Altman, L. C. (1974d). *Ann. N.Y. Acad. Sci.* **256,** 386–406.

Snyderman, R., Blaylock, B., and Pike, M. C. (1975a). *Fed. Proc., Fed. Amer. Soc. Exp. Biol.* **34,** 4374.

Snyderman, R., Pike, M. C., McCarley, D., and Lang, L. (1975b). *Infec. Immunity* **11,** 488–492.

Stecher, V. J., and Sorkin, E. (1972). *Int. Arch. Allergy Appl. Immunol.* **43,** 879–886.

Stroud, R. M., Shin, H. S., and Shelton, E. (1973). *In* "Immune Response at the Cellular Level" (T. Zacharia, ed.), pp. 161–211. Dekker, New York.

Tempel, T. R., Snyderman, R., Jordan, H. V., and Mergenhagen, S. E. (1970). *J. Periodontol.* **41,** 3/71–12/80.

Till, G., and Ward, P. A. (1973). *J. Immunol.* **111,** 299.

Wahl, S. M., Altman, L. C., Oppenheim, J. J., and Mergenhagen, S. E. (1974a). *Int. Arch. Allergy Appl. Immunol.* **46,** 768–784.

Wahl, S. M., Iverson, G. M., and Oppenheim, J. J. (1974b). *J. Exp. Med.* **140,** 1631–1645.

Wahl, S. M., Wilton, J. M., Rosenstreich, D. L., and Oppenheim, J. J. (1975). *J. Immunol.* **114,** 1296–1301.

Waldmann, T. A., Strober, W., and Blaese, R. M. (1972). *Ann. Intern. Med.* **77,** 605–628.

Ward, P. A. (1968). *J. Exp. Med.* **128,** 1201–1221.

Ward, P. A., and Berenberg, J. L. (1974). *N. Engl. J. Med.* **290,** 76–80.

Ward, P. A., and Hill, J. H. (1970). *J. Immunol.* **104,** 535–543.

Ward, P. A., Cochrane, C. G., and Müller-Eberhard, H. J. (1965). *J. Exp. Med.* **122,** 327–346.

Ward, P. A., Lepow, I. H., and Newman, L. J. (1968). *Amer. J. Pathol.* **52,** 725–736.

Ward, P. A., Remold, H. G., and David, J. R. (1969). *Science* **163,** 1079–1081.

Ward, P. A., Remold, H. G., and David, J. R. (1970). *Cell. Immunol.* **1,** 162–174.

Wilkinson, P. C. (1974). *In* "Chemotaxis and Inflammation" (P. C. Wilkinson, ed.), pp. 33–53. Churchill, London.

Wilkinson, P. C., Borel, J. F., Stecher-Levin, V. J., and Sorkin, E. (1969). *Nature (London)* **222,** 244–247.

Wissler, J. H., Stecher, V. J., and Sorkin, E. (1972). *Int. Arch. Allergy Appl. Immunol.* **42,** 722–747.

Yoshida, A., Watanabe, S., and Morris, J. (1970). *Proc. Nat. Acad. Sci. U.S.* **67,** 1600–1607.

Zbar, B., Wepsic, H. T., Rapp, H. J., Stewart, L. C., and Borsas, T. (1970). *J. Nat. Cancer Inst.* **44,** 701–717.

Zigmond, S. H., and Hirsch, J. G. (1973). *J. Exp. Med.* **137,** 387–410.

14

Cellular and Molecular Aspects of Chemotaxis of Macrophages and Monocytes

P. C. Wilkinson

I. Introduction 350
II. Locomotion of Different Types of Macrophage 350
III. Modes of Macrophage Migration 351
  A. Random Migration Not Chemically Stimulated 351
  B. Chemokinesis 351
  C. Chemotaxis 351
IV. Recognition of Chemotactic Factors at the Cell Membrane 353
  A. Denaturation 354
  B. Conjugation of Side Groups to Proteins 354
V. Intracellular Events following Interaction of the Chemotactic Factor with the Cell Membrane 356
  A. Contractile Events 356
  B. Metabolic Activation 358
VI. Differential Effects of Bacterial Toxins on Locomotion of Neutrophils and Macrophages 358
VII. Recognition in Chemotaxis, Phagocytosis, and Other Macrophage Functions 360
  A. Phagocytosis 360
  B. Macrophage Activation 360
VIII. Antigen-Specific Chemotaxis 361
IX. Conclusions 363
References 363

I. INTRODUCTION

In this chapter, I shall discuss some recent approaches to an understanding of the molecular and cellular biology of chemotaxis and locomotion of macrophages, responses that enable these cells to reach sites of infection or tissue damage. Cellular aspects of chemotaxis of macrophages and other phagocytic cells have only recently become a subject of interest, since earlier research in this field was directed more to the identification of the various chemotactic factors in inflammation than to the analysis of the cell's response to them.

The technique used in the majority of studies of macrophage chemotaxis in recent years has been the micropore filter method introduced by Boyden (1962) and modified variously since. The technique which I use (Wilkinson, 1974a) is similar in principle to that described by Snyderman and Mergenhagen (Chapter 13), with the difference that a cellulose ester filter of 8 μm pore size and 150 μm thickness is used and that cell migration is estimated by measuring the distance migrated by the leading front of cells during a fixed time interval (Zigmond and Hirsch, 1973) and not by counting the number of cells that have reached the lower surface of the filter.

In addition to the Boyden technique, direct observation of migrating macrophages under the microscope in the presence or absence of chemical stimuli is a valuable and little used method from which a good deal may be learned. The morphological changes in cells responding to stimuli and their method of locomotion can best be studied in this way.

II. LOCOMOTION OF DIFFERENT TYPES OF MACROPHAGE

"Free" or motile macrophages from whatever source are capable of responding to chemoattractants. Alveolar macrophages, peritoneal macrophages, whether from induced exudates or from the normal peritoneal cavity, and blood monocytes all respond to the same stimuli. The response of the human blood monocyte is very predictable from day to day. This may not be the case for exudate macrophages, which are sometimes unresponsive to locomotor stimuli, possibly because they are in a period of inertia after responding to the inducing agent that brought them into the peritoneum. We have recently observed that hepatic Kupffer cells, if freed from hepatocytes and prepared as a single cell suspension with EDTA and trypsin, are capable of migrating in Boyden chambers. The classification of macrophages into fixed and free forms may therefore reflect a temporary influence of their environment rather than an irreversible differentiation.

III. MODES OF MACROPHAGE MIGRATION

Since there exists a good deal of confusion about the ways in which macrophages and other phagocytes migrate, and a tendency to use the word chemotaxis loosely, it is worth discussing what is meant by chemotaxis before proceeding further. Macrophage migration may take any one of the forms listed below.

A. Random Migration Not Chemically Stimulated

Cells in the absence of a chemical stimulus migrate slowly and randomly. This migration can be observed in balanced salt solutions with or without added protein. It should be noted that "normal" serum contains substances that accelerate macrophage migration and is therefore not a suitable negative control medium in which unstimulated locomotion can be studied (Wilkinson *et al.*, 1969; Borel and Sorkin, 1969).

B. Chemokinesis

Keller and Sorkin (1966) showed by photomicrographic tracing that leukocytes placed on a slide in a medium containing serum activated with aggregated γ-globulin moved randomly, but considerably more than cells placed in an inert medium. This was in the absence of a gradient, and the cells were responding to the absolute concentration of a chemoattractant—presumably complement—in the absence of any concentration differences. This chemically enhanced nondirectional locomotion is called chemokinesis. All chemotactic factors so far studied enhance chemokinetic migration under nongradient conditions, a point that is implicit in the rest of this chapter. The dose–response curve for leukocytes responding to such factors under nongradient conditions in filters reaches a peak at an optimum concentration and then falls away as the concentration is raised further (Zigmond and Hirsch, 1973).

C. Chemotaxis

Chemotaxis has been defined by McCutcheon (1946) as "a reaction by which the direction of locomotion of cells or organisms is determined by substances in their environment." The word therefore defines an orientation of movement rather than the movement itself. When macrophages are placed in a gradient of a chemotactic substance, they respond by migrating toward the source of the gradient. In Boyden chambers the gradient is set up across the width of the micropore filter into which the cells migrate. However it cannot then be assumed that this migration is chemotactic. The cells may be responding, not to the gradient, but to the absolute local concentration of the factor in their environment, i.e., by chemokinesis. Chemotaxis has been most satisfactorily distinguished from chemokinesis using the slide and coverslip technique. Zigmond and Hirsch (1973) showed that neutrophil leukocytes placed in a chemotactic gradient and observed directly become oriented with a flattened, hyaline leading edge facing the gradient source and a knoblike tail at the rear. Most of the cells then migrate in the direction of the gradient. Zigmond (1974) has shown that leukocytes can detect concentration differences across their own length. They may possess multiple membrane sites that can interact with chemotactic factors and therefore distinguish concentration differences between their two poles. Macrophages also can be observed to take up an elongated morphology in chemotactic gradients with an anterior hyaline membrane and a tail that may contain retraction fibers that adhere to the substratum. An oriented chemotactic response for macrophages can also be demonstrated in Boyden chambers and distinguished from chemokinetic movement by varying the concentrations of attractant above and below the filter, so that the cells are moving either in a positive gradient, a negative gradient, or no gradient. The calculations necessary to establish whether migration through filters is, or is not, chemotactic are given by Zigmond and Hirsch (1973).

Chemotactic factors, therefore, both accelerate the movement of cells (kinesis) probably by activating energy-providing metabolic systems and contractile systems in the cell and, in gradients, cause that movement to be oriented (taxis). In a gradient where more chemoattractant molecules "hit" the front portion of cell membrane than the rear, the cell will move forward. If the number of "hits" is distributed evenly over the cell, the cell may move the same overall distance, but at random.

The distinction of chemotaxis from chemokinesis is important. First, it is likely that microtubule integrity is essential for orientation of movement but not for the movement itself (see Section V,A). Second, one of the difficulties of demonstrating chemotaxis *in vivo* has been that several workers studying the migration of leukocytes in living tissues have observed that this migration is enhanced in injured sites, but they could not show that it was directional (Allison *et al.*, 1955; Harris, 1960; Cliff, 1966). They were usually observing the migration of cells from vessels close to the site of a microinjury, perhaps near the center of any gradient. In living tissues, gradients are likely to be upset by tissue movements, and it is, therefore, an advantage for phagocytes to move by chemokinesis where the gradient is poor or disturbed, but also, where there is a good gradient, to be able to sense and home in on its source. Buckley (1963) made microinjuries at a sufficient distance from the nearest vessel for him to be able to observe cells moving directionally through the tissues toward it. An important aspect of chemotaxis in the development of lesions *in vivo* is that cells become trapped at the center of a gradient, since as soon as they move away they come under the influence of the gradient again and are attracted back in.

IV. RECOGNITION OF CHEMOTACTIC FACTORS AT THE CELL MEMBRANE

Mononuclear phagocytes migrate in response to numerous chemotactic factors, including C5a and lymphocyte-derived factors (Snyderman and Mergenhagen, Chapter 13), α- and β-caseins (Wilkinson, 1972), and factors derived from chronic granuloma-forming bacteria such as the *Corynebacterium parvum* group (Wilkinson *et al.*, 1973a,b) and *Listeria* spp. (R. J. Russell, unpublished). Some of these factors, e.g., C5a, also attract neutrophils but others, such as the corynebacterial factor, are macrophage-specific. Most of the factors so far described are proteins or peptides. The corynebacterial factor is a phospholipid (Section VII). The factors are so diverse in structure and origin that it is extremely unlikely that there is any structural feature common to them all. This implies of course that there cannot be any "chemotaxis receptor" of a sterically defined type (such as an antibody-combining site) with which they react at the cell surface. Since we are then faced with a problem of an identical cellular response to a very diverse group of molecules, it is necessary to find some common physicochemical basis that allows these factors to initiate a locomotor response, while, at the same time, numerous other molecules that the cell meets evoke no response from it. We have published several studies exploring recognition in chemotaxis (Wilkinson and McKay, 1971, 1972; Wilkinson, 1973a, 1974b). The data presented in those papers mostly concerned neutrophils. Contemporaneous but previously unpublished studies of macrophages that revealed a similar pattern of recognition are described below.

Because, at the time we began our study, little was known of the structure of chemotactic factors from complement and other sources, we decided that the most fruitful approach would be to modify the structure of proteins that were normally present in the environment of the phagocytic cells but which were not chemotactic, and to see what sort of modification would induce a chemotactic response to them. These modifications are discussed below.

A. Denaturation

Table I shows that human serum albumin (HSA) that has been denatured with alkali is more chemotactic for macrophages than native HSA. This acquisition of chemotactic activity is not due to polymerization or aggregation. Sephadex-fractionated monomer fractions are as chemotactic as or, usually, more chemotactic than polymer fractions. The chemotactic effect results from changes in the structure of the monomeric molecule. These molecules show physicochemical evidence of unfolding as measured by the increase in their specific viscosity (Wilkinson and McKay, 1971), by increased surface activity (Wilkinson, 1974b), and by difference spectroscopy (Wilkinson, 1973b). Similarly hemoglobin and myoglobin molecules (Wilkinson, 1973a) can be unfolded by removing the heme group from the globin molecule by acid–acetone treatment at —20°C. The unfolded globin molecule then becomes chemotactic. This unfolding of heme proteins is fully reversed simply by adding the heme group back to the globin. When this is done, the globin molecule folds up again fully and at the same time loses chemotactic activity.

When proteins are unfolded, hydrophobic residues, normally packed into the interior of the molecule, become exposed to the aqueous solvent. Such molecules become surface-active and thermodynamically unstable in the bulk phase of aqueous solutions. They, therefore, show an affinity for air–water interfaces (Wilkinson, 1974b), and it is possible that they also show an affinity for the phospholipid bilayer of cell membranes, where they can attain a lower free energy state than is possible in aqueous solution. This can also be tested by conjugating hydrophobic (nonpolar) groups to proteins. These groups ought to make proteins more chemotactically active than analogous unconjugated proteins or those conjugated to polar side groups.

B. Conjugation of Side Groups to Proteins

Table I shows the chemotactic activity for macrophages of proteins conjugated to a variety of side groups. Nonpolar groups, such as tosyl or butyryl groups, conferred on the protein the ability to attract macrophages, and, in general, the more of the side group used for conjugation,

TABLE I

Migration of Mononuclear Phagocytes toward Denatured or Conjugated Proteins

Human blood monocytes		Guinea pig peritoneal macrophages		
Protein at 1 mg/ml	Chemotactic activity[a]	Protein at 1 mg/ml	Conjugating agent and quantity added to 40 mg protein[b]	Chemotactic activity[a]
HSA (native)	1.0	HSA (native)	None	1.0
Heat-denatured HSA	1.6	Tosyl-HSA	Tosyl Cl 1 mg	0.9
Alkali-denatured HSA			Tosyl Cl 4 mg	1.4
Sample I	2.1		Tosyl Cl 10 mg	2.1
Sample II	3.6	Acetyl-HSA	Acetic anhydride 2 mg	1.9
Sample III	2.7	Butyryl-HSA	Butyric anhydride 2 mg	1.6
Butyryl-HSA	2.6	Methyl-HSA	Acid methanol in excess	2.1
Hemoglobin (human)	1.0	Formol-HSA	Formaldehyde (0.05 *M*)	0.8
Globin		Guanidyl-HSA	*O*-Methyl isourea (0.5 *M*)	1.2
Sample I	2.1			
Sample II	2.0			

[a] Chemotactic activity $= \dfrac{\text{migration } (\mu\text{m}) \text{ toward test protein (2 hours 8 } \mu\text{m pore size filter)}}{\text{migration } (\mu\text{m}) \text{ toward native protein (unconjugated HSA or Hb)}}$

[b] Details of the conjugating procedures and protein: sidegroup ratios are given by Wilkinson and McKay (1972).

the more active was the conjugate. Addition of basic guanidyl groups or small groups such as formaldehyde did not make HSA chemotactic.

These results led us to the conclusion that locomotion and chemotaxis of macrophages and neutrophils are probably initiated by hydrophobic interactions between the chemotactic factor and the phospholipid bilayer of the cell membrane. This conclusion is supported by studies suggesting that enzymes and toxins which act on the bilayer can modify the chemotactic response (Section VI). It explains the lack of specificity in chemotactic recognition. Hydrophobic interactions lack the directionality necessary for such structural specificity. The pattern underlying recognition of chemoattractants is to be found at the physicochemical and not at the structural level.

Nothing is yet known about the way complement-derived or other chemotactic factors found in inflammatory lesions interact with cell membranes. Whether they interact in the way proposed here needs to be tested. It is of interest that α- and β-caseins, both of which are chemotactic, are both proteins with an intrinsically high content of nonpolar residues, too high apparently for them all to be packed internally (Waugh *et al.*, 1970), and both of these proteins have high surface activity (Evans *et al.*, 1970; Wilkinson, 1974b).

V. INTRACELLULAR EVENTS FOLLOWING INTERACTION OF THE CHEMOTACTIC FACTOR WITH THE CELL MEMBRANE

A. Contractile Events

How is the sensory event of membrane recognition of a chemotactic factor translated into the motor event of directed locomotion? Possible answers to this question are now beginning to emerge. It begins to look as if the phagocytes should be regarded as "excitable cells" by analogy with a muscle which responds to an impulse from the motor end plate by contracting. In the muscle, contraction is driven by the interaction of myosin with actin, for which energy is supplied in the form of ATP and which is regulated by calcium fluxes across the cell membrane and into and out of the sarcoplasmic reticulum. The molecular biology of macrophage chemotaxis may be remarkably similar in outline. In the case of the macrophage, the initiating stimulus is not a nervous impulse but contact of the cell membrane with a chemoattractant. This contact may increase the permeability of the membrane locally and allow an influx of divalent cations into the cell, either from outside or from an intracellular cation reserve. In neutrophils at rest the intracytoplasmic calcium concentration is low, but increases in membrane permeability are followed by an inflow of calcium and by contractile events (Woodin, 1972). This seems likely also in macrophages but has not been demonstrated directly. Wilkinson (1975a) showed that blood monocyte migration, like neutrophil migration (Becker and Showell, 1972), is depressed but not abolished in media free of Ca^{2+} and Mg^{2+}. Divalent cation ionophores, such as A23187 (Eli Lilly), which assist transfer of divalent cations across membranes, can at low concentrations restore the chemotactic response of Ca^{2+}- and Mg^{2+}-depleted monocytes and neutrophils to normal (Wilkinson, 1975a), perhaps by enabling them to make more efficient use of their own intracellular cation stores. The site of these stores is still unknown. Their action must be to sequester divalent cations and during continued cell movement to allow sequential contraction and relaxation by controlled release of cations into the cytoplasm followed by removal of the cations. If the cytoplasmic calcium concentration remained high, the cell would go into rigor and cease movement.

Macrophages and neutrophils contain microfilaments composed of actomyosin (Bhisey and Freed, 1971; Allison *et al.*, 1971), and, indeed, both actin and myosin have been isolated in pure form from neutrophils (Tatsumi *et al.*, 1973; Stossel and Pollard, 1973). Cytochalasin B, which is believed to disrupt microfilaments, inhibits locomotion of macrophages (Allison *et al.*, 1971) and neutrophils (Becker *et al.*, 1972; Zigmond and Hirsch, 1972). It seems likely that locomotion of these cells is driven by microfilaments, but, since cytochalasin B blocks other functions such as glucose transport in cells, independent evidence is required to confirm this. The microfilament system would be expected to be Ca^{2+}-sensitive and thus to respond to calcium fluxes in the way described above.

Microtubules form a second contractile protein system in macrophages. In oriented migrating macrophages, microtubules are arranged as a cytoskeletal structure in the cytoplasm which maintains the polarized shape of the oriented cell. Bhisey and Freed (1971), and Allison *et al.* (1971), and Allison (1974) showed that the elongated form of migrating macrophages was lost after treatment with colchicine or vinblastine, both agents that specifically depolymerize microtubule proteins. The cells could still move but had lost directionality of movement. Bandmann *et al.* (1974) had similar findings with antitubulin drugs. In Boyden chambers (P. C. Wilkinson, unpublished observations), the chemokinetic migration of human blood monocytes (and neutrophils) is little affected by colchicine, but the cells are much less able to detect a gradient. All these studies seem to be in agreement that microtubules are essential for the cell to orient itself correctly in a gradient but are not required for locomotion itself.

B. Metabolic Activation

A "metabolic burst" accompanies contractile events in leukocytes, and phagocytosis by macrophages is accompanied by an increase in glucose consumption and respiratory rate (Karnovsky *et al.*, 1970). A similar increase in glycolytic and respiratory activity accompanies chemotaxis, at least in neutrophils (Goetzl and Austen, 1974). The locomotor response of macrophages from several sources is blocked by inhibitors of anaerobic glycolysis (Wilkinson *et al.*, 1973a) but is less affected by uncouplers of oxidative phosphorylation, such as dinitrophenol (DNP), suggesting that glycolysis probably forms the major source of energy for macrophage locomotion. Unstimulated macrophages are more sensitive to DNP than stimulated cells. These metabolic changes are accompanied by increased release of hydrolases from lysosomes. Incubation with chemotactic factors, such as casein or anaerobic coryneform bacteria, causes a rise in the activity of acid phosphatase and β-glucuronidase in cultures of human blood monocytes or guinea pig peritoneal macrophages (Wilkinson *et al.*, 1973a), and a proportion of this enzyme is released from the cells into the supernatant medium, probably by exocytosis, as has also been shown for macrophages cultured in the presence of immune complexes (Cardella *et al.*, 1974).

VI. DIFFERENTIAL EFFECTS OF BACTERIAL TOXINS ON LOCOMOTION OF NEUTROPHILS AND MACROPHAGES

Much of the information presented so far in this chapter on the cellular mechanisms of macrophage chemotaxis is equally relevant to neutrophils. Nevertheless certain chemotactic factors are remarkably macrophage-specific, and it is a commonplace finding that the pattern of emigration of the two cell types into lesions is strikingly different. We have recently been studying the effects of a number of highly purified bacterial toxins on the locomotor responses of macrophages and neutrophils (results in preparation for publicaton). Table II shows that the individual toxins have strikingly different effects on the membranes of human blood neutrophils and of human blood monocytes. θ toxin from *Clostridium perfringens* at nontoxic doses inhibits neutrophil migration but not monocyte migration. Conversely, phospholipase C (α toxin) from the same orga-

TABLE II

Effects of Clostridium perfringens Toxins[a] on Migration of Human Blood Cells (Dose Response to Casein)

Cells treated with	Migration towards casein at concentration below filter (μg/ml)			
	100	250	500	1000
Monocytes[b]				
No treatment	N/T[c]	63	75	77
Phospholipase C[d], 100 mU/ml	N/T	31	38	46
θ-toxin,[d] 0.1 HU/ml	N/T	68	70	70
Neutrophils[e]				
No treatment	39	68	75	60
Phospholipase C,[d] 100 mU/ml	35	57	86	70
θ-toxin, 0.1 HU/ml	37	42	44	33

[a] Samples of pure toxin were a gift from Drs. C. J. Smyth and R. Möllby, Bacteriology Institute, Karolinska Institute, Stockholm, Sweden.

[b] Migration in μm in 2 hours, 8 μm filter.

[c] N/T, not tested.

[d] Phospholipase C splits phosphorylcholine from the polar head of phosphatidylcholine and related phospholipids. θ toxin has an affinity for cholesterol in cell membranes (Bernheimer, 1970).

[e] Migration in μm in 75 minutes, 3 μm filter.

nism, also at nontoxic dose levels, has little effect on neutrophil migration but inhibits monocyte migration. Bee venom phospholipase A potentiates migration of neutrophils toward chemattractants (Wilkinson, 1974b) but has no effect on monocytes. These results raise two interesting points. First, they reveal that even though the general nature of the interaction of chemotactic factors with the membranes of the two cell types may be similar, there are probably differences in the detailed architecture of the membrane sites involved. Probes, such as bacterial toxins, with an affinity for specific membrane sites will be useful in pinpointing these differences. Second, the fact that toxins with specific effects on membrane lipids may influence the chemotactic response supports the idea that the chemotactic factors themselves also interact with the phospholipid bilayer and not with exposed surface glycoproteins. Treatment of macrophages with enzymes that attack glycoproteins, such as neuraminidase and other glycosidases, has little effect on locomotion. Trypsin and other proteases reduce locomotion slightly, but this may be because they reduce the ability of the cells to adhere to a substratum.

VII. RECOGNITION IN CHEMOTAXIS, PHAGOCYTOSIS, AND OTHER MACROPHAGE FUNCTIONS

A. Phagocytosis

Chemically directed locomotion of macrophages, phagocytosis, the fusion of lysosomes with phagosomes, and exocytosis of lysosomal hydrolases are probably all triggered contractile events with related molecular mechanisms. Are the membrane interactions involved in recognition of chemotactic factors and in recognition of particles in phagocytosis therefore also similar? Van Oss and his colleagues (van Oss and Gillman, 1972a,b 1973; Thrasher *et al.*, 1973; van Oss *et al.*, 1974) have explored the physicochemical basis for phagocytosis and have proposed that macrophages will only phagocytize particles whose surface is more hydrophobic than the surface of the macrophage itself. Rabinovitch (1970) stated that macrophages do not phagocytize normal erythrocytes but do phagocytize erythrocytes coated with aldehyde groups. We have shown that HSA conjugated to aldehydes, which contain nonpolar side chains, is chemotactic (Wilkinson and McKay, 1972), and the same molecular interaction could be taking place at the cell membrane in the two cases. Furthermore, van Oss and Gillman (1973) and van Oss *et al.* (1974) suggest that, at the physicochemical level, immune recognition by phagocytes is similar to nonimmune recognition, since opsonizing antibody or complement bound to erythrocytes or bacteria increases their surface hydrophobicity and therefore their phagocytosability. They also suggest that the interaction of the Fc fragment of cytophilic immunoglobulin with the phagocyte surface is essentially a hydrophobic one.

To suggest such physicochemical resemblances between membrane activation in chemotaxis and phagocytosis is not, of course, to say anything that helps to explain how the very different sequences of motor events in oriented locomotion and in particle ingestion are controlled.

B. Macrophage Activation

Chemotactic substances, such as casein, are commonly used to induce macrophage-rich exudates in animals. However, following injection of casein, cell numbers in the peritoneum are not sustained for longer than a few days, and long-term macrophage activation is not seen. The macrophages do not become cytotoxic for tumor cells in the way shown by Alexander and Evans (1971), nor do they show an increased ability to kill bacteria. Other chemotactic agents, such as *Mycobacteria,* which attract macrophages in the presence of plasma (Symon *et al.*, 1972), do cause long-term macrophage activation. Since the initial membrane excitation by the two groups of factors is presumably similar, the ability or nonability of chemotactic factors to cause long-term macrophage activation must depend on later events. In certain models of such events, T lymphocytes release macrophage-activating products. However, the bacteria of the anaerobic coryneform group, which do not activate T lymphocytes (Howard *et al.*, 1973), release a macrophage-specific chemotactic factor (Wilkinson *et al.*, 1973a,b) and also cause long-term macrophage activation. These organisms incite formation of a macrophage granuloma at the site of injection (Pinckard *et al.*, 1968) and enhance clearance of carbon from the circulation in mice (Halpern *et al.*, 1964). In the guinea pig, they raise antibody levels, mainly of γ_1-globulin, to antigens injected with them but have little effect on delayed hypersensitivity (O'Neill *et al.*, 1973). There is considerable current interest in the ability of these organisms to induce regression of tumors (Woodruff and Boak, 1966; Halpern *et al.*, 1966; also see reviews in Halpern, 1975), which appears to be mediated directly by activated macrophages. We have purified a macrophage chemotactic factor from these anaerobic corynebacteria (Russell *et al.*, 1975). It is a chloroform-soluble phospholipid, active at concentrations of less than 1 μg/ml, and containing little or no carbohydrate or peptide as judged by its infrared spectrum. Its ability to stimulate other macrophage functions is under study. Fauve and Hevin (1974) have recently reported that a similar phospholipid extract from the same group of organisms, when injected into mice, enhances resistance to infections with *Listeria monocytogenes* and other organisms and that this enhancement is macrophage-mediated. It remains to be seen whether these phospholipids are one and the same.

VIII. ANTIGEN-SPECIFIC CHEMOTAXIS

Jensen has suggested that immune reactions occurring on the surface of a phagocytic cell might induce a chemotactic reaction in that cell (Jensen and Williams, 1973; Jensen and Esquenazi, 1975). His evidence was derived from experiments with neutrophils in which *inter alia* cytophilic antibody-coated neutrophils were shown to migrate toward specific antigen. Complement was required but not as a source of chemotactic factor. It was suggested that when diffusing molecules of antigen met the complementary cell-bound antibody, the immune reaction between them at the cell surface induced migration of the cell in the gradient of diffusing antigen.

Rosa Vasquez, R. J. McInroy, and myself have recently studied the migration of guinea pig macrophages coated with guinea pig cytophilic anti-HSA serum. Table III shows an enhancement of migration of these macrophages toward HSA but not toward other proteins. This phenomenon requires both cell-bound antibody and a serum factor other than antibody, but this factor is stable to heat and to cobra venom, so its relation to complement remains to be determined. It is interesting that cytophilic antibody-coated cells show reduced migration to *denatured* HSA. Nonspecific recognition (of denaturation) has been replaced by specific recognition (of antigen). This could be either because the denatured HSA reacts with the cytophilic antibody rather than with the cell surface or because cytophilic antibody competes for the cell site to which denatured HSA normally binds. If antigen acts as a chemoattractant by binding to cell-bound antibody, it would appear to activate the cell membrane by a different mechanism from the one described above. However it must

TABLE III

Effect of Cytophilic Anti-HSA on Migration of Guinea Pig Peritoneal Macrophages toward HSA

	Migration (μm in 2 hours in 12 μm filters) toward				
Treatment of macrophages[a] (all from unimmunized guinea pigs)	Gey's solution (negative control)	HSA 1 mg/ml	BSA 1 mg/ml	HGG 1 mg/ml	Alkali-denatured HSA 1 mg/ml
Untreated macrophages	31	32	36	28	68
Macrophages treated with guinea pig anti-HSA	31	46[b]	37	30	54
Macrophages treated with guinea pig anti-SRBC	30	32			53
Macrophages treated with normal guinea pig serum	31	31			63

[a] Macrophages were incubated for 1 hour at 4°C with the appropriate antiserum then washed free of unattached serum proteins before being placed in chemotaxis chambers. The protein solutions were placed below the filter.

[b] The increase in migration toward specific antigen is fairly small, probably because the available combining sites on the cell surface soon become filled. *In vivo* there would be a likelihood of renewal of these sites and thus of further migration.

be remembered that the membrane-activating event is taking place, not at the antigen-binding site, but at the Fc receptor site. Thus, antigen-induced Fc clustering or conformational changes in Fc might cause the required permeability changes in the bilayer. The idea that macrophages can borrow specific recognition for their migratory responses is an intriguing one that should open up all sorts of new possibilities.

IX. CONCLUSIONS

It begins to seem that monocytes and macrophages in locomotion are excitable cells in the same way as muscle cells. When chemoattractants interact with the cell membrane, they may allow an influx of divalent cations into the cytoplasm either from outside or from storage vesicles within the cell. Regulated cation fluxes may control the contraction and relaxation of microfilaments that are the locomotor organs of the cell. The microtubules are also necessary to orient the cell's movement. Chemoattractants may possess appropriate physicochemical properties (e.g., increased hydrophobicity and surface activity) that allow them to penetrate into the phospholipid bilayer by nonpolar bonding and thus to increase the ion permeability of the cell membrane. This mechanism is in essence similar in mononuclear phagocytes and in neutrophils, but preliminary experiments indicate that there are differences between the two cell types in the membrane-binding sites for chemoattractant molecules.

ACKNOWLEDGMENT

Part of the work described in this paper was supported by the Medical Research Council.

REFERENCES

Alexander, P., and Evans, R. (1971). *Nature (London), New Biol.* **232,** 76–78.

Allison, A. C. (1974). *Antibiot. Chemother. (Washington, D.C.)* **19,** 191–217.

Allison, A. C., Davies, P., and de Petris, S. (1971). *Nature (London), New Biol.* **232,** 153–155.

Allison, F., Smith, M. R., and Wood, W. B. (1955). *J. Exp. Med.* **102,** 655–668.

Bandmann, U., Rydgren, L., and Norberg, B. (1974). *Exp. Cell Res.* **88,** 63–73.

Becker, E. L., and Showell, H. J. (1972). *Z. Immunitätsforsch.* **143,** 466–476.

Becker, E. L., Davis, A. T., Estensen, R. D., and Quie, P. G. (1972). *J. Immunol.* **108,** 396–402.

Bernheimer, A. W. (1970). *In* "Microbial Toxins" (S. J. Ajl, S. Kadis, and T. C. Montie, eds.), Vol. 1, pp. 183–212. Academic Press, New York.

Bhisey, A. N., and Freed, J. J. (1971). *Exp. Cell Res.* **64,** 419–429.
Borel, J. F., and Sorkin, E. (1969). *Experientia* **25,** 1333–1335.
Boyden, S. V. (1962). *J. Exp. Med.* **115,** 453–466.
Buckley, I. K. (1963). *Exp. Mol. Pathol.* **2,** 402–417.
Cardella, C. J., Davies, P., and Allison, A. C. (1974). *Nature* (*London*) **247,** 46–48.
Cliff, W. J. (1966). *J. Exp. Med.* **124,** 543–556.
Evans, M. T. A., Mitchell, J., Mussellwhite, P. R., and Irons, L. (1970). *Advan. Exp. Med. Biol.* **7,** 1–22.
Fauve, R. M., and Hevin, B. (1974). *Proc. Nat. Acad. Sci. U.S.* **71,** 573–577.
Goetzl, E. J., and Austen, K. F. (1974). *J. Clin. Invest.* **53,** 591–599.
Halpern, B. N., ed. (1975). "*Corynebacterium parvum:* Applications in Experimental and Clinical Oncology." Plenum, New York.
Halpern, B. N., Prévot, A. R., Biozzi, G., Stiffel, C., Mouton, D., Morard, J. C., Bouthillier, Y., and Decreusefond, C. (1964). *J. Reticuloendothel. Soc.* **1,** 77–96.
Halpern, B. N., Biozzi, G., Stiffel, C., and Mouton, D. (1966). *Nature* (*London*) **212,** 853–854.
Harris, H. (1960). *Bacteriol. Rev.* **24,** 3–15.
Howard, J. G., Scott, M. T., and Christie, G. H. (1973). *Immunopotentiation, Ciba Found. Symp.* pp. 101–120.
Jensen, J. A., and Williams, D. (1973). *Nouv. Rev. Fr. Hematol.* **13,** 899.
Jensen, J. A., and Esquenazi, V. (1975). *Nature* (*London*) **256,** 213–215.
Karnovsky, M. L., Simmons, S., Glass, E. A., Shafer, A. W., and d'Arcy Hart, P., (1970). *In* "Mononuclear Phagocytes" (R. van Furth, ed.), pp. 103–120. Blackwell, Oxford.
Keller, H. U., and Sorkin, E. (1966). *Immunology* **10,** 409–416.
McCutcheon, M. (1946). *Physiol. Rev.* **26,** 319–336.
O'Neill, G. J., Henderson, D. C., and White, R. G. (1973). *Immunology* **24,** 977–995.
Pinckard, R. N., Weir, D. M., and McBride, W. H. (1968). *Clin. Exp. Immunol.* **3,** 413–421.
Rabinovitch, M. (1970). *In* "Mononuclear Phagocytes" (R. van Furth, ed.), pp. 299–315. Blackwell, Oxford.
Russell, R. J., McInroy, R. J., Wilkinson, P. C., and White, R. G. (1975). *Behring. Inst. Mitt.* **57,** 103–109.
Stossel, T., and Pollard, T. D. (1973). *J. Biol. Chem.* **248,** 8288–8294.
Symon, D. N. K., McKay, I. C., and Wilkinson, P. C. (1972). *Immunology* **22,** 267–276.
Tatsumi, N., Shibata, N., Okamura, Y., Takeuchi, K., and Senda, N. (1973). *Biochim. Biophys. Acta* **305,** 433–444.
Thrasher, S. G., Yoshida, T., van Oss, C. J., Cohen, S., and Rose, N. R. (1973). *J. Immunol.* **110,** 321–326.
van Oss, C. J., and Gillman, C. F. (1972a). *RES, J. Reticuloendothel. Soc.* **12,** 283–292.
van Oss, C. J., and Gillman, C. F. (1972b). *RES, J. Reticuloendothel. Soc.* **12,** 497–502.
van Oss, C. J., and Gillman, C. F. (1973). *Immunol. Commun.* **2,** 415–419.
van Oss, C. J., Gillman, C. F., and Neumann, A. W. (1974). *Immunol. Commun.* **3,** 77–84.
Waugh, D. F., Creamer, L. K., Slattery, C. W., and Dreschner, G. W. (1970). *Biochemistry* **9,** 786–795.
Wilkinson, P. C. (1972). *Experientia* **28,** 1051–1052.
Wilkinson, P. C. (1973a). *Nature* (*London*) **244,** 512–513.

Wilkinson, P. C. (1973b). *In* "Future Trends in Inflammation" (G. P. Velo, D. A Willoughby, and J. P. Giroud, eds.), pp. 125–134. Piccin, Padua.
Wilkinson, P. C. (1974a). "Chemotaxis and Inflammation." Churchill-Livingstone, Edinburgh.
Wilkinson, P. C. (1974b). *Nature (London)* **251,** 58–60.
Wilkinson, P. C. (1975a). *Exp. Cell Res.* **93,** 420–426.
Wilkinson, P. C. (1975b). *Nature (London)* **255,** 485–487.
Wilkinson, P. C., and McKay, I. C. (1971). *Int. Arch. Allergy Appl. Immunol.* **41,** 237–247.
Wilkinson, P. C., and McKay, I. C. (1972). *Eur. J. Immunol.* **2,** 570–577.
Wilkinson, P. C., Borel, J. F., Stecher-Levin, V. J., and Sorkin, E. (1969). *Nature (London)* **222,** 244–247.
Wilkinson, P. C., O'Neill, G. J., McInroy, R. J., Cater, J. C. and Roberts, J. A. (1973a). *Immunopotentiation, Ciba Found. Symp. pp.* 121–140.
Wilkinson, P. C., O'Neill, G. J., and Wapshaw, K. (1973b). *Immunology* **24,** 997–1006.
Woodin, A. M. (1972). *In* "The Staphylococci" (J. O. Cohen, ed.), pp. 281–299. Wiley, New York.
Woodruff, M. F. A., and Boak, J. L. (1966). *Brit. J. Cancer* **20,** 345–355.
Zigmond, S. H. (1974). *Nature (London)* **249,** 450–452.
Zigmond, S. H., and Hirsch, J. G. (1972). *Exp. Cell Res.* **73,** 383–393.
Zigmond, S. H., and Hirsch, J. G. (1973). *J. Exp. Med.* **137,** 387–410.

15

Lymphocyte–Macrophage Interactions and Macrophage Activation in the Expression of Antimicrobial Immunity *in Vivo*

Robert V. Blanden, Andrew J. Hapel, Peter C. Doherty, and Rolf M. Zinkernagel

I. Introduction 367
II. Generation of Effector T Cells 369
A. Origin 369
B. Induction 370
C. Kinetics 372
D. Regulation 373
E. Migration 374
F. Memory 375
III. Mechanisms of T Cell- and Macrophage-Mediated Immunity to Infection 375
A. Cytotoxicity 375
B. Recruitment of Monocytes 381
C. Activation of Macrophages 389
D. Interferon 394
IV. Conclusions 395
References 397

I. INTRODUCTION

Over the last 15 years or so, it has become increasingly clear that lymphocytes collaborate with macrophages in the process of recovery from, and subsequent resistance to, certain infectious diseases. A wide variety of infections caused by viruses, bacteria, fungi, and protozoan or metazoan parasites have now been studied with varying degrees of success, in terms of unravelling the nature of the lymphocyte–macrophage interactions responsible for immunity (World Health Organization, 1973). Here we will deal with only a portion of this immense field, but our intention nonetheless is to illustrate the general pattern of evidence that is emerging. We will restrict ourselves primarily to mechanisms involving thymus-derived (T) lymphocytes, and not thymus-independent (B) lymphocytes, i.e., to cell-mediated immunity* (CMI), not antibody-mediated immunity and to certain intracellular bacterial and viral infections that provide useful examples.

At this point it is appropriate to introduce the idea that a single basic theme is common to many different immunological effector mechanisms or reactions including CMI, namely, immunologically specific events trigger "preprogrammed," nonspecific sequelae. For example, acute phenomena, such as anaphylaxis and Arthus reactions, and allergic reactions, such as hay fever and urticaria, are triggered by the interaction between antigen and specific antibodies of a particular class in a particular location. This interaction results in the release of pharmacologically active agents whose inflammatory effects are unrelated to the kind of antigen that caused their release. Similarly, it seems that antigen-specific effector T lymphocytes,† upon stimulation with the appropriate antigen, release chemical mediators of CMI (World Health Organization, 1973); these substances have a wide variety of biological effects, including the attraction and activation of macrophages,‡ which are unrelated to the specificity of the stimulating antigen. Recent evidence reviewed elsewhere in this book suggests that B cells, as well as T cells, may produce some of these factors, but the overwhelming weight of evidence clearly shows that T cells§ are essential for triggering normal manifestations of CMI *in vivo* (World Health Organization, 1973; Blanden, 1974a; Doherty and Zinker-

* "Cell-mediated immunity" is used in this chapter to describe a broad group of immunological phenomena that appear to require specific effector T lymphocytes and to be independent of free antibodies. This includes phenomena previously referred to as "cellular immunity" or "cellular resistance."

† The terms "effector T lymphocytes" or "effector T cells" are used instead of "sensitized lymphocytes," simply because, in our view, they convey better the idea that such cells are functionally important in controlling infectious diseases.

‡ "Activated macrophages" are defined in this chapter as macrophages possessing enhanced nonspecific microbicidal activity.

§ T cells active in CMI are the only T cell class considered in this chapter. Helper T cells may well be a separate T cell class because of evidence reviewed elsewhere (Blanden, 1974a) and for theoretical reasons (Bretscher, 1974). Whether cytotoxic T cells are a subset separate from T cells which recruit or activate macrophages is to our knowledge, not resolved.

nagel, 1975a). We intend to present support for the view that effector T cells operate to control infection by circulating in blood, by recognizing "specific" antigens emanating from foci of infection, and by causing (probably via soluble factors) the recruitment and activation of blood monocytes. Thus there would be assembled in foci of infection a collection of cells capable of specific and nonspecific cytotoxicity, phagocytic, bactericidal, or virucidal effects. These cells could be augmented further in antiviral action by interferon.

In some laboratories, interaction between lymphocytes and macrophages has been shown to result in apparently specific antiviral (McFarland, 1974) or antitumor (Evans *et al.*, 1972; Lohmann-Matthes and Fischer, 1973) activity in macrophages. The nature of the factor(s) conferring specificity and the biological significance of these findings have yet to be completely elucidated. Some aspects of these problems are discussed in this volume by Epstein (Chapter 8), Lohmann-Matthes (Chapter 18), and Evans and Alexander (Chapter 21), but the findings differ from the bulk of evidence currently available from infectious disease studies.

Some of what we say is of necessity speculative, since we are mainly confined to discussing events *in vivo* which are potentially of great complexity. Before discussing T lymphocyte–macrophage interaction in terms of effector mechanisms against pathogens, we will begin with a brief review of events leading to the production of effector T cells and their localization in foci of infection.

II. GENERATION OF EFFECTOR T CELLS

A. Origin

Evidence that precursors of lymphocytes active in CMI are T cells is as follows. Procedures that deplete animals of T cells also depress CMI responses. Furthermore, in mice, which possess T cells identifiable by the cell surface antigen θ, treatment of immune lymphoid cell populations with anti-θ serum and complement abrogates their specific CMI effector functions. This and other evidence establishing an essential role for T cells in triggering manifestations of antiviral and antibacterial immunity is not central to the theme of this chapter and is reviewed in detail elsewhere (World Health Organization, 1973; Blanden, 1974a). However, it is noteworthy that some methods of depleting mice of T cells, viz., neonatal thymectomy (Takeya *et al.*, 1964, 1968) or adult thymectomy, lethal irradiation, and bone marrow protection (ATXBM) (Blanden and Langman, 1972; Zinkernagel *et al.*, 1974; Zinkernagel and Blanden, 1975) may result in the activation of both free and fixed (littoral) macrophages. Nude (athymic) mice may also possess activated macrophages (Zinkernagel and Blanden, 1975; Cheers and Waller, 1975). The reasons for this phenomenon are not known. Perhaps it reflects direct stimulation of macrophages by bacterial products emanating from abnormal gut flora or absence of a homeostatic mechanism regulating macrophage activity which is normally exerted by virgin T cells or the thymus.

The presence of activated macrophages in T cell-depleted mice may falsely deny the importance of T cells in the normal process of recovery from primary infection (Blanden and Langman, 1972; Zinkernagel *et al.*, 1974). For example, it can delay or prevent infection of target organs by blood-borne infectious agents and/or slow down proliferation of the agent in lesions to the point where the reduced numbers of T cells, or other types of antibody-dependent mechanisms that may never contribute to the normal recovery process, could be given time to develop to effective levels.

B. Induction

Immunologists interested in infectious diseases have known for many years that the efficient induction of CMI (i.e., generation of effector T cells) requires living vaccines or the use of Freund-type adjuvants. Killed vaccines or purified antigen preparations are far less efficient. This constitutes one of the most important practical problems in immunoprophylaxis of infectious diseases and the related problem of immunotherapy of cancer. While it remains essentially unsolved at the cellular and molecular levels, recent findings have begun at least partly to explain it. As detailed in other chapters of this book, antigen processed by macrophages, or presented on the surface membranes of lymphoid cells or macrophages, or perhaps complexed with certain cell product(s) appears to stimulate T cells more efficiently than free antigen (Unanue, 1972; Katz and Unanue, 1972; Kapp *et al.*, 1973; Pierce *et al.*, 1974) (see Pierce and Kapp, Chapter 1; Mosier, Chapter 2; Basten and Mitchell, Chapter 3). In fact, it may be questionable if free, native antigen ever stimulates T cells directly, since it can rarely be excluded that the triggering antigen is bound to a "presenting" cell or cell product or has been modified as a consequence of interaction with cells. Furthermore, recent studies on infection of mice with lymphocytic choriomengitis (LCM) virus (Zinkernagel and Doherty, 1974a,b), ectromelia virus (Gardner *et al.*,

1975), and the bacterium *Listeria monocytogenes* (Zinkernagel, 1974) suggest strongly that effector T cells in these systems have receptors for antigen which are not specific for virus-specified or bacterial products alone, but which recognize antigens produced by the action of host cell genes as well as the genome of the infectious agent. These antigens could be major transplantation antigens of the infected host which are modified in a specific way as a consequence of infection. Alternatively, host cell genes concerned with regulating expression of histocompatibility antigens may specifically modify antigenic products of viruses and bacteria (Garon and Moss, 1971; Cook and Stoddart, 1973). The basis for this contention will be covered in more detail in Sections III,A–III,C. We mention the idea here because it leads to the generalization that in mammals and birds, at least, cell membranes (or possibly particular components of them coded within gene complexes controlling major transplantation antigens) are essential for efficient antigen presentation to precursor T cells. If this is true, we suggest further that living infectious agents residing and replicating within macrophages (and also lymphoid cells in the case of certain viruses) achieve this efficient form of antigen presentation to T cells far more readily than killed vaccines or purified antigens.

There is evidence from studies on graft versus host reactions (Cantor and Asofsky, 1972) and generation of alloantigen-reactive cytotoxic T cells *in vitro* (Wagner, 1973) that this simple two-cell model for induction of CMI (i.e., one cell, perhaps a macrophage, presenting antigen in a suitable form to a precursor T cell) is not sufficient for an optimal response and that collaboration between different classes or subsets of T cells is also required. These T cell subsets are usually referred to as T_1 and T_2 (Raff and Cantor, 1971). To this point, there is no indication that T–T collaboration is essential for optimal response to infection.

Another aspect of the induction problem worthy of discussion is antigen dose. Small doses of nonreplicating antigens are capable of inducing CMI as illustrated by the early work of Salvin (1958) and the more recent examples by Parish (1971) and Lagrange *et al.* (1974). The theory of Bretscher (1974) would also predict CMI induction with very large antigen doses as well as very small ones. The route of injection of antigen and its persistence are also potentially important; for example, antigen injected subcutaneously would reach the draining lymph nodes in at first increasing and then decreasing concentrations as a function of time after injection. More remote nodes would receive less antigen than closer ones. Factors of this kind may explain the production of CMI, expressed as delayed-type hypersensitivity (DTH) reactions in the foot, after subcutaneous doses of sheep red cells (SRBC) which are far greater than the optimal intravenous does (Lagrange *et al.*, 1974). Freund-type adjuvants, in addition to nonspecifically recruiting macrophages to sites of antigen deposition, may also operate via the mechanisms of slow antigen release from within water in oil emulsions.

We can visualize the inductive stimulus of living infectious agents in this context as providing many "point sources" of antigen (the early foci of infection) distributed through various tissues including lymphoid tissue. At some point, either close to or more remote from these sources, depending on the size of the focus or the rate of antigen release from it or the time for which it has been established, antigen concentration should be theoretically optimal for T cell induction (Bretscher, 1974). We reiterate that by "antigen" in this context we do not mean native antigen but some product of the combined action of the genome of both host and infectious agent.

C. Kinetics

T cells active against infectious agents in rodent models appear in lymphoid tissues or central lymph within 3 days after infection (Blanden, 1974a). In the case of acute infections caused by intravenous (i.v.) injection of ectromelia virus or *Listeria monocytogenes,* the agent multiplies in the spleen for 2 to 3 days and is then rapidly eliminated over the following 2 to 3 days. Maximum numbers of effector T cells are present in the spleen 5–6 days after infection (Mackaness, 1969; North, 1973; Gardner *et al.*, 1974a; Blanden *et al.*, 1975a) and then a rapid decline occurs, presumably reflecting reduced production and increasing egress of effector cells into blood. Kinetics with other acute infections caused by Sindbis virus (McFarland, 1974), Venezuelan equine encephalomyelitis virus (Rabinowitz and Adler, 1973; Rabinowitz and Proctor, 1974), and Murray Valley encephalitis virus (Doherty and Hapel, 1975) appear similar. With more chronic infections (e.g., tuberculosis) the kinetics are considerably slower. There is evidence from the work of North (1973), McGregor and Logie (1973), and Lefford *et al.* (1973) that effector T cells are the progeny of dividing precursors that presumably have been triggered specifically by antigen as outlined above, although the amount of proliferation and differentiation required for an individual cell to acquire effector activity is not known. However, recent studies have shown that many effector T cells of other specificities (e.g., reactive to alloantigens) appear in lymphoid tissues in small numbers (Gardner *et al.*, 1975; Blanden *et al.*, 1975a) during the response, possibly as a consequence of mitogenic factors released by T cells triggered specifically by antigen. Thus, immune cell populations must be regarded as mixtures of clones of many different specificities. Those directed against the infectious agent, while being the most prominent in functional tests, may comprise 5% or less of the total cell populaton in the spleen (Gardner *et al.,* 1974b).

D. Regulation

Little is known about the regulation of effector T cell production in the response to infection. The simplest regulatory mechanism would be elimination of antigen. For example, acute infections are characterized by more rapid production and more rapid disappearance of both antigen and effector T cells than chronic infections. This suggests that the production of effector cells may be required to be driven by antigen for at least some time. Thus, in the acute intravenous infections of mice caused by ectromelia virus or *Listeria monocytogenes* mentioned in Section II,C the infectious agent that provides the antigenic stimulus is progressively eliminated from the spleen from the third day after infection, and effector cell numbers in the spleen also decline after day 6. *Mycobacterium tuberculosis,* on the other hand, grows in lymphoid tissues for 14 days or so and then slowly declines, and effector cell production is similarly sustained (Lefford *et al.,* 1973). The response to LCM virus appears to be a little slower than the responses to ectromelia virus or *L. monocytogenes,* with maximum effector T cell levels occurring in the spleen about 7 days postinfection (Doherty and Zinkernagel, 1974). If these cells are transferred to an infected, lethally irradiated, histocompatible recipient, they appear to proliferate further under the influence of the antigenic stimulus present in the immunosuppressed recipient (Zinkernagel and Doherty, 1974b; Doherty and Zinkernagel, 1975a). This also suggests that the maintenance of effector cell proliferation depends upon sustained antigenic stimulation. However, all of the foregoing evidence does not distinguish between continuing proliferation in cells induced early in infection and continuous induction of fresh precursors over the time interval for which antigen is available. Whether or not there is a built-in physiological limit to the number of cell divisions performed by responding T cells is not known.

Other feedback mechanisms of the type involving receptor blockade by specific immune complexes as suggested by Mackaness *et al.* (1974) for the response to sheep erythrocytes (SRBC), suppressor T cells (Basten and Mitchell, Chapter 3), or activated macrophages (Nelson, Chapter 9; Keller, Chapter 19) are of unknown significance in regulation of the response to infection, although a role for activated macrophages is consistent with the evidence reviewed in this chapter.

E. Migration

Both direct and indirect evidence suggests that effector T cells enter the blood after their generation in lymphoid tissues and are thus available to enter foci of infection in target organs. There are both specific and nonspecific mechanisms by which their entry to lesions may be achieved. The specific mechanism depends upon the recognition of antigen, presumably on the surface membranes of cells lining the vasculature adjacent to foci of infection, by specific receptors on the T cell surface. This would result in the arrest of bloodborne T cells and their subsequent migration out of the blood vessel into the focus. The importance of this mechanism is clearly illustrated by events in the liver lesion of mousepox (ectromelia virus infection), which remain as necrotic foci of hepatic parenchyma cells, uninvaded by inflammatory cells over the first 2 to 3 days after infection, until effector T cells are present (Blanden, 1971a,b). Injection of labeled immune lymphoid cells into infected recipients has revealed a degree of specific localization of these cells in liver lesions (as compared with suitable controls) over the succeeding 20 hours, together with progressive recruitment of blood monocytes from the nonimmune, infected recipient (Blanden, 1974a). Another dramatic example can be found in the lethal inflammatory response seen in meninges, choroid plexus, and cerebrospinal fluid (CSF) of mice infected intracerebrally with LCM virus. In this case, the virus itself is noncytopathic and provokes no damage or inflammatory response in infected tissues. The onset of lethal inflammation coincides temporally with maximum levels of effector T cells in the spleen and their appearance in the blood (Doherty and Zinkernagel, 1974; Zinkernagel and Doherty, 1973). Furthermore, effector T cells are present in high concentrations in the CSF of moribund mice (Zinkernagel and Doherty, 1973). Similar events occur in mice infected intracerebrally with ectromelia virus; in this example, specific effector T cells appear in CSF on day 4 after infection and appear to be in the blood by day 3 (Hapel and Gardner, 1974).

The second mechanism depends upon effector T cells possessing an affinity for inflamed sites which is immunologically nonspecific and which is not yet explained at the molecular level (Koster and McGregor, 1970, 1971; McCluskey and Werdelin, 1971). This mechanism could operate whenever the focus of infection is itself intrinsically inflammatory, as with listeriosis (Mackaness, 1962) and other bacterial infections and as a sequel to the specific mechanism described above.

The fate of effector T cells has not been clearly determined. Obviously, those entering a focus of rampant infection could be easily destroyed, either as a consequence of infection by virus, toxic effects of bacteria, or phagocytosis by macrophages. Some may be lost from the body through migration into the lumen of the gut or alveoli. Some may simply die, while others may persist as memory cells.

F. Memory

The simplest model for memory in CMI is that a portion of the effector T cell population survives as a memory cell population, probably after dedifferentiation from blast cells back to small lymphocytes that become part of the recirculating, slowly dividing, long-lived pool of small lymphocytes. Whether this simple model is correct is unknown. Memory may be simply a reflection of increased numbers of T cells of the appropriate specificity, or it may also involve a qualitative change in inductive requirements and response characteristics. Comprehensive answers to these questions are unavailable as yet in infectious disease systems. However, the marked similarities between effector T cells induced by viral infection and in response to alloantigens suggest that the studies of Cerottini *et al.* (1974) and McDonald *et al.* (1974) may illustrate some common features of T cell memory. These studies are consistent with the simplest model, outlined above, but suggest further that following primary stimulation and differentiation to effector status, T cells may be refractory to secondary stimulation for some days until they have again dedifferentiated (perhaps to small lymphocytes). They may then persist for several months. Evidence from an *in vitro* system for eliciting T cell memory in ectromelia virus infection (Gardner and Blanden, 1975) is consistent with the interpretation of Cerottini *et al.* (1974) and McDonald *et al.* (1974).

III. MECHANISMS OF T CELL- AND MACROPHAGE-MEDIATED IMMUNITY TO INFECTION

A. Cytotoxicity

1. Introduction

That T lymphocytes may exert cytotoxic effects is now very well established (Cerottini and Brunner, 1974). Such effects have been demonstrated in a wide varietey of *in vitro* systems using tumor cells of many different types, fibroblasts, lymphocytes, or lymphoblasts (Cerottini and Brunner, 1974), and macrophages (Zinkernagel and Doherty, 1974a) as target cells. These cells were sometimes transformed or infected by oncogenic viruses (Lavrin *et al.*, 1973; Leclerc *et al.*, 1973); others were infected by cytopathic viruses, e.g., ectromelia (Gardner *et al.*, 1974b), Sindbis (McFarland, 1974), Murray Valley encephalitis (MVE) (Doherty and Hapel, 1975), or a noncytopathic virus (LCM) (Cole *et al.*, 1973; Zinkernagel and Doherty, 1973; Doherty *et al.*, 1974). This suggests strongly that T cells exert cytotoxic mechanisms to which few, if any, cells are intrinsically resistant and points to potentially broad biological significance. It is now apparent that T cells kill target cells as a consequence of contact promoted by specific recognition of antigens on the surfaces of target cells by receptors for antigen on the T cell membrane without production of detectable soluble cytotoxic factors (Cerottini and Brunner, 1974; Henney, 1973; Henney *et al.*, 1974). Whether this receptor is immunoglobulin or not is controversial. Furthermore, it now appears that the antigens recognized by T cells on the surfaces of virus-infected target cells may not be simply virus specified, but may involve the major transplantation antigen systems of the host cell (Zinkernagel and Doherty, 1974b). Thus, immune T cells from inbred mice will recognize and kill virus-infected target cells only if donors of T cells and target cells share genes in the major histocompatibility antigen system of mice (the *H-2* gene complex) (Zinkernagel and Doherty, 1974a,b; Doherty and Zinkernagel, 1975b; Gardner *et al.*, 1975). The essential genes map in the K or *D* regions of the *H-2* complex, and thus appear to be either closely linked to, or identical to, private H-2 specificities (Blanden *et al.*, 1975b). Immune response (*Ir*) genes or Ia specificities, which are located in the *I* region, public specificities, non-*H-2* background, or *M* locus, are not essential (Doherty and Zinkernagel, 1975b; Gardner *et al.*, 1975; Blanden *et al.*, 1975b). This phenomenon has been clearly shown using LCM (Zinkernagel and Doherty, 1974a,b; Doherty and Zinkernagel, 1975b) and ectromelia viruses and several different target cell types. Published data from systems involving murine sarcoma virus (Lavrin *et al.*, 1973; Leclerc *et al.*, 1973) are suggestive, as is evidence from experiments with Rous sarcoma virus in chickens (Wainberg *et al.*, 1974). Evidence from other species, including man, will be eagerly awaited. The effect of the *H-2* complex also holds true *in vivo* and will be dealt with in later sections.

Macrophages are extremely useful as target cells for *in vitro* cytolytic assays, constituting a readily available source of autochthonous cells that can be infected with a variety of viruses. Using this technique we have shown that, at least so far as LCM is concerned, outbred mouse strains behave essentially as if they are inbred (Zinkernagel and Doherty, 1975). Furthermore, there is no cross-reactivity between different outbred strains with inbred mice or with xenogeneic target cells (Zinkernagel and Doherty, 1975) (Table I). Killing of xenogeneic virus-infected target

TABLE I

Seven Day LCM-Immune Mouse Lymphoid Cells Assayed on Xenogeneic Inbred or Outbred LCM-Infected Target Cells

CBA/H spleen cells	Target[a] cell	Fluorescent anti-LCM staining[b]	% ^{51}Cr release: LCM-infected	% ^{51}Cr release: Normal
Immune	Vero	+++	18.9 ± 1.1	19.2 ± 0.7
Normal	(monkey)		21.4 ± 1.2	
Immune	HeLa	+++	18.7 ± 1.0	19.6 ± 0.8
Normal	(human)		16.4 ± 1.7	
Immune	BHK-21	+++	16.6 ± 0.5	14.7 ± 0.9
Normal	(hamster)		16.7 ± 0.4	
Immune	L cell	++	74.5 ± 1.2	26.1 ± 0.7
Normal	(mouse H-2^k)		26.7 ± 1.1	
Immune	Outbred	N.T.	30.7 ± 1.9	31.3 ± 3.0
Normal	(mouse macrophages)		31.1 ± 2.5	

Outbred[c] spleen cells	Target cell	Fluorescent anti-LCM staining	% ^{51}Cr release: LCM-infected	% ^{51}Cr release: Normal
Immune	Outbred[d]	N.T.	65.7 ± 2.2	30.1 ± 1.0
Normal	(mouse macrophages)		27.1 ± 1.7	
Immune	L cell	++	17.4 ± 1.2	14.1 ± 2.1
Normal	(mouse H-2^k)		15.1 ± 1.1	

[a] Infected with WE3-LCM for 24–48 hours.
[b] Hyperimmune rabbit anti-LCM plus goat anti-rabbit Ig coupled with fluorescein.
[c] Assayed at 30:1 for 12 hours at 37°C.
[d] Walter and Eliza Hall Institute multicolored mice. This colony has been maintained as closed outbred colony for 20 years at the Australian National University.

cells by immune cell populations is possibly the province of "K" cells (Ramshaw, 1975; Rager-Zisman and Bloom, 1974).

2. Analysis of the Requirement for H-2 Compatibility

Two mutually exclusive hypotheses have been proposed to explain the requirement for H-2 compatibility between cytotoxic T cells and virus-infected target cells (Zinkernagel and Doherty, 1974a,b; Doherty and Zinkernagel, 1974). First, that genes in the *H-2* gene complex code for a physiological interaction system, which operates in addition to recognition of viral antigen by a specific T cell receptor. The second possibility, the "altered self" model, is that the T cell receptor is specific for virus-induced modification of *H-2* components. This may be thought of as some complex of viral and H-2 structures, or as more long-range alteration of the H-2 antigens themselves, perhaps reflecting modified glycoprotein synthesis (Cook and Stoddart, 1973).

Two separate lines of evidence favor the altered self hypothesis. First, competitive inhibition experiments *in vitro* (de Landazuri and Herberman, 1972) demonstrate that unlabeled competitor target cells have to

TABLE II

LCM-Specific Cytotoxic Activity of 7-Day Immune[a,b] Spleen Cells

	Added competitors	% ^{51}Cr release[c]			
		L cells (H-2^k)		P815 (H-2^d)	
		Infected	Normal	Infected	Normal
CBA/H × BALB/c F1 (H-$2^{k/d}$)	O	68.5 ± 1.0	14.1 ± 1.1	90.7 ± 1.8	14.7 ± 0.7
	9 LCM-L[d]	23.2 ± 0.2[f]	—	74.4 ± 0.8[e]	—
	9 LCM-P815	52.2 ± 0.9[e]	—	47.2 ± 0.3[f]	—
C3H.OH (H-$2^{d/k}$)	O	58.4 ± 1.1	14.2 ± 1.5	59.6 ± 1.1	15.3 ± 0.7
	9 LCM-L	17.7 ± 0.6[f]	—	35.2 ± 0.8[e]	—
	9 LCM-P815	12.0 ± 0.7[e]	—	16.9 ± 0.4[f]	—

[a] Modified from Zinkernagel and Doherty (1975) with permission of *Journal of Experimental Medicine.*

[b] Mice were injected with 1000 LD_{50} of WE3 of LCM. Normal spleen cells on infected targets released from 13.1 ± 0.3 to 18.7 ± 0.7. Assayed on labeled LCM-infected L cells or P815. Competitive inhibition of ^{51}Cr release by unlabeled infected L cells or P815.

[c] ^{51}Cr release was determined by assaying lymphocytes at 20:1 for 12 hours at 37°C (Zinkernagel and Doherty, 1974c). Results are expressed as means ±SEM for 4 replicates.

[d] Ratio of unlabeled competitor:labeled LCM-infected target cells 9:1.

[e] Significantly less ($p < 0.01$) than without cold competitor cells, but this is due to steric hindrance, as the same decrease is obtained by adding any uninfected cold competitor at 9:1 (Zinkernagel and Doherty, 1975).

[f] Significantly less ($p < 0.001$) than without cold competitor cells or than with H-2 incompatible LCM-infected cold competitor cells.

be *H-2 K* or or *H-2 D* compatible with both immune T cells and labeled target cells to cause decrease in ^{51}Cr release (Table II). The mutual interaction model would predict that H-2 compatibility of the competitor with the T cell alone (but not with the target) would be sufficient for competitive inhibition. Second, it has been shown that 7 day LCM-immune cells proliferate after transfer into immunosuppressed, LCM-infected recipients as described above. If the mutual interaction model was correct, it would be expected that F_1 ($H\text{-}2^{k/d}$) or C3H.OH ($H\text{-}2^{k/d}$) immune T cells could proliferate in either $H\text{-}2^k$ or $H\text{-}2^d$ recipients to produce increased cytotoxicity against both $H\text{-}2^k$ and $H\text{-}2^d$ targets. However, these *in vivo* proliferation experiments clearly show that F_1 ($H\text{-}2^{k/d}$) or C3H.OH ($H\text{-}2^{k/d}$) proliferate in $H\text{-}2^k$ recipients to produce increased cytotoxicity only against infected $H\text{-}2^k$ targets, but not against $H\text{-}2^d$ targets and vice versa (Table III). Thus, T cells are apparently specifically reactive to virus-altered *H-2 K* or *H-2 D*. Homozygous mice apparently possess T cells of at least two specificities, sensitized to modified

TABLE III

Cytotoxic T Cell Activity in Lymphoid Tissue of Irradiated LCM-Infected Recipients Dosed with LCM-Immune Spleen Cells 3 Days Previously[a,b]

		% ^{51}Cr release[c]			
		L-929 ($H\text{-}2^k$)		P-815 ($H\text{-}2^d$)	
Donors	Recipients	Infected	Normal	Infected	Normal
CBA/H × BABL/c F1	BALB/c	21.2 ± 1.2[d,e]	18.5 ± 1.2	78.0 ± 1.2[f]	26.9 ± 3.1
CBA/H × BALB/c F1	CBA/H	84.9 ± 0.9[f]	25.5 ± 2.1	29.8 ± 0.8[g]	22.7 ± 2.1
C3H.OH	CBA/H	48.3 ± 0.3[f]	21.9 ± 1.2	25.8 ± 1.5[e]	23.8 ± 3.1

[a] Modified from Zinkernagel and Doherty (1975) with the permission of *Journal of Experimental Medicine*

[b] Donor mice were injected i.v. with 2000 LD_{50} of WE3 LCM virus and killed after 7 days. Recipient mice were irradiated (850 R) 24 hours previous and dosed with 10^5 LD_{50} of WE3 LCM 6 hours prior to cell transfer.

[c] Target cells were overlaid at a ratio of 30:1 and incubated for 10 hours at 37°C. Means ±SEM of 4 replicas.

[d] Significance of value on infected target cells versus normal target cells.

[e] Not significant.

[f] $p < 0.001$.

[g] $p < 0.05$.

self antigens coded at, or near to, *H-2 K* or *H-2 D*. The alternative is some form of genetic control, in addition to allelic exclusion, of physiological recognition structure(s) coded in the *K* or *D* region. This seems extremely improbable.

If the altered self concept is correct F_1 mice may, therefore, be considered to generate effector T cells of at least four different specificities, recognizing antigens associated with *H-2 K* or *H-2 D* of each parental haplotype. Such a mechanism for increasing the range of T cell responsiveness may be invoked to explain selective advantage of both gene duplication and heterozygosity (with resultant high level polymorphism, which is observed) within the *H-2* gene complex. Selection for heterozygotes would thus operate in the absence of positive evolutionary pressure favoring any particular *H-2* gene. This hypothesis is in accord both with present knowledge of H antigen systems (Zinkernagel and Doherty, 1975) and with Bodmer's modification of the Jerne argument for generation of immunological diversity (Jerne, 1971; Bodmer, 1972).

3. *Significance of T Cell-Mediated Cytotoxicity in Control of Infection*

What is the likelihood of cytotoxic T cells acting alone, contributing to the control of viral infection *in vivo*? This question cannot, of course, be answered definitively. All we can offer is a theoretical discussion of possibilities. First, it seems certain that cytotoxic T cells do enter foci of infection from the blood according to evidence outlined in the section on migration. Second, most virus-infected target cells employed appear to be intrinsically susceptible to T cell attack, and individual cytotoxic T cells seem capable of killing a number of target cells in succession by a one-hit process (Cerottini and Brunner, 1974; Gardner *et al.*, 1974b; Zinkernagel and Doherty, 1974a). The foregoing evidence suggests that cytotoxic T cells would indeed kill virus-infected cells in foci of infection. In order to halt virus replication and spread, however, they would need to kill target cells before assembly of progeny virus within them. Thus, T cell-recognizable virus-induced changes in the infected cell membranes would need to occur early after infection. With some viruses, this does happen. Ectromelia-infected L cells, for example, become susceptible to immune T cell attack about 3 hours postinfection, yet normally remain intact for more than 20 hours after infection (N. A. Bowern and R. V. Blanden, unpublished data, 1975). Furthermore, vaccinia virus, a poxvirus closely related to ectromelia, is assembled mainly within the cytoplasm of infected cells. Very little progeny virus is released by budding from infected cell membranes early after infection; most remains within the debris of the infected cell after its death (Smith and Sharp, 1960). If ectromelia-infected cells *in vivo* behaved this way, cytotoxic T cells could be a significant virostatic mechanism. The elimination of infectious virus produced prior to the advent of the T cell response and residing in necrotic tissue in the focus would require active virucidal mechanisms, e.g., ingestion and destruction by macrophages (Blanden, 1971b). This seems to be a sequel to the presence of T cells within lesions, as described in Section III,B.

Since it is clear that macrophages infected with either LCM virus or ectromelia virus are killed by virus-specific effector cells *in vitro* (Zinkernagel and Doherty, 1974a; Blanden *et al.*, 1975b), it seems conceivable, even likely, that this could happen *in vivo,* but its biological significance is not known.

To our knowledge, there is no evidence concerning the killing by T cells of target cells infected with bacteria or with bacterial antigens bound to their membranes. Since virus-infected macrophages are so killed and since many bacteria parasitize macrophages, it seems quite possible that this could occur, and it is readily testable using, for example, macrophages infected with *Mycobacteria.* However, it seems likely that T cell-mediated cytotoxicity is less important in controlling bacterial infection than viral infection.

B. Recruitment of Monocytes

1. Significance of an Antimicrobial Mechanism in Vivo

Chemotaxis of macrophages is covered elsewhere in this volume (Snyderman and Mergenhagen, Chapter 13; Wilkinson, Chapter 14). The ability of effector T cells to attract blood monocytes to foci of infection appears to be one of their most important functions in certain viral and bacterial infections. The evidence that this phenomenon occurs *in vivo* will be reiterated here. First, immune lymphoid cell populations depleted of T cells (by treatment with anti-θ serum and complement, for example) lose the ability to transfer protection to recipient animals (Blanden, 1971a; Lane and Unanue, 1972; Blanden and Langman, 1972; Mims and Blanden, 1972; North, 1973). Second, mononuclear phagocytes appear in foci of infection as a sequel to immune T cell injection, and this influx coincides temporally with clearance of infection (Blanden, 1971a,b).

Local migration of adjacent fixed macrophages into lesions seems less important than recruitment of monocytes from blood for the following reasons. First, many of the macrophages that appear in lesions during the course of primary infection, or as a sequel to adoptive immunization with immune T cells, can be labeled with tritiated thymidine injected *before* infection (North, 1970; Blanden, 1974a). This implies that they are derived from a multiplying pool of precursors and thus fits the known pattern of monocyte production described in detail by Volkman (Chapter 12). Second, prior irradiation of recipients of immune T cells or treatment with drugs, such as cyclophosphamide, that eliminate dividing cells significantly impairs the expression of immunity (Tripathy and Mackaness, 1969; Blanden, 1971a; McGregor and Koster, 1971). This evidence is consistent with a role for radiosensitive recipient components in the immune mechanism, presumably the dividing precursors of monocytes. However, it does not exclude the possibility that local proliferation of fixed macrophages may also make a significant contribution. The elegant experiments of North (1970) are the best indication that blood monocytes are sufficient, without participation of cells derived from fixed macrophage proliferation. North subjected the livers of mice, with the rest of the body shielded, to a dose of irradiation that dramatically impaired expression of immunity if given to unshielded mice. Subsequent infection with *Listeria monocytogenes* showed no impairment in expression of antibacterial mechanisms in the irradiated livers of shielded mice, thus clearly implicating a radiosensitive component that entered the liver postinfection. Together with the preceding evidence, this leaves little doubt that blood monocytes are the major source of macrophages in liver lesions. Presumably events in other target organs are similar.

Theoretically, there are two major questions dictating the importance of T cell-triggered monocyte recruitment to the control of infection. First, is the infectious agent destroyed after ingestion by normal macrophages, or does it survive and multiply? Second, is the lesion nonspecifically attractive to monocytes in the absence of specific effector T cells? Analysis of this issue is illustrated by two examples given below. Liver lesions of mousepox are not attractive to monocytes in the absence of effector T cells. Thus, mice with depressed T cell responses caused by graft versus host reactions (GVHR) die of liver damage due to unchecked growth of ectromelia virus in liver parenchyma, which remains virtually free of inflammatory cells until death (Blanden, 1971b). In contrast, mice with GVHR are resistant to listeriosis (Blanden, 1969, 1971b). This can be explained by the finding that *Listeria* lesions are intrinsically inflammatory and are heavily invaded by monocytes within 1 or 2 days after infection (Mackaness, 1962), before the advent of effector T cells. Since GVHR also cause activation of macrophages to enhanced bactericidal activity (Blanden, 1969), mice with GVHR do not require a T cell response and recover from listeriosis, despite profound immunosuppression (Blanden, 1969, 1971b). We should point out here that *Listeria* organisms can survive and multiply within normal mouse macrophages (Mackaness, 1962), and macrophage activation as defined here and covered in detail in the next section is, therefore, required for control of infection. Ectromelia virus, on the other hand, while capable of infecting normal mouse macrophages, is nonetheless relatively unproductive in these cells (Roberts, 1964), i.e., as a cell population, infected macrophages produce fewer progeny infectious particles than they ingested (Blanden, 1971b). Thus, cycles of infection confined to macrophages would result in ever-decreasing amounts of infectious virus. Phagocytosis and destruction of virus in liver and spleen lesions would thus explain the dramatic fall in virus titers in these organs 24 hours after adoptive immunization with immune T cells (Blanden, 1971a). Activated macrophages can be found in ectromelia-infected mice, but not until the process of recovery is virtually completed (Blanden and Mims, 1973). Furthermore, activated macrophages are only marginally superior to normal in terms of their refractoriness to infection with ectromelia virus *in vivo* (Blanden, 1971b). Thus, to summarize, in the case of mousepox, T cell-mediated monocyte recruitment appears to be esssential for recovery, macrophage activation being nonessential; conversely, recovery from listeriosis requires T cell-triggered macrophage activation, whereas recruitment of sufficient monocytes into lesions may occur by immunologically nonspecific mechanisms. The example of listeriosis probably illustrates events in a number of bacterial infections in which CMI is demonstrably important, e.g., salmonellosis, brucellosis, and tuberculosis (Mackaness, 1964; Mackaness *et al.*, 1966; Blanden *et al.*, 1966, 1969; Collins *et al.*, 1966). Whether the importance of monocyte recruitment extends to viral infections other than mousepox is not clear, since it has received little detailed attention. As outlined above, this mechanism would be important when macrophages are resistant to viral infection and when little nonspecific inflammation occurs in lesions. More quantitative information is required on both of these questions. Additional complexity arises from findings that growth of mouse hepatitis virus in macrophages may be determined by a single dominant gene in the host (Bang and Warwick, 1960) or by the virulence of the virus strain (Burns and Allison, 1975). Furthermore, herpesvirus infection of mouse macrophages is dependent on the age of the mouse (Johnson, 1964; Hirsch *et al.*, 1970; Stevens and Cook, 1971).

Superficially, it appears that CMI may help to control infections caused by poxviruses (Blanden, 1970, 1971a,b; Hirsch *et al.*, 1968), arenaviruses (Mims and Blanden, 1972; Volkert *et al.*, 1974; Cole *et al.*, 1974; Johnson and Cole, 1975), herpesviruses (Ennis, 1973; World Health Organization, 1973), measles virus, varicella virus, and cytomegalovirus (World Health Organization, 1973; Allison, 1974).

Recent studies on infection of mice with Bebaru virus (a togavirus) point strongly to virus clearance from the brain being dependent upon mechanisms involving T cells and macrophages. Intracerebral (i.c.) inoculation of Bebaru virus into adult CBA mice results in nonfatal meningitis and encephalitis. The inflammatory response can be quantitated by counting cells in cerebrospinal fluid (CSF). Following i.c. inoculation virus titers increase in brain until day 2 or day 3, then decrease sharply at a time when many mononuclear cells are found in CSF but no antibody is found in serum (Fig. 1).

Virus titers are enhanced in anti-thymocyte serum (ATS)-treated mice but not in ATXBM mice on day 3 (Table IV). One possible explanation for this is that T cells enhance the phagocytic and virucidal capacity

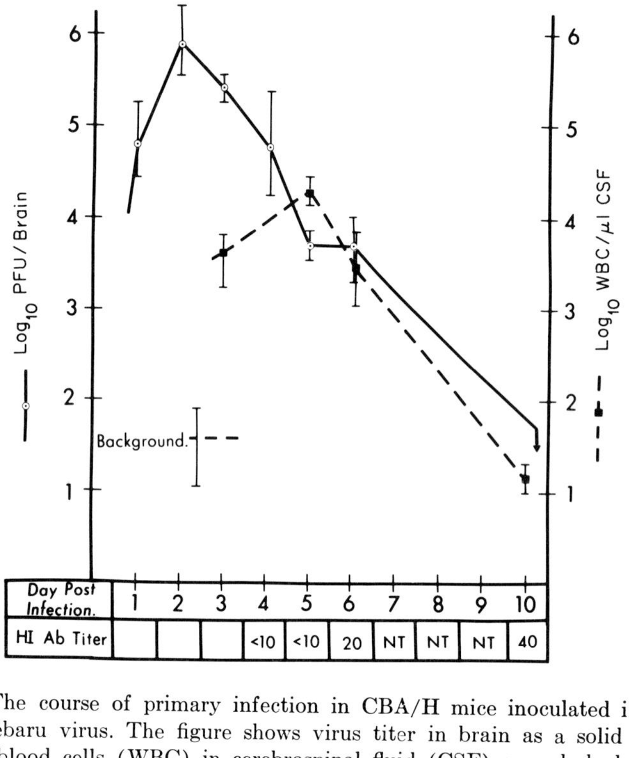

Fig. 1. The course of primary infection in CBA/H mice inoculated i.c. with 10^5 PFU of Bebaru virus. The figure shows virus titer in brain as a solid line graph and white blood cells (WBC) in cerebrospinal fluid (CSF) as a dashed line. Error bars enclose one standard deviation. Hemagglutination inhibiting (HI) antibody titers are given as the reciprocal of the dilution of serum resulting in 50% inhibition. NT, not tested. The arrow on the virus titer graph indicates that the titer on day 10 was below the detection level of the assay system. The total range in numbers of leukocytes found per μl of CSF in normal mice is illustrated by the word background and a horizontal dashed line transversed by an error bar.

TABLE IV

Virus Titers[a] in Brains of ATS-Treated,[b] ATXBM, and Normal Mice 3 and 6 Days after i.c. Inoculation of 10^3 PFU of Bebaru Virus[c]

Day postinfection	Mice used and treatment		
	Normal	ATXBM	ATS
3	3.2 ± 0.2	3.2 ± 0.4	5.5 ± 0.2[e]
6	<1.8[d]	3.5 ± 0.2	3.6 ± 0.2

[a] Expressed as mean $\log_{10}$ PFU/brain, ±1 SE from groups of five mice.
[b] ATS was given in 0.2 ml aliquots 6 and 2 days before infection.
[c] Modified from Hapel (1975).
[d] Significantly smaller titers in ATS-treated or ATXBM mice on the same day ($p < 0.01$).
[e] Significantly greater titers in ATXBM or normal mice on the same day ($p < 0.01$).

TABLE V

Numbers of Mononuclear Cells in Cerebrospinal Fluid of ATS-Treated, ATXBM, or Normal Mice 6 Days after i.c. Inoculation of 10^3 PFU of Bebaru Virus[a]

Mice used and treatment	Numbers of monocytes[c] per μl CSF
Normal	4.3 ± 0.1[d]
ATXBM	2.9 ± 0.3
ATS[b]	2.1 ± 0.3

[a] Modified from Hapel (1975) with the permission of *Scandinavian Journal of Immunology*.
[b] ATS was given in 0.2 ml aliquots 6 and 2 days before infection.
[c] Expressed as the mean value obtained from groups of five mice ($\log_{10}$/μl of CSF ±1 SE).
[d] Significantly greater cell numbers in CSF of AT × BM or ATS-treated mice.

of macrophages but that nonspecific activation of macrophages in ATXBM mice overcomes this T cell requirement. On day 6 postinfection, inflammation is abolished and virus persists in ATS-treated or ATXBM mice (Table IV). In normal, control infected mice, inflammatory cells are very numerous in CSF (Table V), and virus has been completely eliminated at this time (Table IV). Immune cell transfers into infected ATXBM mice confer protection (assessed by reduction of virus titers in brain 1 and 2 days after cell transfer), but similar cells have much less effect in brains of cyclophosphamide-treated mice (Table VI). The protective effect is abolished by treating transferred cells with anti-θ serum and complement and is therefore T cell-dependent (Table VI). As transferred cells do not function in cyclophosphamide-treated mice, dividing host accessory cells seem to be required to effect virus clearance; these cells could be monocyte precursors. B cells (anti-θ-treated immune spleen cells) do not confer protection on ATXBM mice, and antibody

TABLE VI

Titers of Virus in Brains of Normal, ATXBM, and Cyclophosphamide-Treated Mice after Transfer of 4 × 10⁷ Normal or Immune Spleen Cells on Days 1 and 2 after Infection[a]

Day post-infection	Bebaru virus ($\log_{10} \pm$ SE)/brain[b]			Cells given on days 1 and 2
	Normal	Cyclophosphamide	ATXBM	
1	3.1 ± 0.2	3.1 ± 0.2	2.8 ± 0.1	4×10^7 normal spleen cells
2	7.1 ± 0.5	5.7 ± 0.3	5.6 ± 0.1	
3	7.6 ± 0.1	7.1 ± 0.2	6.2 ± 0.3	
2	NT[c]	6.4 ± 0.5	2.2 ± 0.2[e]	4×10^7 immune spleen cells
3	NT	5.9 ± 0.2[d]	2.1 ± 0.2[e]	
2	NT	7.3 ± 0.2	7.5 ± 0.2	4×10^7 anti-θ-treated immune spleen cells
3	NT	7.8 ± 0.1	7.1 ± 0.2	

[a] Modified from Hapel (1975) with permission of *Scandinavian Journal of Immunology*.

[b] Five mice were used per group. Virus titers are expressed as $\log_{10}$ PFU/brain, ±1 SE.

[c] NT, not tested.

[d] Significantly less than the normal or cyclophosphamide-treated mice that were given normal spleen cells ($p < 0.01$).

[e] Significantly less than all other groups ($p < 0.01$).

production is not enhanced in recipients of immune spleen cells (by day 3 after infection). In summary, this evidence suggests that the process of recovery involves T cells that interact with monocytes or macrophages to effect virus clearance. Since macrophages cannot be infected *in vitro* with Bebaru virus, it would be obviously advantageous to recruit monocytes into infected foci.

Further evidence for this scheme was obtained by studying recruitment of monocytes into CSF using immune spleen cells separated into Ig-bearing (Ig-positive) (B cell rich) and Ig-negative (T cell rich) populations (Parish *et al.*, 1975). Such cells were inoculated into cyclophosphamide-treated infected mice that had previously received large numbers of normal spleen and bone marrow cells as a monocyte source. Only Ig-negative cells or unseparated spleen cells were capable of triggering a rapid influx of mononuclear cells into CSF, which could be measured 2 days after cell transfer. Anti-θ and complement treatment abolished the ability of

TABLE VII

Role of Ig-Positive and Ig-Negative Cells in Reconstruction of Inflammatory Cell Counts in CSF of Immunosuppressed Mice Infected with Bebaru Virus[a,b]

Transferred spleen cells	WBC/μl of CSF ($\log_{10} \pm$ SE)[c] 2 days after cell transfer
2×10^7 Ig + immune cells	3.0 ± 0.2
2×10^7 Ig − immune cells	3.8 ± 0.1[c]
4×10^7 immune cells	3.8 ± 0.2
4×10^7 normal cells	2.9 ± 0.1
4×10^7 immune cells $\times$ anti-θ and complement	2.5 ± 0.1

[a] Modified from Hapel (1975) with the permission of the *Scandinavian Journal of Immunology*.

[b] Separated by the method of Parish *et al.* (1975). Mice were given cyclophosphamide i.p. (0.25 mg/gm dry weight) 1 day before infection and 6 hours after infection by i.c. inoculation of virus. One and 2 days after the second dose of cyclophosphamide they received 3×10^7 normal spleen cells plus 4×10^7 normal bone marrow cells. On the next 2 days they received immune or normal spleen cells. Two days after the first immune cell transfer or 1 day after the second immune cell transfer, monocytes in CSF were counted.

[c] Not significantly different from counts obtained in mice receiving 4×10^7 immune spleen cells, but significantly greater than counts obtained in all other groups ($p < 0.01$). SE, standard error, obtained from values in groups of five mice.

unseparated spleen cells to reconstitute inflammation in this system (Table VII). The specificity of the transferred population was demonstrated using immune cells from donors immunized with viruses with similar or widely differing antigenic specificities (Table VIII). Only Ross River virus- or Bebaru virus-immune cells were effective in reconstituting the inflammatory process in the test mice. Other immune spleen cell populations were far less efficient in reconstituting inflammation. Sindbis- and ectromelia-immune spleen both had slight but significant effects in elevating inflammation above that found in control mice. Although both Ross River and Bebaru virus are in the Semliki Forest virus (SFV) complex, SFV-immune spleen did not reconstitute inflammation. Bebaru virus and Ross River virus are both in the same subgroup of this complex and cross-react at the serological level (Theiler and Downs, 1973), while SFV is in a different subgroup. It, therefore, appears that T cells do not readily distinguish between closely related viruses (e.g., Ross River and Bebaru)

TABLE VIII

Specificity of Reconstitution of Inflammatory Cell Counts in the CSF of Immunosuppressed Mice Infected with Bebaru Virus[a,b]

Immune cells transferred	Mononuclear cells/μl of CSF ($\log_{10} \pm$ SE)	
	Day 2	Day 3
Bebaru[c]	3.0 ± 0.1	3.6 ± 0.1
Ross River[d]	3.1 ± 0.1	3.6 ± 0.1
SFV	2.2 ± 0.1	2.6 ± 0.1
Sinbis	2.1 ± 0.1	2.9 ± 0.1
Kunjin	1.4 ± 0.1	2.5 ± 0.1
MVE	NT	2.3 ± 0.1
Ectromelia	1.7 ± 0.1	2.9 ± 0.1
Non immune	1.7 ± 0.1	2.5 ± 0.1

[a] Modified from Hapel (1975) with the permission of the *Scandinavian Journal of Immunology.*

[b] Mice were prepared as described in Table VII. CSF cells were counted 2 and 3 days after the first transfer of immune spleen cells.

[c] Identical to Ross River and significantly greater than all other groups.

[d] Significantly higher than all other groups except Bebaru. Groups of 5 mice were used throughout and results expressed as mean $\log_{10} \pm 1$ SE.

but do distinguish between slightly greater antigen differences (e.g., SFV and Bebaru).

2. *Nature of Antigen Recognized by T Cells*

The theme pervading this section is that effector T cells recognize specific antigen(s) within foci of infection and either directly or indirectly cause the release of immunologically nonspecific factor(s) chemotactic for macrophages. Evidence for T cell specificity in terms of the infectious agent is not extensive but seems rigorous (Mackaness, 1969; Blanden, 1971a). As with cytotoxic T cells, recent evidence suggests that the antigens recognized in foci of ectromelia (Blanden, 1974b; Blanden *et al.*, 1975c) or LCM (Zinkernagel and Doherty, 1974b; Doherty and Zinkernagel, 1975a) infection *in vivo* are not solely virus-specified, but are virus-induced specific modifications of host cell transplantation antigens coded within the *H-2* gene complex. Table IX indicates that transfer of antiviral activity by immune spleen cells (in which effector T cells are essential) only operates when donors and recipients share one H-2 haplotype. The failure of allogeneic cells to have an effect is not logically explained by rejection, since only 24 hours elapse between cell transfer and virus titration in recipient organs, F_1 hybrid cells operated in parental strain recipients, and similar findings are obtained in cytotoxicity assays *in vitro* (Zinkernagel and Doherty, 1974a,b; Doherty and Zinkernagel, 1975b; Gardner *et al.*, 1975; Blanden *et al.*, 1975b). The simplest explanation is based on the analysis in Section III,A,2, i.e., that effector T cells respond only to "altered self" antigens and not to virus-specified antigens alone. Thus, immune T cells would fail to recognize virus-infected foci in allogeneic recipients, no chemotactic factors would be produced in the foci, and the monocytes crucial for clearance of infection would not be recruited to the lesions. These data are also convincing evidence of the insignificance of B cells producing antibody to virus-specified antigens in the early events in recovery.

C. Activation of Macrophages

1. *Introduction*

Reference to "macrophage activation" has already been made repeatedly throughout this chapter. Theoretically, macrophage activation in one form or another is essential for recovery from any infectious disease in which the agent can survive or multiply within normal macrophages. Clear evidence of its importance is available from studies on

TABLE IX

Restriction of Transfer of Antiviral Activity with Ectromelia-Immune Spleen Cells to Syngeneic or Semiallogeneic Recipients[a,b]

Experiment	Spleen cell donors		Recipients	
	Strain	Status	Strain	$\log_{10}$ PFU/spleen[c]
1	C57BL/6	Normal	CBA/H	6.40 ± 0.05
		Immune		6.49 ± 0.10
	C57BL/6	Normal	C57BL/6	5.32 ± 0.20
		Immune		<2.0[d]
	C57BL/6	Normal	CBA/H × C57BL/6(F1)	5.58 ± 0.19
		Immune		<2.0[d]
2	CBA/H	Normal	CBA/H	7.06 ± 0.10
		Immune		5.28 ± 0.22[d]
	CBA/H	Normal	C57BL/6	4.97 ± 0.35
		Immune		5.77 ± 0.22
	CBA/H	Normal	CBA/H × C57BL/6(F1)	6.55 ± 0.22
		Immune		5.24 ± 0.40[e]
3	CBA/H × C57BL/6(F1)	—	CBA/H	5.77 ± 0.16
		Immune		<3.0[c]
	CBA/H × C57BL/6(F1)	—	C57BL	5.40 ± 0.17
		Immune		<3.0[d]

[a] Modified from Blanden *et al.* (1975c) with the permission of the *Australian Journal of Experimental Biology and Medical Science.*

[b] From donors immunized i.v. with 2 × 10⁴ PFU of attenuated virus 6 days previously, 5 × 10⁷ viable cells per recipient were injected i.v. 24 hours after infection of recipients i.v. with 6 × 10⁴ PFU of virulent virus.

[c] Mean ± standard error of the mean in groups of 4–5 mice: spleens harvested 24 hr after cell transfer.

[d] Significantly less than controls, $p < 0.001$.

[e] Significantly less than controls, $p < 0.02$.

listeriosis, brucellosis, tuberculosis, and salmonellosis cited above. In this section we will briefly review recent work on the lymphocyte–macrophage interactions which lead to macrophage activation.

A major advance in the understanding of the importance of CMI and macrophage activation during recovery from infectious diseases was made by Mackaness (1962). He studied the time course of bacterial growth in mouse spleen and liver following i.v. inoculation of sublethal amounts of *Listeria monocytogenes*. He established a clear precedent by measuring not only numbers of bacteria in target organs but also the development of humoral immunity (measured by assaying serum for antibody), cell-mediated immunity (measured by DTH reactions), and activation of macrophages (measured by their bactericidal activity *in vitro*). Control of bacterial growth in spleen coincided temporally with activation of macrophages and development of DTH (about 4 days postinfection) but not with development of humoral immunity, which was detected 3 days later. Thus a convincing argument was assembled to support the role of macrophages in recovery from listeriosis and to suggest a close relationship between DTH and macrophage activation. As outlined previously effector T cells responsible for both antibacterial mechanisms and DTH can be demonstrated in mice 3–4 days after infection with *L. monocytogenes* at a time when Mackaness could first detect macrophage activation and DTH (North, 1973; Youdim *et al.*, 1973; Zinkernagel *et al.*, 1974).

Evidence for a causal relationship between effector T cells and activation of macrophages is now consolidating, but the precise mechanisms are not yet defined. A brief review of this area follows.

Two important conclusions regarding macrophage activation triggered by T cells may be drawn from the work of Krahenbuhl and Remington (1971) and Remington *et al.* (1972). Immune spleen cells from guinea pigs chronically infected with *Toxoplasma gondii* were cultured with normal guinea pig peritoneal macrophages in the presence or absence of *Toxoplasma* antigen. Only those macrophages in cultures containing immune spleen cells and *Toxoplasma* antigen acquired enhanced resistance to *Toxoplasma* infection. Such cells simultaneously acquired resistance to *Listeria monocytogenes* infection. If one accepts that *Listeria* and *Toxoplasma* do not contain cross-reacting antigens, then these experiments demonstrate the following.

a. Activation of macrophages requires lymphocyte-dependent specific antigen recognition.

b. As a result of this, macrophages may acquire a nonspecific increase in their microbicidal properties. Similar conclusions can be drawn from the results of Simon and Sheagren (1971, 1972).

Using *Mycobacterium tuberculosis,* Patterson and Youmans (1970) demonstrated that cultures of immune spleen cells when mixed with virulent *M. tuberculosis* bacilli *in vitro* produced a dialyzable substance that enhanced the ability of macrophages to digest homologous intracellular bacteria, but nonspecific expression of the antibacterial qualities of the macrophages was not examined.

Simon and Sheagren (1972) have demonstrated that immune lymphocytes, obtained from the peritoneal exudate of guinea pigs with DTH to bovine γ-globulin (BGG), could be stimulated with BGG *in vitro* to produce macrophage migration inhibitory factor (MIF) in supernatant fluids. The ability of guinea pig macrophages to kill *Listeria monocytogenes* was not enhanced by treatment with MIF. This finding, using a nonpathogenic antigen, suggests that MIF alone is not capable of "activating" macrophages.

In systems of this type there are no published data, at least to our knowledge, which rigorously point to T cells synthesizing a soluble macrophage activating factor. J. Mauel and R. Behin (personal communication, 1973) have abrogated the macrophage activating capacity of immune mouse lymphoid cells with anti-θ treatment, which clearly establishes T cell dependence, but does not exclude the involvement of other ancillary cells.

Lymphocyte–macrophage interaction has also been reported to give rise to antigen-specific macrophages (McFarland, 1974; Rabinowitz and Proctor, 1974; Tompkins *et al.*, 1970; Avila *et al.*, 1972). The possibility that these phenomena involve T cell-dependent production by B cells of small amounts of antibody cannot be excluded. In other *in vitro* (Cole and Ward, 1973) or *in vivo* (Rager-Zisman and Allison, 1973) tests, very small amounts of antibody have been shown to confer specific bactericidal or virucidal activity, respectively, on macrophages. A role for a specific T cell product is, therefore, unknown. The significance of these phenomena in infectious disease systems *in vivo* is also not known.

2. *Nature of Antigen Recognized by T Cells*

We have argued previously that T cell-triggered macrophage activation rather than monocyte recruitment seems to be crucial for control of listeriosis. Sections II,E and III,A, evidence was presented to support the idea that effector T cells in the circulation recognize antigens in foci of infection, thus leading to their localization in the foci where their local activities bring about control of infection. The antigens responsible for T cell stimulation and ultimate production of monocyte chemotactic factors, appeared to be specifically "altered self" antigens. Recent studies by Zinkernagel (1974), outlined below, show that this may also be the case for T cells responsible for macrophage activation.

Listeria-immune spleen cells from F_1 (H-$2^{k/b}$) mice protect both parental type recipients very efficiently, but are much less efficient in H-2 incompatible recipients (Table X). The requirement for H-2 compatibility for transfer of maximal protection may operate at either of two points in the above-mentioned sequence. As in the LCM and ectromelia systems, T cells may recognize *Listeria*-"altered self" antigens and, therefore, be triggered to cause macrophage activation only by an identical cell surface alteration, which would be present only in H-2 compatible recipients. Alternatively, the putative soluble factors produced by T cells may only be able efficiently to activate H-2 compatible macrophages. There is only weak precedence for this second explanation in the species specificity of MIF (Youngner and Salvin, 1973) or interferon (Merigan, 1964; Baron *et al.*, 1964).

3. Biochemical Basis

The biochemical mechanisms by which macrophages acquire increased microbicidal activity under the influence of effector T cells is not yet clear. However, there has been considerable study of antimicrobial mechanisms in phagocytes, blood monocytes, and macrophages. Unfortunately many authors have not been rigorous in distinguishing between different phagocytes, so much of the data available comes from studies of mixed cell populations. Phagocytes may be activated by minor perturbations in the cytoplasmic membrane. Such perturbations as pinocytosis activate the hexose monophosphate shunt with associated shifts in NADP + NADPH:NAD + NADH ratios in guinea pig or human

TABLE X

Protective Effect of 6 Day Listeria-Immune or Normal Spleen Cells Transferred into Semiallogeneic or Allogeneic Recipients Infected with 5 × 10³ Bacteria 2 Hours Previously[a,b]

Donor	Recipient (H-2 type)	Log_{10} viable bacteria count[c]	
		Immune cells	Normal cells
CBA/H × C57B1	CBA/H × C57B1(k/b)	3.12 ± 0.21[d]	5.71 ± 0.15
$H\text{-}2^{k/b}$	CBA/H (k)	3.31 ± 0.27[d]	6.10 ± 0.19
	C57B1 (b)	1.97 ± 0.15[d]	5.03 ± 0.10
	BALB/c (d)	4.67 ± 0.20[e]	5.45 ± 0.20

[a] Modified from Zinkernagel (1974) with the permission of *Nature*.
[b] Donors were infected with 5 × 10³ *L. monocytogenes*.
[c] Mean ± SEM of groups of five mice.
[d] Significance of immune cells versus normal cells. $p < 0.01$.
[e] Significance of immune cells versus normal cells. $p > 0.01$.

peripheral blood leukocytes (Paul *et al.*, 1970; Sbarra *et al.*, 1971) in which the most numerous cell is the granulocyte. Ultimately these metabolic changes result in increased H_2O_2 production, which is utilized by myeloperoxidase in the presence of an oxidizable cofactor (iodide, bromide, chloride, or thiocyanate) to inactivate microorganisms. Myeloperoxidase-containing subcellular organelles can be prepared semiquantitatively and their activity against various bacteria assayed *in vitro* in the presence of H_2O_2 and halide ions. A wide variety of bacteria can be killed by this technique (Sbarra *et al.*, 1971) but only when both the peroxidase system and H_2O_2 are present. Viruses (Belding *et al.*, 1970) and fungi (Lehrer and Cline, 1969) can sometimes be inactivated by this system. Although iodide is preferred by some authors for *in vitro* experiments, chloride is the most likely cofactor of the myeloperoxidase-H_2O_2 system *in vivo*. The concentration of iodide necessary for optimal antimicrobial activity is at least six times greater than the amount normally found in blood, while chloride concentrations that are effective *in vitro* are readily obtained *in vivo* (Oser, 1965, Zgliczynski *et al.*, 1968). Sbarra *et al.* (1971) have suggested that decarboxylation and deamination of amino acids to aldehydes, which are potent antimicrobial agents (Wilson and Miles, 1964) may be important in inactivating ingested organisms. Myeloperoxidase (from human leukocytes) has been shown to catalyze such reactions at pH 5.3 in the presence of H_2O_2 and chloride ions (Zgliczynski *et al.*, 1968). The surface of the microorganism and the phagocytic cell both have substrates, such as amino acids and fatty acids, that could give rise to aldehydes.

In order to get efficient killing of bacteria there must be direct contact with myeloperoxidase (Paul *et al.*, 1970). Physical separation of the bacteria from myeloperoxidase using a dialysis bag results in significantly less bactericidal activity (Sbarra *et al.*, 1971). Thus it may be that peroxidative activity is directed principally at the ingested organism, possibly at free carboxyl and amino groups on the bacterial cell wall (Salton, 1964).*

D. Interferon

While interferon may be produced in infections other than viral infections, we will consider it only in the latter context. In a focus of viral

* The biochemical basis of the microbicidal capacity of macrophages is indeed poorly understood, and the essential biochemical differences between normal and activated macrophages are even less clear. For a more extended discussion, see Nelson (1969, 1972) and for reasons for scepticism about the significance of the myeloperoxidase/halide system, see Cline (1970)—Ed.

infection containing infected cells, lymphocytes, and macrophages, there are many potential sources of interferon. The conventional sources are virus-infected cells. It has been claimed that relatively pure macrophage cultures also produce interferon *in vitro* (Hirsch *et al.*, 1970; Subrahmanyan and Mims, 1970; Smith and Wagner, 1967; Acton and Myrvik, 1966). Since the initial discovery of Glasgow (1966), it has also become apparent that interferon may be produced by immune lymphocyte populations after specific antigenic stimulation. Such interferon seems different from virus-induced interferon in that it is acid unstable (Salvin *et al.*, 1973). Production of interferon by lymphocytes is reviewed in this volume by Epstein (Chapter 8).

Whatever its source, in our view the crucial points concerning interferon are the following.

a. It is virostatic, not virucidal.

b. Is it produced rapidly enough and in sufficient quantities in a focus of infection to retard virus production and spread of infection?

c. What are the sensitivities of various cell types to the action of interferons from these various sources?

There is little or no quantitative information on the questions posed above to provide a basis for firm conclusions on the importance or otherwise of interferon in CMI-dependent recovery from primary viral infection. Since it is demonstrable in a wide variety of systems derived from many different species, it seems reasonable on teleological grounds to say that it has been retained throughout evolution because it is useful enough to confer a selective advantage. Because we are not aware of substantial evidence contrary to the idea that the normal course of events is for immunologically recognized foci of infection to be invaded rapidly by monocytes (macrophages), which are capable of very efficient phagocytosis and destruction of many viruses, we suggest that a possible role of lymphocyte-produced interferon is to protect macrophages from those viruses capable of infecting them. Thus, interferon would be to viral infection what macrophage activation is to bacterial infection. This suggestion is readily testable.

IV. CONCLUSIONS

We have emphasized the concept that antigen presentation on cell membranes, or antigen presented in some manner controlled by genes within major histocompatibility systems, is mandatory for efficient induction of effector T cells leading to a CMI response. At this time, the concept is supported by a limited amount of data from experimental systems involving infection of mice with LCM or ectromelia viruses or *Listeria monocytogenes*. If studies of other infectious or oncogenic agents in a variety of host species further support this concept, it could provide a basis for fruitful investigation of the cellular and molecular requirements for T cell induction, the nature of T cell receptors for antigen, and the library of T cell receptor specificities in normal animals. This in turn could lead to a more rational approach to practical problems of immunoprophylaxis and immunotherapy.

There is convincing evidence that effector T cells are generated rapidly in lymphoid tissues during the response to infection, leave these tissues, circulate in blood, recognize specific antigens in sites of infection, and localize at these foci. They then appear to cause, either directly or indirectly, the recruitment of blood monocytes to the lesions and their differentiation to activated macrophages. As defined here, activated macrophages have enhanced phagocytic and microbicidal powers that are immunologically nonspecific, although their development seems to be triggered by a specific interaction between effector T cells and antigen. Activated macrophages kill intracellular parasites that are capable of survival and growth within normal macrophages. Interferon produced by lymphocytes may be regarded as a supplementary mechanism serving a similar function to macrophage activation, i.e., it could protect macrophages from infection by certain viruses that would otherwise multiply within them. Evidence for *specific* antimicrobial activity of macrophages, specificity being conferred either directly or indirectly by effector T cells, is not reviewed in detail here. In our view, the need for such mechanism(s) in lesions where macrophage activation would inevitably occur is not obvious, but the precise nature and origin of the factor(s) conferring specificity are of considerable interest.

Many questions have yet to be answered; some of the more obvious of these are listed here.

a. What factors regulate T cell responses?

c. What is the nature of T cell memory?

d. Are different T cell subsets responsible for recruitment of monocytes, activation of macrophages, and cytotoxicity?

e. Does activation of macrophages depend directly upon a soluble T cell product, or is the process more complicated, e.g., are ancillary cells or products involved?

f. What are the precise mechanisms by which macrophages activated by T cells kill ingested bacteria, viruses, or other parasites?

g. What is the relative potency of (T) lymphocyte interferon, compared with other interferons, in terms of protecting macrophages from viral infection?

h. Are all activated macrophages the same, or is there some element of specificity, not necessarily immunological, in their antiparasitic activity?

i. Do activated macrophages acquire their characteristic changes, viz., increased phagocytic and microbicidal powers simultaneously or not, i.e., can one property be acquired without the other?

j. How many different pathways may lead to macrophage activation, e.g., what mechanisms are involved in T cell-depleted mice?

REFERENCES

Acton, J. D., and Myrvik, Q. N. (1966). *J. Bacteriol.* **91,** 2300–2304.

Allison, A. C. (1974). *Transplant. Rev.* **19,** 3–55.

Avila, F. R., Schultz, R. M., and Tompkins, W. A. F. (1972). *Infec. Immunity* **6,** 9–16.

Bang, F. B., and Warwick, A. (1960). *Proc. Nat. Acad. Sci. U.S.* **46,** 1065–1075.

Baron, S., Babar, S., and Buckler, C. E. (1964). *Science* **145,** 814–817.

Belding, M. E., Klebanoff, S. J., and Ray, C. G. (1970). *Science* **167,** 195–196.

Blanden, R. V. (1969). *Transplantation* **7,** 484–497.

Blanden, R. V. (1970). *J. Exp. Med.* **132,** 1035–1054.

Blanden, R. V. (1971a). *J. Exp. Med.* **133,** 1074–1089.

Blanden, R. V. (1971b). *J. Exp. Med.* **133,** 1090–1103.

Blanden, R. V. (1974a). *Transplant. Rev.* **19,** 56–88.

Blanden, R. V. (1974b). *In* "Progress in Immunology II" (L. Brent and J. Holborow, eds.), Vol. 4, pp. 117–125, North-Holland Publ., Amsterdam.

Blanden, R. V., and Langman, R. E. (1972). *Scand. J. Immunol.* **1,** 379–391.

Blanden, R. V., and Mims, C. A. (1973). *Aust. J. Exp. Biol. Med. Sci.* **51,** 393–398.

Blanden, R. V., Mackaness, G. B., and Collins, F. M. (1966). *J. Exp. Med.* **124,** 585–599.

Blanden, R. V., Lefford, M. J., and Mackaness, G. B. (1969). *J. Exp. Med.* **129,** 1079–1107.

Blanden, R. V., Gardner, I. D., and Bowern, N. A. (1975a). In preparation.

Blanden, R. V., Doherty, P. C., Dunlop, M. B. C., Gardner, I. D., Zinkernagel, R. M., and David, C. S. (1975b). *Nature (London)* **254,** 269–270.

Blanden, R. V., Bowern, N. A., Pang, T. E., Gardner, I. D., and Parish, C. R. (1975c). *Aust. J. Exp. Biol. Med. Sci.* **53,** 187–195.

Bodmer, W. F. (1972). *Nature (London)* **237,** 139–145.

Bretscher, P. A. (1974). *Cell. Immunol.* **13,** 171–195.

Burns, W. H., and Allison, A. C. (1975). *Progr. Med. Virol.* (in press).

Cantor, H., and Asofsky, R. (1972). *J. Exp. Med.* **135,** 764–779.

Cerottini, J.-C., and Brunner, K. T. (1974). *Advan. Immunol.* **19,** 67–132.

Cerottini, J.-C., Engers, H. D., McDonald, H. R., and Brunner, K. T. (1974). *J. Exp. Med.* **140,** 703–717.

Cheers, C., and Waller, R. (1975). *J. Immunol.* **115,** 844–847.

Cline, M. J. (1970). *Infec. Immunity* **2,** 156–161.

Cole, B. C., and Ward, J. R. (1973). *Infec. Immunity* **7,** 691–699.

Cole, G. A., Prendergast, R. A., and Henney, C. S. (1973). *In* "Lymphocytic Choriomeningitis Virus and Other Adenoviruses" (F. Lehmann-Grube, ed.), pp. 61–72. Springer-Verlag, Berlin and New York.

Cole, G. A., Prendergast, R. A., Johnson, E. D., and Henney, C. S. (1974). *RES, J. Reticuloendothel. Soc.* **15,** 29a (abstr.).

Collins, F. M., Mackaness, G. B., and Blanden, R. V. (1966). *J. Exp. Med.* **124,** 601–619.

Cook, G. M. W., and Stoddart, R. W. (1973). *In* "Surface Carbohydrates of the Eukaryotic Cell," pp. 257–270. Academic Press.

de Landazuri, M. O., and Herberman, R. B. (1972). *J. Natl. Cancer Inst.* **49,** 147–154.

Doherty, P. C., and Hapel, A. K. (1975). In preparation.

Doherty, P. C., and Zinkernagel, R. M. (1974). *Transplant. Rev.* **19,** 89–120.

Doherty, P. C., and Zinkernagel, R. M. (1975a). *J. Immunol.* **114,** 30–33.

Doherty, P. C., and Zinkernagel, R. M. (1975b). *J. Exp. Med.* **141,** 502–507.

Doherty, P. C., Zinkernagel, R. M., and Ramshaw, I. A. (1974). *J. Immunol.* **112,** 1548–1552.

Ennis, F. A. (1973). *J. Infec. Dis.* **127,** 632–638.

Evans, R., Grant, C. K., Cox, H., Steele, K., and Alexander, P. (1972). *J. Exp. Med.* **136,** 1318–1322.

Gardner, I. D., Bowern, N. A., and Blanden, R. V. (1974a). *Eur. J. Immunol.* **4,** 63–67.

Gardner, I. D., Bowern, N. A., and Blanden, R. V. (1974b). *Eur. J. Immunol.* **4,** 68–72.

Gardner, I. D., Bowern, N. A., and Blanden, R. V. (1975). *Eur. J. Immunol.* **5,** 122–127.

Garon, G. F., and Moss, B. (1971). *Virology* **46,** 233–246.

Glasgow, L. A. (1966). *J. Bacteriol.* **91,** 2185–2191.

Hapel, A. J. (1975). *Scand. J. Immunol.* **3,** 311–319.

Hapel, A. J., and Gardner, I. (1974). *Scand. J. Immunol.* **3,** 311–319.

Henney, C. S. (1973). *Transplant. Rev.* **17,** 37–70.

Henney, C. S., Gaffney, J., and Bloom, B. R. (1974). *J. Exp. Med.* **140,** 837–852.

Hirsch, M. S., Nahmias, A. J., Murphy, F. A., and Kramer, J. H. (1968). *J. Exp. Med.* **128,** 121–130.

Hirsch, M. S., Zisman, B., and Allison, A. C. (1970). *J. Immunol.* **104,** 1160–1165.

Jerne, N. K. (1971). *Eur. J. Immunol.* **1,** 1–9.

Johnson, E. D., and Cole, G. A. (1975). *J. Exp. Med.* **141,** 866–881.

Johnson, R. T. (1964). *J. Exp. Med.* **133,** 19–38.

Kapp, J A., Pierce, C. W., and Benacerraf, B. (1973). *J. Exp. Med.* **138,** 1121–1132.

Katz, D. H., and Unanue, E. R. (1972). *J. Exp. Med.* **137,** 967–990.

Koster, F. T., and McGregor, D. D. (1970). *Science* **167,** 1137–1139.

Koster, F. T., and McGregor, D. D. (1971) *J. Exp. Med.* **133,** 864–876.

Krahenbuhl, J. L., and Remington, J. S. (1971). *Infec. Immunity* **4,** 337–344.

Lagrange, P. H., Mackaness, G. B., and Miller, T. E. (1974). *J. Exp. Med.* **139,** 528–542.

Lane, F. C., and Unanue, E. R. (1972). *J. Exp. Med.* **135,** 1104–1112.

Lavrin, D. H., Herberman, R. B., Nunn, M., and Soares, N. (1973). *J. Nat. Cancer Inst.* **51,** 1497–1508.

Leclerc, J. C., Gomard, E., Plata, F., and Levy, J. P. (1973). *Int. J. Cancer* **11,** 426–432.

Lefford, M. J., McGregor, D. D., and Mackaness, G. B. (1973). *Immunology* **25,** 703–715.

Lehrer, R. I., and Cline, M. J. (1969). *J. Clin. Invest.* **48,** 1478–1488.
Lohmann-Matthes, M., and Fischer, H. (1973). *Transplant. Rev.* **17,** 149–171.
McCluskey, R. T., and Werdelin, O. (1971). *Proc. Int. Convoc. Immunol., 2nd, 1970* pp. 197–206.
McDonald, H. R., Engers, H. D., Cerottini, J.-C., and Brunner, K. T. (1974). *J. Exp. Med.* **140,** 718–730.
McFarland, H. F. (1974). *J. Immunol.* **113,** 173–180.
McGregor, D. D., and Koster, F. T. (1971). *Cell. Immunol.* **2,** 317–325.
McGregor, D. D., and Logie, P. S. (1973). *J. Exp. Med.* **137,** 660–674.
Mackaness, G. B. (1962). *J. Exp. Med.* **116,** 381–406.
Mackaness, G. B. (1964). *J. Exp. Med.* **120,** 105–120.
Mackaness, G. B. (1969). *J. Exp. Med.* **129,** 973–992.
Mackaness, G. B., Blanden, R. V., and Collins, F. M. (1966). *J. Exp. Med.* **124,** 573–583.
Mackaness, G. B., Lagrange, P. H., Miller, T. E., and Ishibashi, T. (1974). *J. Exp. Med.* **139,** 543–559.
Merigan, T. C. (1964). *Science* **145,** 811–813.
Mims, C. A., and Blanden, R. V. (1972). *Infec. Immunity* **6,** 695–698.
Nelson, D. S. (1969). "Macrophages and Immunity." North-Holland Publ., Amsterdam.
Nelson, D. S. (1972). *CRC Crit. Rev. Microbiol.* **1,** 353–384.
North, R. J. (1970). *J. Exp. Med.* **123,** 521–534.
North, R. J. (1973). *J. Exp. Med.* **138,** 342–355.
Oser, B. L., ed. (1965). "Hawk's Physiological Chemistry," 14th ed. p. 978 McGraw-Hill, New York.
Parish, C. R. (1971). *J. Exp. Med.* **134,** 21–47.
Parish, C. R., Kirov, S. M., Bowern, N., and Blanden, R. V. (1975). *Eur. J. Immunol.* **4,** 808–815.
Patterson, R. J., and Youmans, G. P. (1970). *Infec. Immunity* 1, 600–603.
Paul, B. B., Jacobs, A. A., Stranes, R. R., and Sbarra, A. J. (1970). *Infec. Immunity* **2,** 414–418.
Pierce, C. W., Kapp, J. A., Wood, D. D., and Benacerraf, B. (1974). *J. Immunol.* **112,** 1181–1189.
Rabinowitz, S. G., and Adler, W. H. (1973). *J. Immunol.* **110,** 1345–1353.
Rabinowitz, S. G., and Proctor, R. A. (1974). *J. Immunol.* **112,** 1070–1077.
Raff, M. C., and Cantor, H. (1971). *In* "Progress in Immunology" (B. D. Amos, ed.), p. 83. Academic Press, New York.
Rager-Zisman, B., and Allison, A. C. (1973). *J. Gen. Virol.* **19,** 339–451.
Rager-Zisman, B., and Bloom, B. R. (1974). *Nature* (*London*) **251,** 542–543.
Ramshaw, I. A. (1975). *Infec. Immunity* **11,** 766–769.
Remington, J. S., Krahenbuhl, J. L., and Mendenhall, J. W. (1972). *Infec. Immunity* **6,** 829–834.
Roberts, J. A. (1964). *J. Immunol.* **92,** 837–842.
Salton, M. R. J. (1964). *In* "Bacterial Cell Wall," pp. 101, 188, and 254. Amer. Elsevier, New York.
Salvin, S. B. (1958). *J. Exp. Med.* **107,** 109–124.
Salvin, S. B., Youngner, J. S., and Lederer, W. H. (1973). *Infec. Immunity* **7,** 68–75.
Sbarra, A. J., Jacobs, A. A., Strauss, R. R., Paul, B. B., and Mitchell, G. W. (1971). *Amer. J. Clin. Nutr.* **24,** 272–281.
Simon, H. B., and Sheagren, H. N. (1971). *J. Exp. Med.* **133,** 1377–1389.

Simon, H. B., and Sheagren, J. N. (1972). *Infec. Immunity* **6**, 101–103.
Smith, K. O., and Sharp, D. G. (1960). *Virology* **11**, 519–532.
Smith, T. J., and Wagner, R. R. (1967). *J. Exp. Med.* **125**, 559–577.
Stevens, J. G., and Cook, M. L. (1971). *J. Exp. Med.* **133**, 19–38.
Subrahmanyan, T. P., and Mims, C. A. (1970). *RES, J. Reticuloendothelial Soc.* **7**, 32–42.
Takeya, K., Mori, R., and Namato, K. (1964). *Proc. Jap. Acad.* **41**, 769–771.
Takeya, K., Mori, R., and Imaizumi, N. (1968). *Nature (London)* **218**, 1174.
Theiler, M., and Downs, W. G. (1973). *In* "The Arthropod-borne Viruses of Vertebrates," p. 113. Yale Univ. Press, New Haven, Connecticut.
Tompkins, W. A. F., Zarling, J. M., and Rawls, W. E. (1970). *Infec. Immunity* **2**, 783–790.
Tripathy, S. P., and Mackaness, G. B. (1969). *J. Exp. Med.* **130**, 17–30.
Unanue, E. R. (1972). *Advan. Immunol.* **15**, 95–165.
Volkert, M., Marker, O., and Bro-Jorgensen, K. (1974). *J. Exp. Med.* **139**, 1329–1343.
Wagner, H. (1973). *Science* **181**, 1170–1172.
Wainberg, M. A., Markson, Y., Weiss, D. W., and Daljanski, F. (1974). *Proc. Nat. Acad. Sci. U.S.* **71**, 3565–3569.
Wilson, G. S., and Miles, A. A., eds. (1964). "Principles of Bacteriology and Immunity," 5th ed., p. 164. Williams & Wilkins, Baltimore, Maryland.
World Health Organization. (1973). *World Health Organ., Tech. Rep. Ser.* **519**.
Youdim, S., Stutman, O., and Good, R. A. (1973). *Cell. Immunol.* **6**, 98–109.
Youngner, J. S., and Salvin, S. B. (1973). *J. Immunol.* **111**, 1914–1922.
Zgliczynski, J. M., Stelmaszyska, T., Ostrowski, M., Naskalski, J., and Sznajd, J (1968). *Eur. J. Biochem.* **4**, 540–547.
Zinkernagel, R. M. (1974). *Nature (London)* **251**, 230–233.
Zinkernagel, R. M., and Blanden, R. V. (1975). *Experientia* **31**, 591–593.
Zinkernagel, R. M., and Doherty, P. C. (1973). *J. Exp. Med.* **138**, 1266–1269.
Zinkernagel, R. M., and Doherty, P. C. (1974a). *Nature (London)* **248**, 701–702.
Zinkernagel, R. M., and Doherty, P. C. (1974b). *Nature (London)* **251**, 547–548.
Zinkernagel, R. M., and Doherty, P. C. (1974c). *Scand. J. Immunol.* **3**, 287–294.
Zinkernagel, R. M., and Doherty, P. C. (1975). In preparation.
Zinkernagel, R. M., Blanden, R. V., and Langman, R. E. (1974). *J. Immunol.* **112**, 496–501.

16

Macrophage Activation by Lymphocyte Mediators and Studies on the Interaction of Macrophage Inhibitory Factor (MIF) with Its Target Cell

John R. David and Heinz G. Remold

I. Introduction 401
II. Macrophage Activation by Lymphocyte Mediators .. 403
A. Changes Occurring in Activated Macrophages ... 403
B. Characterization of Macrophage Activating Factor 411
C. Kinetics of Activation 412
D. Macrophages Activated by Culture Directly with Lymphocytes and Antigen 413
III. Interaction of MIF with the Macrophage 414
A. Cell Surface Carbohydrates and MIF Action 414
B. Macrophage-Associated Esterases in MIF Action 418
IV. Biologically Active Substances Produced by Macrophages 421
V. Conclusion 423
References 423

I. INTRODUCTION

Considerable information reviewed in this volume illustrates the crucial role of the macrophage both in the induction of the immune response and as a powerful effector cell. In the latter capacity, macrophages ingest and dispose of a variety of organisms, kill tumor cells, and participate in a number of immunopathologic processes. It has been known for some time that macrophages obtained from immune animals have altered morphology and metabolism and exhibit an enhanced ability to deal with a number of microorganisms (Metchnikoff, 1905; Lurie, 1964; Mackaness, 1964; Suter and Ramseier, 1964). Such macrophages are said to be activated. More recent studies suggest that *in vivo* activation of macrophages requires the interaction of specifically sensitized T lymphocytes with the appropriate antigen (Mackaness, 1969; Lane and Unanue, 1972). This is dealt with in detail in Chapter 15.

The question arises as to how the interaction of lymphocytes with antigen leads to the activation of macrophages. Ever since the discovery that sensitized lymphocytes produce a soluble material—migration inhibitory factor (MIF), which affects the behavior of macrophages (David, 1966; Bloom and Bennett, 1966; Dumonde *et al.*, 1969)—we have thought that such lymphocyte mediators might also activate macrophages. In the past few years, our laboratory and others have accumulated considerable evidence that corroborates this hypothesis. The following will be a brief review of studies which demonstrate that lymphocyte mediators can indeed activate macrophages. In addition, studies on the interaction of MIF with macrophages will also be discussed.

Most of these studies were carried out using guinea pig cells. Casein-induced peritoneal exudates were plated on petri dishes, and monolayers of adherent cells, predominantly macrophages, were obtained (Nathan *et al.*, 1971). An irritant is required, since only a few macrophages, which survive only poorly in culture, are obtainable from the peritoneal cavity when no irritant is used. The macrophage monolayers were incubated for varying periods of time in tissue culture medium containing lymphocyte mediators. The mediators were produced by incubating lymph node lymphocytes from guinea pigs sensitized with *o*-chlorobenzoyl bovine γ-globulin (OCB-BGG) with that antigen for 24 hours (Remold *et al.*, 1970). Control cultures were not stimulated by antigen. After incubation, the cells were removed by centrifugation, and antigen was added to the control supernatant. In some studies, lymphocytes were stimulated by the mitogen concanavalin A instead of antigen (Remold *et al.*, 1972). In most experiments described, the supernatants were chromatographed on Sephadex G-100 columns, and fractions rich in MIF and its control counterpart were used (Remold *et al.*, 1972). In some experiments, human blood monocytes and human lymphocytes were also used (Rocklin *et al.*, 1974). Recently, it has been possible to activate macrophages in suspension culture (Churchill *et al.*, 1975).

First, the changes that appear to reflect alterations in the macrophage membrane will be described, then other metabolic and functional changes, and finally, the enhanced ability of such mediator-activated macrophages to deal with microorganisms and tumor cells (see Table I).

TABLE I

Activation of Macrophages by Lymphocyte Mediators

Increase in adherence to glass
Increase in ruffled membrane activity
Increase in phagocytosis of some particles (dead *Mycobacterium*) but decrease in others (aggregated hemoglobin)
Increase in membrane enzyme adenylate cyclase
Increase in incorporation of glucosamine
Decrease in electron-dense surface material
Increase in pinocytosis of colloidal gold
Increase in glucose oxidation through hexose monophosphate shunt
Increase in cytoplasmic enzyme lactic dehydrogenase
Decrease in lysosomal enzyme acid phosphatase, cathepsin D, β-glucuronidase
Increase in number cytoplasmic granules
Production of collagenase
Enhanced bacteriostasis to *Listeria*
Enhanced tumoricidal activity

II. MACROPHAGE ACTIVATION BY LYMPHOCYTE MEDIATORS

A. Changes Occurring in Activated Macrophages

1. Increased Macrophage Adherence to Glass or Plastic

Macrophages incubated in MIF-rich Sephadex G-100 fractions were found to stick much better to dishes after 3 days of incubation, as assessed by numbers of macrophages remaining (Nathan *et al.*, 1971). Similar findings using mediators from rabbits were found by Mooney and Waksman (1970). Although this adherence is usually seen best after 3 days of culture, it occasionally is seen earlier. Recently, it has been found that macrophages incubated in mediator-rich fractions in suspension culture for 24 hours will subsequently exhibit increased adherence when cultured in petri dishes for 1 hour. This rapid adherence is analogous to that seen when mouse macrophages are activated *in vivo* and then plated *in vitro* (Mackaness, 1970). Human blood monocytes incubated in human MIF-rich fractions also show enhanced adherence (Rocklin *et al.*, 1974).

2. Increased Ruffled Membrane Movement

A marked increase in ruffled membrane movement was observed after 3 days of culture using time-lapse cinematography (Nathan *et al.*, 1971) (Fig. 1). Macrophages cultured in MIF-rich media also spread out much

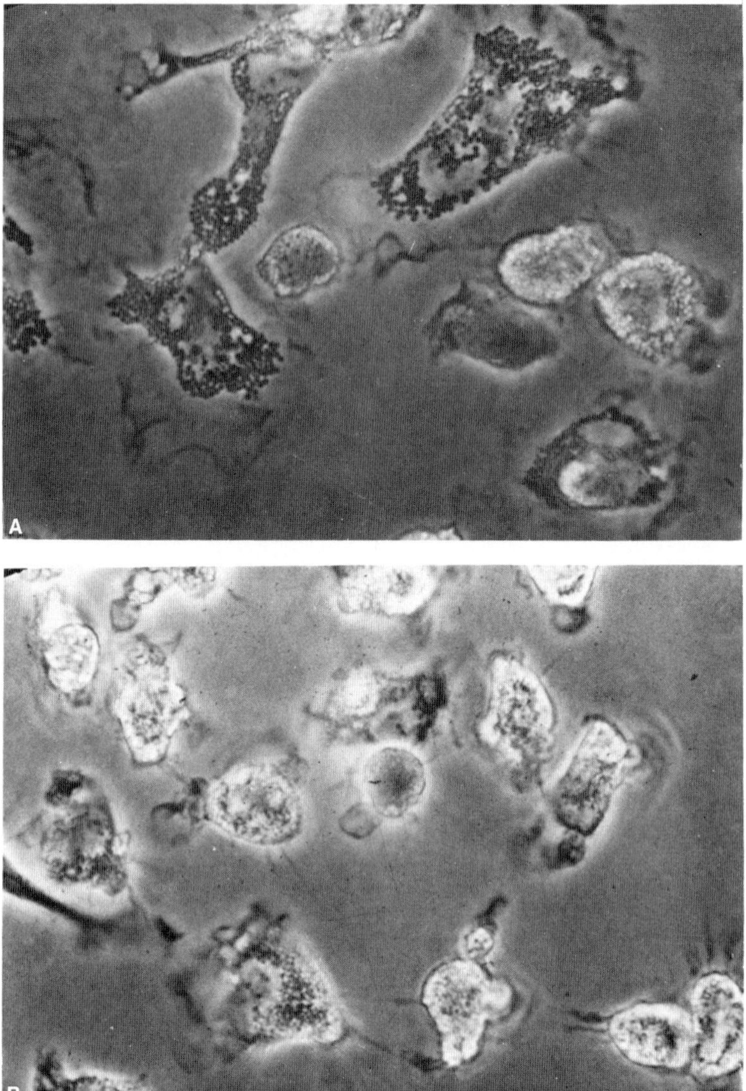

Fig. 1. Macrophages after 72 hours cultured in MIF-rich supernatant Sephadex fractions (A) and in control fraction (B). Macrophages incubated with lymphocyte mediators are more spread out and have more active ruffled membranes and more granules. (From studies cited in Nathan *et al.*, 1971.)

more than those in the control media. It is noteworthy that such increased spreading was also seen when the periphery of a fan of cells inhibited from migrating from a capillary tube by antigen was examined (David and Haber, 1969). Increased ameboid movement has also been reported (Mooney and Waksman, 1970). On the other hand, early after incubation with mediators, it has been found that cells may spread less (Fauve and Dekaris, 1968; Salvin *et al.*, 1971).

3. *Phagocytosis*

Enhancement of both the rate and extent of phagocytosis of dead *Mycobacteria* was observed (Nathan *et al.*, 1971). However, this was not seen with all particles studied. There was only a slight increase in phagocytosis of starch particles. In contrast, Remold and Mednis (1972) found a decrease in phagocytosis of denatured aggregated hemoglobin by macrophages preincubated in MIF-rich Sephadex fractions compared to controls. Furthermore, the amount of denatured hemoglobin sticking to the macrophage, and thus recovered after pronase treatment, was also less on activated than control cells. Neta and Salvin (1971) reported a decrease in phagocytosis of *Candida albicans* by mediator-activated macrophages. Hoff (1975) noted that mouse macrophages that had been activated *in vivo* by injection of mice with BCG or *Trypanosoma cruzi* showed a decrease in ability to take up *T. cruzi* as compared to control macrophages. These results suggest that the membrane of the activated macrophages is altered leading either to increased or to decreased phagocytosis depending upon the surface properties of the particle.

4. *Pinocytosis*

Meade *et al.* (1974) have reported that guinea pig macrophages incubated with mediator-rich supernatants take up more radioactive gold than controls. Maximum uptake was seen after 20–30 hours of incubation.

5. *Increase in the Membrane Enzyme Adenylate Cyclase*

The activity of this plasma membrane bound enzyme was studied by Remold-O'Donnell and Remold (1974). Specific adenylate cyclase activity was increased at 24 and 48 hours relative to zero time and decreased at 72 hours in all cultures. Of note, at 24 and 48 hours, specific activity of adenylate cyclase was 30% greater in macrophages incubated with MIF-rich fractions than in controls (Remold-O'Donnell and Remold,

1974) (see Fig. 2). Indomethacin (3×10^{-6} *M*) reduced this difference significantly, suggesting a role for prostaglandins. The addition of MIF-rich fractions to macrophage homogenates did not increase adenylate cyclase activity. Thus, the action of MIF-rich fractions on adenylate cyclase requires prolonged incubation with intact cells. The change in activity of this enzyme precedes several other changes observed in mediator-activated macrophages.

6. *Increase in Incorporation of Glucosamine*

Hammond and Dvorak (1972) reported that when peritoneal exudate cells from sensitized guinea pigs were cultured with antigen, there was an increase in glucosamine incorporation. Further studies suggested this was incorporated into the membrane structures. Normal macrophages incubated in mediator-rich supernatants also show an increase in incorpo-

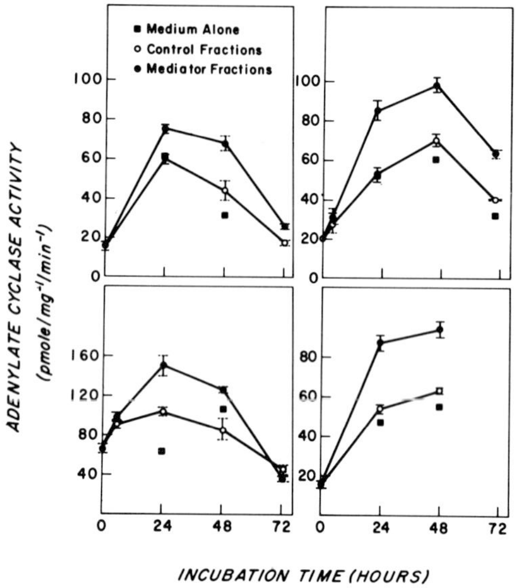

Fig. 2. The enhancement of macrophage adenylate cyclase by products of activated lymphocytes. Effect of lymphocyte mediator-containing fraction, control fraction, and culture medium alone on the adenylate cyclase activity of guinea pig peritoneal macrophages in 4 experiments. Specific activities shown with solid error bars are the mean ± SE of quadruplicate determinations. Specific activity shown with dashed error bars are the mean ± the range of duplicates. Solid squares are the mean of duplicates. Note that under all three incubation conditions adenylate cyclase activity is increased at 24 and 48 hours over the zero time values and that macrophages incubated with mediator fraction show consistently higher activities. (From Remold-O'Donnell and Remold, 1974, with permission from Williams & Wilkins).

ration of glucosamine. This group has also described a decrease in the electron-dense surface material of macrophages that have been activated by lymphocyte mediators (Dvorak *et al.*, 1972).

7. Glucose Oxidation

Macrophages incubated in MIF-rich fractions as well as whole supernatants show a fourfold increase in glucose-1-C oxidation through the hexose monophosphate shunt when compared to cultures incubated in control fractions or supernatants (Nathan *et al.*, 1971). Increase in the cytoplasmic enzyme lactic dehydrogenase has also been observed (Remold and Mednis, 1972).

8. Lysosomal Enzymes and Intracellular Granules

Remold and Mednis measured the activity of acid phosphatase, cathepsin D, and β-glucuronidase in macrophage monolayers after 0, 24, 48 and 72 hours of incubation of MIF-rich and control fractions. Although no differences were observed during the first 2 days, a consistent decrease in the specific activity of these three enzymes (measured as activity per cell DNA) in the MIF-treated cultures compared to control was found on the third day (Remold and Mednis, 1972). Further, the loss of enzyme activity could not be readily explained. No corresponding increase in enzyme activity was found in the supernatant fluid. The serum used did not inhibit enzyme activity. Testing of macrophage homogenates kept at 37°C for 3 days showed that the enzymes were stable under these conditions. The loss of these three lysosomal enzymes does not correlate with any decrease in lysosomal granules. On the contrary, by both phase and electron microscopy, more granules are seen in the activated macrophages.

An explanation for the decrease in lysosomal enzyme activity observed in macrophages activated by MIF-rich fractions remains to be found. Possibly, there is a decrease in lysosomal enzyme synthesis in favor of the synthesis of other substances.

9. Collagenase

The macrophages' versatility in contributing to the pathogenesis of certain inflammatory states is illustrated by recent findings that demonstrate that mediator-activated macrophages secrete collagenase into the medium (Wahl *et al.*, 1975). Maximum production was found after 48 hours and continued for several days. Both antigen- and mitogen-stimulated lymphocytes produced supernatants that caused macrophages to produce this enzyme. Cycloheximide prevented the mediator-induced production of collagenase by macrophages, indicating that this increase in collagenase activity depends on active protein synthesis in the macrophage.

10. Enhanced Macrophage Bacteriostasis

Having found that MIF-rich fractions altered the function of normal macrophages in a number of ways, studies were carried out to determine if macrophages activated in this manner would also demonstrate an enhanced yet nonspecific capacity to handle microorganisms, such as *Listeria monocytogenes*. The problems encountered in the preliminary studies are discussed elsewhere (Leibowitch and David, 1973). Fowles *et al.* (1973) found that macrophages incubated for 3 days in MIF-rich fractions exhibited a two- to tenfold enhanced bacteriostasis compared with controls, with no antibiotics present.

It was important to determine whether the enhanced macrophage bacteriostasis in the MIF-treated monolayers was a consequence of the greater number of macrophages in these cultures than in controls. To compensate for the enhanced adherence of macrophages in MIF-rich cultures, fewer peritoneal exudate cells were initially plated in dishes that were to receive MIF-rich fractions. The results of this experiment are seen in Fig. 3. The control monolayers contained an average of 53 μg of macrophage protein before infection and contained 3499 viable *Listeria* per μg as measured 10 minutes after infection. Twenty-two hours later, the monolayers had lost 60% of their protein, and there was a 47-fold increase in viable *Listeria* per μg protein. The MIF-treated monolayers had less macrophages to start with, 29 μg, and contained 5281 bacteria per μg macrophage protein. In contrast to controls, however, the monolayers had maintained their cell number after 22 hours of infection, having lost only 9% of their protein, and growth of *Listeria* was limited to fourfold. Thus, despite there being less macrophages in MIF-treated monolayers and more *Listeria* per macrophage at the beginning of the experiment, bacteriostasis in these cultures was enhanced ten times over controls; no antibiotics were present at any time.

That the bacteriostatic effect was exerted by the activated macrophages themselves, and not by the different media in which they were cultured, is shown by the fact that, in separate experiments, *Listeria* cultured without cell monolayers grew equally well in MIF-rich or control fractions (Fowles *et al.*, 1973).

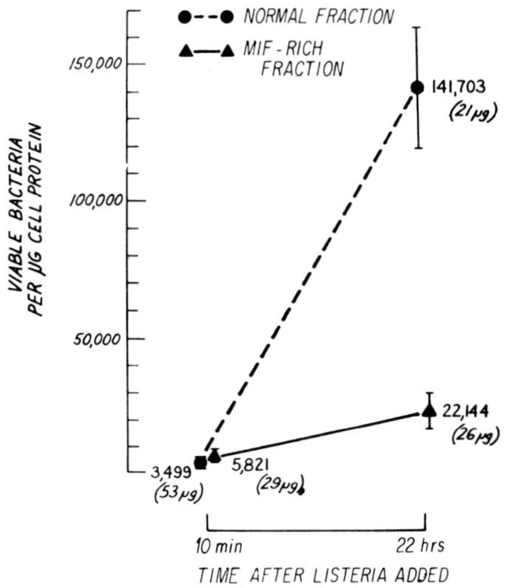

Fig. 3. Enhanced macrophage bacteriostasis induced by 72 hours of preincubation with MIF-rich fractions even under conditions when there are less macrophages present at the time of infection in this group than in the controls. Peritoneal exudate cells were initially plated so that, at the time of infection, there were about half as many macrophages in the MIF-treated monolayers than in the controls; despite this, MIF-treated monolayers were still markedly bacteriostatic compared to controls. Details are described in the text. The points represent mean and SE of triplicate cultures ($p < 0.03$). Italicized numbers in parenthesis represent micrograms of macrophage protein, and other numbers represent number of viable *Listeria monocytogenes*. (Data from Fowles *et al.*, 1973).

Macrophages incubated for only 24 hours with MIF-rich fractions exhibited enhanced bacteriostasis only in one-fourth of the experiments. Others have reported that supernatants from either stimulated lymphoid cells, mixed lymphocyte cultures, or mixed stimulated spleen cells and macrophage cultures enhance resistance to a number of organisms (Patterson and Youmans, 1970; Godal *et al.*, 1971; Krahenbuhl and Remington, 1971; Anderson and Remington, 1974). Whereas in some instances, the relationship between the antigen inducing the lymphocyte mediator and the antigenicity of the organism being killed by the macrophage need bear no relationship, in other cases, the specificity of the lymphocyte sensitivity must be identical to the organisms used (Borges and Johnson, 1975). Furthermore, the production of mediator in the latter case appears to have different kinetics than in the former case. This suggests that several different mechanisms are involved as is seen in studies on the killing of tumor cells by macrophages. A comparison of bacteriostasis by mediator-activated macrophages with macrophage activation by direct contact with lymphocytes and antigen is made below.

11. Tumor Killing by Macrophages Activated by Lymphocyte Mediators

The tumoricidal capacity of macrophages activated by lymphocyte mediators was studied in a syngeneic strain 2 guinea pig tumor system by Piessens *et al.* (1975). Monolayers of normal strain 2 macrophages were incubated for 3 days in unfractionated MIF-rich and control supernatants from OCB-BGG-stimulated guinea pig lymphocytes. Tumor cells labeled with [^{3}H]thymidine were then added, and cytotoxicity was determined after 24 hours of cocultivation by comparing the number of adherent tumor cells remaining in dishes containing similar numbers of activated and control macrophages. This is a true reflection of cytotoxicity, as 90% of the radioactivity that is released from the monolayer is non-cell-associated.

The macrophages that had been preincubated in MIF-rich supernatants were toxic for line 1 hepatoma cells in 23 of 29 experiments. The cytotoxicity ranged from 17 to 72% (mean 38%). Such macrophages were also cytotoxic for MCA-25 fibrosarcoma in 5 of 5 experiments, with percent kill ranging from 20 to 74% (mean 31%). On the other hand, such activated macrophages did not kill either syngeneic fibroblasts or kidney cells. Tumor cells adhered equally well to both activated and control macrophages when measured after just 2 hours of cocultivation (see Fig. 4). In addition, activation could be induced by supernatants devoid of lymphotoxin activity, suggesting that the effect was not due to this mediator absorbed to macrophages.

The observation that macrophages activated by lymphocyte mediators kill syngeneic tumor cells but not normal cells is consistent with the previous findings of Hibbs *et al.* (1972) and Hibbs (1972), who reported that activated macrophages obtained from mice immunized with a number of different microorganisms kill transformed cells but not their normal counterparts, whereas macrophages from nonimmunized mice kill neither cell type. Since activated macrophages exhibit certain membrane changes, such as increased ruffled membrane movement, increased spreading, and increased adenylate cyclase activity, as well as other changes (Hammond and Dvorak, 1972; Dvorak *et al.*, 1972), it is tempting to speculate that membrane alterations possibly analogous to those found between normal and transformed cells might be present between normal and activated macrophages. Such surface changes might lead activated macrophages to recognize or have a greater affinity for the altered tumor cell membrane

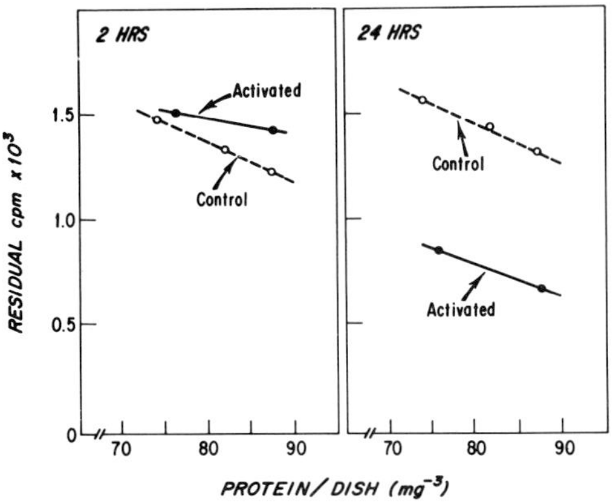

Fig. 4. Initial adherence of labeled line 1 hepatoma cells to monolayers of control and activated macrophages. Residual radioactivity adherent to macrophage monolayers is plotted as a function of the number of macrophages (as micrograms of protein/dish) present at the time of addition of tumor cells. Macrophages were preincubated for 3 days with mediator-rich ("activated") and control lymphocyte supernatants. After 2 hours, the tumor cells adhered equally well to both types of monolayers. At 24 hours, the activated macrophages are cytotoxic for the tumor cells. Each point represents the mean of triplicate determinations. (From Piessens *et al.*, 1975, with permission from The Williams & Wilkins Co.)

leading to interaction and subsequent killing of the tumor cell (for further discussion, see Keller, Chapter 19).

In more recent studies, it was shown that macrophages incubated for 24 hours in suspension culture also showed enhanced capacity of killing syngeneic tumor cells. Mediator-rich fractions free of antigen were capable of enhancing macrophage cytotoxicity. Further, trypsinization of the activated macrophages did not diminish their cytotoxic potential (Churchill *et al.*, 1975). These findings—that mediators induced by antigens non-cross-reacting with the tumor antigen are effective, that antigen need not be present, and that trypsinization does not alter the cytotoxicity—differentiate this type of enhanced macrophage function from that produced by the specific macrophage arming factor described by Evans and Alexander (Evans *et al.*, 1972, 1973) and others (Lohmann-Matthes *et al.*, 1973; Pels and Den Otter, 1974) (see Chapter 21).

B. Characterization of Macrophage Activating Factor

The macrophage activating factor elutes from Sephadex G-100 with molecules between 68,000–25,000 daltons, with peak activity between 55,000–35,000 (Nathan *et al.*, 1973). This is the same fraction that contains peak activity of guinea pig MIF, chemotactic factor for macrophages, and lymphotoxin (Coyne *et al.*, 1973; Ward *et al.*, 1972). Further studies showed that the active fractions' ability to enhance both cell adherence and glucose oxidation was destroyed by incubation with neuraminidase, a procedure that also destroys guinea pig MIF but does not affect chemotactic factor or lymphotoxin (Coyne *et al.*, 1973; David, 1971). This finding, along with the observation that the macrophage activating factor after isopycnic centrifugation in CsCl is recovered in a band with a buoyant density slightly greater than albumin, as is MIF but not the other two mediators, indicates that, with the present techniques, it is indistinguishable from MIF and may be the same material (Nathan *et al.*, 1973). Human macrophage activating factor is also the same size as human MIF (Rocklin *et al.*, 1974) and differs from human lymphotoxin, chemotactic factor, and leukocyte inhibitory factor (LIF) (Kolb and Granger, 1968; Altman *et al.*, 1973; Rocklin, 1974).

C. Kinetics of Activation

The kinetics of macrophage activation depend upon the particular function that is being assessed, the culture conditions, and, as will be discussed below, whether lymphocytes themselves are present or not. A number of activities can be seen after 24 hours of incubation as monolayers, such as increases in adenylate cyclase activity, pinocytosis, collagenase secretion, and, at times, adherence. Changes in glucose oxidation and phagocytosis usually take 48–72 hours. In early studies, Nathan *et al.* (1973) showed that the MIF-rich fractions need not be present in the early period of incubation. The data suggested that the latent period required for macrophages to manifest response to activating factor consisted of two stages: In the first, the macrophages were refractory to the influence of the activating factor but underwent changes to render them receptive. In the second, they responded to the activating factor. More recently, it has been shown that activation in suspension culture rather than monolayer culture may shorten the latent period *vis-à-vis* macrophage tumor cytotoxicity (Churchill *et al.*, 1975) and enhanced adherence (W. H. Churchill, W. F. Piessens, and J. R. David, unpublished observation). The reasons for the difference in latent periods when assessing various manifestations of macrophage activation and differing culture conditions require further study. It is interesting that the presence of lymphocytes with the macrophages during activation not only shortens the latent period, but, as concerns macrophage resistance to *Listeria,* also appears to turn a bacteriostatic activity into a bactericidal one (Leibowitch and David, 1973; Simon and Sheagren, 1971).

D. Macrophages Activated by Culture Directly with Lymphocytes and Antigen

In their experiments on cellular immunity, Simon and Sheagren first took peritoneal exudates from protein purified derivative of tuberculin (PPD) or BGG sensitized guinea pigs (exudates that contained *both* sensitized lymphocytes and macrophages) and incubated them directly with specific antigen for 24 hours. The resulting monolayers of macrophages, when washed and infected with *Listeria monocytogenes* were bactericidal for the bacteria compared to cultures that had been preincubated without antigen (Simon and Sheagren, 1971). In subsequent experiments, sensitive lymphocytes obtained from lymph nodes (Leibowitch and David, 1973) or peritoneal exudates (Simon and Sheagren, 1972) when added to normal macrophages with antigen resulted in macrophage monolayers that exhibited enhanced bactericidal capacity for *Listeria*. An example of bactericidal activity by macrophages which had been activated by the preincubation with OCB-BGG sensitized lymphocytes and specific antigen is seen in Fig. 5. Recent experiments suggest that the lymphocytes involved in this type of *in vitro* reaction are T lymphocytes (Krahenbuhl *et al.*, 1973). In addition to exhibiting enhanced bactericidal activity at 24 hours, such lymphocyte-activated macrophages also exhibit some enhanced adherence (Leibowitch and David, 1973).

The differences between activation of macrophages by the direct presence of lymphocytes and antigen and that brought about by lymphocyte mediators are the following. First, in the presence of lymphocytes and antigen, macrophages show enhanced bactericidal activity and some increased cell adherence after 24 hours of incubation rather than 3 days. The latent period is thus shortened, and we have preliminary evidence that it can be shortened even further. Second, the degree of bactericidal activity is greater than the bacteriostasis manifested by macrophages activated by lymphocyte mediators alone.

The evidence clearly shows that macrophages can be activated by lymphocyte mediators. It is not known why lymphocytes themselves have a greater influence on macrophages than their mediators. They may produce essential factors that are more labile than mediators such as MIF. Alternatively, direct contact between the lymphocyte and macrophage may be required for more effective bactericidal activity in some cases. Anatomic interaction between lymphocytes and macrophages has been documented (Salvin *et al.*, 1971; Sharp and Burwell, 1960; Schuenberg *et al.*, 1974; McFarland *et al.*, 1966; Lipsky and Rosenthal, 1973) and is discussed by Rosenthal *et al.* (Chapter 6). Further work is required to document whether such a mechanism is contributing to the

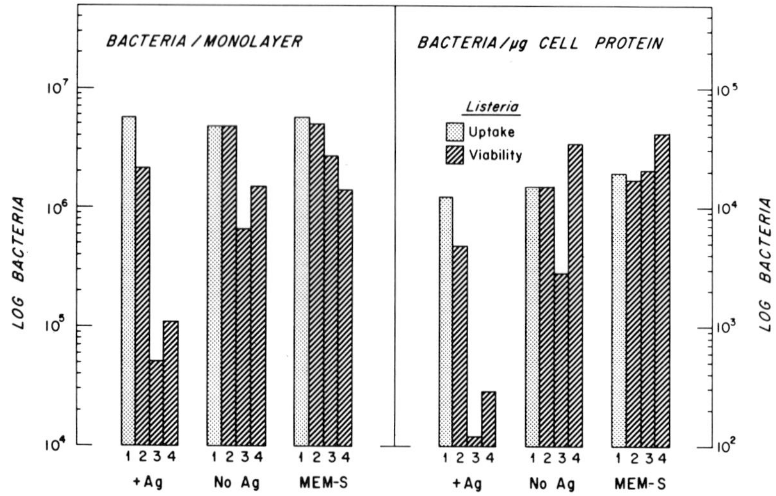

Fig. 5. Enhancement of listericidal capacity of macrophages by stimulated lymphocytes. Monolayers of normal macrophages were incubated with sensitized lymphocytes and antigen (+Ag), or without antigen (no Ag), or without lymphocytes or antigen (MEM-S) for 22 hours. The monolayers were then infected with radiolabeled *Listeria monocytogenes* for 10 minutes, the monolayers washed and further incubated in culture medium. Sampling was carried out at 10 minutes and 4 and 24 hours after the bacteria were added. In each group of 4 bars, numerals represent, respectively, 1, uptake of radiolabeled *Listeria* in 10 minutes; 2, 3, and 4, viable *Listeria* at 20 minutes and 4 and 22 hours after infection. Each bar figures the average of duplicate monolayers plotted on a $\log_{10}$ scale at 22 hours. Control monolayers (no Ag) yielded 120 times more bacteria per µg cell protein than experimental monolayers (+Ag). (From Leibowitch and David, 1973, with permission from the Institut Pasteur).

enhancement of macrophage function that characterizes the activated macrophages.

III. INTERACTION OF MIF WITH THE MACROPHAGE

A. Cell Surface Carbohydrates and MIF Action

Let us turn now to another facet of lymphocyte–macrophage interactions, namely, the mechanism underlying the interaction of one lymphocyte mediator, MIF, with the macrophage. Early studies suggest that the surface of the macrophage plays an important role in the interaction with MIF; when peritoneal exudate cells from sensitized animals were trypsinized and then placed in capillary tubes, they were no longer inhibited from migrating by antigen (David *et al.*, 1964). Subsequently, it was found that trypsinized macrophages no longer responded to MIF (David and David, 1972; Remold, 1972; Leu *et al.*, 1972; Bartfeld and Atoynatan, 1969). They regained their ability to respond after 12–24 hours of preincubation in culture medium. Similarly, macrophages incubated with pronase no longer respond to MIF (Remold, 1972). The reversibility of the protease effect is consistent with the regeneration of surface receptors, as well as with other possible repair mechanisms. These findings suggest that certain surface proteins, probably glycoproteins, are essential for the MIF response because trypsin only affects the outer cell surface structures of cells (Kraemer, 1971).

There is increasing evidence for the importance of carbohydrates on the surface of cells. The first hint that carbohylrate groups were involved with MIF–macrophage interactions was the finding that neuraminidase destroyed MIF activity, indicating that sialic acid groups were crucial for it to function (Remold and David, 1971). MIF might also interact with the macrophage in a similar way to a lectin, via cell surface carbohydrates. If this were so, specific monosaccharides should prevent the interaction of MIF with the macrophage. To test for this possibility, guinea pig peritoneal macrophages were incubated with MIF in the presence of α-L-fucose, α-D-mannose, α-D-glucose, β-D-galactose, and *N*-acetyl-β-D-glucosamine. α-L-Fucose consistently blocked the action of MIF, whereas the other sugars had no effect (Remold, 1973). Further experiments showed that this effect on MIF was reversible, i.e., when MIF was incubated with fucose and then the sugar removed by dialysis, the MIF was still active; similarly, if macrophages were incubated with fucose and then the sugar removed by washing, they responded normally to MIF. The fucose had to be present throughout the period of incubation to exert its effect.

In further studies, the investigations were carried out to determine whether the effect of L-fucose was on MIF or on the macrophage. Two situations could be possible. L-Fucose could compete with MIF for a fucose-binding site on the macrophage. In this case, fucose would be part of the MIF molecule, and removal of fucose from MIF would result in a loss of activity. Second, L-fucose on the surface of macrophages could play an essential role as part of a receptor for MIF. In this case, the removal of fucose from the macrophage would result in the loss of its responsiveness. To investigate these two possibilities, MIF or macrophages were incubated with L-fucosidase, an enzyme that cleaves L-fucose from oligosaccharides (Carlsen and Pierce, 1972). This enzyme was prepared from rat epididymides and contains a little galactosidase and *N*-acetylglucosaminidase activity, but no neuraminidase and proteinase activity which could destroy MIF activity or affect macrophages.

When MIF was incubated for 1 hour with this enzyme, its activity was not destroyed. This was not due to an inhibitor present in the MIF preparation because 90% of the L-fucosidase activity could be recovered after incubation with MIF. In contrast, when macrophages were incubated for 1 hour with L-fucosidase, they no longer responded to MIF (Fig. 6).

These experiments strongly suggest that L-fucose, probably on the macrophage surface, is essential for the MIF response. Further experiments indicated that the effect of the enzyme preparation indeed was due to α-L-fucosidase. It is known that α-L-fucosidase is inhibited by the pres-

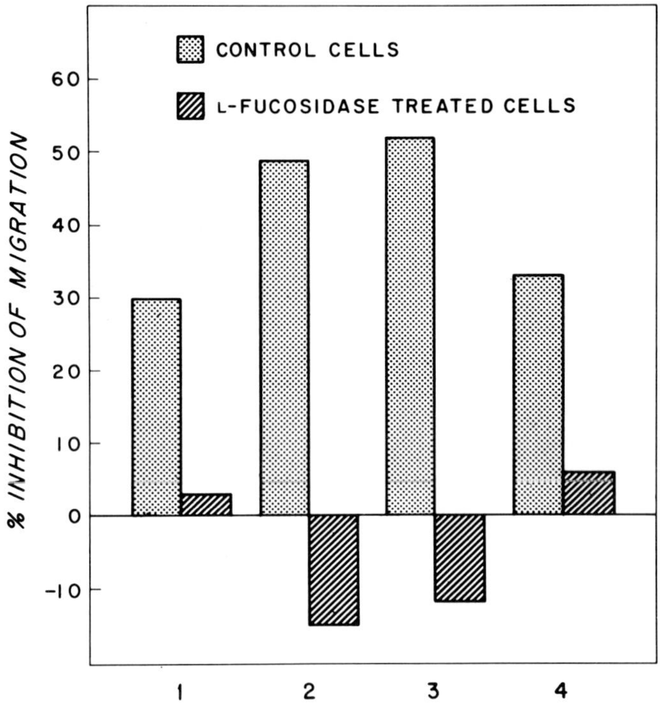

Fig. 6. Effect of L-fucosidase on macrophages. Numbers on the abscissa indicate different experiments. Cells were incubated for 1 hour with L-fucosidase and without enzyme (control cells), washed, and incubated for a second hour in concentrated MIF or control fractions 40 μl/ml. The cells were then washed, made up in capillary tubes, and percent inhibition of migration assessed at 7–12 hours. The amounts of L-fucosidase in experiments 1–4 were 32, 111, 111, and 85 U/ml. Note that L-fucosidase abolished the ability of macrophages to respond to MIF in every case. (From Remold, 1973, with permission from The Rockefeller University Press).

ence of appropriate amounts of α-L-fucose. When macrophages were incubated with α-L-fucosidase in the presence of L-fucose, no effect of the enzyme on macrophages could be found. This suggests the specific action of α-L-fucosidase being responsible for the abolition of the MIF effect.

Furthermore, macrophages which were incubated for 1 hour with MIF and 0.1 M fucose and then washed were not inhibited from migrating as compared to control cells where fucose was absent, further supporting the probability that fucose plays a part as a receptor for MIF. If fucose was simply necessary for a macrophage–macrophage interaction *following* the action of MIF, the experimental cells in the studies above should have been inhibited after washing away the fucose, as were the controls (H. G. Remold, unpublished observations).

In conclusion, we assume that the effect of L-fucose is at the cell surface, which is supported by the findings of others that most of the L-fucose of mammalian cells appears to be on the surface (Atkinson and Summers, 1971) and that L-fucose plays a role in cell surface interaction (Lloyd *et al.*, 1968; Cox and Gesner, 1965) with other cells. The possibility that L-fucose enters the macrophage and acts intracellularly has not been ruled out, but it appears very unlikely.

In the studies described above, the concentration of L-fucose (0.1 *M*) necessary to prevent MIF activity was high. This would be explained if the involved binding sites were more extended, and showed a higher affinity for a glycoprotein containing L-fucose than for L-fucose alone. For example, it has been shown that the lectin concanavalin A interacts more strongly with a disaccharide D-mannose $\alpha(1 \rightarrow 2)$-D-mannose and the trisaccharide D-mannose $\alpha(1 \rightarrow 2)$-D-mannoside (So and Goldstein, 1968). Further, fucose in solution is mainly in the β form, whereas the α form is biologically active.

Our studies using affinity chromatographic techniques further suggest that MIF binds poorly to fucose itself. When MIF was passed through ε-aminocaproyl-L-fucosamine Sepharose columns, no activity was retained when compared to MIF passed through control Sepharose columns. Further, no MIF activity could be subsequently eluted from the columns with 0.1 *M* L-fucose (J. R. David and H. G. Remold, unpublished results). These findings are at variance with those of Fox and MacSween who reported that they could successfully absorb MIF with ε-aminocaproyl-L-fucosamine columns (Fox and MacSween, 1974).

It should be mentioned here that a material from fetal calf serum which inhibits the migration of guinea pig macrophages can be inhibited by 0.1 *M* L-fucose, bovine submaxillary mucin, and blood group substances A and H. Human type O erythrocytes can absorb this factor from fetal calf serum, as can aminocaproylfucosyl Sepharose (Fox *et al.*, 1974). The relationship of this factor to MIF produced by sensitized and stimulated lymphocytes is not known.

Further studies are required for a better understanding of the role of L-fucose in the macrophage interaction, and it will be of interest to determine if L-fucose or glycoproteins containing L-fucose or other sugars affect other manifestations of lymphocyte–mediator interactions with macrophages, both *in vitro* and *in vivo*.

B. Macrophage-Associated Esterases in MIF Action

In studies carried out to isolate the macrophage receptor for MIF, in which trypsin was used to remove potential receptors from the surface and soybean trypsin inhibitor to neutralize the trypsin, it was found quite by accident that soybean trypsin inhibitor itself markedly enhanced the action of MIF (Remold, 1974). This lead to a further analysis of the sequence of MIF–macrophage interaction. Macrophages incubated with diisopropyl fluorophosphate (DFP) or soybean trypsin inhibitor, both specific esterase inhibitors, showed an increased response to subthreshold doses of MIF (Remold, 1974) (Fig. 7). The effect of DFP was dose-, time-, and temperature-dependent, i.e., an increase in dose, the incubation time, or the incubation temperature gave increased enhancement of MIF activity. On the other hand, pretreatment of guinea pig MIF itself or serum with DFP (that was then removed by dialysis) did not alter the MIF response (Remold, 1974; David and Becker, 1974). These findings

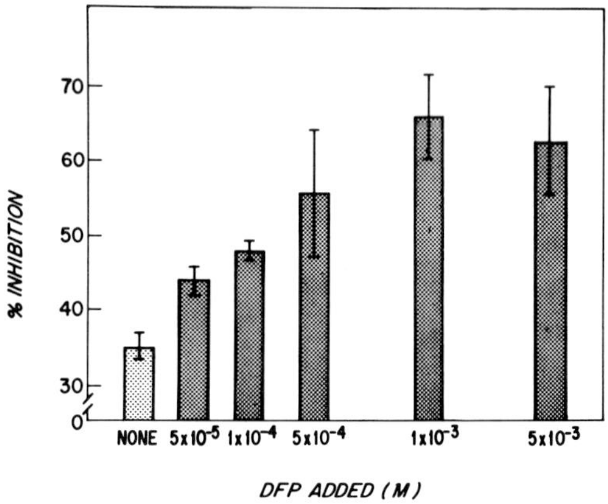

Fig. 7. Effect of DFP on macrophages. Peritoneal exudate cells from strain 13 guinea pigs were incubated with the concentrations of DFP indicated on the abscissa for 1 hour at 37°C, washed, and assayed with 12 μl/ml concentrated MIF or control fraction. The columns represent the mean of three experiments; the standard error is indicated. (From Remold, 1974, with permission from Williams & Wilkins).

suggest that a macrophage-associated esterase inhibits the effect of MIF and that the enzyme is present in the active form. When the esterase is inhibited, the MIF effect is increased.

Recently, experiments were carried out to determine whether plasma esterase inhibitors, which might interact with macrophages *in vivo,* could enhance the activity of MIF (Remold and Rosenberg, 1974, 1975). When guinea pig macrophages were incubated with increasing amounts of α_2-macroglobulin, anti-thrombin-III, α_1-anti-trypsin, or C1 esterase inhibitor, then extensively washed and incubated with subthreshold doses of MIF, a significant enhancement of MIF activity could be observed. It should be noted that the esterase inhibitors themselves were not inhibitory at the concentrations (10–200 μg/ml) used. This effect was specific for plasma esterase inhibitors because incubation of macrophages with a variety of other proteins, such as RNase, myoglobin, IgM, and transferrin, caused no enhancement of MIF activity.

In further experiments, the effect of heparin on the MIF enhancement by anti-thrombin-III was investigated. In previous studies by Rosenberg and Damus (1973), it was shown that addition of heparin to anti-thrombin-III accelerates the action of these inhibitors on thrombin by increasing the rate of formation of the anti-thrombin-III–thrombin complex without influencing its stability, probably by making the active sites more accessible to the active center of the enzyme. Experiments employing anti-thrombin-III in our system demonstrate that the enhancing effects of anti-thrombin-III on MIF activity was not accelerated but was abrogated by the presence of heparin.

In order to explain these results, it was postulated that heparin might compete for a specific macrophage binding site for anti-thrombin-III. It has been shown previously that lysyl residues on anti-thrombin-III are responsible for the heparin binding of this molecule and that this binding site can be abolished by pretreatment with *o*-methylisourea (OMISU), leading to the guanidination of the lysyl groups. Such modified OMISU-anti-thrombin-III was tested in the MIF enhancing system. There was no difference in enhancing activity of unmodified and modified anti-thrombin-III. These experiments showed that guanidination does not affect the enhancing capacity of MIF, suggesting that the effect of heparin is not due to the blocking of a specific receptor on the macrophage but rather most likely to a charge effect; the highly negatively charged heparin–anti-thrombin-III complex might be repelled from the negatively charged macrophage surface.

Studies on the active site of the macrophage-associated esterase were undertaken. A number of experiments suggest that the active site of the macrophage-associated esterase is different from the active site of trypsin or thrombin. When soybean trypsin inhibitor or anti-thrombin-III were treated with 2,3-butanedione, which abolishes the activity of soybean trypsin inhibitor on trypsin and of anti-thrombin-III on thrombin by altering the arginyl residues (Huang and Tang, 1972; Foster and Harrison, 1974) in the active sites, no effect on the MIF enhancing capacity of these inhibitors could be observed. A difference of the active sites of soybean trypsin inhibitor and of anti-thrombin-III affecting the macrophage esterase from that affecting trypsin or thrombin, respectively, is therefore likely, since the specificity of the active site of the esterase is reflected by that of the esterase inhibitors (Laskowski and Sealock, 1971).

Experiments carried out with pure plasma esterase inhibitors, such as anti-thrombin-III, strongly suggest that the macrophage esterase is on the surface of the cell. Such large inhibitors should not get into the cell, and, if they did, they would in all likelihood be broken down. Recent studies further indicate that enzymes on the surface of the macrophage can modulate the cells' response to MIF. These studies employed diazotized sulfanilic acid (DSA), a compound that diazotizes a number of amino acids, especially tyrosine, and which has been used as a cell surface marker (Berg, 1969). Macrophages were incubated for $\frac{1}{2}$ hr at 0°C (to exclude pinocytosis) with various concentrations of DSA and the MIF response determined. These experiments showed that 10^{-4} to 10^{-6} *M* DSA enhanced the response of the macrophage to MIF significantly (H. G. Remold, unpublished results).

Further experiments showed that DSA did indeed only interact with the cell surface and did not enter the cell. The activity of glutamic-oxalacetic transaminase (GOT), a cytoplasmic enzyme that is highly sensitive to DSA because of the presence of tyrosine in its active site (Christen and Riordan, 1970), was monitored. It could be shown that macrophages incubated as above, then washed and homogenized, showed normal GOT activity. However, if DSA was present at the time of homogenization, GOT activity was completely abolished (H. G. Remold, unpublished results). This indicates that at biologically active concentrations DSA does not enter the cell in appreciable amounts, and that its MIF enhancing action on the cells arises from its interacting with the cell surface and not with the internal substances. These experiments taken together strongly point to the existence of enzymes on the macrophage which modulate the cell's response to MIF and may well prove to be the basis of control mechanisms between these mediators and the cell (Fig. 8). Some associated esterases have been involved in the control of several other biological processes, including the chemotaxis of polymorphonuclear leukocytes (Ward and Becker, 1967), the histamine re-

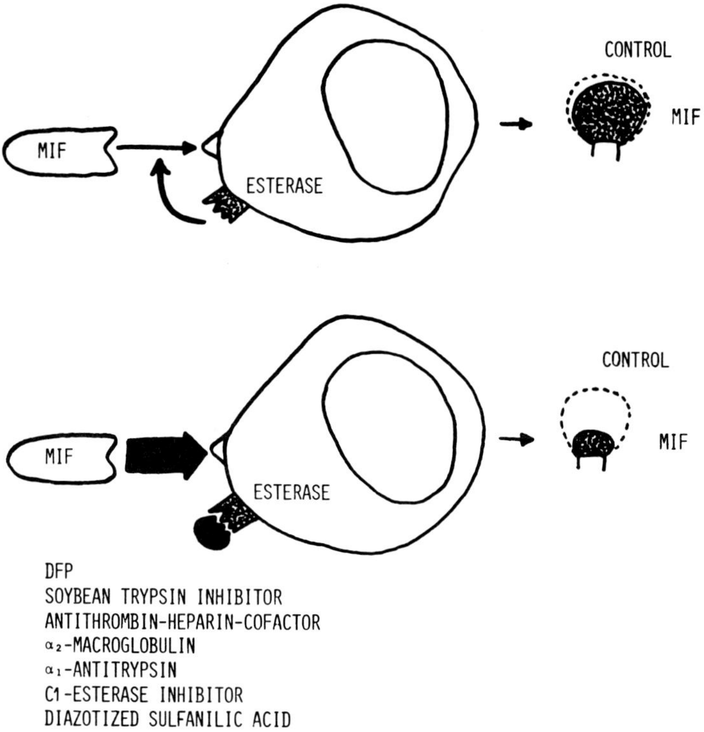

Fig. 8. A model for the action of a macrophage-associated esterase on MIF is shown. When low doses of MIF are used, only minimal inhibition of migration is seen as in the top figure. When the macrophages have been preincubated with a number of esterase inhibitors or with diazotized sulfanilic acid, which alters surface substances, the effect of MIF is marked enhanced as in the lower figure. [From data from Remold (1974), Remold and Rosenberg (1975), and H. G. Remold (unpublished results).]

lease of mast cells (Becker and Austen, 1964), and erythrophagocytosis (Pearlmann *et al.*, 1969).

IV. BIOLOGICALLY ACTIVE SUBSTANCES PRODUCED BY MACROPHAGES

So far we have focused our attention on events that occur when lymphocyte mediators interact with macrophages and the subsequent alterations of the cell's morphology, metabolism, and function. It is important, however, that we not overlook the fact that macrophages can also exert an effect by producing a number of biologically active substances. Although the production, characterization, and action of all these substances will not be reviewed here, it seems pertinent to note a few of them.

Mouse macrophages synthesize and secrete considerable quantities of lysozyme (Gordon *et al.*, 1974a). It is of note, however, that macrophages that have been activated by the *in vivo* injection of thioglycollate do not make much more of this enzyme than normal macrophages. The amount of lysozyme made by macrophages activated by lymphocyte mediators is not known.

Adherent cells obtained from mouse spleen and bone marrow cells, following stimulation with lipopolysaccharide, phytohemaglutinin (PHA), or Con A, produce a macromolecule, termed lymphocyte activating factor (LAF), that potentiates the response of mouse T cells to PHA (Gery and Waksman, 1972). A similar factor has recently been found in media obtained from cultures of mouse macrophages (Calderon and Unanue, 1975). Media obtained from cultures of adherent cells have also been found to have an effect on antibody production and lymphocyte thymidine incorporation (Hoffman and Dutton, 1971; Bach *et al.*, 1970) (see Nelson, Chapter 9). These factors may contribute to the macrophages' role in the induction of a variety of immune responses discussed in detail elsewhere in this volume. In regard to this, it is of interest that macrophages are required for the production of MIF by guinea pig lymphocytes (Nelson and Leu, 1975); the possible role of a macrophage mediator in this case should also be considered.

Activated macrophages, obtained from mice injected with thioglycollate, produce a plasminogen activator *in vitro* (Unkeless *et al.*, 1974), whereas normal macrophages do not. This plasminogen activator has a molecular weight of 48,000–26,000 daltons and thus resembles the enzyme released by virally transformed fibroblasts. Of interest, macrophages obtained from mice that have been injected with lipopolysaccharide produce only one-tenth the plasminogen activator *in vitro* as that made by cells from thioglycollate stimulated mice; however, the endotoxin stimulated cells can be triggered by a phagocytic stimulus to produce large amounts of plasminogen activator (Gordon *et al.*, 1974b). Whether or not this enzyme is also made by macrophages activated by lymphocyte mediators remains to be determined. The production of plasminogen activator may be an important function of the macrophage because this enzyme results in the formation of plasmin, a potent protease. Plasmin plays a part in complement activation and kinin formation and, as has been shown in *in vitro* studies, may influence the properties of other cells (Ossowski *et al.*, 1973). However, because plasminogen can be activated by a variety of nonspecific processes, one wonders whether the activation of plasminogen is the primary physiologic function of the protease synthesized by macrophages. Macrophages can also be induced to produce a number of other biologically active substances, including some that break down collagen (Wahl *et al.*, 1975), kill bacteria (Bast *et al.*, 1974), or lyse cells (Pincus, 1967; Nelson *et al.*, 1974). Undoubtedly there should be considerable progress in the next few years in the enumeration and characterization of biologically active substances produced by macrophages and the assessment of their part in reactions of immunity and hypersensitivity.

V. CONCLUSION

The studies that have been discussed here indicate that lymphocyte mediators play a significant role in the activation of macrophages. Such activated macrophages exhibit a number of functional changes when compared to their normal counterparts, many of which are reflected in alteration of the macrophage plasma membrane. Such cells exhibit enhanced bacteriostasis and tumoricidal capacity as well as the production and secretion of biologically active substances. In certain circumstances, such activated macrophages demonstrate a nonspecific increase in ability to handle microorganisms and tumor cells; in others there appears to be a specificity requirement between the antigen sensitivity of the lymphocyte used to produce the mediator and the action of the macrophage on the microorganism or tumor cell. Thus, several different mechanisms and different mediators appear to be involved.

Studies on the action of one mediator, MIF, indicate that carbohydrate groups are crucial in its interaction with macrophages. Furthermore, enzymes on the surface of the macrophage are capable of modulating the macrophage response to this lymphocyte mediator. Hopefully, further study of such control mechanisms will provide better understanding of the fascinating interrelationships between lymphocytes, mediators, and macrophages.

ACKNOWLEDGMENT

Research supported by United States Public Health Service Grants AI 07685, AI 10921, AI 12110, RR 05669, and Contract NIH-NOI-CB 33896.

REFERENCES

Altman, L. C., Snyderman, R., and Oppenheim, J. J. (1973). *J. Immunol.* **110,** 801–810.

Anderson, S. E., and Remington, J. S. (1974). *J. Exp. Med.* **139,** 1154–1174.

Atkinson, P. H., and Summers, D. F. (1971). *J. Biol. Chem.* **246,** 5162–5175.

Bach, F. H., Alter, B. J., Solliday, S., Zoschke, D. S., and Janis, M. (1970). *Cell. Immunol.* **1,** 219–227.

Bartfeld, H., and Atoynatan, T. (1969). *Proc. Soc. Exp. Biol. Med.* **130,** 497–501.
Bast, R., Cleveland, R., Littman, B., Zbar, B., and Rapp, H. (1974). *Cell. Immunol.* **10,** 248–259.
Becker, E. L., and Austen, K. F. (1964). *J. Exp. Med.* **120,** 491–506.
Berg, H. C. (1969). *Biochim. Biophys. Acta* **183,** 65–78.
Bloom, B. R., and Bennett, B. (1966). *Science* **153,** 80–82.
Borges, J. S., and Johnson, W. D. (1975). *J. Exp. Med.* **141,** 483–496.
Calderon, J., and Unanue, E. (1975). *Nature (London)* **253,** 359–361.
Carlsen, R. B., and Pierce, J. G. (1972). *J. Biol. Chem.* **247,** 23–32.
Christen, P., and Riordan, J. F. (1970). *Biochemistry* **15,** 3025–3034.
Churchill, W. H., Piessens, W. F., Sulis, C. A., and David, J. R. (1975). *Fed. Proc., Fed. Amer. Soc. Exp. Biol.* **34,** 991 (abstr.).
Cox, R. P., and Gesner, B. M. (1965). *Proc. Nat. Acad. Sci. U.S.* **54,** 1571–1579
Coyne, J. A., Remold, H. G., Rosenberg, S. A., and David, J. R. (1973). *J. Immunol.* **110,** 1630–1637.
David, J. R. (1966). *Proc. Nat. Acad. Sci. U.S.* **56,** 72–77.
David J. R. (1971). *Fed. Proc., Fed. Amer. Soc. Exp. Biol.* **30,** 1730.
David, J. R., and Becker, E. L. (1974). *Eur. J. Immunol.* **4,** 287–289.
David, J. R., and David, R. A. (1972). *Progr. Allergy* **16,** 300–449.
David, J. R., and Haber, E. (1969). *In* "Cellular Recognition. 4th Developmental Workshop 1968," (R. I. Smith and R. A. Good, eds.), pp. 227–227. Appleton, New York.
David, J. R., Lawrence, H. S., and Thomas, L. (1964). *J. Exp. Med.* **120,** 1189–1200.
Dumonde, D. C., Wolstencroft, R. A., Panayi, G. S., Matthew, M., Morley, J., and Howson, W. T. (1969). *Nature (London)* **224,** 38–42.
Dvorak, A. M., Hammond, M. E., Dvorak, H. F., and Karnovsky, M. J. (1972). *Lab. Invest.* **27,** 561–574.
Evans, R., Grant, C. K., Cox, H., Steele, K., and Alexander, P. (1972). *J. Exp. Med.* **136,** 1318–1322.
Evans, R., Cox, H., and Alexander, P. (1973). *Proc. Soc. Exp. Biol. Med.* **143,** 256–259.
Fauve, R. M., and Dekaris, D. (1968). *Science* **160,** 795–796.
Foster, M. C., and Harrison, J. H. (1974). *Biochem. Biophys. Res. Commun.* **58,** 263–267.
Fowles, R. E., Fajardo, I. M., Leibowitch, J. L., and David, J. R. (1973). *J. Exp. Med.* **138,** 952–964.
Fox, R. A., and MacSween, I. M. (1974). *Immunol. Commun.* **3,** 375–389.
Fox, R. A., Gregory, D. S., and Feldman, J. D. (1974). *J. Immunol.* **112,** 1867–1872.
Gery, I., and Waksman, B. H. (1972). *J. Exp. Med.* **136,** 143–155.
Godal, T., Rees, R. J. W., and Lamvik, J. O. (1971). *Clin Exp. Immunol.* **8,** 625–637.
Gordon, S., Todd, J., and Cohn, L. (1974a). *J. Exp. Med.* **139,** 1228–1248.
Gordon, S., Unkeless, J. C., and Cohn, Z. A. (1974b). *J. Exp. Med.* **140,** 995–1010.
Hammond, M. E., and Dvorak, H. F. (1972). *J. Exp. Med.* **136,** 1518–1532.
Hibbs, J. B. (1972). *Science* **180,** 868–870.
Hibbs, J. B., Lambert, L. H., and Remington, J. S. (1972). *Science* **177,** 998–1000.
Hoff, R. (1975). *J. Exp. Med.* **142,** 299–311.
Hoffman, M., and Dutton, R. W. (1971). *Science* **172,** 1047–1048.
Huang, W. Y., and Tang, J. (1972). *J. Biol. Chem.* **247,** 2704–2710.
Kolb, W. P., and Granger, G. A. (1968). *Proc. Nat. Acad. Sci. U.S.* **61,** 1250–1255.
Kramer, P. M. (1971). *In* "Biomembranes" (L. A. Monson, ed.). Vol. I, pp. 67–190. Plenun, New York.

Krahenbuhl, J. L., and Remington, J. S. (1971). *Infec. Immunity* **4,** 337–343.

Krahenbuhl, J. L., Rosenberg, L. T., and Remington, J. S. (1973). *J. Immunol.* **111,** 992–995.

Lane, F. C., and Unanue, E. R. (1972). *J. Exp. Med.* **135,** 1104–1112.

Laskowski, M., Jr., and Sealock, R. W. *In* "The Enzymes" (P. D. Boyer, ed.), 3rd ed., Vol. 3, Academic Press, New York.

Leibowitch, J. L., and David, J. R. (1973). *Ann. Immunol. Inst. Pasteur* **124c,** 441–464.

Leu, R. W., Eddeston, A. L. W. F., Hadden, J. W., and Good, R. A. (1972). *J. Exp. Med.* **136,** 589–603.

Lipsky, P. E., and Rosenthal, A. S. (1973). *J. Exp. Med.* **138,** 900–924.

Lloyd, K. O., Kabat, E. A., and Licerio, E. (1968). *Biochemistry* **7,** 2976–2990.

Lohmann-Matthes, M. L., Ziegler, F. G., and Fischer, H. (1973). *Eur. J. Immunol.* **3,** 56–58.

Lurie, M. B. (1964). "Resistance to Tuberculosis: Experimental Studies in Native and Acquired Defensive Mechanisms." Harvard Univ. Press, Cambridge, Massachusetts.

McFarland, W., Heilman, D. H., and Moorhead, J. R. (1966). *J. Exp. Med.* **124,** 851–857.

Mackaness, G. B. (1964). *J. Exp. Med.* **120,** 105–120.

Mackaness, G. B. (1969). *J. Exp. Med.* **129,** 973–992.

Mackaness, G. B. (1970). *In* "Infectious Agents and Host Reactions" (S. Mudd, ed.). pp. 62–75. Saunders, Philadelphia, Pennsylvania.

Meade, C. J., Lachmann, P. J., and Brenner, S. (1974). *Immunology* **27,** 227–239.

Melsom, H., Kearny, G., Gruca, S., and Seljelid, R. (1974). *J. Exp. Med.* **140,** 1085–1096.

Metchnikoff, E. (1905). "Immunity in Infective Disease." Cambridge Univ. Press, London and New York.

Mooney, J. J., and Waksman, B. H. (1970). *J. Immunol.* **105,** 1138–1145.

Nathan, C. F., Karnovsky, M. L., and David, J. R. (1971). *J. Exp. Med.* **133,** 1356–1376.

Nathan, C. F., Remold, H. G., and David, J. R. (1973). *J. Exp. Med.* **137,** 275–290.

Nelson, R. D., and Leu, R. W. (1975). *J. Immunol.* **114,** 606–609.

Neta, R., and Salvin, S. B. (1971). *Infec. Immunity* **4,** 697–702.

Ossowski, L., Quigley, J. P., Kellerman, G. M., and Reich, E. (1973). *J. Exp. Med.* **138,** 1056–1064.

Patterson, R. J., and Youmans, G. P. (1970). *Infec. Immunity* **1,** 600–603.

Pearlmann, D. S., Ward, P. A., and Becker, E. L. (1969). *J. Exp. Med.* **130,** 745–764.

Pels, E., and Den Otter, W. (1974). *Cancer Res.* **34,** 3089–3094.

Piessens, W. F., Churchill, W. H., and David, J. R. (1975). *J. Immunol.* **114,** 293–299.

Pincus, W. B. (1967). *Res. J. Reticuloendothel. Soc.* **4,** 122–139.

Remold, H. G. (1972). *Transplant. Rev.* **10,** 152–176.

Remold, H. G. (1973). *J. Exp. Med.* **138,** 1065–1076.

Remold, H. G. (1974). *J. Immunol.* **112,** 1571–1577.

Remold, H. G., and David, J. R. (1971). *J. Immunol.* **107,** 1090–1098.

Remold, H. G., and Mednis, A. (1972). *Fed. Proc., Fed. Amer. Soc. Exp. Biol.* **31,** 753 (abstr.).

Remold, H. G., and Rosenberg, R. D. (1974). *Fed. Proc., Fed. Amer. Soc. Exp. Biol.* **33,** 745 (abstr.).

Remold, H. G., and Rosenberg, R. D. (1975). *J. Biol. Chem.* (in press).

Remold, H. G., Katz, A. B., Haber, E., and David, J. R. (1970). *Cell. Immunol.* **1,** 133–145.

Remold, H. G., David, R. A., and David, J. R. (1972). *J. Immunol.* **109,** 578–586.

Remold-O'Donnell, E., and Remold, H. G. (1974). *J. Biol. Chem.* **249,** 3622–3627.

Rocklin, R. E. (1974). *J. Immunol.* **112,** 1461–1466.

Rocklin, R. E., Winston, C. T., and David, J. R. (1974). *J. Clin. Invest.* **53,** 559–564.

Rosenberg, R. D., and Damus, P. S. (1973). *J. Biol. Chem.* **248,** 6490–6505.

Salvin, S. B., Sell, S., and Nishio, J. (1971). *J. Immunol.* **107,** 655–662.

Schoenberg, M. D., Mumaw, V. R., Moore, R. D., and Weisberger, A. S. (1964). *Science* **143,** 964–965.

Sharp, J. A., and Burwell, R. G. (1960). *Nature (London)* **188,** 474–475.

Simon, H. B., and Sheagren, J. N. (1971). *J. Exp. Med.* **133,** 1371–1389.

Simon, H. B., and Sheagren, J. N. (1972). *Cell. Immunol.* **4,** 163–174.

So, L. L., and Goldstein, I. L. (1968). *J. Biol. Chem.* **243,** 2003–2008.

Suter, E., and Ramseier, H. (1964). *Advan. Immunol.* **4,** 117–173.

Unkeless, J., Gordon, S., and Reich, E. (1974). *J. Exp. Med.* **139,** 834–850.

Wahl, L. M., Wahl, S. M., Mergenhagen, S. E., and Martin, G. R. (1975). *Science* **187,** 261–262.

Ward, P. A., and Becker, E. L. (1967). *J. Exp. Med.* **125,** 1001–1020.

Ward, P. A., Remold, H. G., and David, J. R. (1972). *Cell. Immunol.* **1,** 162–174.

17

Secretion of Macrophage Enzymes in Relation to the Pathogenesis of Chronic Inflammation

Philip Davies and Anthony C. Allison

I. Introduction 428
II. The Origin and Turnover of Cells in Sites of Chronic Inflammation 428
III. *In Vitro* Studies on the Role of Macrophages in Chronic Inflammation 430
A. The Secretion of Hydrolytic Enzymes by Macrophages 433
B. The Selective Release of Acid Hydrolases by Macrophages 435
C. The Direct Interaction of Substances with Macrophages to Cause Chronic Inflammation of a Nonimmunological Nature 438
D. The Release of Macrophage Lysosomal Enzymes by Products of Immune Reactions 443
E. Secretion of Neutral Proteinases by Macrophages 445
F. Secretion of Lysozyme by Macrophages 447
IV. What Is the Contribution of Hydrolytic Enzyme Secretion to Chronic Inflammation? 448
V. Other Products of Macrophages 451
A. The Secretion of Pyrogen by Macrophages 451
B. The Secretion of Prostaglandins by Macrophages 451
C. The Generation of Inflammatory Mediators by Secretory Products of Macrophages 453
VI. Interactions and Modulating Factors 454
A. Factors Produced during Acute Exacerbations of Chronic Inflammation Which May Influence Macrophage Function 454

B. The Interaction of Macrophages and Fibroblasts at Sites of Chronic Inflammation 455
C. Pharmacological Modification of Macrophages at Sites of Chronic Inflammation 456
References 457

I. INTRODUCTION

Although chronic inflammatory lesions are heterogeneous, we have presented evidence that macrophages always play an essential role in their pathogenesis (Allison and Davies, 1974). Macrophages can interact with at least four other cell types in the generation of chronic inflammatory lesions: T lymphocytes, B lymphocytes, K cells (antibody-dependent cytotoxic cells), and fibroblasts. In addition polymorphonuclear leukocytes, blood platelets, and basophils may influence the function of macrophages during the initiation or in acute exacerbations of chronic inflammatory lesions. The relative prominence of each cell type varies in different types of chronic inflammation, and interactions between the cells are still poorly understood.

Chronic inflammatory lesions may arise by the direct interaction of the inflammatory agent with macrophages or, more often, after an immunological response involving either or both T and B cells. The participation of lymphocytes, K cells, and fibroblasts in chronic inflammation has been discussed elsewhere (Allison and Davies, 1974). Here we limit discussion to direct effects of agents inducing inflammation on macrophages and ways in which products of lymphocytes may stimulate macrophages to release mediators relevant to the pathogenesis of chronic inflammation. Also discussed are recent observations on how the products of stimulated macrophages may affect the function of lymphocytes and fibroblasts.

Macrophages are usually thought of as phagocytic cells, the enzymes of which act within the cells. However, research carried out during the past few years has established that macrophages have major secretory functions. In addition to substantial amounts of hydrolytic enzymes, macrophages secrete biologically active products whose chemical nature is still poorly defined. Some of the secretory products, e.g., lysozyme, can be described as constitutive, whereas others are secreted only when the macrophages have been suitably stimulated.

II. THE ORIGIN AND TURNOVER OF CELLS IN SITES OF CHRONIC INFLAMMATION

From observations of [^{3}H]thymidine and carbon labeling, Spector *et al.* (1965) concluled that nearly all the mononuclear cells in inflammatory reactions are derived from blood monocytes, which show a high rate of DNA synthesis. Volkman and Gowans (1965) found that after injection of [^{3}H]thymidine-labeled bone marrow cells, labeled mononuclear cells appear in impressions of damaged skin, whereas this did not occur after injection of labeled lymphocytes. Similar results have been obtained in the more complex types of inflammation induced by Freund's complete and incomplete adjuvants (Spector and Willoughby, 1968).

Chronic inflammatory reactions are maintained by sustained migration of mononuclear phagocytes, mitotic division of macrophages in lesions, and the long life span of the cells. The relative importance of these mechanisms varies in granulomas induced by different agents. A measure of turnover rate is obtained by prelabeling an animal's leukocytes with [^{3}H]thymidine before the onset of inflammation. The macrophages in the lesion initially show a high proportion of labeled cells; the rate at which this figure declines reflects the entry of unlabeled cells into the lesion. In most granulomas this decline is fairly rapid, but the fall after carrageenan administration is much slower (Ryan and Spector, 1969). The entry of freshly labeled transferred leukocytes is rapid into high turnover lesions, such as induced by *Bacillus pertussis* vaccine or Freund's incomplete adjuvant, but slow in low turnover reactions due to carrageenan.

Another way to estimate the dependence of a granuloma on a regular supply of circulating cells is to destroy the source of these cells by radiation of the bone marrow, while preserving the mitotic activity in the granulomas by shielding. High turnover granulomas induced by *B. pertussis* or BCG are rapidly depleted of cells, while the carrageenan granuloma is barely affected (Ryan and Spector, 1970).

Division of mononuclear phagocytes can be measured by counting the cells in a granuloma with nuclei labeled after a single pulse of [^{3}H]thymidine. The uptake of a pulse of labeled thymidine is greater in high turnover granulomas than in those with low turnover (Ryan and Spector, 1969). Some of the [^{3}H]thymidine incorporation is local; normally about 4% of macrophages on subcutaneous coverslips incorporate a single pulse of label, whereas when separated from a fresh supply of immigrating cells, 25% of macrophages incorporate label in a 30 minute period.

Macrophage populations that normally undergo little division, e.g., from the peritoneum, multiply freely when transferred to an inflammatory environment (Ryan and Spector, 1970). In lesions with very high turnover rates, e.g., the *B. pertussis* granuloma, nearly all the cells incorporating thymidine are new arrivals, whereas in carrageenan granulomas most are long established residents. Such granulomas contain cells labeled by a single pulse of thymidine several weeks beforehand, indicating their longevity. Some macrophages remain in such lesions for months, dividing infrequently and incorporating [^{3}H]uridine into nuclear and cytoplasmic RNA (Ryan and Spector, 1969).

The factors favoring chronicity of inflammatory lesions are not fully understood. One factor is certainly the persistence, often within cells, of the agent inducing the response (see Spector *et al.*, 1968; Page *et al.*, 1974a,b). Quantitative analysis of the degradation of bacteria not inducing granulomas shows that they are completely broken down and eliminated, whereas granuloma-inducing bacteria are not (Spector *et al.*, 1970).

Considering immunological mechanisms, equivalence of antibody with antigen in the formation of immune complexes leads to granuloma formation as opposed to transient inflammation (Spector and Heesom, 1969). Cell-mediated immune responses probably contribute to some types of granuloma formation, but a range of experimental granulomas develop normally or in a quantitatively modified form in thymectomized animals (Rothwell and Spector, 1972).

From observations of skin coverslips and cells in diffusion chambers incorporating [^{3}H]thymidine, Mariano and Spector (1974) concluded that inflammatory giant cells are formed by fusion of newly arrived macrophages with macrophages already *in situ*, many of which are dividing.

III. *IN VITRO* STUDIES ON THE ROLE OF MACROPHAGES IN CHRONIC INFLAMMATION

Macrophages were one of the first cell types to be established in primary culture (Carrel and Ebeling, 1926), and subsequently such cultures have been used for the study of a wide variety of phenomena in cell biology (for review, see Gordon and Cohn, 1973). After their release from bone marrow, macrophages still retain considerable capacity for protein synthesis and metabolic and functional plasticity. They show a wide variety of biochemical and functional responses to different stimuli (Table I) when cultured *in vitro*. The use of terms such as activation and stimulation for these different processes has caused semantic confusion, and we suggest that such terms should only be used with reference to a specified stimulus and the response to it. The definition of biochemical responses accompanying functional responses and vice versa will also clarify the ways in which macrophages respond to different stimuli.

However, little attention has been paid to their interaction with substances that induce, or are associated with, chronic inflammatory lesions. We would like to suggest that this is explained in part by the activity of macrophages as secretory cells, a function that would be difficult to

TABLE I

Some in Vitro Biochemical and Functional Responses of Macrophages

Stimulus	Biochemical responses	Reference
Phagocytosis; products of activated lymphocytes (cell-mediated immunity)	Increased metabolism by the hexose monophosphate pathway	Karnovsky *et al.* (1970) Nathan *et al.* (1971)
Phagocytosis or pinocytosis of degradable substrates	Transient increase in lysosomal enzyme levels	Axline and Cohn (1970)
Anti-cellular antibody (bovine serum, pinocytosis)	Prolonged increase in lysosomal enzyme levels	Cohn (1970)
Phagocytosis or pinocytosis of nondegradable substrates	Increased cholesterol and phospholipid synthesis	Werb and Cohn (1971)
Nondigestible streptococcal cell walls, immune complexes	Increased cellular levels of lysosomal and cytoplasmic enzymes, selective exocytosis of lysosomal hydrolases	Davies *et al.* (1974a) Cardella *et al.* (1974)
Phagocytosis by macrophages from mice stimulated by thioglycolate and other agents	Secretion of plasminogen activator	Gordon *et al.* (1974a)
Endotoxin	Secretion of collagenase	Wahl *et al.* (1974)
Endotoxin	Secretion of pyrogen	Bodell (1974)
Phagocytosis	Secretion of pyrogen	Denarillo *et al.* (1974)
Hydrocortisone	Induction of haemoxygenase	Gemsa *et al.* (1973)
Growth in conditioned medium, transformation by SV40	DNA synthesis, mitosis	Mauel and Defendi (1971a,b)

Stimulus	Functional responses	Reference
Anti-cellular antibody (bovine serum), polyanions	Increased macropinocytosis and lysosome formation	Cohn (1970)
Pinocytosis of nondegradable substrates	Accumulation of secondary lysosomes	Cohn (1970)
Macrophages from infected animals (cell-mediated immunity)	Increased adhesion, spreading, phagocytosis, motility, killing of *Listeria*, nonspecific killing of tumor cells	Mackaness (1970) Stubbs *et al.* (1973) Hibbs *et al.* (1972)
Products of activated lymphocytes (cell-mediated immunity)	Increased adhesion, spreading, motility, phagocytosis	Nathan *et al.* (1971)
Products of lymphocytes + antigen (arming factors)	Inhibition of tumor cell growth	Evans and Alexander (1970)
In vitro stimulation with endotoxin or double-stranded RNA	Inhibition of tumor cell growth	Alexander and Evans (1971)
In vivo peptone injections or worm infestation; culture *in vitro*	Inhibition of tumor cell growth	Keller (1973)
Culture *in vitro*	Acquisition of capacity to lyse erythrocytes by contact	Melsom and Seljelid (1973)

TABLE II

Biologically Active Secretory Products of Macrophages

Product	Source	Stimulus for production or release	Reference
Lysosomal hydrolases	Mouse peritoneal	Zymosan	Weissman *et al.* (1971a)
	Mouse peritoneal	Dental plaque	Page *et al.* (1973)
	Mouse peritoneal	Group A streptococcal cell walls	Page *et al.* (1974a) Davies *et al.* (1974a)
	Mouse peritoneal	Immune complexes	Cardella *et al.* (1974)
	Mouse peritoneal	Asbestos	Davies *et al.* (1974b)
	Guinea pig alveolar	Zymosan	Ackerman and Beebe (1974)
	Mouse peritoneal	Human lymphocyte activation products	Pantalone and Page (1975)
	Mouse peritoneal	Carrageenan	Davies *et al.* (1975)
Plasminogen activator	Mouse peritoneal	Thioglycolate *in vivo*	Gordon *et al.* (1974a)
	Human peripheral blood monocytes	Phagocytosis *in vitro*	Unkeless *et al.* (1974)
Collagenase	Guinea pig peritoneal	Endotoxin	Wahl *et al.* (1974)
Lysozyme	Mouse peritoneal	None	Gordon *et al.* (1974b)
	Human peripheral blood monocytes	None	
Pyrogen	Human peripheral blood monocytes	Endotoxin	Bodell (1974)
	Human peripheral blood monocytes	Phagocytosis	Denarillo *et al.* (1974)
Prostaglandins	Guinea pig peritoneal macrophages	Lymphocyte activation products	Bray *et al.* (1974)
Colony stimulating factor	Human peripheral blood monocytes	None	Chervenick and LoBuglio (1972)
	Human peripheral blood monocytes	Endotoxin	Eaves and Bruce (1974)
	Human peripheral blood monocytes	Polyinosinic–polycytidylic acid	Ruscetti and Chervenick (1974)
Cytolytic factor for syngeneic and for allogeneic erythrocytes	Mouse peritoneal	Culture *in vitro*	Melsom and Seljelid (1973)
Stimulant of T cell response to mitogen	Human peripheral blood monocytes and other macrophages	Endotoxin	Gery and Waksman (1972)
Stimulant of antibody production by B cells in nu/nu mice	Peritoneal macrophages of nu/nu mice	Proteose peptone *in vivo*	Schrader (1973)
Stimulant of antibody production by B cells in mice	Human peripheral blood leucocytes	None	Wood and Gaul (1974)
Inhibitor of lymphocyte transformation	Mouse peritoneal macrophages	*In vivo* endotoxin	Nelson (1973)
Inhibitor of fibroblast proliferation	Mouse peritoneal macrophages		Calderon *et al.* (1974)
Stimulant of polymorph migration	Human peripheral blood monocytes	Hydrocortisone	Stevenson (1974)

demonstrate *in vivo*. It has become increasingly clear in recent years that macrophages secrete many products *in vitro* (see Table II). Several of these products have been discussed in detail in other chapters and will not be mentioned further here. The release of these products has been observed under a wide variety of conditions, but only a few studies of secretion induced by substances associated with chronic inflammation have been carried out.

A. The Secretion of Hydrolytic Enzymes by Macrophages

Secretion of hydrolytic enzymes by macrophages can account for extensive tissue damage during chronic inflammation (see Table III). These enzymes can be divided into at least three classes, defined by the conditions under which release occurs.

1. Acid Hydrolases

Acid hydrolases are rapidly released in large amounts when macrophages are exposed to substances known to induce chronic inflammation. This is not a general response of macrophages to extracellular substances (Davies *et al.,* 1974a). The endocytosis of digestible substrates and those that are biologically unreactive does not result in selective extracellular release of acid hydrolases. Enzymes secreted in this way are almost certainly derived from a performed store contained in lysosomes. Studies with Group A streptococcal cells walls (Davies *et al.,* 1974a) and dental plaque (Page *et al.,* 1973) have shown, however, that lysosomal enzyme release continues for up to 72 hours after exposure to the stimulating agent, suggesting that at least some of this enzyme is newly synthesized. This possibility is supported by observations that higher levels of acid hydrolases are seen in cultures exposed to stimulating agents for 72 hours than in control cultures (Page *et al.,* 1973; Davies *et al.,* 1974a).

2. Neutral Proteinases

The recent studies of Gordon and his colleagues have demonstrated the ability of macrophages to secrete several neutral proteinases that may play an important role in both the destructive and reparative phases of the chronic inflammatory process. The enzymes include plasminogen activator (Unkeless *et al.,* 1974; Gordon *et al.,* 1974a), collagenase, and elastase (S. Gordon, personal communication, 1974). In addition Wahl *et al.* (1974) have shown that the secretion of collagenase from guinea pig peritoneal macrophages can be induced by either endotoxin or the prod-

TABLE III

Degradation of Tissue Components by Hydrolytic Enzymes Occurring in Macrophages

Enzyme	Enzyme source	Tissue component	Reference	Identification in macrophages
Acid hydrolases				
Cathepsin B1	Liver	Collagen	Burleigh (1973)	C. Finlay, P. Davies, and A. C. Allison (unpublished observations)
	Liver	Proteoglycan	Morrison *et al.* (1973)	
Cathepsin C	Liver	Hormones	McDonald *et al.* (1971)	C. Finlay, P. Davies, and A. C. Allison (unpublished observations)
Cathepsin D	Polymorphonuclear	Basement membranes	Cochrane and Aikin (1966)	Cohn and Wiener (1963)
	Liver	Proteoglycan	Barrett (1969)	
	Spleen	Thyroglobulin	Weigle *et al.* (1969)	
Acid proteinase (probably cathepsin D)	Spleen, inflammed synovium	Immunoglobulin	Fehr *et al.* (1970)	
	Rabbit peritoneal and pulmonary macrophages	C5	Snyderman *et al.* (1972)	
Hyaluronidase	Liver	Proteoglycan	Weissmann and Spilberg (1968)	Goggins *et al.* (1968)
Neutral proteinases				
Collagenase	Polymorphonuclear leukocyte	Collagen	Lazarus *et al.* (1968)	Wahl *et al.* (1974)
Elastase	Polymorphonuclear leukocytes	Elastin, proteoglycan	Janoff and Zeligs (1968)	Janoff (1972)
Plasminogen activator	Macrophages	Plasminogen		Unkeless *et al.* (1974)

ucts of stimulated T lymphocytes. The factors promoting the secretion of these enzymes will be discussed in detail below, but it is already clear (P. Davies and A. C. Allison, unpublished observations) that these enzymes are not secreted under conditions in which lysosomal acid hydrolases are released after exposure of macrophages to some chronic inflammatory stimuli.

3. *Lysozyme*

Lysozyme is secreted constantly by macrophages regardless of the culture conditions (Gordon *et al.*, 1974b) (see Section III,F).

B. The Selective Release of Acid Hydrolases by Macrophages

Acid hydrolases stored in the lysosomes of macrophages may contribute to tissue damage at sites of chronic inflammation. Cohn and Wiener (1963) established that acid hydrolases are present in macrophage lysosomes, and it is now clear that a wide range of these enzymes are present in lysosomes at high specific activity (Table III). Before describing *in vitro* studies on the release of acid hydrolases by inflammatory stimuli, it is relevant to mention the behavior of macrophages cultured *in vitro* and their responses to various substances.

The capacity of mononuclear phagocytes to undergo marked morphological changes both *in vivo* (Ebert and Florey, 1939) and during *in vitro* culture (Lewis, 1925; Carrel and Ebeling, 1926; Weiss and Fawcett, 1953) is well established. Biochemical studies of three different types of mononuclear phagocytes indicated that levels of cellular protein and enzymes varied considerably, depending on their site of origin and the stimuli to which they had been exposed *in vivo* (Cohn and Wiener, 1963; Cohn and Benson, 1965; Saito and Suter, 1965). Subsequently Cohn and his collaborators established optimal conditions for the culture of mouse peritoneal macrophages (Cohn and Benson, 1965) and carried out extensive studies on the properties of these cells *in vitro* (for reviews, see Cohn, 1968, 1970; Gordon and Cohn, 1973). It is clear that although they rarely undergo mitosis, macrophages synthesize large amounts of protein.

Moreover, the levels of cellular constituents are very responsive to changes in the extracellular environment. Macrophages cultured in the presence of high concentrations of newborn calf serum show striking increases in the levels of various cellular constituents, with lysosomal enzyme levels showing the most dramatic increases. These increases were associated with the formation of many pinosomes that accumulated within the macrophages (Cohn, 1966). It was later found that the stimulation of pinocytosis was due to activity of a macroglobulin, normally present in newborn calf serum, with activity against surface components of the macrophage and other murine cells (Cohn and Parks, 1967). Subsequent studies showed that many anionic substances, including some proteins, polypeptides, polysaccharides, nucleic acids, and nucleotides, also stimulate the accumulation of pinocytic vesicles in macrophages. It is not known what biochemical changes occur in cells after stimulation of pinocytosis by these substances. Recent studies in our laboratory, using radioactive colloidal gold as a marker of pinocytosis, have shown the majority of the pinocytic activity of macrophages to occur by the formation of small vesicles not visible by light microscopy. Unlike macropinocytosis, this process is insensitive to the effect of cytochalasin B (Allison *et al.*, 1971; Wills *et al.*, 1972) and inhibitors of oxidative phosphorylation (Allison and Davies, 1975).

Although the association remains to be proved definitively, it seems that the stimulation of macrophage pinocytosis by high levels of newborn calf serum is the cause of the increased levels of lysosomal enzymes seen in these cells. This is thought to result from the formation of a large number of secondary lysosomes and digestion of ingested substrates, stimulating the formation of further primary lysosomes. Similarly, the phagocytosis of digestible substances, such as sheep red blood cells and aggregated γ-globulin, induces an increase in the levels of lysosomal enzymes in macrophages. Axline and Cohn (1970) reported that the ingestion of nondigestible particles did not result in any increase in lysosomal enzyme levels, although Cohn and Ehrenreich (1969) had stated earlier that the accumulation of nondigestible sugars such as sucrose also resulted in higher cellular levels of lysosomal enzymes. Regardless of the effect of these substances on intracellular levels of acid hydrolases, there was no extracellular release of acid hydrolases from cells either during or after their uptake. It is to be noted, however, that none of the substances used by this group have been shown to induce chronic inflammatory lesions after administration *in vivo*.

Weissmann *et al.* (1971a) investigated the phenomenon of selective release of acid hydrolases from polymorphonuclear leukocytes and macrophages during the phagocytosis of zymosan. They found release of lysosomal enzymes from both cell types without any change in cell viability as determined by dye exclusion tests and cytoplasmic enzyme determinations. On the other hand, they showed that endocytosis of sheep red blood cells did not induce selective release of acid hydrolases from macrophages. It is notable that zymosan contains glucans with marked inflammatory activity (McCandless, 1965), but it is not known whether these are responsible for the selective release of acid hydrolases.

As we have already described, it is clear that many macrophages are present in chronic inflammatory lesions of both nonimmunological and immunological origin. We and others have, therefore, investigated the effects of nonimmunogenic materials eliciting chronic inflammation and certain lymphocyte products on macrophages cultured *in vitro,* paying particular attention to the behavior of the lysosomal system. Our findings show that several substances with a recognized capacity to cause chronic inflammation induce the selective release of lysosomal enzymes from mouse peritoneal macrophages *in vitro.* The cells that respond in this way remain viable, as determined by several different criteria, so that enzyme release continues over prolonged periods. The mechanism by which these agents release acid hydrolases is not known. It is possible that their interaction with the macrophage results in the generation of mediators, such as cleavage products of complement components (Goldstein and Weissmann, 1974), with the capacity to induce selective release of acid hydrolases. In marked contrast, inert substances do not cause the release of lysosomal enzymes so that there is a correlation between the capacity of substances to cause chronic inflammation and to induce release of lysosomal enzymes from macrophages in culture.

This information leads us to suggest that the release of acid hydrolases from macrophages may mediate tissue damage in chronic inflammatory lesions of both immunological and nonimmunological origin, as outlined schematically in Figs. 1 and 2. Furthermore, the interactions of inflammatory substances with macrophages or lymphocytes may also lead to the release of neutral proteinases. Indeed, Wahl *et al.* (1974) have already shown that both endotoxin and lymphocyte activation products stimulate the synthesis and release of collagenase by macrophages, while Gordon *et al.* (1974a) have shown that macrophages stimulated *in vivo* by inflammatory agents secrete plasminogen activator when cultured *in vitro.*

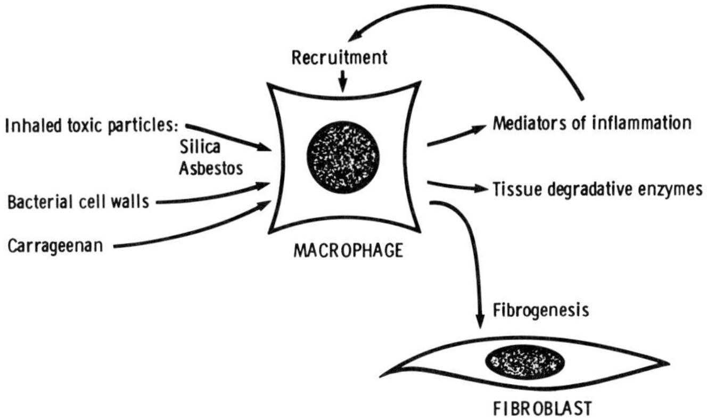

Fig. 1. Schematic representation of the direct effects of inflammatory materials on macrophages.

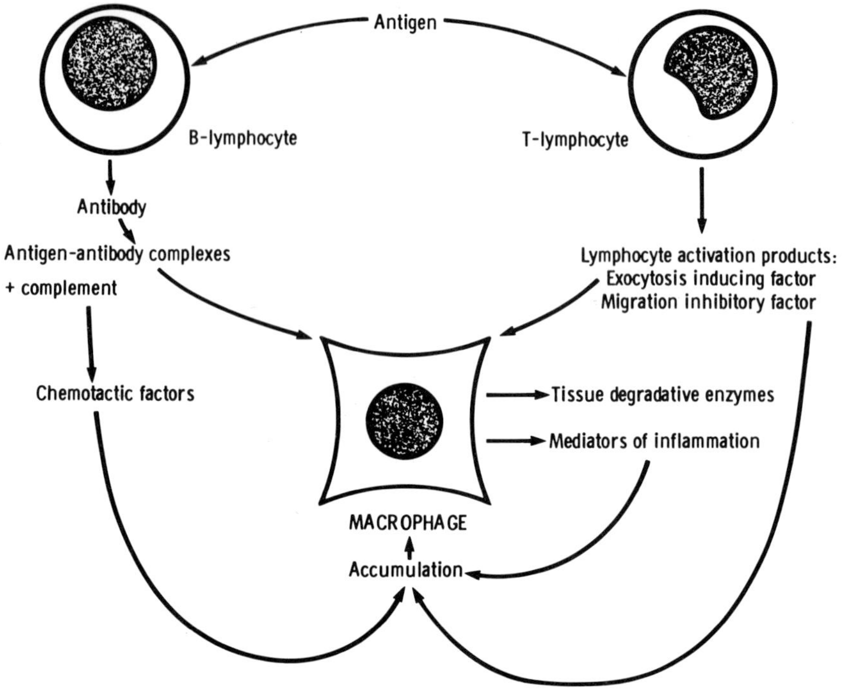

Fig. 2. Schematic representation of the interaction of macrophages with the products of lymphocytes to produce chronic inflammation.

C. The Direct Interaction of Substances with Macrophages to Cause Chronic Inflammation of a Nonimmunological Nature

1. Group A Streptococcal Cell Walls

The association of Group A streptococci with a number of diseases, including rheumatic fever, is well established (Wannamaker and Matsen, 1972; Ginsburg, 1972). Several factors produced by these organisms have been shown to cause inflammatory changes. In addition a type-specific C-mucopolysaccharide–peptidoglycan complex (PPG) from Group A streptococcal cell walls causes chronic inflammatory lesions, in which macrophages are the predominant cells, after single injections at various sites (Schwab *et al.*, 1959; Ginsburg, 1972; Page *et al.*, 1974a). The cell wall material is extremely resistant to the action of lysosomal enzymes (Ayoub and McCarty, 1968) and persists for many months at sites of chronic inflammation. The granulomatous lesion does not appear to have an immunopathological basis but is due to direct effects of PPG on macrophages, as shown with cultures of these cells (Davies *et al.*, 1974a;

Page *et al.*, 1974a). After exposure to PPG, macrophages undergo rapid and marked morphological changes that persist for many days. These include a two- to fourfold increase in cell size, an increase in the number of lysosomes as shown by vital staining with acridine orange, and an increase in ruffled membrane activity. These changes are brought about by concentrations of PPG ranging from 1 to 10 μg/ml. Macrophages cultured in the presence of 15–50 μg/ml of PPG show comparable increases in size, but they tend to become more rounded and the cytoplasm exhibits more prominent but fewer vacuoles. These cells show no loss of viability as determined biochemically by estimations of lactate dehydrogenase levels or morphologically by the capacity to hydrolyze fluorescein dibutyrate (Davies *et al.*, 1974a).

The cells showed two to threefold increases in protein levels. There are also considerable changes in the levels and distribution of various cellular enzymes. Exposure to doses of PPG in the range of 1–15 μg/ml for 72 hours resulted in marked increases in the cellular levels of nonlysosomal enzymes, such as lactate dehydrogenase and leucine-2-naphthylamidase. There are also smaller increases in cellular levels of lysosomal enzymes such as β-glucuronidase. At these relatively low concentrations of PPG, there is no detectable release of any enzymes from the cells into the culture medium. However, addition of PPG to cultures in amounts ranging from 15 to 50μg/ml did induce the release of lysosomal enzymes from viable macrophages in a dose- and time-dependent manner. As shown in Fig. 3, up to 80% of cellular β-glucuronidase is released by macrophages into the culture medium on exposure to 50 μg/ml PPG. The release proceeds rapidly, with much of the enzyme being redistributed within 6 hours of exposure to PPG.

2. *Homogenates of Dental Plaque*

Dental plaque is a mixed bacterial growth on the sheltered areas of the teeth of humans and experimental animals. It contains numerous microorganisms of various types. There is substantial evidence that plaque is the primary etiological agent involved in the pathogenesis of chronic periodontitis. Plaque sterilized by irradiation causes very similar changes to those seen with PPG when added to cultures of macrophages (Page *et al.*, 1973). Plaque in doses of 5 to 50 μg/ml causes a rapid and massive redistribution of acid hydrolases from the cells into the culture medium. Although no net increase in acid hydrolase levels was detected in cultures exposed to plaque for 24 hours, there were significant increases in the levels of β-glucuronidase in cultures exposed to concentrations of plaque greater than 10 μg/ml for 72 hours (Fig. 4). This suggests that the continuous depletion of intracellular lysosomal enzyme serves as a stimulus

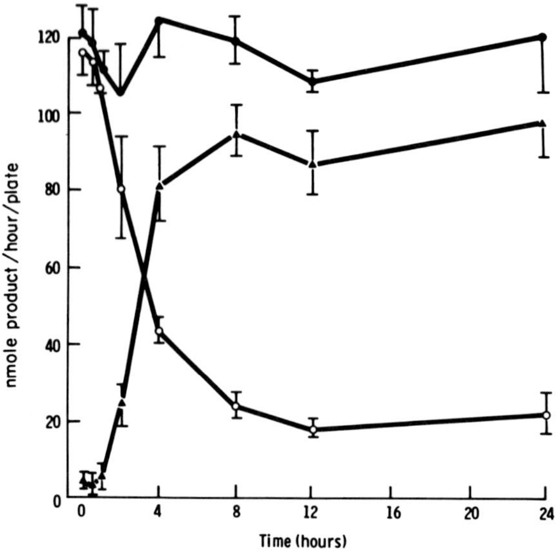

Fig. 3. The effect of PPG (50 μg/ml) on β-glucuronidase activity in cultures of mouse peritoneal macrophages (●——●), in the cells (○——○), and in the culture medium (▲——▲) at time intervals over a time period of 24 hours. (Reprinted with permission from Davies *et al.*, 1974a.)

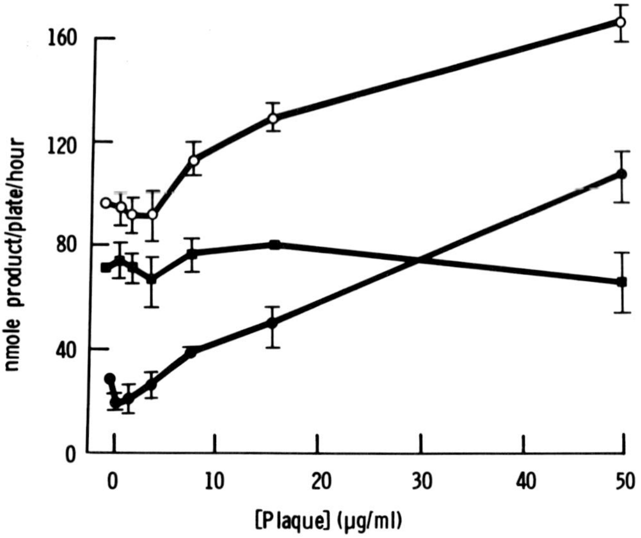

Fig. 4. The levels of β-glucuronidase in cultures of mouse peritoneal macrophages exposed to various concentrations of dental plaque for 72 hours. ●——● denotes enzyme activity in the culture medium, ■——■ denotes cellular levels, and the total amount of enzyme in the cultures is shown by ○——○. (Reprinted with permission from Page *et al.*, 1973.)

for the replacement of enzyme released into the culture medium. These changes also occur in the absence of any detectable cell death. The plaque constituents responsible for this effect are not known, although subsequent studies (Page *et al.*, 1974b) have shown that sterile homogenates of *Actinomyces viscosus* have a similar effect to plaque. This is a gram-positive anaerobic filamentous microorganism that has the capacity to induce severe chronic inflammatory periodontal disease in monoinfected germ-free rodents. It is also found in high concentrations in human periodontal pockets.

3. *Carrageenan*

Carrageenan, a mixture of sulfated D-galactose and 3,6-dehydro-D-galactose, induces chronic inflammation in experimental animals, such as guinea pigs (Robertson and Schwartz, 1953) and rats (Benitz and Hall, 1959). Recent experiments in our laboratory indicate that certain preparations of carrageenan also induce intense chronic inflammatory lesions after intramuscular injection in mice (Davies *et al.*, 1975). It is also clear that the same preparations of carrageenan induce selective release of acid hydrolases from macrophages. The accumulation of enzymes in the medium is both time- and dose-dependent. Enzyme release is delayed in comparison with the particulate stimuli discussed above, approximately 10 hours elapsing before significant amounts of acid hydrolases above control levels are detected in the culture medium. This may be accounted for by the solubility of carrageenan, which means that it enters cells by pinocytosis, a less rapid process than phagocytosis. We have compared three commercially available preparations of carrageenan for their ability to induce chronic inflammation *in vivo* and selective release of lysosomal enzymes *in vitro*. Native undegraded carrageenan (Gelcarin HMR, Marine Colloids) produces an intense chronic inflammatory reaction after intramuscular injection, as well as inducing the greatest increase in selective release of acid hydrolases. In contrast the calcium salt of carrageenan (Sigma Chemical Company) has negligible inflammatory activity and lacks the ability to induce selective release of acid hydrolases, while the potassium salt of carrageenan shows intermediate activity in both tests. Structure–activity relationships show that λ-carrageenan, a linear polymer of D-galactose with α-1,3 linkages and sulfated on the fourth carbon, has the greatest activity. κ-Carrageenan, containing alternate units of 4-sulfated D-galactose and 3,6-anhydro-D-galactose with α-1,3 and β-1,4 linkages, possesses lower inflammatory activity. The correlation of the inflammatory activity of purified preparations of the various forms of carrageenan with their activity on macrophages should give further information on the relevance of selective release of lysosomal enzymes in chronic inflammation. Such a study of the purified ι, κ, and λ forms of carrangeenan is in progress.

4. Inhaled Cytotoxic Particles

The most common route of entry into the body of cytotoxic particles is by inhalation into the lungs. The toxic effects of such particles result in a number of lung diseases known collectively as the pneumoconioses (Spencer, 1968). Many of the pneumoconioses are characterized by a chronic inflammatory lesion that has an immunological or nonimmunological basis depending on the nature of the inhaled material.

It is accepted that the initial event after inhalation of toxic particles is their phagocytosis by macrophages in the pulmonary alveoli (Allison, 1968). Failure of the macrophages to digest or remove the particles from the lungs results in a chronic inflammatory process leading to irreversible damage. *In vitro* studies of the interaction of toxic particles, such as silica and asbestos, with mononuclear phagocytes has demonstrated the cytotoxic effects of these substances (Allison *et al.*, 1966; Allison, 1971). Although asbestos is less cytotoxic than silica, recent work has shown that small amounts of asbestos fibers induce the selective release of lysosomal enzymes from cultured mononuclear phagocytes (Table IV) (Davies *et al.*, 1974b). The release of lysosomal enzymes is accompanied by marked increases in cellular levels of lactate dehydrogenase (Davies *et al.*, 1974b). Extracellular levels of lactate dehydrogenase do not increase, in-

TABLE IV

Redistribution of β-Galactosidase from Mouse Peritoneal Macrophages Exposed to Asbestos[a]

Concentration asbestos (μg/ml)	Enzyme levels (nmole *p*-nitrophenol released/culture/hour)			% enzyme in culture medium
	Total	Cells	Medium	
0	170 ± 9	157 ± 1	16 ± 5	9.4 ± 2.7
2	171 ± 4	149 ± 5	23 ± 2	13.3 ± 1.3
5	159 ± 13	138 ± 12	21 ± 2	13.4 ± 0.7
10	155 ± 16	125 ± 13	31 ± 3	19.8 ± 0.7
25	163 ± 7	108 ± 6	55 ± 4	33.7 ± 2.3
50	164 ± 9	78 ± 4	89 ± 3	54.3 ± 3.0

[a] Protease–peptone cultured macrophages exposed to different concentrations of asbestos for 24 hours in culture. U.I.C.C. standard chrysolite.

dicating that the cultures have remained viable. Morphological observations show that the mononuclear phagocytes have phagocytized most of the asbestos fibers and contain an increased number of vacuoles, which are probably secondary lysosomes. At the higher doses of asbestos (25–50 μg/ml) the cells tend to form clusters, but the majority retain the cytoplasmic extensions characteristic of normal mononuclear phagocytes.

The cytotoxic effects of silica on mononuclear phagocytes *in vitro* are well documented (Allison *et al.*, 1966), but it is not known whether the particles induce selective release of acid hydrolases in a manner similar to that induced by asbestos. Recent studies in this laboratory show that silica does not release acid hydrolases from macrophages without concomitant cell death (Davies and Allison, 1975).

The differing effects of asbestos and silica on mononuclear phagocytes *in vitro* are of interest in view of the proposed differences in the ways by which they interact with membranes (Allison, 1976). Silica is thought to cause cell death by disrupting the phospholipid components of membranes which form hydrogen bonds with the phenolic hydroxyl groups of silicic acid that are rigidly arranged on the surfaces of particles. On the other hand, asbestos is thought to disturb membranes in a nonlytic fashion by the interaction of its magnesium groups with membrane glycoproteins. Such an interaction may lead to the formation of protein clusters in membranes. Since asbestos induces selective release of lysosomal enzymes from mononuclear phagocytes, it is of interest that clustering of membrane proteins also accompanies the exocytosis of mucocysts by *Tetrahymena pyriformis* (Satir *et al.*, 1973).

Cytotoxic particles, such as silica and asbestos, are useful tools for the study of chronic inflammation. The *in vitro* studies described above show clearly that the responses of macrophages to the two particles differ. These differences may in turn reflect the distinct pathogenesis of the two diseases (Spencer, 1968); asbestos inhalation induces an intense cellular reaction and diffuse fibrosis, while silica inhalation is followed by nodular fibrosis.

D. The Release of Macrophage Lysosomal Enzymes by Products of Immune Reactions

The products of both T and B lymphocytes have many effects on macrophages. Both tissue macrophages (Berken and Benacerraff, 1966) and human peripheral blood monocytes (Huber *et al.*, 1968) have Fc receptors for immune complexes containing either IgG or IgM antibodies (for review, see Shevach *et al.*, 1973). The binding site for immune complexes on human mononuclear phagocytes displays a specificity for the γ_1 and γ_3 subclasses of human IgG (Huber and Wagner, 1974). The endocytosis of immune complexes by macrophages has been studied by Steinman and Cohn (1972), who reported that aggregates of horseradish peroxidase and the corresponding antibody were taken up and degraded within secondary lysosomes of mouse peritoneal macrophages.

1. The Release of Acid Hydrolases from Macrophages Exposed to Immune Complexes

Immune complexes are deposited at sites of chronic inflammation in several common diseases, including rheumatoid arthritis and certain types of glomerulonephritis. The injection of immune complexes formed at antigen excess causes an acute inflammatory response (Cochrane and Weigle, 1958). These lesions resolve rapidly without any appreciable residue of mononuclear cells, indicating that there is no onset of chronic inflammation. However, the intradermal injection of immune complexes formed at equivalence into rats results in a chronic inflammatory lesion characterized by many macrophages containing residual immune complexes (Spector and Heesom, 1969). There is considerable evidence showing that immune complexes interact with polymorphonuclear leukocytes *in vitro* to cause selective release of acid hydrolases (Henson, 1971; Weissmann *et al.*, 1971a,b; Hawkins, 1971). However, until recently there has been no information concerning this process in macrophages exposed to immune complexes. We have studied the interaction of immune complexes with mouse peritoneal macrophages and found that small amounts of complexes formed at equivalence induce selective release of various acid hydrolases (Cardella *et al.*, 1974). The release increases with time of exposure to complexes over a period of at least 24 hours and is dependent upon the dose of immune complex (Fig. 5). Selective release of lysosomal hydrolases is not seen in cells exposed to antigen or antiserum. Cultures exposed to immune complexes for 24 hours show elevated levels of acid hydrolases compared to control values. This may be due to a cellular response to a digestible substrate (see Axline and Cohn, 1970) or may result from the depletion of the cellular pool of lysosomal enzymes. Preliminary studies show that selective release of acid hydrolases occurs in cultures of macrophages exposed to immune complexes containing an excess of either antigen or antibody.

2. The Selective Release of Acid Hydrolases from Macrophages Exposed to the Products of Stimulated T Lymphocytes

The exposure of T lymphocytes to specific antigens or nonspecific mitogens results in the release of several biologically active macromolecules (David and David, 1972), a number of which influence macrophage function (see Allison and Davies, 1974). Pantalone and Page (1975) have

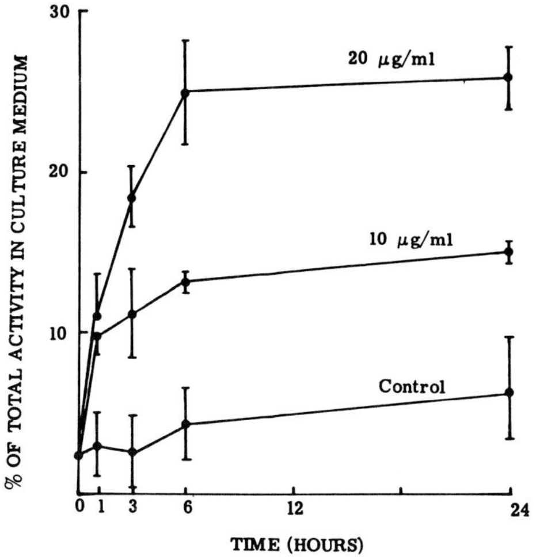

Fig. 5. The time and dose dependence of the release of β-glucuronidase from macrophages exposed to bovine serum albumin–anti-bovine serum albumin immune complexes. The lower line indicates release in control cultures, while the upper two lines indicates the response to complexes containing 10 and 20 μg/ml of antigen. (Reprinted with permission from Cardella *et al.*, 1974.)

incubated mouse peritoneal macrophages with culture media from human peripheral blood leukocytes incubated with phytohemagglutinin or sensitized lymphocytes stimulated with antigen. The macrophages show elevated levels of both lysosomal and nonlysosomal enzymes, and selective release of acid hydrolases was observed without any detectable loss of cell viability. It is not clear whether the selective release of lysosomal enzyme described above is caused by factors of the type described by Ruddle and Waksman (1968), Granger and Williams (1968), and David and David (1972) or by previously undescribed factors. Mononuclear phagocytes are resistant to the cytotoxic effects of lymphotoxin (David and David, 1972), although this does not exclude the possibility that lymphotoxins may cause selective release of lysosomal enzymes. This *in vitro* phenomenon may form the basis of tissue damage seen in delayed hypersensitivity where factors released from T lymphocytes lead to the recruitment of macrophages into the site of inflammation and their immobilization there, with subsequent release of acid hydrolases.

E. Secretion of Neutral Proteinases by Macrophages

1. *Collagenase*

The presence of collagenase at sites of both acute and chronic inflammation has been reported. It is likely that collagenase found at sites of acute inflammation is derived from polymorphonuclear leukocytes, which have been shown to contain the enzyme (Lazarus, 1973). However, collagen breakdown is most evident during chronic inflammation, when relatively few polymorphonuclear leukocytes are present. Although these lesions usually contain many macrophages, it was not until very recently that the presence of collagenase within these cells was demonstrated. Senior *et al.* (1972) and Robertson *et al.* (1973) demonstrated the presence of this enzyme in alveolar macrophages. Recent work by Wahl *et al.* (1974) has shown the production and secretion of large amounts of collagenase by macrophages maintained in tissue culture. These workers have shown that guinea pig peritoneal exudate macrophages exposed to bacterial lipopolysaccharide in culture produce considerable amounts of collagenase over a period of several days. It is clear that the enzyme was newly synthesized by the macrophages, since its appearance in the culture medium was inhibited by cycloheximide. It is also notable that no collagenase activity was detected in freshly isolated cells after detergent lysis or freeze-thawing. The appearance of the collagenase was delayed for at least 24 hours after the addition of the lipopolysaccharide, and cultures maintained in the absence of lipopolysaccharide did not show any detectable collagenase activity during 5 days of culture. It was found that the lipid A fraction was the most active of the lipopolysaccharide components in inducing synthesis and release of collagenase. The glycolipid portion was less active than the lipid A, while the lipid-free polysaccharide fraction induced only low levels of collagenase production and secretion. The macrophage collagenase resembles other collagenases in many respects. It is inhibited by serum and EDTA and was found to cleave native collagen molecules into three-fourth and one-fourth portions. It is not known whether stimulated macrophages synthesize collagenase as such or in the form of proenzyme, as reported in other tissues. Wahl *et al.* (1974) have also shown that sensitized lymphocytes treated with specific antigen or with concanavalin A release a factor or factors that stimulate macrophages to produce collagenase. It is, therefore, clear that both bacterial constituents and the products of immunological reactions can stimulate macrophages to release collagenase, which can in turn degrade collagen and therefore account for some aspects of tissue damage observed during chronic inflammatory processes.

Further analyses of the effects of lymphocyte activation products on macrophages may show the release of other less well-defined mediators of chronic inflammation. It is already known that lymphocyte activation products have a number of effects on macrophage function (David and David, 1972; Allison and Davies, 1974), but the secretory activity of such stimulated cells has not yet been thoroughly investigated.

2. Plasminogen Activator

The enzymatic cleavage of plasminogen to form the enzyme plasmin is of considerable relevance to inflammatory processes, since not only does plasmin degrade fibrin, the final product of the blood coagulation cascade, but it can also act upon several other substrates to generate inflammatory mediators. These include the Hageman factor, which is the initial component of the blood coagulation system. The activation of the Hageman factor not only leads to blood coagulation but also to the generation of kinins that are derived by the hydrolysis of plasma protein substrates by the enzyme kallikrein, which can be generated from its precursor by the action of activated Hageman factor (Cochrane *et al.,* 1974). In addition, plasmin can act upon the fifth component of complement to generate a chemotactic factor for both polymorphonuclear leukocytes and macrophages. Interest in plasminogen activator has recently been stimulated by the observations that the enzyme is released by mouse embryo fibroblasts after transformation by oncogenic viruses (Unkeless *et al.* 1973), whereas untransformed cells show minimal release of this enzyme. Recent studies by Unkeless *et al.* (1974) and Gordon *et al.* (1974a) have shown also that macrophages that have been stimulated in certain ways will secrete large amounts of plasminogen activator. It was found that mouse macrophages obtained after intraperitoneal injection of thioglycolate broth secrete large amounts of plasminogen activator when cultured. This is in marked contrast to macrophages from unstimulated mice which do not synthesize or secrete this enzyme. *In vivo* stimulation with agents, such as endotoxin, calf serum, BCG, or mineral oil, induces the *in vitro* secretion of much smaller amounts of plasminogen activator than thioglycollate. However, if cells stimulated *in vivo* by these agents are exposed to phagocytic stimuli, such as latex beads, *in vitro* their secretion of plasminogen activator is greatly enhanced. Other phagocytic stimuli besides latex beads act as efficient inducers of plasminogen activator secretion from stimulated macrophages *in vitro,* although nondigestible materials are more efficient in this respect than digestible substrates, such as *Micrococcus lysodeikticus,* heat aggregated γ-globulin, or peroxidase–anti-peroxidase immune complexes. The production and secretion of plasminogen activator by stimulated macrophages continues for periods of up to 9 days, as was observed when *Micrococcus lysodeikticus* was added to cultures obtained from mice injected intraperitoneally with endotoxin.

F. Secretion of Lysozyme by Macrophages

Lysozyme is a low molecular weight, cationic protein, which hydrolyses *N*-acetylmuramic–β-1,4-*N*-acetylglucosamine linkages in bacterial cell walls. High concentrations of lysozyme are found in both polymorphonuclear leukocytes and in rabbit alveolar macrophages. In the polymorphonuclear leukocyte, the enzyme is largely particulate, being found in both azurophilic and specific granules of this cell. The early studies of Cohn and Wiener (1963) showed that BCG-induced rabbit alveolar macrophages released a large fraction of their intracellular lyzozyme during phagocytosis. Large amounts of this enzyme accumulate in both serum and urine of humans and experimental animals suffering from monocytic leukemia. Recent studies by Gordon *et al.* (1974b) have shown that both mouse peritoneal macrophages and human peripheral blood monocytes synthesize and secrete substantial amounts of lysozyme *in vitro*. This enzyme is a major secretory product of both macrophages and monocytes, since its daily production represents 0.5 to 2.5% of the total cell protein (Gordon *et al.*, 1974b). The enzyme is secreted under a wide variety of conditions, is not drastically changed by the presence or absence of serum in the culture medium, and is not stimulated either by phagocytosis or the introduction of its substrate *Micrococcus lysodeikticus*. Secretion *in vitro* begins after a lag period, but then continues for as long as 17 days. Macrophages secrete the equivalent of their cellular pool of lysozyme in a period between 5 and 8 hours, and this secretion can be almost completely abolished in the presence of an inhibitor of protein synthesis, such as cycloheximide. The secretion of lysozyme seems to be restricted to macrophages, since other cell types, such as epithelioid cell lines, fibroblasts, and lymphocytes, do not secrete lysozyme. Although polymorphonuclear leukocytes release their intracellular store of lysozyme when cultured, there is no evidence of synthesis of new enzyme by these cells.

At present there is little to suggest that lysozyme secreted by macrophages influences the course of chronic inflammatory reactions. It has, however, been suggested recently (Howell *et al.*, 1974) that lysozyme affects the stability of aggregates of proteoglycans in cartilage matrix. It was shown that lysozyme degrades proteoglycans from 60 S to 12–16 S aggregates, thereby rendering them more susceptible to the action of neutral proteinases and cathepsin D.

IV. WHAT IS THE CONTRIBUTION OF HYDROLYTIC ENZYME SECRETION TO CHRONIC INFLAMMATION?

Although it is now apparent that macrophages secrete a variety of hydrolytic enzymes *in vitro*, there is little information on the activity of these enzymes at sites of chronic inflammation. It remains to be demonstrated whether macrophage secretion of netural proteinases and lysozyme is affected by exposure to inflammatory stimuli. Studies on the induction of collagenase secretion *in vitro* (Wahl *et al.*, 1974) suggest that this enzyme is released under conditions that differ from those leading to the release of lysosomal enzymes (Allison *et al.*, 1973). Another approach will be to study the behavior *in vitro* of macrophages derived from sites of inflammation. It is possible that induction of the secretion of certain enzymes may require conditions not available in culture, including the proximity of other cell types and their secretory products.

If the secretion of the various classes of hydrolytic enzymes occurs at sites of chronic inflammation, their contribution to the pathogenesis of the lesion must be considered. This problem can only be answered by defining the extracellular milieu into which these enzymes are released. Since most lysosomal enzymes function optimally at acid pH, determination of the acidity of the extracellular environment in chronic inflammatory lesions at various stages of evolution would be useful. Acid hydrolases are released most rapidly and abundantly from macrophages during the first 24 hours after exposure to inflammatory agents, and it will also be important to determine the turnover rate of these cells at sites of chronic inflammation (Ryan and Spector, 1970). In lesions with high macrophage turnover rates, release of greater quantities of hydrolases would be expected.

Another factor in the extracellular environment that may restrict hydrolytic enzyme activity is the presence of various inhibitors in tissue fluids. Several well-characterized inhibitors of proteinases occur in blood plasma (for review, see Davies, 1976), and these are known to penetrate into extravascular spaces in variable amounts. However, there is little information on the levels of these inhibitors at sites of chronic inflammation, where increases of vascular permeability would raise their levels. Plasminogen activator and elastase are serine proteinases and are, therefore, susceptible to α-1-trypsin inhibitor, which shows 90% of the trypsin inhibitor capacity of plasma, while collagenase and cathepsins B1 and D are susceptible to inhibition by α-2-macroglobulin. The balance between the concentrations of proteinases and these inhibitors may determine the activity of these enzymes at sites of chronic inflammation. The state of the vasculature in the lesion would be important, with sites containing relatively few blood vessels allowing greater activity to extracellular proteinases.

It is already apparent that the conditions under which macrophages secrete neutral proteinases differ from those required for acid hydrolase release. Accordingly, it can be speculated that macrophages secrete acid hydrolases and neutral proteinases at different stages of their life span at chronic inflammatory sites. For example, acid hydrolases may be secreted during the early, destructive phase of the process, while plasminogen activator and collagenase secretion is more prominent during the reparative phase when they mediate fibrinolysis and modulate fibrogenesis, respectively. The variety of ways by which macrophages can respond to various stimuli under different conditions (Allison and Davies, 1974) also suggests that macrophages possess the functional flexibility to secrete various enzymes at different times.

The nature of the releasing stimulus affects the extracellular fate of secreted enzymes. For example, if acid hydrolases are secreted during unsuccessful attempts to phagocytize a nondigestible substrate, it is possible that the enzymes are released at sites where cells are in close apposition to connective tissue surfaces. This would result in a trapping of enzymes, thereby maintaining their concentration, protecting them from extracellular inhibitors, such as those derived from blood plasma, and possibly creating a local environment where the pH is lowered by generation of lactic acid. An example of where such a situation may exist is in experimental arthritis induced by injection of antigen into the joints of previously immunized animals (Cooke *et al.*, 1972). In this type of arthritis, the majority of antigen persists in collagenous tissues of the joint, such as articular cartilage. The antigen probably exists in the form of immune complexes, since it is associated with immunoglobulin and C3. Since it was seen in the surface layer of articular cartilage, it would be accessible to inflammatory cells in invading pannus. Macrophages at these sites would bind to the immune complexes via their Fc receptors, and, if the complex were immobilized, lysosomal enzymes could be released directly onto the complex and its surrounding cartilage by a mechanism similar to that described by Henson (1971) for polymorphonuclear leukocytes. The nonphagocytic release of lysosomal enzymes by macrophages is already established (Temple *et al.*, 1973). Guinea pig peritoneal macrophages exposed to antibody-coated chicken erythrocytes in the presence of cytochalasin B selectively release a large proportion of their lysosomal enzymes in the absence of any detectable phagocytosis.

The mechanism by which neutral proteinases are released from macrophages is unknown; indeed it is not yet clear whether they are secreted from lysosomes or a separate granule population. Nichols and Bainton (1973) have shown that human monocytes contain at least two distinct granule populations, one of which appears to be typical lysosomes, containing several histochemically identifiable acid hydrolases. The presence of neutral proteinases in these two granule populations remains to be investigated. These enzymes are particularly susceptible to the activity of plasma proteinase inhibitors, so that they would be expected to be active at sites where proteinase inhibitors are present in small amounts or where proteinases are only slowly removed, resulting in the accumulation of enzyme in amounts exceeding the neutralizing capacity of local inhibitors. For example, elastase released from macrophages into alveolar spaces of the lungs of individuals suffering from pneumoconiosis may damage elastic tissue, since the enzyme cannot readily cross the alveolar basement membrane. This possibility is emphasised by the greatly increased occurrence of chronic obstructive pulmonary disease in individuals who are deficient in α-1-trypsin inhibitor. Similarly a fibrotic inflammatory lesion may be poorly vascularized, thereby decreasing local concentrations of plasma proteinase inhibitors and allowing greater activity of locally secreted neutral proteinases, such as plasminogen activator and collagenase, to aid the resolution of the lesion.

V. OTHER PRODUCTS OF MACROPHAGES

A. The Secretion of Pyrogen by Macrophages

It is now accepted that the interaction of exogenous pyrogenic materials, such as endotoxin and other bacterial products, with host phagocytic cells stimulates these cells to release pyrogenic materials that act on the hypothalamus to produce fever. Human blood leukocytes have two distinct pyrogenic molecules, one produced by polymorphonuclear leukocytes, while the second is released from monocytes (Denarillo *et al.*, 1974). Monocytes secrete 20 times as much pyrogen as polymorphonuclear leukocytes after exposure to heat-killed *Streptococcus albus*. Denarillo *et al.* (1974) have concluded that monocytes may not make any major contribution to total pyrogen production, since polymorphonuclear leukocytes present in buffy coat preparations suppress the secretion of pyrogen by monocytes. Bodell (1974) has shown that pyrogen is not spontaneously secreted by human monocytes even after 5 days in culture. On the other hand, stimulation of these cells by either endotoxin or a phagocytic stimulus resulted in production of pyrogen within 4 hours, which then continued for at least 24 hours. The initiation and continuation of pyrogen secretion could be depressed by puromycin, an inhibitor of protein synthesis. The secretory activity of monocytes may, therefore, be responsible in part for the pyrexia that is a common feature of inflammatory disease.

B. The Secretion of Prostaglandins by Macrophages

Prostaglandins can act as both humoral mediators of inflammation and as regulators of various cells involved in this process (for reviews, see

Morley, 1974; Bourne *et al.*, 1974). There is now evidence that polymorphonuclear leukocytes, platelets, and macrophages release prostaglandin-like substances during their participation in inflammatory reactions. During phagocytosis, polymorphonuclear leukocytes produce PGE_2-like activity (Higgs and Youlten, 1972), while platelets release PGE and after exposure to various aggregating agents (Smith *et al.*, 1973). Both these cell types are involved in acute inflammatory responses, and some of the changes characteristic of this process may be mediated by prostaglandins. Anderson *et al.* (1971) have suggested that lysosomal enzymes may stimulate prostaglandin synthesis at sites of inflammation. This suggestion was based on the close correlation observed between acid phosphatase and β-glucuronidase levels with prostaglandin levels at sites of carrageenan-induced inflammation in rats. They postulated that polymorphonuclear leukocytes release hydrolases, including phospholipases, which generate arachadonic acid, a precursor required by the prostaglandin synthesis system. Anderson *et al.* (1971) did not study the carrageenan lesions for more than 24 hours, so that the possible role of macrophages in prostaglandin generation remains unresolved. It is known, however, that macrophages contain several phospholipases (Franson and Waite, 1973), liberation of which might increase the synthesis of certain prostaglandins. Indeed, Bray *et al.* (1974) have provided evidence that macrophages secrete E-type prostaglandin-like material when exposed to products of stimulated lymphocytes. Morley (1974) suggests that prostaglandin secreted in this way may play at least two roles in the inflammatory process. The first is to mediate some of the humoral changes, such as increased vascular permeability, pain production, erythema, chemotaxis of polymorphonuclear leukocytes, and platelet aggregation. Second, he suggests that these prostaglandins may have effects that limit the extent of the inflammatory process. Evidence is presented that PGE_1 can inhibit the production of lymphocyte activation products by stimulated lymphocytes, thereby limiting the production of factors active on macrophages to induce chronic inflammation. Conceivably, the release of such factors by macrophages may limit the secretory activity of these cells. It is well established that high doses of prostaglandins can reduce the release of inflammatory mediators from cell types, such as platelets, basophils, and polymorphonuclear leukocytes.

Nonsteroid anti-inflammatory drugs are efficient inhibitors of prostaglandin synthesis in various cellular systems. Morley (1974) suggests that nonsteroid antiinflammatory drugs have an ameliorative but not curative effect in chronic inflammatory diseases, such as rheumatoid arthritis, since they fail to inhibit completely synthesis of mediators, such as lymphocyte activation products, which stimulate macrophages to exert their tissue-damaging effects in these diseases. Moreover, lymphocytes may become resistant to the effects of prostaglandins secreted by macrophages in diseases, such as rheumatoid arthritis, providing an alternative explanation for the inefficiency of nonsteroid antiinflammatory agents.

C. The Generation of Inflammatory Mediators by Secretory Products of Macrophages

Proteinases secreted by macrophages under various conditions may act on a variety of humoral substrates to generate factors that may contribute to the progress of the chronic inflammatory process.

1. Chemotactic Factors

Macrophages have been shown to respond to chemotactic stimuli of various types (Ward, 1968; Wilkinson *et al.*, 1969; Ward *et al.* 1970; Snyderman *et al.*, 1971) (see Snyderman and Mergenhagen, Chapter 13). Synderman *et al.* (1971) showed that a factor chemotactic for macrophages could be generated by the action of trypsin on highly purified guinea pig C5. It was shown that this chemotactic activity was mediated by C5a, a fragmentation product of the fifth component of complement. Further studies by Snyderman *et al.* (1972) showed that an acid proteinase, with properties similar to those of cathepsin D, could also generate the chemotactic factors with physical properties similar to C5a when incubated with purified guinea pig C5. This is a potentially important mechanism for the prolongation of a chronic inflammatory response, whereby macrophage acid proteinases cleave C5 to produce C5a, which in turn attracts more macrophages into the inflammatory site. It is not yet known whether neutral proteinases secreted by macrophages (Gordon *et al.*, 1974a) have the ability to cleave C5 to produce chemotactic factors.

2. Generation of Kinins

Greenbaum and co-workers (Greenbaum, 1972) have described structurally distinct peptides showing the biological properties of bradykinin. These peptides are formed by the action of lysates of polymorphonuclear leukocytes or alveolar macrophages on partially purified plasma kininogen. These kinins, designed leukokinin-PMN and leukokinin-M (Chang *et al.*, 1972) are formed by incubation at low pH, suggesting that lysosomal acid proteinases may be involved, but experiments with subcellular fractions so far carried out are insufficient to establish this point. Additional studies with well-characterized lysosomal and other proteinases from PMN and macrophages should be undertaken to ensure that these enzymes can generate kinins.

3. *Prostaglandins*

The possible role of released phospholipases in formation of prostaglandins has already been discussed.

4. *Activation of Hageman Factor*

It is now well established that the Hageman factor lies at the crossroads of the blood coagulation, complement, and fibrinolytic systems (Cochrane *et al.*, 1974). High priority should be given to determining whether this important extracellular substrate is susceptible to the activity of any proteinases released by macrophages.

VI. INTERACTIONS AND MODULATING FACTORS

A. Factors Produced during Acute Exacerbations of Chronic Inflammation Which May Influence Macrophage Function

The mechanisms mediating the transition of an acute inflammatory response into a chronic one are not understood. Macrophages may be attracted into acute inflammatory sites by products of the activity of enzymes released by polymorphonuclear leukocytes and platelets or by products of stimulated lymphocytes into sites of delayed hypersensitivity reactions. It is already known that polymorphonuclear leukocytes contain a neutral proteinase that cleaves the fifth component of complement to produce a product, C5a, which is chemotactic for both polymorphonuclear leukocytes and macrophages (Snyderman *et al.*, 1969, 1971; Ward and Newman, 1969). Some PMN's discharge their granules and soon die in sites of lesions, and others rapidly move on, leaving the macrophages behind. Other products of polymorphonuclear leukocytes and platelets might also affect the function of macrophages. For example, the effect on macrophage function of cationic proteins found in abundance in both cell types (Zeya and Spitznagel, 1963; Nachman *et al.*, 1970) is unknown. There is already suggestive evidence (Ward, 1968) that the cationic peptides of lysosomal fractions of rabbit polymorphonuclear leukocytes are chemotactic for macrophages from the same species. Polymorphonuclear leukocytes release a substance showing chemotactic activity against this cell type (Zigmond and Hirsch, 1973) which should be tested for its chemotactic activity for macrophages.

The activity of substances derived from cells involved in acute inflammatory reactions may assume importance when chronic inflammatory responses are complicated by acute exacerbations, as occurs in rheumatoid arthritis. Although the products of these cells might not contribute directly to tissue damage, they may stimulate macrophages present at the site to secrete mediators, such as hydrolytic enzymes, which cause tissue damage. In addition, the products of cells involved in acute exacerbations of chronic inflammation would generate chemotactic factors that would recruit more macrophages into the site of chronic inflammation.

Exacerbations of immune responses, provoked by an increased amount or reexposure to an immunogen, involving B or T lymphocytes, may also influence the behavior of macrophages at sites of chronic inflammation. Antibody production by B cells results in the formation of immune complexes that interact with macrophages in the way we have described, and likewise with polymorphonuclear leukocytes, which are also attracted to the site of their formation by certain products of the activated complement sequence. The products of stimulated T cells will attract more macrophages to the site of inflammation (Ward *et al.*, 1970), stimulate their activities in various ways (David and David, 1972; Allison and Davies, 1974), and induce the release of acid hydrolases (Pantalone and Page, 1975).

B. The Interaction of Macrophages and Fibroblasts at Sites of Chronic Inflammmation

Pneumoconiosis induced by the inhalation of silica provides the best example of an inflammatory lesion in which fibroblasts and macrophages are present almost exclusively. The lesion is characterized by extensive fibrosis, and it has been suggested that the stimulus to collagen synthesis is derived from macrophages. As we have mentioned above, if macrophages ingest silica in sufficient amounts cell death soon follows. We have noted, however, that uptake of small doses of silica which do not cause detectable cell death result in significant increases in cellular size and the levels of nonlysosomal enzymes, such as leucine-2-napthylamidase and lactate dehydrogenase, in cultured macrophages. It will be interesting to examine further the effect of these doses of silica on macrophages from the point of view of induction of collagen synthesis by fibroblasts. It is possible that fibrogenic factors are released by macrophages under these conditions rather than after cell death. A report by Heppleston and Styles (1967) that macrophage cultures exposed to silica particles release a fibrogenic factor has not been confirmed by others (Harington *et al.*, 1973). It is clear, however, that further studies under favorable conditions may allow the demonstration of a fibrogenic factor released by macrophages exposed to silica.

There are also indications that fibroblast products may influence the function of macrophages. Mauel and Defendi (1971a) have reported that macrophages grown in conditioned medium from mouse fibroblasts show DNA synthesis within 24 to 48 hours of exposure. Similar mitogenic factors released from fibroblasts may account for the incorporation of thymidine into DNA by a small proportion of macrophages *in vivo* and also by macrophage polykaryons formed at sites of chronic inflammation (Mariano and Spector, 1974).

C. Pharmacological Modification of Macrophages at Sites of Chronic Inflammation

Although it is clear that macrophages are sensitive to the effects of steroids and other drugs (Thompson and van Furth, 1970, 1973; Dale *et al.*, 1974) before their arrival at sites of chronic inflammation, only little is known of the sensitivity of cells that are present at inflammatory sites. There is evidence that steroids can interfere with the effects of lymphocyte activation products (Lockshin, 1972; Weston *et al.*, 1972; Balow and Rosenthal, 1973) on macrophages so that steroids may influence the function of macrophages at sites of chronic inflammation of the immune type.

Wiener *et al.* (1972) have reported the inhibition of phagocytosis of heat-aggregated human serum albumin and *Salmonella typhimurium* by high concentrations of hydrocortisone in excess of 1×10^{-4} *M*. These doses are far in excess of pharmacological doses of this steroid so that the relevance of this information is doubtful. An earlier report by Wiener and Marmary (1969) stated that hydrocortisone in amounts as low as 1.4×10^{-7} *M* inhibited the increase in cellular levels of acid phosphatase and cathepsin seen in mouse peritoneal macrophages cultured *in vitro*. On the other hand, unpublished work from our laboratory shows that even lower concentrations of dexamethasone and hydrocortisone, in the range 1×10^{-8} *M* to 1×10^{-6} *M* increase cellular levels of acid glycosidases such as β-glucuronidase, β-galactosidase and *N*-acetyl-β-D-glucosaminidase. It is, therefore, evident that a thorough evaluation of the effect of steroids on the levels of lysosomal enzymes in macrophages is required, and their effect on the release of these enzymes should also be examined.

Very recently Ringrose *et al.* (1975) have reported that steroid antiinflammatory drugs, such as dexamethasone, prednisolone, and hydrocortisone, inhibit the selective release of acid hydrolases from macrophages caused by the phagocytosis of zymosan particles. The response showed a biphasic concentration dependence, the maximum inhibitory activity being seen at between 3×10^{-6} and 3×10^{-7} *M*.

The intracellular changes leading to the release of secretion products from macrophages are not known, but it is likely that the microtubule–microfilament system is involved (for review, see Allison, 1973). Studies on the release of inflammatory mediators from blood platelets, polymorphonuclear leukocytes, basophils, and mast cells (for reviews, see Bourne *et al.*, 1974; Kaliner and Austen, 1974) show that cyclic nucleotides can modify the secretory activity of these cells. Exogenously added or elevated cellular levels of cyclic adenosine 3′,5′-monophosphate are associated with inhibition of mediator release, while increased extracellular or intracellular levels of cyclic guanosine 3′,5′-monophosphate usually results in enhanced mediator release. There is some evidence that these nucleotides exert their activity, at least in part, by modifying microtubule and microfilament function, but the precise nature of these interactions remains to be elucidated.

In contrast to the large body of work on effect of cyclic nucleotides and substances that influence their cellular levels on the release of inflammatory mediators from other cell types, there are very few reports on the possible role of these substances in modifying the secretory activity of macrophages. Weissmann *et al.* (1971a) reported that cyclic adenosine 3′,5′-monophosphate inhibited the release of acid hydrolases from mouse peritoneal macrophages exposed to zymosan. A recent report by Ringrose *et al.* (1975) shows that high concentrations of cyclic adenosine 3′,5′-monophosphate, prostaglandin E, and papaverine give a slight inhibition of zymosan-induced enzyme release. On the other hand, Ackerman and Beebe (1975) have found that cyclic nucleotides and agents affecting their intracellular levels do not influence the release of acid hydrolases from guinea pig alveolar macrophages. It is not clear whether these differences are due to species differences, the tissue sources, or both.

The possibility that the function of macrophages at sites of chronic inflammation may be modified by pharmacological agents remains to be investigated in detail. The effects of conventional steroid and nonsteroid antiinflammatory drugs, as well as those influencing cellular levels of cyclic nucleotides, should be examined for their effects on the secretory activity of macrophages.

REFERENCES

Ackerman, N. R., and Beebe, J. R. (1974). *Nature (London)* **247,** 475–477.
Ackerman, N. R., and Beebe, J. R. (1975). *J. Pharmacol. Exp. Ther.* (in press).
Alexander, P., and Evans, R. (1971). *Nature (London), New Biol.* **232,** 76–78.
Allison, A. C. (1968). *Sci. Basis Med.* pp. 18–30.

Allison, A. C. (1971). *Arch. Intern. Med.* **128,** 131–139.
Allison, A. C. (1973). *Locomotion Tissue Cells, Ciba Found. Symp.* Vol. 14, New Ser., pp. 109–148.
Allison, A. C. (1976). *In* "Respiratory Defense Mechanisms" (J. D. Brain and L. L. Reid, eds.). (in press).
Allison, A. C., and Davies, P. (1974). *In* "Future Trends in Inflammation" (G. P. Velo, D. A. Willoughby, and J. P. Giroud, eds.), pp. 449–480. Piccin, Padua.
Allison, A. C., and Davies, P. (1975). *In* "Mononuclear Phagocytes" (R. van Furth, ed.), pp. 487–504 Blackwell, Oxford.
Allison, A. C., Harington, J. C., and Birbeck, M. (1966). *J. Exp. Med.* **124,** 141–153.
Allison, A. C., Davies, P., and De Petris, S. (1971). *Nature (London), New Biol.* **232,** 153–155.
Allison, A. C., Davies, P., and Page, R. C. (1973). *J. Infec. Dis.* Suppl. **128,** S212–S219.
Anderson, A. J., Brocklehurst, W. E., and Willis, A. J. (1971). *Pharmacol. Res. Commun.* **3,** 13–19.
Axline, S. G., and Cohn, Z. A. (1970). *J. Exp. Med.* **131,** 1239–1260.
Ayoub, E. M., and McCarty, M. (1968). *J. Exp. Med.* **127,** 833–851.
Balow, J. E., and Rosenthal, A. S. (1973). *J. Exp. Med.* **137,** 1031–1041.
Barrett, A. J. (1969). *In* "Lysosomes in Biology and Pathology" (J. T. Dingle and H. B. Fell, eds.), Vol. 2, pp. 245–312. North-Holland, Publ., Amsterdam.
Benitz, K. F., and Hall, L. M. (1959). *Proc. Soc. Exp. Biol. Med.* **102,** 442–445.
Berken, B., and Benaceraff, B. (1966). *J. Exp. Med.* **123,** 119–144.
Bodell, P. (1974). *J. Exp. Med.* **140,** 954–965.
Bourne, H. R., Lichtenstein, L. M., Melmon, K. L., Henney, C. S., Weinstein, Y., and Shearer, G. M. (1974). *Science* **184,** 19–28.
Bray, M. A., Gordon, D., and Morley, J. (1974). *Brit. J. Pharmacol.* **52,** 453P.
Burleigh, M. C. (1973). *Trans. Biochem. Soc.* **1,** 380–381.
Calderon, J., Williams, R. T., and Unanue, E. R. (1974). *Proc. Nat. Acad. Sci. U.S.* **71,** 4273–4277.
Cardella, C. J., Davies, P., and Allison, A. C. (1974). *Nature (London)* **247,** 46–48.
Carrel, A., and Ebeling, A. H. (1926). *J. Exp. Med.* **44,** 285–305.
Chang, J., Freer, R., Stella, R., and Greenbaum, L. M. (1972). *Biochem. Pharmacol.* **21,** 3095–3106.
Chervenick, P. A., and LoPuglio, A. F. (1972). *Science* **178,** 164–166.
Cochrane, C. G., and Aikin, B. S. (1966). *J. Exp. Med.* **124,** 733–752.
Cochrane, C. G., and Weigle, W. O. (1958). *J. Exp. Med.* **108,** 591–604.
Cochrane, C. G., Revak, S. D., Wuepper, K. D., Johnston, A., Morrison, D. C., and Ulevitch, R. (1974). *Advan. BioSci.* **12,** 237–248.
Cohn, Z. A. (1966). *J. Exp. Med.* **124,** 557–571.
Cohn, Z. A. (1968). *Advan. Immunol.* **9,** 163–214.
Cohn, Z. A. (1970). *In* "Mononuclear Phagocytes" (R. van Furth, ed.), pp. 121–132. Blackwell, Oxford.
Cohn, Z. A., and Benson, B. (1965). *J. Exp. Med.* **121,** 153–170.
Cohn, Z. A., and Ehrenreich, B. A. (1969). *J. Exp. Med.* **129,** 201–225.
Cohn, Z. A., and Parks, E. (1967). *J. Exp. Med.* **125,** 1091–1104.
Cohn, Z. A., and Wiener, E. (1963). *J. Exp. Med.* **118,** 991–1008.
Cooke, T. D., Hurd, E. R., Ziff, M., and Jasin, H. E. (1972). *J. Exp. Med.* **135,** 323–338.
Dale, D. C., Fauci, A. S., and Wolff, S. M. (1974). *N. Engl. J. Med.* **291,** 1154–1158.

David, J., and David, R. A. (1972). *Progr. Allergy* **16,** 300–449.
Davies, P. (1976). *In* "Plasma Proteins" (A. C. Allison, ed.), Vol. 2. Plenum, New York (in press).
Davies, P., and Allison, A. C. (1975). *In* "Proceedings of the 50th Anniversary Meeting of the Society of Experimental Biology." Pergamon, Oxford.
Davies, P., Page, R. C., and Allison, A. C. (1974a). *J. Exp. Med.* **139,** 1262–1281.
Davies, P., Allison, A. C., Ackerman, J., Butterfield, A., and Williams, S. (1974b). *Nature (London)* **251,** 423–425.
Davies, P., Allison, A. C., Dym, M., and Cardella, C. J. (1975). *In* "Infection and Immunology in the Rheumatic Diseases" (D. C. Dumonde, ed.). Blackwell, Oxford (in press).
Denarillo, C. A., Goldin, N. P., and Wolff, S. M. (1974). *J. Exp. Med.* **139,** 1369–1381.
Eaves, A. C., and Bruce, W. R. (1971). *Cell Tissue Kinet.* **7,** 19–30.
Ebert, R. H., and Florey, H. W. (1939). *Brit. J. Exp. Pathol.* **20,** 342–356.
Evans, R., and Alexander, P. (1970). *Nature (London)* **228,** 620–622.
Fehr, K., LoSpalluto, J., and Ziff, M. (1970). *J. Immunol.* **105,** 973–983.
Franson, R. C., and Waite, M. (1973). *J. Cell Biol.* **56,** 621–627.
Gemsa, D., Woo, C. H., Fudenberg, H. M., and Schmid, R. (1973). *J. Clin. Invest.* **52,** 812–822.
Gery, I., and Waksman, B. (1972). *J. Exp. Med.* **136,** 143–155.
Ginsburg, I. (1972). *J. Infec. Dis.* **126,** 294–340 and 419–456.
Goggins, J. F., Lazaruz, G. S., and Fullmer, H. M. (1968). *J. Histochem. Cytochem.* **13,** 688–692.
Goldstein, I., and Weissmann, G. (1974). *J. Immunol.* **113,** 1583–1588.
Gordon, S., and Cohn, Z. A. (1973). *Int. Rev. Cytol.* **36,** 171–214.
Gordon, S., Unkeless, J. C., and Cohn, Z. A. (1974a). *J. Exp. Med.* **140,** 995–1010.
Gordon, S., Todd, J., and Cohn, Z. A. (1974b). *J. Exp. Med.* **139,** 1228–1248.
Granger, G. A., and Williams, T. (1968). *Nature (London)* **218,** 1253–1254.
Greenbaum, L. (1972). *Amer. J. Pathol.* **68,** 613–623.
Harington, J. S., Ritchie, M., King, P. C., and Miller, K. (1973). *J. Pathol.* **109,** 21–37.
Hawkins, D. (1971). *J. Immunol.* **107,** 344–352.
Henson, P. M. (1971). *J. Exp. Med.* **134,** Suppl., 114S–135S.
Heppleston, A. G., and Styles, J. A. (1967). *Nature (London)* **214,** 521–522.
Hibbs, J. B., Jr. (1972). *Science* **177,** 998–1000.
Higgs, G. A., and Youlten, L. J. F. (1972). *Brit. J. Pharmacol.* **44,** 330P–331P.
Howell, D. S., Altman, R. D., Pita, J. C., and Kuettner, K. (1974). *J. Rheumatol.* **1,** Suppl. 1., 31.
Huber, H., and Wagner, M. (1974). *In* "Activation of Macrophages" (W.-H. Wagner and H. Hahn, eds.), Workshop Conf. Hoescht, Vol 2, pp. 54–62. Excerpta Med. Found., Amsterdam.
Huber, H., Polley, M. J., Linscott, W. D., Fudenberg, H. H., and Muller-Eberhard, H. J. (1968). *Science* **162,** 1281.
Janoff, A. (1972). *Amer. J. Pathol.* **68,** 579–591.
Janoff, A., and Zeligs, J. D. (1968). *Science* **161,** 702–704.
Kaliner, M., and Austen, K. F. (1974). *Biochem. Pharmacol.* **23,** 763–771.
Karnovsky, M. L., Simmons, S., Glass, E. A., Shafer, A. W., and D'Arcy Hart, P. (1970). *In* "Mononuclear Phagocytes" (R. van Furth, ed.), pp. 103–120. Blackwell, Oxford.
Keller, R. (1973). *J. Exp. Med.* **138,** 625–644.

Lazarus, G. S. (1973). *In* "Lysosomes in Biology and Pathology" (J. T. Dingle, ed.), Vol. 3, pp. 338–364. North-Holland Publ., Amsterdam.

Lazarus, G. S., Brown, R. S., Daniels, J. R., and Fullmer, H. M. (1968). *Science* **159,** 1483–1485.

Lewis, M. R. (1925). *Bull. Johns Hopkins Hosp.* **36,** 361–375.

Lockshin, M. D. (1972). *Experientia* **28,** 571–572.

McCandless, E. L. (1965). *Ann. N.Y. Acad. Sci.* **118,** 867–882.

McDonald, J. K., Callahan, P. X., Ellis, S., and Smith, R. E. (1971). *In* "Tissue Proteinases" (A. J. Barrett and J. T. Dingle, eds.), pp. 69–107. North-Holland Publ., Amsterdam.

Mackaness, G. B. (1970). *In* "Mononuclear Phagocytes" (R. van Furth, ed.), pp. 461–477. Blackwell, Oxford.

Mariano, M., and Spector, W. G. (1974). *J. Pathol.* **113,** 1–19.

Mauel, J., and Defendi, V. (1971a). *Exp. Cell Res.* **65,** 377–385.

Mauel, J., and Defendi, V. (1971b). *J. Exp. Med.* **134,** 335–350.

Melsom, H., and Seljelid, R. (1973). *J. Exp. Med.* **137,** 807–820.

Morley, J. (1974). *Prostaglandins* **8,** 315–326.

Morrison, R. I. G., Barrett, A. J., Dingle, J. T., and Prior, D. (1973). *Biochim. Biophys. Acta* **302,** 411–419.

Nachman, R. L., Weksler, B., and Ferris, B. (1970). *J. Clin. Invest.* **49,** 274–281.

Nathan, C. F., Karnovsky, M. L., and David, J. R. (1971). *J. Exp. Med.* **133,** 1356–1376.

Nelson, D. S. (1973). *Nature (London)* **246,** 306–307.

Nichols, B. A., and Bainton, D. F. (1973). *Lab. Invest.* **29,** 27–40.

Page, R. C., Davies, P., and Allison, A. C. (1973). *Arch. Oral Biol.* **18,** 1481–1495.

Page, R. C., Davies, P., and Allison, A. C. (1974a). *Lab. Invest.* **30,** 568–581.

Page, R. C., Davies, P., and Allison, A. C. (1974b). *RES, J. Reticuloenthol. Soc.* **15,** 413–438.

Pantalone, R., and Page, R. C. (1975). *Proc. Nat. Acad. Sci. U.S.* (in press).

Ringrose, P. S., Parr, M. A., and McLaren, M. (1975). *Biochem. Pharmacol.* **24,** 607–614.

Robertson, P. B., Shru, K. W., Vail, M. S., Taylor, R. E., and Fullmer, H. M. (1973). *J. Dent. Res.* **52,** 189.

Robertson, W. Van B., and Schwartz, B. (1953). *J. Biol. Chem.* **201,** 689–696.

Rothwell, T. L. W., and Spector, W. G. (1972). *J. Pathol.* **108,** 15–21.

Ruddle, N. H., and Waksman, B. H. (1968). *J. Exp. Med.* **128,** 1255–1265.

Ruscetti, F. W., and Chervenick, P. A. (1974). *J. Lab. Clin. Med.* **83,** 64–72.

Ryan, G. B., and Spector, W. G. (1969). *J. Pathol.* **99,** 139–151.

Ryan, G. B., and Spector, W. G. (1970). *Proc. Roy. Soc., Ser. B* **174,** 269–292.

Saito, K., and Suter, E. (1965). *J. Exp. Med.* **121,** 739–749.

Satir, B., Schooley, C., and Satir, P. (1973). *J. Cell Biol.* **56,** 153–176.

Schrader, J. W. (1973). *J. Exp. Med.* **138,** 1466–1480.

Schwab, J. J., Cromartie, W. J., and Robertson, B. S. (1959). *J. Exp. Med.* **109,** 43–54.

Senior, R. M., Bielefeld, D. R., and Jeffrey, J. J. (1972). *Clin. Res.* **20,** 88.

Shevach, E. M., Jaffe, E. S., and Green, I. (1973). *Transplant. Rev.* **16,** 3–28.

Smith, J. B., Ingerman, C., Kocsis, J. J., and Silver, M. J. (1973). *J. Clin. Invest.* **52,** 965–969.

Snyderman, R., Shin, H. S., Phillips, J. K., Gewurz, H., and Mergenhagen, S. E. (1969). *J. Immunol.* **103,** 413–422.

Snyderman, R., Shin, H. S., and Hausman, M. H. (1971). *Proc. Soc. Exp. Biol. Med.* **138,** 387–390.

Snyderman, R., Shin, H. S., and Dannenberg, A. M. (1972). *J. Immunol.* **109,** 896–898.

Spector, W. G., and Heesom, N. (1969). *J. Pathol.* **908,** 31–39.

Spector, W. G., and Willoughby, D. A. (1968). *J. Pathol. Bacteriol.* **96,** 389–399.

Spector, W. G., Walters, M. N. I., and Willoughby, D. A. (1965). *J. Pathol. Bacteriol.* **90,** 181–192.

Spector, W. G., Heesom, N., and Stevens, J. E. (1968). *J. Pathol. Bacteriol.* **96,** 203–213.

Spector, W. G., Reichhold, N., and Ryan, G. B. (1970). *J. Pathol.* **101,** 339–354.

Spencer, H. (1968). "Pathology of the Lung," 2nd ed., p. 434. Pergamon, Oxford.

Steinman, R. M., and Cohn, Z. A. (1972). *J. Cell Biol.* **55,** 616–634.

Stevenson, R. D. (1974). *Clin. Exp. Immunol.* **17,** 601–606.

Stubbs, M., Kuhner, A. V., Glass, E. A., David J. R. and Karnovsky, M. L. (1973). *J. Exp. Med.* **136,** 537–542.

Temple, A., Loewi, G., Davies, P., and Howard, A. (1973). *Immunology* **24,** 66 655–670.

Thompson, J., and van Furth, R. (1970). *J. Exp. Med.* **131,** 429–442.

Thompson, J., and van Furth, R. (1973). *J. Exp. Med.* **137,** 10–21.

Unkeless, J. C., Tobia, A., Ossowski, L., Quigley, J. P., Rifkin, D. B., and Reich, E. (1973). *J. Exp. Med.* **137,** 85–111.

Unkeless J. C., Gordon, S., and Reich, E. (1974). *J. Exp. Med.* **139,** 834–850.

Volkman, A., and Gowans, J. L. (1965). *Brit. J. Exp. Pathol.* **46,** 62–70.

Wahl, L. M., Wahl, S. M., Mergenhagen, S. E., and Martin, G. R. (1974). *Proc. Nat. Acad. Sci. U.S.* **71,** 3598–3601.

Wannamaker, L. W., and Matsen, J. M. (1972). "Streptococci and Streptococcal Diseases. Recognition, Understanding, and Management." Academic Press, New York.

Ward, P. A. (1968). *J. Exp. Med.* **128,** 1201–1221.

Ward, P. A., and Newman, L. J. (1969). *J. Immunol.* **102,** 93–99.

Ward, P. A., Remold, H. G., and David, J. R. (1970). *Cell. Immunol.* **1,** 162–174.

Weigle, W. O., High, G. J., and Nakamura, R. M. (1969). *J. Exp. Med.* **130,** 243–262.

Weiss, L. P., and Fawcett, D. W. (1953). *J. Histochem. Cytochem.* **1,** 47–65.

Weissmann, G., and Spilberg, I. (1968). *Arthritis Rheum.* **11,** 162–169.

Weissmann, G., Dukor, P., and Zurier, R. B. (1971a). *Nature (London), New Biol.* **231,** 131–135.

Weissmann, G., Zurier, R. B., Spieler, P. T., and Goldstein, I. M. (1971b). *J. Exp. Med.* **134,** Suppl., 149S–165S.

Werb, Z., and Cohn, Z. A. (1971). *J. Exp. Med.* **134,** 1570–1590.

Weston, W. L., Mandel, M. J., Krueger, G. G., and Claman, H. N. (1972). *J. Invest. Dermatol.* **59,** 345–348.

Wiener, E., and Marmary, Y. (1969). *Lab. Invest.* **21,** 505–511.

Wiener, E., Marmary, Y., and Curelaru, Z. (1972). *Lab. Invest.* **26,** 220–226.

Wilkinson, P. C., Borel, J. F., Stecher-Levin, V. J., and Sorkin, E. (1969). *Nature (London)* **222,** 244–247.

Wills, E. D., Davies, P., Allison, A. C., and Haswell, A. D. (1972). *Nature (London), New Biol.* **240,** 58–60.

Wood, D. D., and Gaul, S. L. (1974). *J. Immunol.* **113,** 925–933.

Zeya, H. I., and Spitznagel, J. K. (1963). *Science* **142,** 1085–1087.

Zigmond, S. H., and Hirsch, J. G. (1973). *J. Exp. Med.* **137,** 387–410.

18

Induction of Macrophage-Mediated Cytotoxicity

Marie-Luise Lohmann-Matthes

I. Introduction 464
II. Macrophage-Mediated Cytotoxicity in Allograft Rejection 464
A. *In Vivo* Evidence for Macrophage Involvement in Graft Destruction 464
B. *In Vitro* Experiments to Assess the Role of Macrophages in Allograft Rejection 467
III. Cytotoxic Macrophages in Syngeneic Tumor Systems 469
A. Morphology and *in Vivo* Evidence for Macrophage Involvement in Syngeneic Tumor Rejection 469
B. *In Vitro* Experiments to Assess the Role of Cytotoxic Macrophages in Tumor Rejection 471
IV. Macrophage-Mediated Cytotoxicity Induced by Infection with Various Microorganisms 472
V. *In Vitro* Induction of Macrophage-Mediated Cytotoxicity 473
A. Cocultivation Experiments 473
B. Induction of Macrophage-Mediated Cytotoxicity by Culture Supernatants 475
C. Specificity of Macrophage-Mediated Cytotoxicity 477
D. Attempts at Chemical Characterization of Macrophage Cytotoxicity Factor 480
VI. Summary and Conclusions 481
References 484

I. INTRODUCTION

The cellular infiltrate at the site of a cell-mediated immune reaction consists largely of mononuclear cells (Gell and Hinde, 1951; Waksman, 1963; Volkman and Gowans, 1965). The mononuclear phagocytes (macrophages) have been shown to be attracted to the reaction site and activated by soluble products of sensitized lymphocytes that have contacted the antigen. It has been demonstrated that sensitized lymphocytes attract macrophages by means of a chemotactic factor, described by Ward *et al.* (1971), arrest these macrophages by MIF activity (David, 1966), and finally activate them (Mooney and Waksman, 1970; Godal *et al.*, 1971; Evans *et al.*, 1972; Lohmann-Matthes *et al.*, 1973). Some of the soluble mediators that act on other cells have been proved to be T cell products (Schimpl and Wecker, 1972; Evans *et al.*, 1972; Lohmann-Matthes *et al.*, 1973) (see Rosenstreich and Oppenheim, Chapter 7; Epstein, Chapter 8). The secretion of these mediators during the course of a T cell sensitization provides the opportunity of an optimal participation of the macrophage system at the site of cell-mediated immune reaction. An interplay between antigen-reactive T cells, antigen, and macrophages may, therefore, play an important role in some cell-mediated immune reactions.

This chapter mainly deals with cytotoxic macrophages in allograft rejection. The role of macrophages in syngeneic tumor systems and in bactericidal systems will be discussed only briefly in order to allow some conclusions to be drawn as to whether similar mechanisms may be responsible for macrophage activation in these three-cell-mediated effector systems. These latter topics will be reviewed elsewhere in this volume (Blanden *et al.*, Chapter 15; Tevethia, *et al.*, Chapter 20; Keller, Chapter 19; Evans and Alexander, Chapter 21). The role of macrophages in the inductive phase (Lonai and Feldman, 1971; Wagner *et al.*, 1972; Ritter, *et al.*, 1975) of cell-mediated immune responses will not be discussed in this context.

II. MACROPHAGE-MEDIATED CYTOTOXICITY IN ALLOGRAFT REJECTION

A. *In Vivo* Evidence for Macrophage Involvement in Graft Destruction

As already mentioned, the histological picture of rejection of a skin or tumor allograft shows an infiltrate of mononuclear cells. A high proportion of these cells have been shown to be bone marrow-derived macrophages (Lubaroff and Waksman, 1968). Giroud *et al.* (1970) grafted C57BL/10 mice with skin of C3H mice and observed a strong macrophage infiltration of the graft bed around days 8 to 12. Gershon *et al.* (1967) demonstrated in an allogeneic tumor system in hamsters that the vast majority of tumor infiltrating cells were macrophages. The peritoneal cavity of animals that have rejected an intraperitoneal inoculum of allogeneic tumor cells contains high numbers of macrophages, about 10- to 50-fold (McIvor and Weiser, 1971) more than in control animals. In this experimental system, the site of allograft rejection is the peritoneal cavity, and the macrophages are taken directly from such site of rejection. They correspond to the infiltrating cells in a solid graft. These peritoneal macrophages from immune mice show increased adherence and spreading as signs of activation. The macrophages infiltrating skin allograft rejection sites are at a similar stage of activation as shown by Poulter *et al.* (1971).

However, the question of the relevance of the macrophage in the effector phase of an allograft rejection is at present still controversial. Giroud *et al.* (1970) obtained rejection of a skin allograft in irradiated mice only when lymph node cells were injected together with bone marrow cells. Lymph node cells alone did not accomplish rejection. Bone marrow cells alone were effective, most probably because some mouse strains do have a comparatively high proportion of T cells in the bone marrow (Cerottini *et al.*, 1970). These results could be interpreted as evidence for cooperative action between T cells present in the lymph node and macrophages present in the bone marrow. Similar conclusions were drawn by Rouse and Wagner (1972). They injected cortisone-resistant thymocytes (CRT) immune to Balb/c mice into CBA mice that had been thymectomized and grafted with Balb/c skin. Complete rejection was observed on day 12. If they did the same reconstitution experiments in irradiated CBA mice, no graft rejection was obtained. If however the thymectomized, irradiated, and skin-grafted animals were injected with bone marrow cells 4 weeks prior to reconstitution with immune CRT, rejection was achieved.

It has been shown that effector T cells are antigen-reactive cells that are sensitized against foreign transplantation antigens. *In vitro* they exert high cytotoxicity as demonstrated by several groups (reviewed by Cerottini and Brunner, 1974); from the above-mentioned results, one may deduce that *in vivo* T cells need the help of a second cell type provided by the bone marrow.

In contrast to the above discussed cooperation data are reports from Nomoto *et al.* (1970), Lubaroff (1973), and Freedman *et al.* (1972). Gershon *et al.* had demonstrated, as mentioned above, that an allogeneic tumor graft in hamsters was largely infiltrated by macrophages. In later experiments, however, they reported (Nomoto *et al.*, 1970) that the main cell necessary for rejection to occur was a sensitized lymphocyte, whereas macrophages seemed to play a minor role. However, they had to inject as many as 300×10^6 lymph node cells intravenously to prevent subcutaneous growth of the tumors. Since it has been reported (see More *et al.*, 1973) that spleen and lymph nodes of immunized animals contain a much higher proportion of macrophages as compared to controls, it remains to be established whether these 300×10^6 immune lymph node cells contained a considerable number of macrophages and their precursors. (Only experiments in which the tumor allograft and the immune cells are injected at different sites can be taken as correlate for physiological *in vivo* cooperation. If high enough numbers of specifically committed lymphocytes are admixed with allograft cells, destruction will most likely be performed by cytotoxic lymphocytes alone, since such a situation is similar to the *in vitro* assay systems.)

Lubaroff (1973) induced rejection of a skin allograft in a rat system by inoculation of 200×10^6 lymphocytes into tolerant, thymectomized, and irradiated rats grafted with allogeneic skin. Both immune and nonimmune lymphocytes were effective. No acceleration of the reaction was obtained by adding bone marrow cells. Thus bone marrow cells were not needed for rejection to occur in this system. It may be argued that even the nonimmune lymphocyte suspension used for transfer itself already contained a critical number of macrophages and macrophage precursors to replace the function of additional bone marrow cells. However, in view of the results discussed above of Giroud *et al.*, showing that lymph node cells alone were not sufficient, this argument seems rather weak. Freedman *et al.* (1972), using the DBA/2 mastocytoma system, published results that arc partly in line with those of Lubaroff. Although they were unable to protect heavily irradiated C57BL/10 mice against i.p. growth of DBA/2 mastocytes by injecting normal lymph node or spleen cells, they could fully protect such animals by injecting immune cells. Their failure to protect with normal cells may be a question of timing and quantity, since the mastocytes grow extremely rapidly in the irradiated host as compared with a skin allograft. These authors reported, in addition, that they protected irradiated C57BL/10 animals from a subcutaneous DBA/2 mastocytoma inoculum by the i.v. injection of as few as 3 immune CRT to 1 mastocytoma cell. Although they added at the same time 2×10^6 bone marrow cells to allow survival of the animals, their controls show conclusively that the rejection must have been performed by the few immune CRT injected intravenously. These latter results seem to exclude a role for the macrophage as an effector cell, at least in this experimental situation. However, it may also reflect the enormous efficiency of immune CRT in a transfer system against alloantigens. Such a population of CRT is selected for cells responding to the DBA/2 alloantigens and has a much higher lytic efficiency than any lymphocyte population sensitized under *in vivo* host versus graft conditions. Thus these results prove the enormous efficiency of this particular T cell subpopulation, which results in destruction of a tumor allograft without the aid of any other cell type. It does not, however, completely rule out the possibility, as also pointed out by Freedman *et al.*, that during rejection of skin or tumor cells by a simple first set sensitization there may be a role for amplifying mechanisms like cytotoxic macrophages.

There is general agreement that macrophages are present in an allograft bed. Their functional role, however, has not yet been fully elucidated. Dyminski and Argyris (1969) and Sonntag and Müller-Ruchholz (1975) have shown that anti-macrophage serum applied *in vivo* prolongs allograft survival. It may well be, however, that, in immune reactions across strong histocompatibility barriers, sensitized T cells may under certain circumstances be sufficient to perform the cytotoxic reaction. This may especially be the case under experimental conditions where highly cytotoxic T cells are mixed with target cells and injected together. Under conventional rejection conditions of skin or tumor allografts such an extreme concentration of sensitized T cells would never occur at the reaction site. Therefore, it seems possible that sensitized T cells, under optimal experimental conditions, may be autonomous as killer cells. Under less artificial conditions, they might require cooperation with other effector cells for graft rejection to occur.

B. *In Vitro* Experiments to Assess the Role of Macrophages in Allograft Rejection

As shown above, under *in vivo* conditions it is very difficult to obtain conclusive results as to whether one or more different cell populations are involved in graft destruction. Therefore, several groups designed *in vitro* experiments in order to elucidate this crucial question. Convincing data have indeed been presented in several laboratories independently that the sensitized cytotoxic T lymphocyte is autonomous as a cytotoxic killer cell. Golstein and Blomgren (1973) have shown in a series of experiments that effector cell populations depleted of macrophages by various methods fully retain their cytotoxic efficiency. They removed the macrophages present in a spleen cell population either by passages over plastic surfaces or by the magnetic iron method. Both methods resulted in complete macrophage depletion. Wagner *et al.* (1972) did similar experiments and confirmed the absence of functional macrophages in other macrophage-dependent systems such as antibody formation against sheep erythrocytes (SRBC). Such macrophage-depleted spleen cell suspension showed no reduction in cell-mediated cytotoxicity against DBA/2 P815X cells; on the contrary a slight increase was observed as compared with untreated suspensions (Golstein *et al.*, 1972). Similarly, no reduction of cytotoxicity was obtained by the removal of B cells. The observed increase in cytotoxicity was explained by the concentrating effect of T cells, which was obtained by the removal of other cell types. CRT, a population of nearly 100% thymocytes, shows a particularly high lytic efficiency *in vitro* (Wagner, 1971; Lohmann-Matthes and Fischer, 1972). All these results conclusively prove that at least under *in vitro* conditions sensitized T lymphocytes can be autonomous with respect to their killer function.

Several groups have been interested in determining whether other cell types also participate as effector cells in cytotoxic reactions. They reported that peritoneal macrophages from immune animals are cytotoxic to allograft cells *in vitro* (Granger and Weiser, 1964; Lohmann-Matthes *et al.*, 1972; Den Otter *et al.*, 1972). In contrast to the pure T cell systems, where usually short-term cytotoxicity assays are used, macrophage-mediated cytotoxicity can only be observed using test periods of at least 24 hours (Evans and Alexander, 1970; Lohmann-Matthes *et al.*, 1972). This must be taken into account and may partially explain controversial data.

Granger and Weiser (1964) were the first to report that suspensions of peritoneal cells specifically destroyed embryonic fibroblasts *in vitro*. They put droplets of peritoneal exudate cells on fibroblast monolayers and observed that target fibroblasts were destroyed only at those places where specifically sensitized peritoneal exudate cells were administered to relevant target monolayers. Since it is well established that peritoneal lymphocytes are a subpopulation with particularly high cytotoxic capacity (Berke *et al.*, 1972), it cannot be excluded that the destructive effects in Granger and Weiser's experiments were due to the lytic activity of peritoneal lymphocytes. Bennett (1965) has reported successful suppression of tumor growth by the simultaneous injection of peritoneal macrophages from immune donors and tumor cells. However in the light of findings on the mechanism of macrophage-mediated cytotoxicity (see Section V; Evans and Alexander, Chapter 21), one could assume that also in these preparations, some T cells may have survived. These T cells did not account for direct cytotoxicity as checked in detail by Bennett (1965). However, they may supply mediators (produce on contact with antigen) which repeatedly render the macrophages cytotoxic. McIvor and Weiser (1971) reported that macrophage cultures from immune donors had cytostatic effects on target cells; in later experiments they isolated a factor released by immune macrophages which accounted for the cytostatic effects in their experiments. Most other authors, however, agree on a direct cell-mediated effect of lymphocytes or macrophages. It should be noted that McIvor and Weiser used mostly adherently growing cells as target cells. There is some evidence that the susceptibility to supernatant toxins varies widely among different target cells used (Granger, 1970; Cerottini and Brunner 1974).

Recently, more evidence has accumulated concerning the macrophage as a cytotoxic effector cell. We showed that monolayers of alloimmune peritoneal macrophages from which lymphocytes had been carefully removed by various methods (Lohmann-Matthes *et al.*, 1972) showed cytotoxicity against specific target cells. For total lysis an incubation period of 24 hours and a ratio of 20:1 were needed. Target cells in most experiments were DBA/2 P815X cells, similar to those used in most T cell systems. These results were confirmed by Den Otter *et al.* (1972) and by Krahenbuhl and Remington (1974). Gallily (1975) cocultivated macrophages from alloimmune donors with target macrophages from the immunizing strain. Immune macrophages specifically depressed DNA synthesis in target macrophages and also had a cytotoxic effect on the target macrophages as measured by ^{96}Rb uptake on day 4 of the cytotoxic culture.

The many controversial results may be summarized as follows. The antigen-reactive cells in allogeneic sensitization are T lymphocytes. The sensitized T lymphocytes have been proved under *in vitro* conditions to be extremely potent autonomous cytotoxic effector cells. In addition, macrophages from *in vivo* immunized donors have cytotoxic capacity against allogeneic target cells. This macrophage-mediated cytotoxicity was a specific reaction in all experimental situations. Lysis was performed rather slowly as compared with T cell lysis. It remains as yet unclear to what degree macrophage-mediated cytotoxicity contributes to allograft rejection processes *in vivo*.

III. CYTOTOXIC MACROPHAGES IN SYNGENEIC TUMOR SYSTEMS

A. Morphology and *in Vivo* Evidence for Macrophage Involvement in Syngeneic Tumor Rejection

In the previous section we dealt with the role of cytotoxic macrophages in allograft rejection tested *in vivo* and *in vitro*.

There is some parallelism in the experimental results of cell-mediated cytotoxicity in allograft and in syngeneic tumor rejection. This similarity can be demonstrated with respect to morphology of the cellular infiltrate and also by functional criteria. As in other delayed-type hypersensitivity reactions at the site of a rejected tumor, strong macrophage infiltration has been reported. In contrast to allograft rejection, however, the autonomy of cytotoxic T cells seems to be less pronounced in syngeneic tumor systems with weak antigenic differences, whereas cooperation with cytotoxic macrophages appears to play an important role in the rejection of some syngeneic tumors. Gershon *et al.* (1967) demonstrated, as already mentioned, that a lymphoma in hamsters was heavily infiltrated with typical macrophages. A second inoculum of the same tumor, which was destroyed due to concomitant immunity, showed an even stronger accumulation of macrophages. Evans (1973) isolated monolayers of macrophages from rat fibrosarcomas by means of trypsinizing the established tumor. This method resulted in extensive spreading of the macrophages, while the tumor cells stayed in suspension and could thus be separated from the macrophages. Eccles and Alexander (1974) extended these finding by demonstrating that the content of macrophages of a tumor is related to its capacity to metastasize, the more macrophage infiltration, the less development of metastases. This parallels the above cited findings of Gershon that a locally growing tumor, which does not metastasize because of developing concomitant immunity, is heavily infiltrated with macrophages. Data of More *et al.* (1973), showing that immunogenic tumors induce strong macrophage proliferation in the host, fit that concept.

Another approach to identifying the role of macrophages in tumor rejection was used by Zarling and Tevethia (1973a,b). These authors transfered tumor-specific immunity against SV40-transformed tumor cells from an immune animal to a normal recipient. Immunity was transfered by injecting spleen cells from an immune Balb/c mouse to a nonimmune Balb/c recipient. If the recipient animal had been irradiated, transfer of spleen cells did not result in tumor protection. If, however, bone marrow cells were given in addition, complete protection was obtained. Also, tumor cell neutralization was significantly diminished in mice pretreated with silica, an agent known to selectively destroy macrophages. Zarling and Tevethia concluded from these experiments that normal bone marrow-derived macrophages do cooperate *in vivo* with sensitized lymphocytes in the effector phase of tumor rejection. Data of Simes *et al.* (1975) also provide evidence that for tumor suppression to occur a radiosensitive host cell must cooperate with immune lymphocytes, at least when only low numbers of sensitized lymphocytes are available. They used a methylcholantrene-induced sarcoma in CBA mice and measured growth suppression after simultaneous injection of sensitized lymphocytes and tumor cells. However, the authors have not as yet characterized this cooperating radiosensitive host cell.

B. *In Vitro* Experiments to Assess the Role of Cytotoxic Macrophages in Tumor Rejection

Evans and Alexander (1970) reported that peritoneal macrophages from DBA/2 mice, which had been repeatedly immunized with intraperitoneal injections of irradiated DBA/2 L1210 lymphoma cells, were specifically cytotoxic *in vitro* against DBA/2 L1210 cells. Cytotoxicity was measured as growth inhibition of the tumor cells in a 72 hour test. The splenic lymphocytes of the same animals showed no cytotoxicity. Peritoneal lymphocytes or mesenteric lymphocytes were not tested. Recently Seeger and Owen (1974), working with the Moloney mouse sarcoma system, presented evidence that cytotoxic macrophages, although a minor subpopulation of lymph node, accounted for much of the cytotoxic tumor-destroying effect in regressor animals. Using the IUdR method, they demonstrated that unfractionated lymph node cells were highly cytostatic for Moloney virus-transformed tumor cells. When they tested the nonadherent fraction and the total lymph node population separately, they observed that stronger cytostatic effects were performed by the unfractionated cells. After treatment of these unfractionated lymph node suspensions with silica, the cytostatic capacity was greatly reduced, although only 2.5% of the unfractionated cells were shown to be macrophages. If they treated the nonadherent cytotoxic lymphocytes with anti-θ serum and complement, cytotoxity was lost, demonstrating the cytotoxicity in this nonadherent fraction to be T cell-dependent. However, no experiment is reported combining the different methods. In such an experiment, using unfractionated cells, treatment with silica should abolish the macrophage-dependent cytotoxicity, whereas T cell cytotoxicity should be undiminished. This latter cytotoxicity should then be sensitive to anti-θ serum and complement. Such an experiment would conclusively prove the relative contribution of each cell type to tumor rejection. Other authors (Leclerc *et al.*, 1973; Lamon and Wigzell, 1974) could not find any macrophage activity using the same system. This may be partially explained by the fact that macrophage precursor cells, which are not removable by the methods available, may contribute to the cytotoxic action of T cells and non-T cells.

In contrast with the experiments so far mentioned, all dealing with a macrophage contribution to tumor rejection, are the results by Röllinghoff *et al.* (1974). Their data are in summary very much like the results obtained in an allograft situation, which may be due to the strong immunogenicity of the mouse plasmocytoma tumors that they use. Macrophages certainly do not play a very conspicious role in their system; one could, however, put forward some arguments in favor of a possible participation of macrophage also in that system: Immunity could be transfered with immune spleen cells. Treatment with anti-θ serum and complement abrogated the immunizing effect of transferred immune spleen cells. Thus, no protection was obtained in the absence of T cells. Whether protection depended on the presence of host macrophages was not excluded. The cytotoxicity tests *in vitro* used were too short to observe macrophage-mediated cytotoxic effects. Inhibition of subcutaneous growth by peritoneal macrophages in the complete absence of T cells has not been shown as yet. The sensitized T lymphocyte may be absolutely necessary to activate the macrophages continuously to exert cytotoxic effects.

The experiments presented above permit the following conclusions. Macrophage precursor cells undergo transformation and proliferation when an immunogenic syngeneic tumor is transplanted (More *et al.*, 1973). Tumors that do not metastasize are often heavily infiltrated with macrophages. Rejection of tumors may need the presence of two populations, sensitized lymphocytes (presumably T lymphocytes) and radiosensitive bone marrow cells [presumably macrophage precursors that are radiosensitive—the mature macrophage has been shown to be radioresistant by Gallily and Feldmann (1967)]. In contrast with the allograft situation in most systems, sensitized T cells do not seem to be sufficient for tumor growth to be suppressed. Cooperation with cytotoxic macrophages seems necessary, and in some tumor systems macrophages seem to play a predominant role as cytotoxic or cytostatic effector cells. Their cytotoxic activity, however, depends on the presence of sensitized T lymphocytes.

In conclusion, it appears that in tumor immunity as well as in allograft immunity, the pattern of the reaction depends critically on the immunogenicity of the graft used.

IV. MACROPHAGE-MEDIATED CYTOTOXICITY INDUCED BY INFECTION WITH VARIOUS MICROORGANISMS

An interesting finding was reported by Hibbs *et al.* (1972). They found that macrophages of animals, which had resisted a severe infection acquired not only intracellular killing capacity for bacteria but also extracellular killing capacity for target tumor cells. They immunized mice of different strains with either *Toxoplasma, Besnoitia,* or *Listeria* (Krahenbuhl and Remington, 1974). Peritoneal macrophages obtained from animals that had survived the infection were strongly cytostatic for L cells, for adenosarcoma cells, and for lymphoma cells of mice. Macrophages were cytotoxic as long as the sensitizing organisms were present in the animals. The authors interpreted this finding in the following way. Sensitized lymphocytes interact with the sensitizing antigen, in this case an infecting organism. As the result of this interaction, macrophages are activated and rendered nonspecifically cytotoxic against tumor target cells. Mackaness and co-workers (Blanden *et al.*, 1969) had shown that a similar interaction takes place when macrophages are activated to intracellular killing. Recently, it was shown that the interacting lymphocyte was a T cell (Lane and Unanue, 1972; Blanden and Langman, 1972; North, 1973). Hibbs *et al.* noted the relationship between the capacity of activated macrophages either to kill microorganisms intracellularly or tumor target cells extracellularly. Therefore, parallel findings in the bactericidal system will be briefly mentioned in relation to induction of macrophage-mediated cytotoxicity.

Keller demonstrated (1973) (see Chapter 19) that even thioglycolate-induced macrophages show cytostatic effects on tumor cells. However, in the light of the question of activation and specificity of macrophage-mediated killing, which will be discussed in the Section V,C, this may fit into the whole concept.

V. *IN VITRO* INDUCTION OF MACROPHAGE-MEDIATED CYTOTOXICITY

In this section experiments will be discussed in which normal peritoneal macrophages are activated *in vitro*. This activation may express itself either in increased intracellular killing of microorganisms or in extracellular cytotoxicity against target cells.

In the preceding section several situations were described in which sensitized lymphocytes, sensitizing antigen, and effector macrophages were mixed at the site of a cytotoxic reaction. This is the case in allograft rejection, in tumor rejection, and also in the model of intracellular killing of bacteria. All the studies on the *in vitro* induction of macrophage-mediated cytotoxicity are based in some way on this situation.

A. Cocultivation Experiments

More detailed information on cytotoxic reactions mediated by macrophages was obtained by cocultivation studies, which served as a model for the situation in a peritoneal cavity of an animal after intraperitoneal immunization. Evans and Alexander (1972) mixed sensitized lymphocytes of DBA/2 mice, immunized several times with irradiated 5178Y DBA/2 lymphoma cells, with 5178Y DBA/2 lymphoma cells and normal peritoneal macrophages from untreated DBA/2 mice. Removing the lymphocytes after 24 hours of cocultivation, they obtained macrophage monolayers that they called "armed" and which were specifically cytotoxic for 5178Y DBA/2 target cells. Similar experiments were performed by Zembala *et al.* (1973) in an allogeneic *in vitro* system. They sensitized lymphocytes of one mouse strain for 3 days on allogeneic fibroblasts. When they tested these lymphocytes on day 3 for cytotoxicity in an 8-hour ^{51}Cr release test, no significant cytotoxicity was detectable. This is in line with kinetics of development of T cell cytotoxicity found by other groups (Cohen *et al.* 1971; Lohmann-Matthes *et al.*, 1972). When, however, they mixed normal peritoneal macrophages with these noncytotoxic lymphocytes and tested the mixed cultures in parallel with the cultures with only sensitized lymphocytes, good cytotoxicity was obtained. They attributed this cytotoxicity to a collaboration between the sensitized but not cytotoxic lymphocytes and normal macrophages.

In the bacterial systems, several comparable experiments have been published. In most of the experiments, increased intracellular killing capacity was measured at the end of the activation period, but as has been shown by Hibbs *et al.*, using the same bacterial systems, intracellular killing capacity may coincide with extracellular killing of tumor cells. Therefore, experiments along this line are briefly described. Patterson and Youmans (1970) cocultivated normal mouse macrophages with lymphocytes sensitized against mycobacteria in the presence of mycobacteria. The macrophages were activated and inhibited multiplication of intracellular virulent *Mycobacterium tuberculosis*. Simon and Sheagren (1972) cocultivated normal guinea pig macrophages with bovine γ-globulin (BGG) and BGG-committed lymphocytes and obtained intracellular killing capacity of *Listeria*. Recently, Anderson and Remington (1974) used human peripheral monocytes. They activated the monocyte-derived macrophage to intracellular killing by the admixture of lymphocytes sensitized against *Toxoplasma* and *Toxoplasma* lysate antigen. It must, however, be mentioned that human monocyte-derived macrophages apparently differ broadly in their capacity to kill different microorganisms (Diamond and Bennett, 1973). The same is true for guinea pig and mouse macrophages (Mauel and Behin, 1974). It remains to be demonstrated, whether the finding of Hibbs *et al.* (1972) that infection with *Toxoplasma* and other microorganisms not only induces intracellular killing capacity for microorganisms but also extracellular killing for tumor cells can be generalized for all systems where intracellular killing capacity is induced.

All these cocultivation experiments, which either lead to extracellular killing of tumor targets or to intracellular killing of microorganisms, have in common that macrophages are activated in the presence of sensitized lymphocytes and specific antigen.

In the bacterial systems, all groups agree on the fact that sensitized lymphocytes have no killing capacity themselves. In allogeneic and also in many syngeneic tumor systems, the situation is quite different. In these systems it is very difficult to formally exclude participation of cytotoxic T cells in the cytotoxic reaction of macrophage cultures. Therefore, experimental conditions were chosen in the allogeneic system to exclude cytotoxic lymphocytes completely from the test.

B. Induction of Macrophage-Mediated Cytotoxicity by Culture Supernatants

Macrophage activation may be assumed to take place in two steps. The first step would be an interaction between sensitized lymphocytes and the specific antigen. It is well known that during such an interaction a variety of mediators is liberated, some of which acting directly on macrophages (Ward *et al.*, 1791; David, 1966; Mooney and Waksman, 1970; Godal *et al.*, 1971). Induction of macrophage-mediated cytotoxicity was, therefore, likely also to be a result of lymphocyte mediators acting on macrophages. To test this assumption, C57BL/10 spleen cells from mice sensitized against DBA/2 alloantigens were cocultivated with DBA/2 lymphoma cells at a ratio of 100:1. The culture supernatant was centrifuged and filtered through 0.2 μm filters. We called this material macrophage cytotoxicity factor (MCF) (Lohmann-Matthes *et al.*, 1972). For testing the material the peritoneal cells from individual C57BL/10 mice are distributed into five flat-bottomed glass tubes (approximately 2×10^5 macrophages per tube). After 3 hours of incubation, the adherent cells are washed, and incubated for 24 hours with fresh medium and the factor to be tested. After this time, the cultures are washed and incubated for further 24 hours with ^{51}Cr-labeled target cells at an effector to target cell ratio of 10:1. Release of ^{51}Cr is determined from the counts in the centrifuged cell pellet and in the supernatant

$$\%\ ^{51}\text{Cr released} = \frac{100 \times \text{cpm in supernatant}}{\text{cpm in sediment} + \text{cpm in supernatant}}$$

Specific cytotoxicity is taken as the difference in percent ^{51}Cr release between factor-treated and control incubations. Evans *et al.*, who produced a similar factor in a syngeneic system, called it specific macrophage arming factor (SMAF). These authors measured cytostatic effects on tumor cells by the supernatant-activated macrophages (Evans *et al.*, 1972). The following experiments were performed to show that MCF was produced by T-cells.

1. Pretreatment of sensitized spleen cells with anti-θ serum and complement inhibited the production of MCF.
2. Concentration of T cells by passing sensitized spleen cells several times through cotton wool columns resulted in an increased activity of the MCF produced.
3. MCF is produced under *in vitro* conditions by cortisone-resistant thymocytes sensitized *in vitro* aginst allogeneic cells (Lohmann-Matthes and Fischer, 1973).

The kinetics of induction of macrophage-mediated cytotoxicity are as shown in Table I. Ten to 12 hours are necessary to fully activate the macrophages and 18 hours to obtain complete target cell destruction at a killed to target ratio of 10:1. (Ziegler *et al.*, 1975).

Some properties of MCF are summarized as follows.

a. MCF activates peritoneal macrophages to cytotoxicity.
b. MCF is cytophilic for macrophages.
c. MCF binds to syngeneic and allogeneic macrophages.
d. Cytotoxic macrophages are resistant to 1000 R.
e. MCF is only active if bound to macrophages. No direct toxic effect on tissue culture cells has been observed (Lohmann-Matthes and Fischer, 1973).

Again in the bacterial systems comparable results were obtained. Thus intracellular killing capacity was induced in macrophages with culture supernatant of sensitized lymphocytes and antigen. Krahenbuhl and Remington (1971) activated normal guinea pig macrophages by incubating them for 72 hours with the supernatant of a culture of lymphocytes (sensitized against *Toxoplasma*) and *Toxoplasma*. Patterson and Youmans (1970) incubated mouse macrophages with cell-free filtered supernatants of cultures from lymphocytes (sensitized against mycobacteria) and mycobacteria. The macrophages acquired the capacity to inhibit intracellular multiplication of virulent *Mycobacterium tuberculosis*. Godal *et al.* (1971) reported that supernatants of rabbit mixed lymphocyte cultures activated rabbit blood-derived macrophages to inhibit multiplication of mycobacteria.

TABLE I

Kinetics of the Induction of Macrophage-Mediated Cytotoxicity

Incubation time (hours)	Specific ^{51}Cr release from labeled P815X target cells (%)
Experiment I[a]	
3	0
6	10
12	35
18	38
24	41
Experiment II[b]	
3	5
6	8
12	15
18	35
24	39

[a] Macrophages were incubated for different time periods with MCF and immediately afterward cytotoxicity was tested during 24 hours of incubation with target cells.

[b] Macrophage monolayers, which had been activated 24 hours with MCF, are now incubated for different time periods with labeled target cells.

C. Specificity of Macrophage-Mediated Cytotoxicity

In all the systems mentioned, sensitized lymphocytes secrete activating mediators only upon contact with the specific antigen. Thus specific interaction is needed for the production of MCF. Specificity of the effector phase, however, has only been described in allogeneic systems and in some syngeneic tumor systems (Evans *et al.*, 1972). We (Lohmann-Matthes *et al.*, 1972) described destruction of allogeneic target cells by cytotoxic macrophages which was specific for the target cell used for immunization. Similar results were reported by Evans *et al.* (1972), Den Otter *et al.* (1972), Zembala *et al.* (1973), and Gallily (1975) in the above-mentioned cocultivation experiments. None of these groups has, however, identified the nature of the specificity conveying moiety. In the meantime, a whole variety of specific T cell products with different biological activities has been described by other groups in different system (Feldmann, 1972; Taussig, 1974; Zembala *et al.*, 1975). Also these groups have not yet been able to characterize fully the nature of their specific T cell product. In our hands, the specificity of the cytotoxic reaction was not inhibited by treatment of the cultures with rabbit anti-mouse immunoglobulin nor was it inhibited by preincubation of test macrophages with normal mouse serum (Lohmann-Matthes and Fischer, 1973).

In the bacterial systems dealing with intracellular killing, there is complete agreement on the nonspecificity of the effector phase. Our later experiments in the allogeneic system suggest that most probably two different components are involved: one activating macrophages and in certain circumstances inducing nonspecific effects, and another having specific effects. The following data favor this interpretation.

1. Peritoneal macrophages from mice that have been kept under specific pathogen-free (SPF) conditions give specific killing reactions when incubated with an MCF preparation raised in allogenically immunized mice, which have been kept under identical SPF conditions.
2. If either the producer mice or the macrophage donors have been kept under conventional conditions (although macrophages are absolutely noncytotoxic by themselves), in most experiments nonspecific cytotoxicity is obtained upon incubation with MCF. To explain this finding we suggest that mice, kept under conventional conditions, are continuously exposed to more or less mild infections that result in a preactivation of the macrophages or in production of nonspecific MCF preparations.
3. Similar results are obtained if we deliberately preactivate the macrophages by injecting thioglycolate. Thioglycolate-induced macrophages are also absolutely noncytotoxic by themselves. Incubating them, however, with specific MCF results, in many experiments, in nonspecific cytotoxicity (Lohmann-Matthes and Fischer, 1973).
4. If the mouse colony has overcome a severe infection, we cannot use the mice again, since the test macrophages obtained from the peritoneal cavity of such mice are highly cytotoxic for tumor target cells without any further treatment. We assume that this may correspond to the well-established situation described by Hibbs *et al.* (1972) using defined microorganisms for infections.

These four points are summarized in Table II.

The conclusion is that the previously observed specific effects can only be demonstrated if both producer mice and test mice are kept under extremely clean conditions. Preactivation with either chemical or biological means appears to result in a nonspecific factor effect. We, therefore,

TABLE II

Specificity of the Cytotoxic Reaction of Macrophages

Macrophages	Specific ^{51}Cr release (%) from labeled C57BL/EL4	DBA/2 P815X
SPF mice	0	0
SPF mice incubated with MCF (C57BL/10 anti-DBA/2)	0	39 ± 5
Conventional mice	0	0
Conventional mice incubated with MCF (C57BL/10 anti-DBA/2)	25 ± 5	45 ± 7
Thioglycolate induced	0	0
Thioglycolate induced incubated with MCF (C57BL/10 anti-DBA/2)	30 ± 6	55 ± 8
From mice that overcame an infection	38 ± 12	53 ± 14

assume that under experimental conditions, using SPF mice for production and testing, two components are present in our MCF preparations: one that activates macrophages and seems to be nonspecific and a specific component that establishes close contact between the activated macrophage and the specific target cell leading to destruction of the latter. The specific component could not be replaced by antiserum (Lohmann-Matthes and Fischer, 1973). Preactivation of the test macrophages seems to add to the activation by specific MCF preparations thus partially or completely hiding the specific effects.

Work is in progress to elucidate the nature of this specificity conveying moiety. However, this approach is very complicated by the considerations outlined above. Therefore, we decided to work on characterization of MCF preparations that induced nonspecific cytotoxicity in macrophages. With regard to the human situation, viewing a SPF mouse breeding colony as a highly artificial model, it seems likely that the cytotoxic effector phase in most cases will be a nonspecific reaction. At the production step, however, specific interaction between sensitized lymphocytes and the antigen is necessary (Evans *et al.*, 1972; Lohmann-Matthes *et al.*, 1973); therefore cytotoxicity-inducing factors will be mostly secreted at the reaction site, where they bind to macrophages. Thus, macrophage activity will be restricted to the specific reaction site.

The purification steps described in Section V,D were applied to large batches of MCF preparations inducing nonspecific cytotoxicity (Hall *et al.*, 1975). It was retested and confirmed that the material used was a T cell product.

D. Attempts at Chemical Characterization of Macrophage Cytotoxicity Factor

Preliminary results showed that MCF is inactivated on incubation with trypsin but is not sensitive to pancreatic ribonuclease A treatment (Ziegler *et al.*, 1975). All fractionation procedures are carried out at 4°C. The MCF-containing supernatant (in serum-free Eagle's medium) is first concentrated fivefold by filtration over a Diaflo PM10 membrane (Amicon). The concentrate is then adjusted to pH 7.5 and applied to a 24 × 1.6 cm column of DEAE cellulose equilibrated with 10 m*M* phosphate buffer, pH 7.5; 150 m*M* NaCl; and 10% (v/v) glycerol. It has been found that the presence of glycerol stabilizes MCF activity. The column is washed with the above buffer at a flow rate of 70 ml/hour, and the breakthrough peak containing nonspecific MCF activity is collected. After concentration as above, the sample is applied to a 100 × 1.3 cm column of Sephadex G-100, and eluted at a flow rate of 7 ml/hour. The activity is obtained in a single peak (molecular weight approximately 30,000) and, after concentration, may be purified further on a 40 × 1.3 cm calibrated column of Sephadex G-75 in the DEAE-cellulose column buffer. Nonspecific MCF elutes from this column with a molecular weight of 28,000 ± 5000. The concentrated active material is filtered (0.2 μm Millipore) and stored in small aliquots at −70°C. It is stable for several months under these conditions. In the absence of glycerol, however, all activity is lost on freezing and thawing (Fig. 1).

By these fractionation procedures we obtain about 18-fold purification. There is no significant loss of activity following the DEAE-cellulose step. We analyzed the purified fraction of MCF by polyacrylamide gel electrophoresis in the presence of sodium dodecyl sulfate (SDS). Several bands are visible after staining with Coomassie brilliant blue.

These experiments show that we have isolated and partially purified a T lymphocyte mediator, molecular weight ~30,000, which activates macrophages to exert nonspecific cytotoxicity toward target tumor cells. The next question arising was, whether we had in fact been purifying one of the macrophage migration inhibitory factor (MIF) fractions and were only using a different test system. For this reason the material was sent to Dr. Sorg (Sorg and Bloom, 1972) to test if for MIF activity. The results obtained so far indicate that the material does indeed have MIF activity.

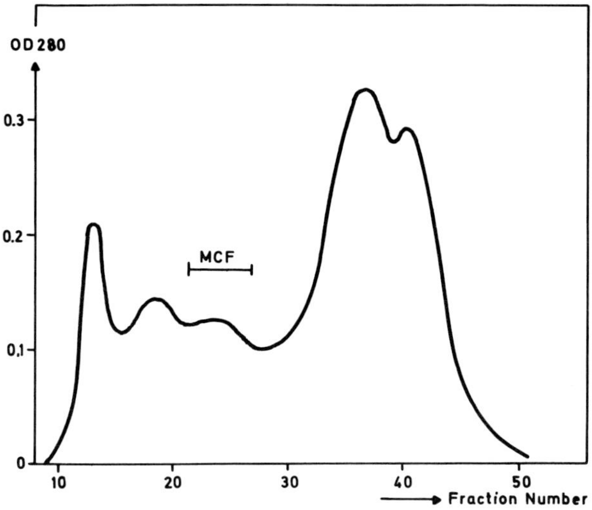

Fig. 1. Purification of MCF on Sephadex G-100. Following chromatography on DEAE-cellulose MCF is purified by gel filtration on Sephadex G-100 as described in the text. MCF activity is only detectable in the region marked on the figure.

Evans and Grant (1972) have also done fractionation experiments on Biogel columns. They found activity peaks at molecular weight 300,000 and 50,000. Whether these results are due to aggregated material remains to be established.

VI. SUMMARY AND IMPLICATIONS

Cytotoxic reactions of mouse peritoneal macrophages against tumor target cells *in vitro* were described. It was shown that macrophages are activated and induced to be cytotoxic for tumor target cells by a product of sensitized T cells secreted in the presence of the sensitizing antigen. This factor, MCF, binds to syngeneic and allogeneic macrophages, rendering them cytotoxic. Cytotoxic macrophages that have destroyed target cells in tissue culture can be rendered cytotoxic again by another incubation with MCF. The same culture of macrophages can thus destroy several target tumor cell populations (Lohmann-Matthes and Fischer, 1973). Macrophage precursors from the bone marrow are radiosensitive. The mature cytotoxic macrophage, however, is a radioresistant cell (Lohmann-Matthes *et al.*, 1972). The fact that the macrophage is radioresistant, that it can be rendered cytotoxic several times, and that it may be most effectively recruited from the pool of quickly dividing bone-marrow precursors favors the idea that it may be a very potent cytotoxic effector cell.

Experiments were reported on chemical characterization of MCF produced in an allogeneic mouse system. The material used activated macrophages and induced nonspecific cytotoxicity. It was shown to elute from Sephadex G-75 in one fraction with molecular weight ~30,000 and proved to be stable if kept at —70°C. MIF activity could be demonstrated in this fraction.

It was also shown that using comparable experimental conditions, i.e., cocultivation of lymphocytes sensitized against a microorganism and antigenic material of the infecting microorganism in the presence of macrophages, activation of macrophages to intracellular killing was obtained. Activation was also obtained by incubating normal macrophages with supernatants of cultures of sensitized lymphocytes with the bacterial antigens. It was further shown that macrophages from animals, which overcame an infection with microorganisms, not only acquired intracellular killing capacity but also extracellular cytotoxicity for tumor target cells.

In both systems activation of macrophages requires an interaction of sensitized T cells with the specific antigen. From the evidence presented it seems likely that a general reaction occurs in both systems: Normal macrophages are activated by a mediator secreted by sensitized T lymphocytes in the presence of the sensitizing antigen. The activation may be manifest either as intracellular killing capacity of microorganisms or as extracellular killing of tumor target cells. It is an appealing, but unproven, idea that the same mechanism and probably the same T lymphocyte mediator may account for macrophage activation in both systems of cell-mediated killing.

In allogeneic mouse systems and some syngeneic mouse tumor systems specific target cell killing has been described. However, the expression of this specificity depends on the SPF state of the animals and therefore lacks reliability and reproducibility. Cytotoxicity effected by macrophages from animals which have overcome a severe infection is always nonspecific. Intracellular killing of microorganism is also a nonspecific event.

Two major questions will be looked at in the near future: The first one is to test our suggestion that the fractionated material activates macrophages not only to extracellular cytotoxicity but also to intracellular killing of microorganisms. The mononuclear phagocyte system can readily be activated to proliferation (Metcalf, 1971; Pluznik *et al.*, 1972), thus providing higher numbers of potential effector cells. Therefore, such generalized effector mechanisms would be of special interest. In animals chronically exposed to mild infections, the material described may be continuously produced, thus leading to a state of chronic preactivation of macrophages. This preactivation may supply a subthreshold dose of macrophage activation, which allows the macrophages at the site of severe reaction to respond with higher sensitivity to locally produced MCF. This preactivation of macrophages may thus guarantee a better protection by providing sensitive macrophages, which are readily activated to extracellular or intracellular killing. In animals under sterile conditions, mild otherwise insignificant infections and otherwise suppressed tumor growth may have deleterious effects. This would concur with the suggestion of active stimulation of the mononuclear phagocyte system.

The second point of interest is the question of whether tumor cell material, which is bound to activated and cytotoxic macrophages, may be of increased immunogenicity with respect to the development of delayed-type hypersensitivity. Zbar *et al.* (1971) and recently Hawrylko and Mackaness (1974) have shown that tumor cells injected into a site of BCG reaction are not only suppressed in their growth but also might cause development of systemic immunity. The BCG granuloma is characterized by an accumulation of T cells and macrophages. Seeger and Oppenheim (1972) demonstrated that the antigen DNP-ovalbumin if presented bound to macrophages induced delayed-type hypersensitivity rather than antibody production (see Oppenheim and Seeger, Chapter 5). The same has been shown by Pearson and Raffel (1971) using SRBC as antigen. Rouse and Wagner (1972) reported that sensitization against subcellular mouse alloantigen was only obtained in the presence of macrophages. They discuss a collaboration between macrophages and T lymphocytes in the process of antigen presentation and recognition. Thus, at the site of allograft or tumor rejection, cytotoxic and activated macrophages kill target cells and may present antigenic determinants of the killed cells on their surface. Such processed antigenic material may increase the T cell response. This may be of special importance in the case of weak antigens.

Thus, further work must be done on the collaboration of T lymphocytes and macrophages both in the induction and in the effector phase of a cell-mediated reaction. Also, the relative importance of contributions by macrophages in different cell-mediated reactions must be clearly defined. Although resistance to some infections is exclusively effected by macrophages activated by T cell mediators, no final conclusions can yet be drawn as to which cytotoxic effector cell population predominates in defense against tumors *in vivo*. This may vary among different tumors and may largely depend on the immunogenicity of a particular tumor. In allogeneic systems, macrophage activation to cytotoxicity does take place. This may, however, be of minor importance in the effector phase, since the sensitized T lymphocytes have a strikingly high efficiency in such situations and may under certain conditions destroy allografts without the collaboration of other cell types.

ACKNOWLEDGMENTS

The excellent technical assistance of Mrs. I. Hulsmann and Mrs. M. Haussman is gratefully acknowledged. This study was supported in part by the Deutsche Forschungsgemeinschaft.

REFERENCES

Anderson, S. E., and Remington, J. S. (1974). *J. Exp. Med.* **139,** 1154–1174.

Bennett, B. (1965). *J. Immunol.* **80,** 656–664.

Berke, G., Sullivan, K., Sullivan, A., and Amos, D. S. (1972). *J. Exp. Med.* **135,** 1334–1350.

Blanden, R. V., and Langman, R. E. (1972). *Scand. J. Immunol.* **1,** 379–391.

Blanden, R. V., Lefford, M. J., and Mackaness, G. B. (1969). *J. Exp. Med.* **129,** 1079–1107.

Cerottini, J. C., Nordin, A. A., and Brunner, K. T. (1970). *Nature (London)* **227,** 72–73.

Cerottini, J. C., and Brunner, K. T. (1974). *Advan. Immunol.* **18,** 67–132.

Cohen, I. R., Globerson, A., and Feldmann, M. (1971). *J. Exp. Med.* **133,** 821–833.

David, J. R. (1966). *Proc. Nat. Acad. Sci.* **56,** 72–77.

Den Otter, W., Evans, R., and Alexander, P. (1972). *Transplantation* **14,** 220–226.

Diamond, R. D., and Bennett, J. E. (1973). *Infec. Immunity* **7,** 231–236.

Dyminski, J. W., and Argyris, B. F. (1969). *Transplantation* **8,** 595–601.

Eccles, S. A., and Alexander, P. (1974). *Nature (London)* **250,** 667–669.

Evans, R. (1973). *J. Nat. Cancer Inst.* **50,** 271–273.

Evans, R., and Alexander, P. (1970). *Nature (London)* **228,** 620–622.

Evans, R., and Alexander, P. (1972). *Immunology* **23,** 615–626.

Evans, R., and Grant, C. K. (1972). *Immunology* **23,** 677–687.

Evans, R., Grant C. K., Cox, H., Steele, K., and Alexander, P. (1972). *J. Exp. Med.* **136,** 1318–1322.

Feldmann, M. (1972). *J. Exp. Med.* **136,** 737–760.

Freedmann, L. R., Cerottini, J. C., and Brunner, K. T. (1972). *J. Immunol.* **109,** 1371–1378.

Gallily, R. (1975). *Cell. Immunol.* **15,** 419–431.

Gallily, R., and Feldmann, M. (1967). *Immunology* **12,** 197–206.

Gell, P. H., and Hinde, I. T. (1951). *Brit. J. Exp. Pathol.* **32,** 516–526.

Gershon, R. K., Carter R. L., and Lane, N. J. (1967). *Amer. J. Pathol.* **51,** 1111–1133.

Giroud, I. P., Spector, W. G., and Willoughby, D. A. (1970). *Immunology* **19,** 857–863.

Godal, T., Rees, R. I. W., and Lamvik, J. O. (1971). *Clin. Exp. Immunol.* **8,** 625–637.

Golstein, P., and Blomgren, H. (1973). *Cell. Immunol.* **9,** 127–141.
Golstein, P., Wigzell, H., Blomgren, H., and Svedmyr, E. A. J. (1972). *J. Exp. Med.* **135,** 890–906.
Granger, G. A. (1970). *Amer. J. Pathol.* **60,** 469–482.
Granger, G. A., and Weiser, R. S. (1964). *Science* **145,** 1427–1429.
Hall, N., Lohmann-Matthes, M.-L., Kuüfermann, L., and Kickhöfen, B., (1975). In preparation.
Hawrylko, E., and Mackaness, G. B. (1974). *J. Nat. Cancer Inst.* **51,** 1683–1688.
Hibbs, J. B., Lambert, L. H., Jr., and Remington, J. S. (1972). *Nature (London)* **235,** 48–50.
Keller, R. (1973). *J. Exp. Med.* **138,** 625–644.
Krahenbuhl, J. L., and Remington, I. S. (1972). *Infec. Immunity* **4,** 337–343.
Krahenbuhl, J. L., and Remington, J. S. (1974). *J. Immunol.* **113,** 507–516.
Lamon, E. W., and Wigzell, H. (1974). *Transplantation* **18,** 368–371.
Lane, F. C., and Unanue, E. R. (1972). *J. Exp. Med.* **135,** 1104–1112.
Leclerc, J. C., Gomard, E., Plata, F., and Levy, J. P. (1973). *J. Nat. Cancer Inst.* **51,** 426–432.
Lohmann–Matthes, M.-L., and Fischer, H. (1972). *Eur. J. Immunol.* **2,** 290–292.
Lohmann-Matthes, M.-L., and Fischer, H. (1973). *Transplantation Rev.* **17,** 150–171.
Lohmann-Matthes, M.-L., Schipper, H., and Fischer, H. (1972). *Eur. J. Immunol.* **2,** 45–49.
Lohmann-Matthes, M.-L., Ziegler, F. G., and Fischer, H. (1973). *Eur. J. Immunol.* **3,** 56–58.
Lonai, P., and Feldman, M. (1971). *Immunology* **21,** 861–867.
Lubaroff, D. M. (1973). *J. Exp. Med.* **138,** 331–341.
Lubaroff, D. M., and Waksman, B. H. (1968). *J. Exp. Med.* **128,** 1425–1435.
McIvor, K. L., and Weiser, R. S. (1971). *Immunology* **20,** 307–313.
Mauel, J., and Behin, R. (1974). *Transplant. Rev.* **19,** 121–146.
Metcalf, D. (1971). *Immunology* **21,** 427–436.
Mooney, J. J., and Waksman, B. H. (1970). *J. Immunol.* **105,** 1138–1145.
More, D. G., Penrose, J. M., Kearney, R., and Nelson, D. S. (1973). *Int. Arch. Allergy Appl. Immunol.* **44,** 611–630.
Nomoto, K., Gershon, R. K., and Waksman, B. H. (1970). *J. Nat. Cancer. Inst.* **44,** 739–749.
North, R. (1973). *J. Exp. Med.* **138,** 342–355.
Patterson, R. I., and Youmans G. P. (1970). *Infec. Immunity* **1,** 600–603.
Pearson, M. N., and Raffel, S. (1971). *J. Exp. Med.* **133,** 494–505.
Pluznik, D. H., Rotter, V., and Scheinman, R. (1972). *RES. J. Reticuloendothel. Soc.* **11,** 154–166.
Poulter, L. W., Bradley, N. J., and Turk, I. L. (1971). *Transplantation* **12,** 40–44.
Ritter, J., Lohmann-Matthes, M.-L., Sonntag, H. G., and Fischer, H. (1975). *Cell. Immunol.* **16,** 153–161.
Röllinghoff, M., Wagner, H., Warner, N. L., and Nossal, G. I. V. (1974). *Isr. J. Med. Sci.* **10,** 1001–1011.
Rouse, B. T., and Wagner, H. (1972). *J. Immunol.* **109,** 1282–1289.
Schimpl, A., and Wecker, E. (1972). *Nature (London), New Biol.* **237,** 15–17.
Seeger, R. C., and Oppenheim, J. I. (1972). *J. Immunol.* **109,** 255–261.
Seeger, R. C., and Owen, C. L. (1974). *Nature (London)* **252,** 420–421.
Simes, R. J., Kearney, D. S., and Nelson, D. S. (1975). *Immunology* **29,** 343–352.

Simon, H. B., and Sheagren, I. N. (1972). *Cell. Imunol.* **4,** 163–174.
Sonntag, H. G., and Müller-Ruchholz, W. (1975). *Z. Immunitaetsforsch.* (in press).
Sorg, C., and Bloom, B. R. (1972). *J. Exp. Med.* **137,** 148–170.
Taussig, M. J., Mozes, E., and Isac, R. (1974). *J. Exp. Med.* **140,** 301–312.
Volkman, A., and Gowans, J. C. (1965). *Brit. J. Exp. Pathol.* **46,** 62–70.
Wagner, H. (1971). *Eur. J. Immunol.* **1,** 498–499.
Wagner, H., and Boyle, W. (1972). *Nature (London)* **240,** 92–94.
Wagner, H., Feldmann, M., Boyle, W., and Schrader, J. W. (1972). *J. Exp. Med.* **136,** 331–343.
Waksman, B. H. (1963). *Lab. Invest.* **12,** 46–57.
Ward, P. A., Offen, C. D., and Montgomery, J. R. (1971). *Fed. Proc., Fed. Amer. Soc. Exp. Biol.* **30,** 1721–1724.
Zarling, J. M., and Tevethia, S. S. (1973a). *J. Nat. Cancer Inst.* **50,** 137–148.
Zarling, J. M., and Tevethia, S. S. (1973b). *J. Nat. Cancer Inst.* **50,** 149–157.
Zbar, B., Bernstein, I. D., and Rapp, H. J. (1971). *J. Nat. Cancer Inst.* **46,** 831–839.
Zembala, M., Ptak, W., and Hanczakowska, M. (1973). *Clin. Exp. Immunol.* **15,** 461–466.
Zembala, M., Asherson, G. L., Mayhew, B., and Krejci, I. (1975). *Nature (London)* **253,** 72–74.
Ziegler, F. G., Lohmann-Matthes, M.-L., and Fischer, H. (1975). *Int. Arch. Allergy Appl. Immunol.* **48,** 182–191.

19

Cytostatic and Cytocidal Effects of Activated Macrophages

R. Keller

I. Introduction 487
II. Nomenclature 488
III. Cytostatic Effects of Activated Macrophages 489
A. Methods 489
B. Effects of Activated Macrophages on Target Cell Proliferation 491
C. Mechanisms of Cytostasis 496
IV. Cytocidal Effects of Macrophages 499
A. Methods 499
B. Cytocidal Tumor Target Alterations following Interaction with Activated Macrophages 500
C. Possible Mechanisms for Cytocidal Target Cell Killing 502
V. The Biologic Relevance of the *in Vitro* Findings 503
VI. Critical Outlook 505
References 507

I. INTRODUCTION

It has been known since the time of Metchnikoff (1905) that phagocytic cells enter areas of inflammation and participate in host defense against microbial pathogens. More recently, macrophages have been established as the ultimate effectors of cell-mediated antibacterial immunity. For the expression of such resistance, macrophages become metabolically altered or "activated" in such a way that they can intracellularly destroy an extensive array of immunologically unrelated microbial pathogens (Blanden *et al.*, 1966). It has become more widely appreciated that mononuclear phagocytes play an important role in pathological processes, such as chronic inflammation, tissue responses to inhaled toxic materials, presentation of antigen to immunocompetent cells, and resistance against intracellular microorganisms. That these macrophages also have profound effects on eukaryotic cells is the most recent development. Such effects can either be immunologically specific or nonspecific and can be induced in a variety of ways (Evans and Alexander, Chapter 21).

This chapter deals with some of the consequences of interaction between nonimmune macrophages and a variety of neoplastic or normal target cells. The information developed is based largely, but not exclusively, on work carried out in the author's laboratory.

II. NOMENCLATURE

The number and kinds of *in vitro* techniques for identifying metabolic or functional alterations and the nature of damage induced in target cells are rather limited, and of these some are not applicable to macrophage–target cell interactions. For example, parameters, such as release of cell-bound ^{51}Cr, uptake of agents normally excluded by intact cells (i.e., dyes such as trypan blue), or expressions of gross and irreversible *cytotoxic* or *cytolytic* membrane defects, may not reveal macrophage-mediated target cell alterations. The macrophage–target cell interaction need not evoke either changes in these particular cytotoxic parameters or phagocytosis of particulate matter but can nonetheless be followed by a marked decrease in the number of target cells; it has therefore been assumed that some other cytocidal mechanism is involved.

In the present work, inhibition of thymidine incorporation and/or target cell proliferation without overt cytolytic or cytotoxic signs is considered to be a purely *cytostatic* effect; interactions accompanied by an increase in ^{51}Cr release, uptake of trypan blue, and/or loss of viability of targets are judged to be *cytolytic* or cytotoxic; interactions followed by a marked decrease in the number of target cells without evident increase in conventional parameters of cytotoxicity or obvious signs of phagocytosis of particulate target cell matter are taken to mean that an as yet unknown *cytocidal* mechanism is responsible for target cell killing.

III. CYTOSTATIC EFFECTS OF ACTIVATED MACROPHAGES

A. Methods

1. Procurement of Macrophages

a. Rat Macrophages. All experiments cited were performed using rat peritoneal cells as effectors unless otherwise indicated. *Normal* or resting macrophages (NM) are obtained from untreated inbred rats of the DA or Lewis strain by seeding peritoneal washouts into plastic petri dishes. After 60 minutes, nonadherent cells are removed by intensive washing. Initially such monolayers consist of approximately 70% mononuclear phagocytes, 15% polymorphonuclear leukocytes, 10% lymphocytes, and a small percentage of eosinophils and mast cells. When the cells are maintained for 15 to 24 hours in modified minimal essential medium supplemented with 10% rat or newborn calf serum and antibiotics, the majority of the nonmacrophage population can be washed off the macrophage monolayer, which is firmly adherent to the dish and shows morphological signs of activation. It is noteworthy that the act of *in vitro* culture of resting mononuclear phagocytes itself gives rise to some activation; accordingly it is difficult to determine reliably in quantitative terms the functional capacities of resting macrophages under *in vitro* culture conditions. *Activated* macrophages (AM) are elicited by intraperitoneal injection of peptone (10 ml 10% peptone per adult DA or Lewis rat). After 3 days, this induced exudate yields a high proportion of adherent cells, the latter consisting almost exclusively (96–99%) of cells exhibiting morphologic and endocytic properties of mononuclear phagocytes (Keller, 1973a).

b. Mouse Macrophages. Mouse peritoneal cells are harvested 5–6 days after intraperitoneal injection of 0.5 ml Freund's complete adjuvant, and macrophage monolayers are prepared as described for rat cells (Keller, 1974a).

2. Target Cell Lines

A variety of syngeneic, allogeneic, and xenogeneic cell lines have been used that are derived from normal and malignant tissues; their origin and characteristics are listed in Table I.

TABLE I

Origin and Growth Characteristics of the Cell Lines Employed

Cell line	Origin	Number of passages *in vitro*	Proliferation (dpm × 100)	
			4 hours	72 hours
Polyoma I	DA rat	70–80	5.5–139	73–1390
Polyoma II	DA rat	3–7	5.6–178	22–1600
Methylcholanthrene	DA rat	30–36	5.3–168	50–1600
Dimethyl-benzanthracene	DA rat	2–4	5–147	28–1700
Methylcholanthrene	Lewis rat	10–17	4–148	197–1750
Normal rat kidney	rat	∞ [a]	6.4–24	31–400
B_{77} Rous sarcoma virus	rat	∞	7.8–17	43–88
Embryonic rat fibroblasts	DA rat	0–3	0.79–1.4	2.6–12.7
		6–12	9.4–15	78–122.5
Adult rat fibroblasts	DA rat	0–3	0.7–2.5	2.6–8.9
Embryonic rat fibroblasts	Lewis rat	0–3	0.7–1.65	10.5–31.5
3T3	Balb/c mouse	∞	7–72	25–1600
SV40 3T3	Balb/c mouse	∞	9–145	60–1600
CHO	Hamster fibroblasts	∞	6.7–69	17–775
Lopez	Human fibroblasts	∞	7–142	12–1700
BT 20	Human adenocarcinoma	∞	7.5–17	21.2–27
SK-mel-1	Human melanoma (suspension)	∞	12–110	650–843
RPMI 7932[b]	Human melanoma	∞	8–100	160–2500
P-815	Mastocytoma DBA/Z mouse (suspension)	∞	10–60	450–2000
Raji[c]	BL[c]	∞	5–55	60–1600
Daudi[c]	BL	∞	3–15	27–1500
Maku[c]	BL	∞	3–11	15–780
Namalwa[c]	BL	∞	5–16	22–1800
F-265[c]	EBV carrier	∞	3–15	18–1400
Molt-4[c]	ALL, EBV-negative	∞	4–10	10–810

[a] ∞, *in vitro* culture was for years.

[b] A gift from Dr. W. D. Terry.

[c] A gift from Dr. G. Klein. BL, Burkitt's lymphoma. F-265 has been derived from a normal donor and is an Epstein-Barr virus (EBV) carrying lymphoblastoid cell line. Molt-4 was derived from acute lymphatic leukemia (ALL) and is EBV-genome negative. Further details on these human lymphoblastoid cell lines are given by Svedmyr *et al.* (1974).

3. Methods Used to Assess Cytostasis

Until recently, the outcome of the interaction between macrophages and target cells has been based mostely on the morphological consequences, i.e. a decrease in number and changes in shape of target cells (Hibbs *et al.*, 1972; Hibbs, 1973) or enumeration of target cells remaining after interaction (Alexander and Evans, 1971; Evans and Alexander, 1973; Holtermann *et al.*, 1973). While these parameters disclose cytocidal, cytolytic, or cytotoxic effects accompanied by a marked diminution in target cell numbers, they are not informative regarding less obvious cytostatic effects. Moreover, such visual methods of evaluating target cell damage are often cumbersome and rather subjective (Takasugi and Klein, 1970; Hellström *et al.*, 1971).

For the assessment of the macrophage effects on target cell proliferation *in vitro*, measurement of the incorporation of a pulse of ^{3}H-labeled thymidine has proved advantageous in its sensitivity and in yielding reproducible and reliable results in *in vitro* systems (Keller, 1973a, 1974b; Olivotto and Bomford, 1974). This approach is feasible because under these *in vitro* culture conditions, macrophages manifest a very low proliferative rate that does not exceed background levels of thymidine incorporation.

Target cells were added to macrophage monolayers (2×10^6 adherent cells), and their residual proliferation measured after varying intervals of effector–target cell interaction by exposure to 1 μCi [^{3}H]thymidine per culture for 60 minutes at 37°C. The cultures were then washed three times with 1.5% perchloric acid and solubilized with hot perchloric acid (Keller, 1973a) to ensure that the radioactive precursor was incorporated into DNA; nucleic acid radioactivity was measured by liquid scintillation counting, and data are reported as disintegrations per minute (dpm). This procedure yielded reproducible results, whereas the transfer of adherent cells that had been removed mechanically or by trypsinization to target cell cultures gave data that were unacceptably variable.

B. Effects of Activated Macrophages on Target Cell Proliferation

1. Effects on Proliferation of Normal and Transformed Target Cells

Extensive investigation has shown that nonspecific stimulation of macrophages as achieved by persistent intracellular infection or by nonspecific stimulation of the mononuclear phagocyte system enables these cells to kill tumor cells in a nonspecific manner (Keller *et al.*, 1971; Alexander and Evans, 1971; Keller and Hess, 1972; Keller, 1973b; Hibbs *et al.*,

1972; Holtermann *et al.*, 1973; Olivotto and Bomford, 1974). *In vitro* studies, in which various syngeneic tumor cell lines were added to macrophage cultures and the rate of thymidine incorporation by tumor cells determined after various intervals, confirmed earlier observations of a striking interaction between AM and targets. At an effector to target cell ratio of 10:1, tumor cell proliferation was invariably promptly and effectively stopped. The finding that incorporation of [^{3}H]uridine was similarly blocked suggested that DNA and RNA synthesis of tumor cells were affected equally by AM. In sharp contrast, NM always exerted a weak and transitory cytostatic effect.

Meanwhile, further studies have demonstrated that incorporation of [^{3}H]thymidine by most of the rapidly replicating cell lines examined, irrespective of whether they were of syngeneic, allogeneic, or xenogeneic origin or showed normal or neoplastic growth characteristics, was similarly inhibited by the presence of AM (Keller, 1974b). At an effector–target cell ratio of 10:1, the performance of target cells expressed as capacity to incorporate [^{3}H]TdR into acid precipitable material is lost progressively (SV40 in 3T3 in Fig. 1). In very slowly proliferating cells, the cytostatic effect is not evident. Proliferation of a few of the thus far examined rapidly replicating cell lines, such as CHO fibroblasts (Fig. 1) and some of the lymphoblastoid cell lines (Section III,B,2), was only moderately inhibited by AM. The reasons for these differences in the

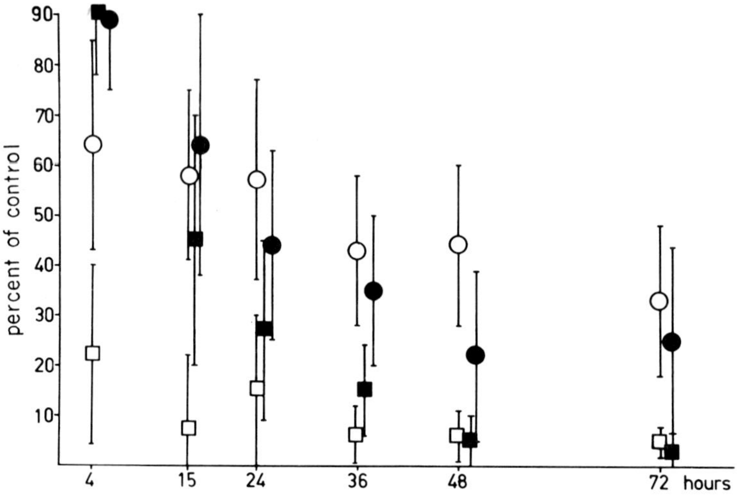

Fig. 1. Kinetics of macrophage-mediated cystostatic (as represented by percent [^{3}H]TdR incorporation, ○, □) and cytocidal (percent of actual cell number in controls, ●, ■) target cell effects. Target cell lines: ○, SV40 3T3 cells; □, CHO fibroblasts.

susceptibility of targets for macrophage-mediated cytostasis are not yet understood.

In experiments with a variety of cell lines, it was shown that effective blockade of target cell proliferation was usually maintained for 60–90 hours, thus attesting to the continuance of the cytostatic effect. However, renewed proliferation was observed occasionally, indicating that macrophage-mediated cytostasis is readily reversible. By supplementing such cultures with additional AM, it was shown that target cells that recovered were not resistant to AM cytostasis but rather had somehow escaped initial interaction with effectors (Keller, 1974a). Parallel morphologic observations indicated that the outcome of the *in vitro* interaction is largely dependent upon the metabolic state of the macrophages and an appropriate ratio of effectors to targets.

The ratio of effector to target cells determines the cytostatic effect. In the majority of experiments with syngeneic, allogeneic, or xenogeneic targets, the presence of AM at a ratio of 1:1 still led to a significant reduction in target cell proliferation. However, at cell ratios of 1:10 to 1:50, enhancement of target cell proliferative capacity was often observed. These observations indicate that, depending on the AM to target cell ratio in the culture, proliferation of normal and transformed cells can be enhanced as well as blocked. These *in vitro* findings provided the initial indication that macrophages had the potential to exert a regulatory function, i.e., the monitoring of cell proliferation.

2. The Influence of AM on Lymphocyte Proliferation

The preceding findings suggested that lymphocyte proliferation *in vitro*, an especially significant and extensively studied example of cell proliferation, should be similarly affected. Indeed, there are a number of reports in the literature that are consistent with such an interpretation (for references see Section IV and Nelson, Chapter 9). In affirming and extending these earlier reports, the following points seem especially noteworthy (Keller, 1975b).

As with other targets examined, lymphocyte proliferation (followed by incorporation of [^{3}H]TdR) is effectively blocked by an appropriate ratio of AM to test cells (10:1 to 1:1). In the presence of a smaller proportion of AM (1:25 to 1:100), stimulation of target cell proliferation often occurred. These profound effects by AM on lymphocyte proliferation *in vitro* are achieved irrespective of whether the DNA synthetic responses were induced by a T cell mitogen such as concanavalin A, by a B cell mitogen such as bacterial lipopolysaccharide, or by an immunologically specific stimulus such as allogeneic lymphocytes. The effector to target cell ratio of 1:1 that is so consistently effective in blocking lymphocyte proliferation only moderately inhibits proliferation of *non-lymphoid* cell lines. Thus, replicating normal lymphoid cells are considerably more susceptible to the macrophage cytostatic effect than are all other normal or transformed (neoplastic) cell types thus far examined. The potency of the cytostatic macrophage effect is further emphasized by the fact that macrophages block either the initiation of or the ongoing lymphocyte proliferation; thus, addition of macrophages during the last 24 hours of culture, i.e., when lymphocyte proliferation induced by mitogen or by allogeneic lymphocytes was already far advanced, also sufficed to produce marked cytostatic effects.

3. *Kinetics of the Cytostatic Process* (Keller, 1973a, 1974a,b)

Study of the kinetics of the cytostatic process revealed that, quite independently of their origin and their growth characteristics, the majority of 24 rapidly replicating cell lines were similarly affected by AM in an effector to target cell ratio of 10:1. Target cell proliferation was depressed to approximately 25% of the control within the first 4 hours, was reduced all the way to background levels within 12 hours, and remained at this base line for the entire observation period of 6 days (SV40 3T3 in Fig. 1). Although this inhibition of proliferation was achieved with every type of rapidly replicating cells examined, there are indications of a quantitative difference in cytostasis on targets from different origin. Replicating normal lymphoid cells are most susceptible (Keller, 1975b). Among the Burkitt cell lines examined (Svedmyr *et al.*, 1974), Raji and Daudi were effectively blocked, whereas proliferation of Namalwa and Maku was only moderately inhibited. Two other lymphoblastoid lines, an Epstein-Barr virus (EBV) carrier (F 265) and an EBV negative cell (Molt-4) were relatively resistant to the macrophage cytostatic effect (Table II).

There are indications of a quantitative difference in macrophage-mediated cytostasis on other types of rapidly replicating targets derived from normal and transformed tissues. For example, proliferation of neoplastic cell lines is consistently fully blocked, whereas in cell lines originally derived from normal tissues (CHO, 3T3; Fig. 1), proliferation often proceeds at a low rate despite the presence of a majority of AM. It is noteworthy that thymidine incorporation is much more inhibited by AM in slowly proliferating *tumor* targets than in slowly proliferating (syngeneic) fibroblasts, indicating that quite apart from rate of replication there are still other significant differences in normal and malignant cells with respect to the macrophage reaction against them (Keller, 1974b).

TABLE II

Differences in Susceptibility of Lymphoblastoid Lines to Macrophage Cytostasis

Time of AM interaction[a]	Residual target cell proliferation (% of control)					
	Raji	Daudi	Namalwa	Maku	F-265	Molt-4
4 hours	7 (±3)	11 (±5)	81 (±11)	56 (±14)	54 (±12)	89 (±13)
15 hours	6 (±5)	4 (±3)	27 (±21)	42 (±16)	45 (±22)	18 (±11)
dpm after 15 hours (control)	60,000	45,000	15,000	6200	12,000	6200

[a] Effector–target cell ratio was 10:1.

The finding that cell lines derived from normal tissues can generally reestablish normal growth following prolonged macrophage cytostasis and the results with lymphocytes support the view that macrophage-mediated blockade of normal cell proliferation is a readily reversible process.

4. Cytostasis as an Effect Unique for Macrophages

Evidence is accumulating that a variety of cell types may, under specified conditions, depress and/or enhance proliferation of other cells (Badger *et al.*, 1974; Cerny, 1974; Hersh *et al.*, 1974). However, the macrophage effects on target cell proliferation appear to be a distinctive category as regards the magnitude of the effects attained. It is appreciated that the macrophage populations obtained for these studies contain a significant number of granulocytes and lymphocytes. These are removed in large part by adherence of macrophages to plastic and extensive washing of such monolayers to remove the nonadherent cells. Nonetheless, additional evidence has been obtained to show that contamining cell types cannot account for these distinctive effects.

Thus, evidence from many directions attests to the nature of the effectors used in these *in vitro* studies, viz., they are radioresistant and show the morphological, functional, and biochemical characteristics of macrophages. Experiments in which functional macrophages were eliminated by an agent specifically toxic, silica, are especially informative. Silica, by itself without discernible effects on target cell proliferation in short-term culture, abolishes macrophage cytostasis. Finally, there is still other evidence favoring this cytostasis as being macrophage-dependent, including modification of target cell ratio and the abolition of cytostatic capacity of macrophage-rich cell populations by removal of adherent cells.

5. *Thymus Independence of Cytostatic Effects*

Activation of normal macrophages seems to be a central requirement for achieving vigorous target cell cytostasis (Section III,C,3). The question arose whether this process in any way involved T lymphocytes, as the soluble mediators they elaborate are known to markedly enhance macrophage functional activities (Nathan *et al.*, 1971, 1973; Fowles *et al.*, 1973). It was, therefore, essential to know whether the presence of exceedingly small numbers of T lymphocytes could in any way be involved in augmenting these macrophage functions. This seems to be ruled out by the finding that adherent peritoneal cells from pathogen-free, congenitally athymic nude mice (activated by Freund's complete adjuvant) were equally capable of reducing target cell proliferation (Keller, 1974a). Thus, the presence of T cells is not required to achieve macrophage-mediated cytostasis. However, it should be emphasized that supernatants from antigen-stimulated lymphocytes effectively enhance macrophage cytostatic potential (R. Keller, unpublished) just as does stimulation of the host with agents such as peptone and endotoxin. In view of the major role now accorded macrophages in collaborative immune responses, it is a reasonable expectation that by elaborating soluble factors consequent to stimulation, this cell type would decisively affect the duration and/or magnitude of the immune reaction.

C. Mechanisms of Cytostasis

1. *Role of Cell to Cell Contact*

Morphologic scrutiny of interaction between AM and target cells consistently revealed close contact, alterations in shape, and a decrease in number of target cells derived from malignant tissues but not of target cells derived from normal tissues (Keller and Jones, 1971; Alexander and Evans, 1971; Hibbs *et al.*, 1972; Keller, 1972, 1973a; Hibbs, 1973; Holtermann *et al.*, 1973).

Various findings, such as the strong parallelism in the appearance of effector–target cell aggregates and inhibition of tumor cell proliferation, the antagonistic action of silica on macrophage-mediated cytostasis for tumor cells, and the failure of 4 hour macrophage culture supernatants and of macrophage lysates to inhibit tumor cell growth, all pointed toward the cell to cell contact phenomenon between functional effectors and targets as essential for attaining cytostasis and tumor cell damage (Keller, 1973a). However, as detailed in Section II,C,2, at least two subsequent observations were not compatible with such a concept.

2. Cytostasis Mediated by a Soluble Macrophage Factor

Some situations were encountered in which cytostasis was effective despite greatly reduced cell to cell contact. Morphologic observations of the interaction between AM and target cells derived from normal tissues did not disclose close cell to cell contact despite effective cytostasis. Moreover, proliferation of rapidly replicating malignant cells growing in suspension culture was also blocked by AM's, despite the considerably reduced opportunity for close contact between effectors and targets in this system. Thus it seemed possible that macrophage-mediated cytostatic action might involve a soluble factor elaborated by these cells.

Subsequently it was found that supernatants from 18–48 hour cultures of peptone-induced, peritoneal rat AM did indeed mediate cytostasis. Thymidine incorporation of all rapidly replicating cell lines examined including syngeneic, allogeneic, or xenogeneic targets, derived from normal and from malignant tissues, as well as lymphocytes was consistently blocked by such macrophage supernatants diluted to a concentration corresponding to an effector to target cell ratio of 10:1 (Keller, 1975b; R. Keller, unpublished). Somewhat similar observations on lymphocyte proliferation have been reported by Nelson (1973), Waldman and Gottlieb (1973), and Calderon *et al.* (1974).

In contrast to the reproducibility with which cytostasis by activated mononuclear phagocytic cells is mediated, results with their soluble supernatants are not as easily reproduced. Nelson (1973) has shown that culture supernatants from mouse macrophages harvested 24–48 hours after endotoxin treatment had high cytostatic activity; but such activity was no longer evident from cells taken at 72 or 96 hours. Our own experience has been that supernatants from peptone-induced rat peritoneal AM taken after 18–48 hours in culture showed mostly high cytostatic activity. However, occasionally such AM supernatants enhance target proliferation.

Macrophages lack thymidine kinase activity and thus contain a sizable thymidine pool that might compete with the label. However, macrophage effects on targets by far exceed this limit. Experiments with a variety of spontaneously replicating target cells, including lymphoblastoid lines, have shown that macrophage-mediated inhibition of thymidine incorporation is accompanied or followed by a decrease in uridine incorporation (Keller, 1973a), a decrease in the number of mitoses (R. Keller, unpublished) and by a standstill or decrease in the number of targets (R. Keller and W. J. Gehring, unpublished). Accordingly, in the present system, it seems reasonably certain that thymidine incorporation actually reflects target cell proliferation.

3. *Functional and Metabolic Requirements for Production of Cytostasis by AM and/or Soluble Mediator*

The reported differences between normal and activated macrophages, as evidenced morphologically in their interaction with targets (Keller, 1973a), in the degree and continuance of cytostatic effects (Keller, 1974a), and in the production of a soluble cytostatic factor (Nelson, 1973; Keller, 1975b), all point to macrophage activation as the critical process for acquiring cytostatic ability. The findings that stimulants triggering macrophage activation inhibit tumor growth *in vivo* (Keller and Hess, 1972; Parr *et al.*, 1973) are consistent with such a concept. Furthermore, macrophages from pathogen-free mice and rats acquire full cytostatic capacity after administration of macrophage-stimulating agents (Keller, 1974a,b), indicating that the acquisition of macrophage cytostasis is not restricted to situations in which macrophage activation occurs secondary to another event, such as infection with facultative intracellular microorganisms. Accordingly, cytostatic potential would seem to be an inherent property of macrophages.

The term "macrophage activation," although widely used, is difficult to express in quantitative, functional, or biochemical terms. A variety of parameters, such as morphology, cellular adherence, pinocytosis, phagocytosis, bactericidal capacity, or biochemical characteristics (e.g., protein synthesis, glucose oxidation, or lysosomal enzyme activity), have been taken individually or collectively to be indicative of the degree of macrophage activation. The fact that these parameters are affected differently during prolonged culture of peptone-induced rat peritoneal macrophages (Keller *et al.*, 1974) makes it doubtful whether all or even the majority really reflect the degree of activation, and whether these classical signs of macrophage activation are in any way related to macrophage-mediated cytostasis. The data can be taken as evidence that the conditions for optimal macrophage activation and/or cytostasis are not yet fully understood.

4. *Relationship of Macrophage Cytostatic Factor to Other Agents Known to Affect Cell Proliferation*

Considerable data now attest to the inherent capacity of macrophage cytostatic factor to inhibit the proliferation of any rapidly replicating cell. This effect seems quite independent of tumor-, cell-, or species-specificity; proliferation of rapidly replicating normal and transformed cells is affected comparably. These properties of the macrophage factor and its destruction at pH 2 (R. Keller, unpublished) can thus be differentiated from those of known inhibitors of cell proliferation, such as interferon (Gresser and Bourali, 1970) or the chalones (Houck, 1973; Bullough, 1973). It has recently been suggested that lysozyme may be important in the surveillance of membranes and may be a mediator of the antitumor functions of macrophages (Osserman *et al.*, 1973). The delayed appearance and low efficiency of lysozyme-mediated cytostasis argue against the notion of the present effects being mediated by this bacteriolytic agent.

IV. CYTOCIDAL EFFECTS OF MACROPHAGES

A. Methods

1. Morphology

To assess the kind and degree of effector–target cell interaction, the morphology of the cultures was followed at varying intervals by phase-contrast microscopy or after fixation with methanol and staining with giemsa.

2. Cytotoxicity

Cytotoxicity was assessed in some of the cell lines that had been labeled with ^{51}Cr (Keller, 1973a, 1974b), or by determining the percentage of cells that had taken up trypan blue.

3. Assessment of Target Cell Numbers

With target cells that were clearly larger in size than effectors, it was possible to enumerate the number of targets remaining in culture at varying intervals of interaction after the cells had been removed by trypsinization.

4. Cloning Experiments

Target cells were cultured for 72 hours in the presence of AM (ratio 1:10), then harvested by trypsinization, washed, and counted. Three hundred target cells were then cultured for 10 days further. Then, incorporation of [^{3}H]TdR and cell numbers were assessed and taken as a measure for target cell viability.

B. Cytocidal Tumor Target Alterations following Interaction with Activated Macrophages

1. Morphology and Cytotoxicity Tests

Interaction of AM with a variety of tumor targets is morphologically characterized by close cell to cell contact, alterations in shape, and a decrease in number of tumor cells. In cultures of AM and targets derived from normal tissues, no such conspicuous signs of effector–target cell interaction were detected (Alexander and Evans, 1971; Keller and Jones, 1971; Hibbs *et al.*, 1972; Keller, 1972, 1973a; Holtermann *et al.*, 1973). These observations have essentially been confirmed on a large number of cell lines derived from normal or from transformed tissues (Keller, 1974b). There is evidence that addition of tumor cells to a monolayer of AM is often followed by an early directed movement of neighboring macrophages onto nearby targets (R. Keller, unpublished). This may lead to the formation of effector–target cell aggregates and the subsequent decrease in the number of targets detectable in the monolayer. The degree of formation of such macrophage–tumor cell aggregates varies considerably from one tumor line to another; consequently study of many more cell lines will be required to establish whether such close effector–target cell interaction is invariably correlated with cytocidal macrophage effects.

The interaction resulting in the disappearance of tumor targets (with a conspicuous absence of cell debris) is a uniform, consistent occurrence, but the underlying basis for this phenomenon is not at all understood. Light and electron microscopic studies (R. Keller and V. T. Bächi, unpublished) have given no further insight into the mechanisms, apart from demonstrating that phagocytosis is not a major component in target cell elimination. Electron microscopy revealed occasional tight junctions between effectors and targets without conspicuous changes in target cell fine structure (Keller, 1975a; R. Keller and V. T. Bächi, unpublished).

As morphological studies have not provided much information, other parameters of cell interaction relating directly to target cell viability were explored. In work with a variety of targets at different intervals of the interaction with effectors, indicators of immune cytotoxicity such as employed in lymphocyte target studies, release of ^{51}Cr or uptake of trypan blue, remained relatively unaffected. It is pointed out, however, that relatively few target cell lines have the requisite qualities for use in assays of lymphocyte-mediated cytotoxicity; consequently, these particular criteria have serious limitations.

2. Progressive Diminution in the Number of Targets

a. Neoplastic Cell Lines. Various authors (Alexander and Evans, 1971; Keller and Jones, 1971; Hibbs *et al.*, 1972; Keller, 1972, 1973a; Holtermann *et al.*, 1973) have shown that interaction with AM results in a progressive and marked reduction in the number of tumor targets in every neoplastic cell line examined. These morphological observations were confirmed by enumerating the number and determining the viability of targets remaining after 72 hours of interaction with AM (Keller, 1974b). Since these experiments were performed in medium supplemented with heat-inactivated (60 minutes, 56°C) rat or calf serum, they suggest that just as for cytostasis, complement is not required for the cytocidal process.

The time course of the cytocidal macrophage effect was followed in a number of tumor cell lines. These studies revealed that the number of tumor cells was not significantly altered during the first 12 hours of interaction with AM but decreased after 24 hours and then gradually declined. After 48–72 hours, tumor cell numbers were always markedly decreased (represented by SV40 3T3 in Fig. 1). Comparison with the time course of macrophage-mediated cytostasis shows that the slope is similar but cytocidal effects become apparent only after 12 to 24 hours.

b. Target Cell Lines Derived from Normal Tissues. Various earlier observations indicating that the conspicuous morphological consequences of AM–target cell interaction, such as close cell-to-cell contact, alterations in shape, and decrease in tumor cell number, were only encountered with tumor targets but not with targets derived from normal tissues (Hibbs *et al.*, 1972; Keller, 1974b) yielded the basis for the concept that the macrophage killer effect is restricted to targets from neoplastic tissues. On the other hand, the aforementioned findings strongly suggest that macrophage-mediated cytostasis affects *all* rapidly replicating cell lines irrespective of their origin and growth characteristics. More recent findings have shown that certain "normal" targets such as CHO fibroblasts (Fig. 1), are markedly diminished in number by the interaction with AM. Studies on a still larger series of cell lines are thus required to decide whether the hitherto often observed marked differences in cytocidal macrophage effects toward targets derived from normal and transformed tissues reflect an inherent macrophage capability or whether this association is actually fortuitous.

3. *Cloning Experiments Disclose Distinction between Macrophage Cytocidal and Cytostatic Effects*

The progressive disappearance of tumor targets with an absence of injured cells or of cell debris is suggestive of a special, most unusual kind of cytocidal process; this was further substantiated by cloning experiments. After interaction with AM for 72 hours syngeneic, allogeneic, or xenogeneic cell lines derived from transformed tissue were often no longer able to reestablish growth, whereas the cloning efficiency of cells derived from normal tissues was only slightly diminished. The data thus attest to the effective killing of tumor targets during this *in vitro* interaction with AM.

4. *Correlation of Cytocidal Effects with Macrophage Activation*

The available evidence suggests that macrophage activation, whatever this entails biochemically, is of central importance both for cytostatic potential and for target cell killing. This provisional conclusion is based largely on morphological grounds, i.e., that close contact between effectors and tumor targets with visual evidence of cell aggregate formation as well as alterations in the shape and decrease in the number of targets were consistently seen with AM but not with resting macrophages (Alexander and Evans, 1971; Hibbs *et al.*, 1972; Keller, 1972, 1973a; Hibbs, 1973, 1974; Holtermann *et al.*, 1973). Similar conclusions were reached from cloning experiments (R. Keller, unpublished).

C. Possible Mechanisms for Cytocidal Target Cell Killing

The mechanisms involved in macrophage cytocidal target cell killing are unknown. Among the hypotheses under consideration, one recently advanced by Hibbs (1974) is of particular interest. He obtained evidence suggesting that the interaction between AM and target cells involved membrane destabilization in both cells favoring local and temporary membrane fusion with consequent direct transfer of the contents of secondary lysosomes of AM into susceptible targets, thus leading to target cell death. Another possibility of nonphagocytic destruction of tumor targets is based on the observations that peroxidase, hydrogen peroxide, and halide ions form a potent system for the intracytoplasmic killing of microbial species (Klebanoff, 1967) and also for extracellular killing of eukaryote cells (Edelson and Cohn, 1973). However, the absence of significant amounts of myeloperoxidase in macrophages (van Furth *et al.*, 1970) is at odds with such a mechanism.

In view of the repeatedly observed close linkage between initially cytostatic and subsequently cytocidal macrophage-mediated effects on targets, the postulate that cytostatic and cytocidal effects could be mediated by low versus high concentrations of the same agent may merit further consideration. It is conceivable that the soluble factor producing cytostatic effects on rapidly replicating cells could attain cytocidal capabilities, especially if it were secreted so as to be focused on a selected area or in a microenvironment of target cell membrane where a very high local concentration could be achieved; this may well be possible when macrophages come into intimate contact with effector cells. Such a hypothesis would become more compelling if it were found that tumor targets (but not normal cells) elaborate a macrophage attracting chemotactic agent.

V. THE BIOLOGIC RELEVANCE OF THE *IN VITRO* FINDINGS

As observations have been made largely in model systems *in vitro,* the question naturally arises whether these results are biologically meaningful or whether they reflect laboratory artifacts. While a definitive answer cannot be given, the available evidence suggests that the morphologic and metabolic alterations observed under culture conditions are physiologically plausible and could reflect processes occurring *in vivo*. Thus, differences in the *in vitro* cytostatic and cytocidal capacities of resting and activated macrophages are marked; actually, in sharp contrast to AM, resting macrophages have little or no potential to kill tumor targets or even to inhibit normal cell proliferation. This is in harmony with *in vivo* conditions where tumors grow unchecked in normal animals, while being inhibited in animals in which macrophages have been activated by infection, immunologic means, or by nonspecific stimulants. This overall correlation between macrophage activation and distinctive effects on tumor targets is further substantiated by the sharply limited duration of these effects both in culture and in animals.

Recognition that macrophage-mediated *cytostasis* affects all rapidly replicating cells thus far examined, quite independent of cell-, species-, or tumor-specificity is a recent development. However, there are reports in the literature suggesting that at least lymphocyte proliferation in the body may be enhanced or blocked depending on the proportion or the degree of activation of macrophages present (Waldman and Gottlieb, 1973). Thus, the presence of an excess of nonimmune macrophages led to inhibition of antibody formation (Perkins and Makinodan, 1965; Parkhouse and Dutton, 1966; Diener *et al.*, 1970), and the response of normal rat spleen cells to endotoxin was reduced by the addition of macrophages (Yoshinaga *et al.*, 1972). Spleen cells from mice injected with *Corynebacterium parvum* (Scott, 1972a,b) or subjected to a graft versus host reaction (Scott, 1972b; Sjöberg, 1973) showed decreased antibody formation and decreased responsiveness to PHA or allogeneic lymphocytes (Scott, 1972a). In contrast to these inhibitory effects, potentiation of the DNA synthetic response of spleen cells by peritoneal exudate cells (Harris, 1965), and of the response of immune lymphocytes to specific antigen (Seeger and Oppenheim, 1970), of thymocytes to PHA (Gery and Waksman, 1972), or of the mixed leukocyte culture reaction (Rode and Gordon, 1974) by macrophages has also been described. All in all, these data lend support to the view that the extent of lymphocyte proliferation *in vivo* in response to immune and nonspecific stimuli could really be determined by the number of macrophages present and their functional activity.

Attempts to demonstrate soluble factors released by macrophages *in vitro* were unsuccessful (Scott, 1972a,b; Keller, 1973a) until very recently (Nelson, 1973; Waldman and Gottlieb, 1973; F. Lejeune personal communication, 1974; Calderon *et al.*, 1974; Keller, 1975b). Gery and Waksman (1972) reported that adherent cells of the macrophage type exposed to endotoxin *in vitro* release a soluble factor that stimulates DNA synthesis by T lymphocytes. Our as yet preliminary data show that a soluble factor released from macrophages during prolonged culture *in vitro,* depending on its concentration, regularly blocks and occasionally enhances proliferation of a large variety of syngeneic, allogeneic, or xenogeneic cells derived from various normal or transformed tissues. Together with other available data (Gery and Waksman, 1972; Nelson, 1973; Waldman and Gottlieb, 1973; Calderon *et al.*, 1974), these observations indicate that the macrophage factors have the potential for playing an important role in the control of cell proliferation in the body.

The extent to which the documented *in vitro cytocidal* macrophage effects reflect the operation of this system in the host will not be easy to assess. First because timing is crucial; and this in turn involves mobilization, activation and number proportionate to tumor cells, etc. There is now considerable evidence that macrophages from animals infected with certain bacterial or parasitic pathogens show considerably enhanced cytocidal ability (Keller *et al.*, 1971; Keller and Jones, 1971; Hibbs *et al.*, 1972; Keller and Hess, 1972; Holtermann *et al.*, 1973; Olivotto and Bomford, 1974). Moreover, macrophage-activating agents, such as endotoxin or double-stranded RNA, which themselves have no direct action on the tumor cells, have been shown to exert marked prophylactic and therapeutic effects on syngeneic murine lymphomas and fibrosarcomas (Parr *et al.*, 1973). However, such macrophage capacities can be blocked or nullified by other agents, such as specific and nonspecific blocking serum factors (Keller, 1973b; Fauve *et al.*, 1974; R. Keller, unpublished). The fact that potent cytostatic and cytocidal effects of AM are exerted at effector–target ratios that seem physiologically attainable further warrants the optimistic view that, in many respects, the *in vitro* systems could reasonably reflect at least some of the *in vivo* potential of the mononuclear phagocytic system.

VI. CRITICAL OUTLOOK

The present findings have confirmed the recently emerging concept that macrophages, quite apart from their long established important role as scavenger cells and in the elimination of microorganisms can, in a partially similar manner, also deeply affect eukaryote cells. These observations indicate that AM interact with targets *in vitro* in a variety of ways and may have the capacities to discriminate between (a) resting and replicating cells and (b) replicating normal versus tumor cells. Both of these *in vitro* capabilities are markedly dependent upon the functional activity ("activation") of macrophages as well as on the actual proportion of effectors to targets.

The *macrophage effects on normal cell proliferation* have been uncovered only very recently; with investigations in progress, interpretation of available data is necessarily speculative. However, results of *in vitro* studies with 24 rapidly replicating target cell lines indicate that the overall susceptibility of targets is apparently quite independent of species (syngeneic, allogeneic, or xenogeneic), cell type (epithelial or lymphoid), growth characteristics (monolayer or suspension), or transformation (normal versus neoplastic tissue). This implies an astonishing and extraordinary distribution of recognition structures and operating at a level quite different from that for specific immune reactivity.

It is noteworthy, however, that cell lines thus far examined exhibit substantial differences in their susceptibility to macrophage-mediated cytostasis. Whereas normal lymphocytes in transformation and syngeneic polyoma-induced, SV40 3T3 or P-815, cells were especially susceptible, other cell lines, e.g., syngeneic DMBA-induced cells, 3T3, CHO, and lymphoblastoid lines Namalwa, Maku, and F-265, were relatively resistant. Lymphocytes stimulated by mitogens or allogeneic lymphocytes were particularly sensitive, and macrophage–lymphocyte ratios of 1:1 generally completely blocked their proliferative response. The differences in susceptibility to cytostasis are presently unexplicable.

The consistent finding that rapidly replicating fibroblasts and lymphocytes are more susceptible to cytostasis than their slowly proliferating counterparts and that lymphoid cells already far advanced in their response to mitogenic stimuli are still susceptible to macrophage cytostasis all point toward the distinctive sensitivity of replicating cells. Increased sensitivity may be linked to a particular phase of the mitotic cycle, but the reported difference in susceptibility to macrophage-mediated cytostasis of a variety of cell lines proliferating at approximately the same rate, makes it clear that the rate of proliferation can be only one of a number of determining factors. Macrophage culture supernatants capable of consistently duplicating the cytostatic capacities of mononuclear phagocytes should greatly facilitate the resolution of some of these issues and, moreover, help to ascertain whether there is a relationship between cytostatic and cytocidal macrophage-mediated effects.

As all authors agree, the second major macrophage effect is on the *viability of target cells.* The mechanism involved and the tumor-specificity of this killing effect remain unresolved. Considering the profound difference in the capabilities manifested by NM and AM, it is evident that the process of macrophage activation carries major biologic implications. The outcome of an *in vivo* encounter between macrophages and tumor targets would, therefore, largely depend on the capacity to mobilize and to activate effectors. The mediators actually involved in such processes *in vivo* are not known, but products such as macrophage migration inhibitory factor should be able to perform both steps in the overall process.

For purely operational reasons, induced peritoneal exudate cells have been chosen for studies performed thus far, but it remains to be seen whether these cells really reflect the potential of macrophages characteristically present in other sites. There are various indications for morphologic and/or functional heterogeneity within the mononuclear phagocytic system (Daems and Brederoo, 1973; Rice and Fishman, 1974; Walker, Chapter 4). The likely existence of differing properties in macrophages obtained from different sites may be taken as a hint that the peripheral blood monocyte might be the cell of choice to assess this issue; as the precursor of the tissue mononuclear phagocyte, the monocyte must have the potential of access to all compartments and thus, given an appropriate environment, to develop any of an array of varied macrophage properties. Accordingly, if cytostatic and cytocidal capacities are, in fact, inherent to the entire mononuclear phagocyte system, the blood monocyte could be expected to exhibit this potential.

Clearly, much remains to be resolved for a satisfactory understanding of the macrophage capacities to interact with and to affect other cell types. While incomplete, the findings reviewed warrant consideration of a major role for the mononuclear phagocytic system in the surveillance against transformed cells and possibly an even broader more basic function in regulation of cell proliferation generally.

ACKNOWLEDGMENTS

The author thanks Dr. Maurice Landy, Schweizerisches Forschungsinstitut Davos, Switzerland, for helpful criticism. This work was supported by the Swiss National Science Foundation, grants 3.516.71 and 3.2340.74.

REFERENCES

Alexander, P., and Evans, R. (1971). *Nature (London), New Biol.* **232,** 76–78.

Badger, A. M., Cooperband, S. R., and Merluzzi, V. J. (1974). *J. Immunol.* **112,** 1435–1443.

Blanden, R. V., Mackaness, G. B., and Collins, F. M. (1966). *J. Exp. Med.* **124,** 585–600.

Bullough, W. S. (1973). *Nat. Cancer Inst., Monogr.* **38,** 5–15.

Calderon, J., Williams, R. T., and Unanue, E. R. (1974). *Proc. Nat. Acad. Sci. U.S.* **71,** 4273–4277.

Cerny, J. (1974). *Nature (London)* **249,** 63–65.

Daems, W. T., and Brederoo, P. (1973). *Z. Zellforsch. Mikrosk. Anat.* **144,** 247–297.

Diener, E., Shortman, K., and Russell, P. (1970). *Nature (London)* **225,** 731–732.

Edelson, P. J., and Cohn, Z. A. (1973). *J. Exp. Med.* **138,** 318–323.

Evans, R., and Alexander, P. (1973). *Nature (London)* **236,** 168–170.

Fauve, R. M., Hevin, B., Jacob, H., Gaillard, J. A., and Jacob, F. (1974). *Proc. Nat. Acad. Sci. U.S.* **71,** 4052–4056.

Fowles, R. E., Tajardo, I. M., Leibowitch, J. L., and David, J. R. (1973). *J. Exp. Med.* **138,** 952–964.

Gery, I., and Waksman, B. H. (1972). *J. Exp. Med.* **136,** 143–155.

Gresser, I., and Bourali, C. (1970). *J. Nat. Cancer Inst.* **45,** 365–376.

Harris, G. (1965). *Immunology* **9,** 529–541.

Hellström, I., Hellström, K. E., Sjögren, H. O., and Warner, G. A. (1971). *Int. J. Cancer* **7,** 1–16.

Hersh, E. M., Melvedie, K. B., and Freireich, E. J. (1974). *Transplantation* **17,** 221–227.

Hibbs, J. B. (1973). *Science* **180,** 868–870.

Hibbs, J. B. (1974). *Science* **184,** 468–471.

Hibbs, J. B., Lambert, L. M., and Remington, J. S. (1972). *Nature (London), New Biol.* **235,** 48–50.

Holtermann, O. A., Klein, E., and Casale, G. P. (1973). *Cell. Immunol.* **9,** 339–352.

Houck, J. C. (1973). *Nat. Cancer Inst., Monogr.* **38,** 1–4.

Keller, R. (1972). *Schweiz. Med. Wochenschr.* **102,** 1148–1151.

Keller, R. (1973a). *J. Exp. Med.* **138,** 625–644.

Keller, R. (1973b). *Brit. J. Exp. Pathol.* **54,** 298–305.

Keller, R. (1974a). *Immunology* **27,** 285–298.

Keller, R. (1974b). *Brit. J. Cancer* **30,** 401–415.

Keller, R. (1975a). *In* "Mononuclear Phagocytes in Immunity, Infection and Pathology" (R. van Furth, ed.), pp. 857–868. Blackwell, Oxford.
Keller, R. (1975b). *Cell. Immunol.* **17,** 542–551.
Keller, R., and Hess, M. W. (1972). *Brit. J. Exp. Pathol.* **53,** 570–577.
Keller, R., and Jones, V. E. (1971). *Lancet* 2, 847–849.
Keller, R., Ogilvie, B. M., and Simpson, E. (1971). *Lancet* **1,** 678–680.
Keller, R., Keist, R., and Ivatt, R. J. (1974). *Int. J. Cancer* **14,** 675–683.
Klebanoff, S. J. (1967). *J. Exp. Med.* **126,** 1063–1078.
Metchnikoff, E. (1905). "Immunity in Infective Diseases." Cambridge Univ. Press, London and New York.
Nathan, C. F., Karnovsky, M. L., and David, J. R. (1971). *J. Exp. Med.* **133,** 1356–1376.
Nathan, C. F., Remold, H. G., and David, J. R. (1973). *J. Exp. Med.* **137,** 275–290.
Nelson, D. S. (1973). *Nature (London)* **246,** 306–307.
Olivotto, M., and Bomford, R. (1974). *Int. J. Cancer* **13,** 478–488.
Osserman, E. F., Klockars, M., Halper, J., and Fishel, R. E. (1973). *Nature (London)* **243,** 331–335.
Parkhouse, R. M. E., and Dutton, R. W. (1966). *J. Immunol.* **97,** 663–669.
Parr, I., Wheeler, E., and Alexander, P. (1973). *Brit. J. Cancer* **27,** 370–389.
Perkins, E. H., and Makinodan, T. (1965). *J. Immunol.* **94,** 765–777.
Rice, S. G., and Fishman, M. (1974). *Cell. Immunol.* **11,** 130–145.
Rode, H. N., and Gordon, J. (1974). *Cell. Immunol.* **13,** 87–94.
Scott, M. T. (1972a). *Cell. Immunol.* **5,** 459–468.
Scott, M. T. (1972b). *Cell. Immunol.* **5,** 469–479.
Seeger, R. C., and Oppenheim, J. J. (1970). *J. Exp. Med.* **132,** 44–65.
Sjöberg, O. (1973). *Clin. Exp. Immunol.* **12,** 365–375.
Svedmyr, E. A., Deinhardt, F., and Klein, G. (1974). *Int. J. Cancer* **13,** 891–903.
Takasugi, M., and Klein, E. (1970). *Transplantation* **9,** 219–227.
van Furth, R., Hirsch, J. G., and Fedorko, M. E. (1970). *J. Exp. Med.* **132,** 794–805.
Waldman, S. R., and Gottlieb, A. A. (1973). *Cell. Immunol.* **9,** 142–156.
Yoshinaga, M., Yoshinaga, A., and Waksman, B. H. (1972). *J. Exp. Med.* **136,** 956–961.

20

Macrophages and the Destruction of Syngeneic Virus-Induced Tumors

Satvir S. Tevethia, Joyce M. Zarling, and Martin H. Flax

I. Introduction 509
II. Antigenicity of Cells Transformed by Oncogenic Viruses 510
A. DNA Virus-Transformed Cells 510
B. RNA Tumor Virus-Transformed Cells 512
III. Immune Response of Syngeneic Host to Virus-Induced Tumors 512
A. Immune Response to DNA Virus-Induced Tumors 512
B. Cellular Immune Response to RNA Virus-Induced Tumors 516
IV. Role of Macrophages in Rejection of Virus-Induced Tumors 518
A. Indirect Evidence 518
B. Direct Evidence: Demonstration of Macrophages in Tumors 525
V. Steps in the Development of Cell-Mediated Immunity and the Mechanism of Rejection of DNA Virus-Induced Tumors 527
References 531

I. INTRODUCTION

Oncogenic viruses differ from one another in nucleic acid content, morphology, mode of replication, host range, ability to cause neoplasia in their natural host, and type of antigens induced in tumor or transformed cells. Invariably, tumors induced by oncogenic viruses (RNA and DNA) are antigenic and induce an immune response in the autochthonous or syngeneic host. The immune response to virus-induced antigens in transformed cells has been used to alter the progression of the neoplastic disease and is directed against cell surface antigens that are responsible for inducing cellular and humoral immune responses. The mechanism of the rejection of virus-induced tumors has been demonstrated to be due to the thymus-dependent cellular immune response, but humoral immunity may also play a role in the tumor host interaction (Herberman, 1974). Thymus derived T cells have been demonstrated to be involved in the rejection of virus-induced tumors and are needed for the generation of other effector cells. The role of T cells in the rejection of highly antigenic allogeneic and syngeneic tumors has been convincingly demonstrated both *in vivo* and *in vitro* (Cerottini and Brunner, 1974). However, evidence is accumulating that uncommitted lymphoid cells (other than T cells) and macrophages may participate in the killing of weakly antigenic syngeneic tumor cells (Zarling and Tevethia, 1973b). This chapter will concentrate on the role of macrophages in the rejection of virus-induced tumors, although reference will be made to the participation of macrophages in the rejection of non-virus-induced tumors. Among the virus-induced tumors, the tumors induced by a DNA virus, SV40, will be discussed in detail, and comparisons will be made with the process involved in the rejection of RNA virus-induced tumors.

II. ANTIGENICITY OF CELLS TRANSFORMED BY ONCOGENIC VIRUSES

A. DNA Virus-Transformed Cells

The antigens present in cells transformed, or tumors induced, by the DNA viruses including papovavirus SV40 are nonvirion in nature but are specifically induced by the transforming virus. These virus-induced nonvirion antigens can be classified into two categories based on their location within the tumor cells: (1) intracellular antigens which are located either in the nucleus or cytoplasm of the transformed cells and (2) cell surface antigens. The intracellular antigens are antigenic in the autochthonous or syngeneic host and induce a humoral immune response only. Intracellular antigens, such as tumor or T antigen, do not play a role in the rejection of virus-induced tumors because of their location in the tumor cells. The presence of these antigens (such as SV40 T antigen) can be used to identify a particular virus to a tumor, since the identical T antigen is induced in SV40 infected monkey cells in which the virus replicates.

Cells transformed *in vitro* or *in vivo* by SV40 undergo alterations in their cell membranes. Some of these changes result in the acquisition of new antigens against which the syngeneic host generates a humoral and/or a cellular immune response (for reviews, see Tevethia and Tevethia, 1975a,b). Perhaps the most important new antigen at the surface of virus-transformed cells is the tumor-specific transplantation antigen (TSTA). TSTA stimulates the development of a cellular immune response in the host, leading to rejection of tumor cells carrying the antigen. TSTA is not a virion antigen. Antiviral antibodies have no effect on the growth of SV40 tumor cells (Khera *et al.*, 1963), and the tumor cells themselves have been shown to be free of the infectious virus and the virion antigens. TSTA present in cells transformed *in vitro* is identical to the antigen in tumor cells; immunization of animals with *in vitro* transformed cells can protect hamsters against a challenge of cells derived from a tumor induced by SV40 and vice versa (Khera *et al.*, 1963). The cross-reactivity of SV40 TSTA is not limited to tumors induced by SV40 within the same animal species. TSTA in SV40 transformed cells of one species cross-reacts with the TSTA in SV40 transformed cells from other species (Girardi, 1965). The TSTA remains stable during the growth of tumor cells either *in vitro* or *in vivo*. However, it has been shown that in the SV40 system, the expression of TSTA at the surface of tumor cells can be altered resulting in immunoresistant cells that escape rejection by an immunized host. These immunoresistant cells retain immunogenicity (Tevethia *et al.*, 1971).

SV40 TSTA is located at the cell surface and has been isolated in soluble form by using 3 *M* KCl and by papain digestion. The activity of the soluble SV40 TSTA was monitored by the *in vitro* macrophage migration inhibition test (Blasecki and Tevethia, 1973). Soluble SV40 TSTA has also been shown to be immunogenic in a syngeneic host (Drapkin *et al.*, 1974). The biochemical nature of TSTA remains unknown.

In addition to TSTA, SV40-transformed cells also possess fetal antigens (Coggin and Anderson, 1974). The presence of these antigens can be demonstrated using either sera from pregnant animals or antisera prepared against fetal tissue. The cross-reacting antigens present in embryonic cells are capable of inducing weak resistance to a challenge of SV40-transformed cells. These conclusions were based on the following observations: (1) Immunization with fetal tissue from midgestational period interrupts primary SV40 tumorigenesis in hamsters and also elicits a state of resistance in adult male hamsters against a challenge of SV40 tumor cells (Coggin *et al.*, 1971; Girardi *et al.*, 1973). (2) Pregnant hamsters develop antibody that is cytostatic for the SV40 tumor cells *in vivo* and sensitized lymphocytes reactive with SV40 tumor cells (Coggin and Anderson, 1974). (3) The fetal antigen from hamster embryos capable of inducing tumor resistance was found not to be species-specific, as mouse and human embryo cells could also elicit resistance (Ambrose *et al.*, 1971a,b).

Reviewing the data published so far, it now appears that during transformation of cells by SV40, the embryonic antigen appears at the cell surface. Indeed, more than one embryonic antigen may be present (Ting *et al.*, 1973). The data also suggest that the embryonic antigens under certain circumstances induce a cellular immune response in the host which may delay the appearance of either primary or transplanted SV40 tumors. The published data strongly suggest, however, that the weakly immunogenic embryonic antigens are distinct from the virus-specific transplantation antigen (TSTA): (a) Immunization of an adult host with either live virus or irradiated tumor cells results in the development of specific cellular immune responses to the TSTA specified by the particular virus (Zarling and Tevethia, 1973a). (b) Specific immunity *in vivo* using irradiated tumor cells is stronger than the immunity induced by the fetal cells (Girardi *et al.*, 1973). (c) Female hamsters do not develop detectable rejection response upon immunization with fetal cells, whereas males can be immunized rather easily to TSTA by either the live virus or by irradiated tumor cells (Girardi *et al.*, 1973).

B. RNA Tumor Virus-Transformed Cells

In contrast to cells transformed by DNA viruses, cells transformed by RNA tumor viruses and infectious virus progeny are released by a budding process without any cytocidal effect on the cell. Under certain circumstances, cells transformed by a sarcoma inducing virus that do not release infectious leukemia helper virus have been demonstrated not to be antigenic in the syngeneic host. However, both avian and murine sarcoma viruses can transform cells from heterologous species, and the transformed cells possess new antigens. As is the case with DNA virus-transformed cells, RNA virus-transformed cells also express embryonic antigens. An excellent review concerning the antigens associated with the surface of cells infected or transformed by RNA viruses has recently been published (Baur, 1974).

III. IMMUNE RESPONSE OF SYNGENEIC HOST TO VIRUS-INDUCED TUMORS

A. Immune Response to DNA Virus-Induced Tumors

Immune responses to SV40-induced tumors in a nonpermissive host has been studied extensively. Hamsters inoculated within 24 hours of birth with live SV40 develop tumors at the site of inoculation after a long latent period (Eddy, 1964). Adult hamsters develop tumors when inoculated with a large dose of virus intravenously (Diamandopoulos, 1973). The animals, before tumor development, synthesize antibodies to SV40-specific surface antigens. These antibodies can be demonstrated in the tumor-resistant animals by the indirect immunofluorescence test (Tevethia *et al.*, 1968a) and by the *in vivo* cytostasis test (Ambrose *et al.*, 1971a,b). Adult animals (hamsters and mice) immunized with live virus or transformed cells also develop antibodies to specific surface antigens that can be measured by the *in vitro* colony inhibition test (Tevethia *et al.*, 1970), cytotoxic test (Wright and Law, 1971), and isotopic antiglobulin test (Ting and Herberman, 1971). The antibodies to surface antigens cannot be demonstrated in tumor bearing animals.

Animals undergoing primary carcinogenesis or adult animals inoculated with the virus or transformed cells develop cellular immune reactivity to SV40-specific transplantation antigen. Such animals are resistant to transplantation of syngeneic SV40 tumor cells (see Butel *et al.*, 1972; Tevethia and Tevethia, 1975a,b). Hamsters undergoing primary SV40 tumorigenesis, when immunized during the latent period with irradiated cells, do not develop tumors (Girardi, 1965; Tevethia *et al.*, 1968b). This phenomenon of immunological reinforcement indicates that the animals undergoing primary carcinogenesis of SV40 do not become tolerant to SV40 TSTA.

The thymus plays a determining role in resistance to viral carcinogenesis. Neonatal thymectomy has been shown to increase incidence of virus-induced tumors in mice (see Herberman, 1974). Similarly, nude mice, which lack T cell functions, are susceptible to polyomavirus oncogenesis as compared to their immunocompetent littlermates (Vandeputte *et al.*, 1974). It has also been demonstrated that virus inoculated thymectomized animals cannot be immunized during the latent period with SV40-transformed cells carrying SV40 TSTA (Girardi and Roosa, 1976). Anti-hamster thymocyte serum, a potent suppressor of cellular immunity, prevented sensitization of animals to SV40 TSTA when administered to hamsters during the period of virus immunization (Tevethia *et al.*, 1968a,b).

Animals bearing a tumor induced by a virus or virus-transformed cells are resistant to the transplantation of either the cells derived from the primary tumor or from tumor induced by cells transformed *in vitro* by the same virus. This concomitant immunity is specific, since the animals bearing tumors induced by a particular virus do not resist the transplantation of cells transformed by another virus or chemical carcinogens. The kinetic studies show that syngeneic mice transplanted with SV40 tumor cells develop concomitant immunity within a few days after transplantation of tumor cells. The rejection of a transplant at a distant site by the tumor bearing host, however, does not have any effect on the progression of primary tumors (Zarling and Tevethia, 1973a).

The cellular basis of resistance to DNA virus-induced tumors has been established by the demonstration that lymph node cells from SV40 virus immunized mice adoptively transfer protection to normal mice against the transplantation of syngeneic SV40 tumor cells. The immune lymphoid cells capable of inhibiting syngeneic SV40 tumor cells have been demonstrated in spleen, lymph nodes, and peritoneal cavity of virus immunized and tumor bearing mice (Zarling and Tevethia, 1973a). The reactivity of lymphocytes immune to SV40 TSTA was specific in nature, since the tumor cells transformed by adenovirus type 7 and a spontaneously oncogenic cell line were not inhibited. Also, lymphocytes from BALB/c mice immune to SV40 TSTA inhibited tumor development by SV40-transformed hamster cells but not by adenovirus-transformed cells in hamsters. The kinetic studies have shown that immune lymphocytes capable of inhibiting SV40 tumor cells *in vivo* appear between 5 and 11 days after the tumor transplantation in mice and between 7 and 14 days in virus immunized mice.

Cellular immune reactivity in SV40 immunized or tumor excised mice can also be demonstrated by the *in vitro* macrophage migration test (Blasecki and Tevethia, 1973, 1975). The peritoneal exudate cells from SV40 immunized mice that had rejected a transplant of syngeneic virus-free tumor cells were inhibited by the soluble TSTA isolated from syngeneic SV40-transformed cells. The data obtained in the macrophage migration test correlated with the *in vivo* tumor inhibitory activity of lymphoid cells.

The presence of lympocytes capable of inhibiting syngeneic tumor cells has also been demonstrated *in vitro* in polyoma and adenovirus tumor systems using a colony inhibition assay and a microcytotoxicity assay. Animals bearing tumors induced by polyomavirus and adenovirus have been shown to possess immune lymphocytes capable of inhibiting syngeneic tumor cells *in vitro* (Hellström and Hellström, 1974).

Not much information is available about the role of various cell types in the rejection of DNA virus-induced tumors. The data showing that thymectomized mice and nude mice, which lack T cell function, do not resist the development of DNA virus-induced tumors indicates that T cells are essential for resistance to viral carcinogenesis. But *in vitro* studies using microcytotoxicity tests have indicated that lymph node cells from thymectomized animals bearing polyomavirus-induced tumors were reactive against polyomavirus-transformed cells *in vitro* (Sjögren and

Borum, 1971). No attempt was made to determine if the reactive cells were really non-T cells. If confirmed, these data would indicate that the effector lymphocytes that are active *in vitro* can be generated *in vivo* in the absence of thymic influence.

Recent work carried out in the author's laboratory (Tevethia *et al.*, 1974) has indicated that T cells are required for the generation of effector lymphocytes capable of inhibiting SV40 tumor cells *in vivo*. BALB/c mice thymectomized, irradiated, and reconstituted (TIR) with syngeneic bone marrow did not develop sensitized lymphocytes upon SV40 immunization. Lymphocytes in the spleens of SV40 immunized TIR mice were unable to inhibit tumor development by SV40 tumor cells *in vivo* (Table I). The SV40 immunized TIR mice were shown to lack θ-positive lymphocytes in their spleens. It was further demonstrated that θ-positive lymphocytes are needed in the rejection of syngeneic SV40 tumor cells in BALB/c mice (Table II). The evidence that θ-positive lymphocytes are needed for tumor cell rejection *in vivo* is twofold: (1) Antisera prepared in AKR mice against θ-antigen shared by BALB/c T cells, when reacted with splenic lymphocytes in the presence of complement, effectively removed lymphocytes capable of inhibiting SV40 tumor cells *in*

TABLE I

Failure to Induce Lymphocytes Immune to SV40 TSTA in TIR Mice[a]

Lymphocyte donors	Donors immunized with	Ratio lymphocyte/ target cells (VLM)	Tumor incidence (%)
Nonthymectomized mice	SV40	100	38
TIR mice	SV40	100	100
Nonthymectomized mice	None	100	88

[a] Normal and TIR mice were immunized twice with 1×10^8 PFU of SV40 subcutaneously at 1-week intervals. One week after immunization, spleen cells were reacted *in vitro* with VLM in a ratio of 100:1 and inoculated into normal adult recipients subcutaneously. The SV40 immunized TIR mice were found to be deficient in θ-positive cells in their spleen. Only 5% of the spleen cells from SV40 immunized TIR mice were killed by anti-θ sera and complement. Nonthymectomized SV40 immunized mice contained 35% θ-bearing lymphocytes. (From Tevethia *et al.*, 1974.)

TABLE II

Requirement for Thymus-Derived θ-Positive Lymphocytes in Inhibition of Tumor Formation by SV40-Transformed Cells (VLM) in BALB/c Mice[a]

Mice immunized with	Treatment of spleen cells	Ratio lymphocytes/ target cells	Target cells	Incidence (%)
SV40	None	100:1	VLM	0
SV40	None	50:1	VLM	0
None	None	100:1	VLM	100
SV40	Anti-C3H (θ) AKR sera + complement	100:1	VLM	75
SV40	Anti-C3H (θ) AKR sera + complement	50:1	VLM	75
SV40	Normal AKR sera + complement	100:1	VLM	0

[a] Spleen cells from normal or immune mice were mixed in a ratio of 100 or 50 lymphocytes to 1 tumor cell, and, after incubation for 30 minutes at 37°C, the mixture was inoculated into adult recipients. In some cases, the spleen cells from immune mice were pretreated with normal or anti-C3H (θ) AKR sera in the presence of complement to eliminate T cells. The treated lymphocytes were tested in the neutralization test for their capability to inhibit SV40 tumors cells (VLM) *in vivo*. The mice were checked for palpable tumors at weekly intervals for 4 weeks postinoculation. The tumor incidence did not change after the fourth week. (From Tevethia *et al.*, 1974.)

vivo. It can also be concluded that the B cells by themselves were incapable of inhibiting tumor cells. (2) Purified T lymphocytes from immune mice are capable of neutralizing tumor cells in syngeneic mice; similar data have also been reported by Howell *et al.* (1974).

B. Cellular Immune Response to RNA Virus-Induced Tumors

Immune response to RNA virus-induced tumors has been recently reviewed by Lamon (1974), and no attempt will be made here to cover all the information available. Of the RNA viruses immune response to murine sarcoma virus (MSV) has been studied in detail both *in vivo* and *in vitro*. The virus rapidly induces tumors in adult animals which spontaneously regress. The regression of MSV-induced tumors is mediated by host immune response, since there is an increased frequency of tumor induction without regression in immunosuppressed adults and adult mice that lack T cell function. Resistance to tumor growth can be induced by transfer of immune lymphoid cells (Lamon, 1974; Herberman, 1974).

Using the *in vitro* technique of microcytotoxicity, the lymphocyte reactivity against MSV tumors has been shown to be mediated by both T as well as B lymphocytes. In mice whose tumors had regressed, only the B lymphocytes were shown to be reactive against the target cells (Lamon *et al.*, 1972). This B cell reactivity was not found to be dependent on the presence of macrophages (Lamon *et al.*, 1973). Kinetic studies have shown that T lymphocytes were also reactive if harvested during early tumor development and soon after regression; B cell activity always accompanied T cell activity. The mechanism of B cell-mediated killing *in vitro* is not known. Recent studies have shown that MSV tumor cells coated with specific antibody reactive against viral antigens could be inhibited by purified unsensitized B cells (Lamon, 1974). Macrophages did not seem to be involved. Whether direct B cell-mediated cytotoxicity is due to the release of small amounts of specific antibody by the sensitized B cells thus allowing other, nonsensitized, B cells to act as killer cells is not known. Antibody-dependent cellular cytotoxicity to other RNA virus-induced tumors has been demonstrated (de Landazuri *et al.*, 1974).

Using a chromium release test, Leclerc *et al.* (1972) have shown that cell-mediated immunity to MSV system is due to the T lymphocytes. Later studies by Plata *et al.* (1973) indicated that only T lymphocytes are reactive in chromium release test, where both T and non-T cells participate in microcytotoxicity test. The participation of T cells in the chromium release test was also confirmed since the reactive cells were susceptible to treatment with antisera to θ antigen in the presence of complement (Herberman *et al.*, 1973).

In vivo studies have indicated that T cells play a definite role in resistance to MSV oncogenesis. Murine sarcoma virus produces progressively growing tumors both in thymectomized mice and in nude mice that lack T cell function (Stutman, 1975). Gorczynski (1974) has recently demonstrated that the reconstitution with T lymphocytes of these mice inoculated with MSV will abrogate virus oncogenesis. Immunoglobulin bearing B lymphocytes had no effect on the oncogenesis by MSV. Reviewing the data on the MSV system, it seems that T lymphocytes are involved in *in vivo* rejection of MSV tumors, whereas both T and B lymphocytes can participate in the *in vitro* destruction of MSV tumor cells.

Recently, it has been found that normal mice of some strains having a low incidence of spontaneous leukemia naturally generate a cell-mediated immune response against antigens associated with leukemia cells, as determined by the ^{51}Cr release assay (Zarling *et al.*, 1975; Kiessling *et al.*, 1975a). In contrast to the findings discussed above that both T and B cells from RNA tumor virus immunized mice are cytotoxic for leukemia and sarcoma cells *in vitro,* neither T nor B cells from normal mice are responsible for the natural killing of leukemia cells *in vitro* (Kiessling *et al.,* 1975b). Depletion of macrophages from spleen cell suspensions from normal mice did not reduce cytotoxic activity for spontaneous AKR leukemia cells (Zarling *et al.,* 1975) or for Moloney virus-induced leukemia cells (Kiessling *et al.,* 1975b). Thus "null" cells may be partially responsible for a cell-mediated type of immune surveillance against leukemia development in mice.

IV. ROLE OF MACROPHAGES IN REJECTION OF VIRUS-INDUCED TUMORS

Classical studies on delayed hypersensitivity and immunity to bacterial and viral infections have clearly established a role for macrophages. Macrophages are involved in these situations as a result of mediators synthesized and released by the T lymphocytes upon interaction with a specific antigen. The manifestation of this cell-mediated immunity depends upon an interaction between the host and the infectious agent (see Blanden *et al.,* Chapter 15). In virus infections, T cell-mediated cytotoxicity, as well as the production of interferon by T cells would affect the outcome of the infections. In the case of bacterial infections, activation of macrophages leads to elimination of the infectious agent.

The evidence is now clear that T lymphocytes alone may bring about the rejection of allogeneic tumors both *in vitro* and *in vivo* (Cerottini and Brunner, 1974). However, there is increasing evidence for the participation of macrophages as effector cells in the rejection of antigenic tumors in syngeneic animals (Levy and Wheelock, 1974). Here, we will discuss the DNA virus (SV40) system in detail and present evidence for the participation of macrophages at the effector level of tumor immunity in SV40 tumor systems.

A. Indirect Evidence

In order to explore this point, a syngeneic SV40 tumor system in BALB/c mice was chosen. BALB/c kidney cells transformed *in vitro* by SV40 that became transplantable in syngeneic adult host were used in this study (Kit *et al.,* 1969; Tevethia and McMillan, 1974). The cells (TU-5) contained SV40-specific tumor (T) antigen and TSTA and were free of infectious virus or virion antigens. Animals bearing tumors induced by TU-5 cells demonstrated specific concomitant immunity and also possessed lymphocytes capable of inhibiting the growth of TU-5 cells and other syngeneic cells transformed by SV40 *in vivo* (Zarling and

Tevethia, 1973a). It has also been established (see Section III,A) that lymphocytes that react with SV40 TSTA resulting in the inhibition of SV40 tumor cells *in vivo* are θ-positive T lymphocytes. Our repeated attempts to utilize an *in vitro* ^{51}Cr release test to demonstrate cytotoxic activity of either spleen cells from TU-5 tumor bearing mice or from mice immunized with X irradiated TU-5 cells or with SV40 were not successful (Table III). Even at a lymphocyte to target cell ratio ranging from 100:1 to 2000:1, no specific release of ^{51}Cr was obtained. Under the same condition, lymphocytes derived from C57B1/6 mice immunized with BALB/c TU-5 tumor cells were cytotoxic to the TU-5 cells. At a ratio of 100 spleen cells to 1 tumor cell, there was 52% specific release of ^{51}Cr from TU-5 cells by the C57B1/6 lymphocytes. The observation that lymphoid cells from BALB/c mice immunized with SV40 or bearing TU-5 tumors neutralize a TU-5 tumor cell *in vivo* when mixed at ratios of 100:1, but do not cause ^{51}Cr release *in vitro* (even at ratios up to 2000:1) suggested either that the lymphocytes directly prevent tumor growth *in vivo* without causing cytolysis or that another cell type is recruited as a result of the tumor cell–lymphocyte interaction.

TABLE III

Effect of Lymphoid Cells from BALB/c Mice Immunized with SV40 and TU-5 Cells on ^{51}Cr Release from SV40-Transformed TU-5 Cells[a]

Mice immunized with	Mouse strain	Source of lymphoid cells	Ratio lymphocyte/ target cells (TU-5)	Percent specific ^{51}Cr release
SV40	BALB/c	Spleen	2000:1	0
SV40	BALB/c	Spleen	1000:1	0
SV40	BALB/c	Lymph node	1000:1	0
TU-5 cells (X-R)	BALB/c	Spleen	1000:1	5
TU-5 cells	C57B1/6	Spleen	500	70
TU-5 cells	C57B1/6	Spleen	100	52

[a] SV40-transformed BALB/c cells (TU-5) were labeled with ^{51}Cr *in vitro* for 12 hours. The labeled cells were brought into single cell suspension by trypsinization, and 1×10^4 cells were reacted with lymphocytes from mice immunized either with SV40 or SV40-transformed BALB/c cells (TU-5) at ratios ranging from 2000:1 to 100:1. After an incubation for 48 hours at 37°C, the cultures were centrifuged, and the radioactivity released from the target cells was counted using the γ counter. The results are expressed as percent specific ^{51}Cr release.

Since ratios of 100:1 and 50:1 were effective in inhibiting the growth of TU-5 cells *in vivo* in the tumor cell neutralization test, experiments were conducted to determine if the ratios lower than 50:1 would bring about tumor growth inhibition. The results obtained (Table IV) show that spleen cells from SV40 immunized mice at ratios as low as 1:1 (lymphocyte–target cell) were effective in preventing the growth of TU-5 cells *in vivo*.

The spleen cells from TU-5 tumor bearing mice also behaved similarly in inhibiting the growth of TU-5 cells at low lymphocytes to target cell ratios. Normal lymphocytes in ratios of 100:1 or 50:1 had no effect on the growth of TU-5 cells. These data obtained in our study indicate that small numbers of immune lymphoid cells are effective in inhibiting tumor growth *in vivo*, whereas large numbers of cells are inactive in the

TABLE IV

Effect of Varying Concentrations and Effect of Irradiation Immune Spleen Cells on Tumor Development by TU-5 Cells in BALB/c Mice[a]

Source of spleen cells	Treatment of spleen cells	Ratio lymphocyte/target cells	Target cells	Tumor incidence (%)
SV40-immunized mice	None	100:1	TU-5[b]	0
TU-5 tumor bearing mice	None	100:1	TU-5	6
TU-5 tumor bearing mice	None	50:1	TU-5	0
TU-5 tumor bearing mice	None	10:1	TU-5	29
TU-5 tumor bearing mice	None	1:1	TU-5	21
TU-5 tumor bearing mice	None	100:1	TUT3 #2[c]	100
Normal mice	None	100:1	TU-5	91
TU-5 tumor bearing mice	500 R	50:1	TU-5	0
TU-5 tumor bearing mice	2000 R	50:1	TU-5	67
TU-5 tumor bearing mice	None	1:1	TU-5	17
TU-5 tumor bearing mice	500 R	1:1	TU-5	40
TU-5 tumor bearing mice	2000 R	1:1	TU-5	83
Normal mice	None	1:1	TU-5	100

[a] Spleen cells from various sources were mixed with target cells in varying ratios and after an incubation at 37°C for 30 minutes, the mixture was inoculated into normal adult BALB/c mice. The animals were watched for tumor development. (From Zarling and Tevethia, 1973b.)

[b] TU-5 cells are SV40 transformed cells which are virus-free but contain SV40 TSTA and T antigens and are transplantable in BALB/c mice.

[c] TUT3 #2 are spontaneously oncogenic cells of BALB/c origin and do not contain SV40-specific antigens.

killing of tumor cells *in vitro*. This is in agreement with previously reported studies by Evans and Alexander (1970), who demonstrated in a syngeneic system that immune lymphocytes from spleen and lymph nodes upon transfer to normal mice confer specific immunity to L5178Y lymphoma cells but that these immune lymphoid cells were not cytotoxic to lymphoma cells *in vitro*. These data have been interpreted to indicate that immune lymphocytes recruit other cell types *in vivo* for the inhibition of tumor growth. The inhibition of tumor cell growth by low ratios of lymphocytes to target cells has also been reported by other workers (Old *et al.*, 1972; Coggin *et al.*, 1967; Gershon *et al.*, 1967a,b; Nomoto *et al.*, 1970; Zbar *et al.*, 1970a,b; Howell *et al.*, 1974). It is difficult to predict accurately what the actual ratio of immune lymphocytes per tumor cell is since not all the lymphocytes from an animal are directed against SV40 TSTA, nor are tumors produced by the inoculation of a single tumor cell. Nonetheless, the actual ratio of immune lymphocyte to tumor cell is less than 1:1 when equal numbers of tumor cells and spleen cells are used, since the *in vivo* inhibition of SV40 tumor cells is initiated by T and not B lymphocytes.

The possibility that immune spleen cells after tumor cell interaction are stimulated and proliferate *in vivo* was ruled out by testing the capacity of irradiated lymphocytes to inhibit tumor cell growth *in vivo*. Immune spleen cells that received 500 R were tested for their ability to prevent tumor development by TU-5 cells in the tumor cell neutralization test. The results in Table IV show that none of the recipients inoculated with spleen cell–tumor cell mixtures at ratios of 100:1 or 50:1 developed tumors regardless of whether the lymphoid cells received 500 R or no irradiation. When immune spleen cells were tested at a ratio of 1 per tumor cell, only 1 of 6 recipients of nonirradiated spleen cells and 2 of the 5 recipients of irradiated (500 R) spleen cells developed tumors. A radiation dose of 2000 R greatly diminished the neutralizing activity of immune spleen cells. There was no difference in tumor incidence between recipients of normal spleen and freeze-thawed immune or irradiated (2000 R) immune spleen cells when mixed at ratios of 50:1 or 1:1. These results demonstrate that immune lymphoid cells that cannot undergo blast transformation and hence mitosis after exposure to 500 R retain their capacity to prevent tumor development *in vivo* and is in agreement with finding that DNA synthesis is not required to exert cytotoxic effects *in vitro* (Cerottini and Brunner, 1974) and that treatment of lymphocytes with doses of mitomycin C, which only prevented DNA synthesis, did not totally abolish the lymphocytes' ability to transfer delayed hypersensitivity. Immune lymphocytes treated with a similar dose of irradiation have shown to transfer delayed hypersensitivity and produce macrophage migration inhibitory factor (MIF) *in vitro* (Salvin and Nishio, 1972). Howell *et al.* (1974) arrived at the same conclusion that proliferation of the sensitized T lymphocyte is not required for inhibition of tumor growth.

The observations that very low concentrations of immune spleen cells were effective in neutralizing tumor cells, even if the lymphoid cells had been irradiated so that they could not undergo mitosis, support the hypothesis that a small number of lymphocytes prevents tumor growth either directly or indirectly by releasing sufficient quantities of a hypothetical cell recruiting factor. The first possibility, that a small number of immune T lymphocytes may actually inhibit all the tumor cell directly, was tested. In experiments recently carried out in the author's laboratory, it was discovered that purified T lymphocytes derived from syngeneic mice immunized to SV40 TSTA were only partially inhibitory to SV40 tumor cells in the *in vitro* microcytotoxicity assay. The percent inhibition of SV40 tumor cells did not increase even at a ratio of 5000 lymphocytes to 1 tumor cell, whereas the same lymphocytes at a ratio of 100:1 or less were inhibitory to SV40 tumor cells *in vivo* (S. S. Tevethia and M. J. Tevethia, unpublished observation). This finding again strengthens the view that immune T lymphocytes upon interaction with TSTA on the SV40 tumor cells may release a mediator that may be responsible for recruiting host cells for the rejection of tumors *in vivo.*

To explore further the possibility of cell cooperation in the rejection of SV40 tumor cells *in vivo,* tumor cell neutralization experiments were performed in newborn mice. In experiments where mice less than 24 hours old were inoculated with spleen cell–tumor cell mixtures, neutralization did not occur even at high ratios. This finding is similar to one reported by Coggin *et al.* (1967), who found the failure of peritoneal exudate cells from SV40 immunized hamsters to prevent tumor growth of admixed SV40 tumor cells in newborn hamsters, suggesting that a cell type that cooperates with the immune lymphocyte is either absent in the newborn animals or nonfunctional. It has been found that newborn mice lack certain macrophage functions (Argyris, 1968).

Neutralization performed in preirradiated (500 R) hosts showed that the tumor cell neutralization by immune lymphocytes is less efficient in mice irradiated 3 days previously with 500 R than in normal mice. The circulating leukocyte count after irradiation had dropped to 20% of the normal value. The data in Table V show that whereas approximately 7% of normal mice inoculated with immune spleen and tumor cells developed tumors, 80% of the irradiated mice inoculated with the same cell mixture developed tumors. These results suggest that the recipient supplies a radiosensitive cell or a cell derived from a radiosensitive precursor

TABLE V

Evidence for Macrophage Participation at the Effector Level Of Tumor Immunity[a]

Source of lymphoid cells	Target cells	Tumor incidence (%) in recipients treated with				
		Untreated (normal)	500 R[b]	700 R[c] (bone marrow treated 3 days before)	700 R (bone marrow treated 14 days before)	Silica treated[d]
Immune	TU-5	7	80	100	10	58
Normal	TU-5	100	100	Not tested	Not tested	Not tested

[a] Spleen cells from TU-5 tumor bearing or normal mice were incubated with TU-5 cells in a ratio of 50:1 for 30 minutes at 37°C and inoculated into adult recipients that received various treatments.

[b] Mice received 500 R ^{60}Co γ radiation 3 days before the experiment.

[c] Mice received 700 R ^{60}Co γ radiation and were reconstituted with 6×10^6 nucleated bone marrow cells. They were used as recipients 3 or 14 days later.

[d] Mice were inoculated intravenously with 3 mg of silica suspended in 0.3 ml isotonic saline 3 days previously.

which aids in tumor cell rejection. It is known that the production of macrophages by bone marrow is radiosensitive and that some of the macrophage functions are radiosensitive (Chen and Schooley, 1970). Using a polyoma tumor system, Sjögren (1964) was able to show only a weak reactivity of immune lymphocytes in the tumor cell neutralization test when the recipients were preirradiated.

In recent experiments by Simes *et al.* (1975) with a methylcholanthrene-induced sarcoma it was found that purified peritoneal exudate lymphocytes from tumor bearing animals had a specific inhibitory effect on the tumor cells when the mixture was inoculated into the footpads of normal mice. At low ratios of lymphocytes to tumor cells (10:1), cooperation between recipient's cells and immune lymphocytes was demonstrated. The helper cell was radiosensitive, or derived from a radiosensitive precursor, and was present in normal peritoneal exudates; it seems likely that it was a macrophage.

To determine if the radiosensitive cells recruited in the recipient to aid in the rejection of SV40 tumor cells is bone marrow derived, a neutralization experiment was done in lethally irradiated bone marrow reconstituted mice. BALB/c mice were irradiated with 700 R and immediately inoculated intravenously with 6×10^6 bone marrow cells. Bone marrow donors had been treated with anti-lymphocyte serum (ALS) 5 days previously to inhibit circulation of thymus-dependent cells to the bone marrow. Tumor cell neutralization experiments were performed 3 to 14 days postirradiation and bone marrow inoculation. The results shown in Table V indicate that immune spleen cells mixed with TU-5 cells at a ratio of 50:1 did not prevent tumor development in mice irradiated and bone marrow inoculated 3 days previously. However, tumor development was prevented in mice irradiated and inoculated with bone marrow cells 14 days before inoculation with tumor cells and immune lymphocytes. The immune spleen cells were effective in preventing tumor formation in sham-irradiated mice. Spleen cells from normal animals had no effect on tumor development by TU-5 cells. These results indicate that bone marrow cells, since they have replicated or differentiated sufficiently in the recipients, can supply irradiated mice with the cell type that cooperates with immune lymphoid cells in tumor cell rejection and agrees with the finding that bone marrow-derived cells are required in the manifestation of delayed hypersensitivity reactions. The macrophage is a bone marrow-derived cell necessary for a delayed-type immune response to be elicited by immune lymphocytes and antigen in irradiated recipients.

These results, although clearly indicating that a bone marrow derived cell cooperates with immune lymphocytes in the killing of syngeneic SV40 tumor cells *in vivo*, could be explained on the basis that since 1×10^5 tumor cells were used in the tumor cell neutralization test, irradiation of the recipients may have decreased the lymphocyte to target cell ratio since more tumor cells may now be capable of initiating a tumor than in unirradiated hosts. The other explanation of the results obtained in our study could be that there may be a primary immune response to the TU-5 cells in the unirradiated host which is eliminated by preirradiation. These possibilities are, however, unlikely. We have recently carried out experiments where the tumor cell neutralization test was carried out at a constant ratio of 100 lymphocytes to 1 target cell, but using an increasing number of target cells. In all cases where the target cell number was varied from 1×10^4 to 1×10^6, a 100:1 ratio of lymphocytes to target cell was inhibitory to tumor cells. The latent period of 1×10^6 tumor cell was less than 1 week. Preirradiation of recipients did not significantly alter the tumor cell producing dose. We have also demonstrated that mixing irradiated TU-5 cells (2×10^6) with unirradiated TU-5 cells (2×10^5) did not affect the tumor producing capacity of TU-5 cells, indicating that the immune response to the nonreplicating tumor cells probably did not play any significant role in tumor formation by TU-5 cells.

Macrophages are bone marrow derived (Volkman and Gowans, 1965).

To determine whether the bone marrow-derived cell that aids in tumor rejection is the macrophage, adult mice were treated with silica, a specific macrophage toxin (Allison *et al.*, 1966). By 24 hours after an intravenous inoculation of 3 mg of silica, macrophages containing large cytoplasmic vacuoles similar to those seen after *in vitro* incubation of macrophages with silica could be detected in peritoneal fluid and occasionally in the blood. By 72 hours the number of macrophages detectable in the peritoneal cavity was markedly depressed, and, at this time, tumor cell neutralization experiments were performed. The results of two separate experiments are shown in Table V. Whereas about 7% of normal recipients of immune spleen cells and TU-5 cells developed tumors, approximately 58% of silica-treated mice inoculated with this mixture developed tumors. These results indicate that tumor cell neutralization by immune lymphoid cells is markedly depressed in mice that have decreased numbers of macrophages as a result of irradiation or silica treatment.

There is evidence suggesting that the macrophage may have the same function in tumor immunity as it has in the manifestation of delayed hypersensitivity. It was shown that the lymphocytes of peritoneal exudates from immune animals were needed in the specific initiation steps of tumor rejection (Zbar *et al.*, 1970b), but that the final steps in the rejection of guinea pigs hepatoma cells were nonspecific, since unrelated tumor cells were killed at the site of rejection of sensitizing tumor cells (Zbar *et al.*, 1970a). That macrophages may be responsible for the final tumor cell killing was subsequently supported by the finding that with the same tumor system it was possible to prevent the development of tumors by local inoculation of a preparation containing MIF activity (Bernstein *et al.*, 1971). *In vitro* studies by Zembala *et al.* (1973) have also demonstrated the requirement of normal macrophages for the destruction of polyomavirus-induced tumors in the presence of sensitized lymphocytes. Thus, it would appear that the efferent limb of cellular immunity to syngeneic SV40 tumor cells may be more like that of delayed hypersensitivity reactions, where the macrophage has been assigned an unequivocal role (Mackaness, 1971; Tubergen and Feldman, 1971; Volkman and Collins, 1971).

B. Direct Evidence: Demonstration of Macrophages in Tumors

Macrophages are often seen at the site of tumor rejection. Histochemical examination showed that the macrophages were activated (Gershon *et al.*, 1967a). Recently, Evans (1972) reported the presence of macrophages in the tumor mass and has isolated them free of tumor cells. In addition, in several primary and transplanted tumors in rats and mice, the macrophage content ranged from 4 to 50% of the total cell population. The content of macrophages in the tumor cell was found to correlate inversely with the capacity of the tumor to metastasize. Eccles and Alexander (1974) have suggested that trapping of macrophages in the tumor mass may be responsible for the decreased delayed hypersensitivity responses to antigens in animals bearing tumors with high macrophage content. We have also shown that mice bearing tumors induced by SV40-transformed cells (TU-5) contain large numbers of macrophages in the tumor mass. The presence of macrophages and histiocytes has also been demonstrated by the histological means.

Morphological studies of the rejection of subcutaneously implanted TU-5 tumor cells revealed the presence of both lymphocytes and histiocytes. These mononuclear cells accumulate in largest numbers along the periphery of the tumor nodule, but also invade the interstices of the tumor mass (Fig. 1). An electron micrograph of a typical histiocyte in such a reaction is illustrated in Fig. 2. Although growth retardation and destruction of the tumor apparently result from the activity of these mononuclear cells, direct injury by these infiltrating cells was not evident.

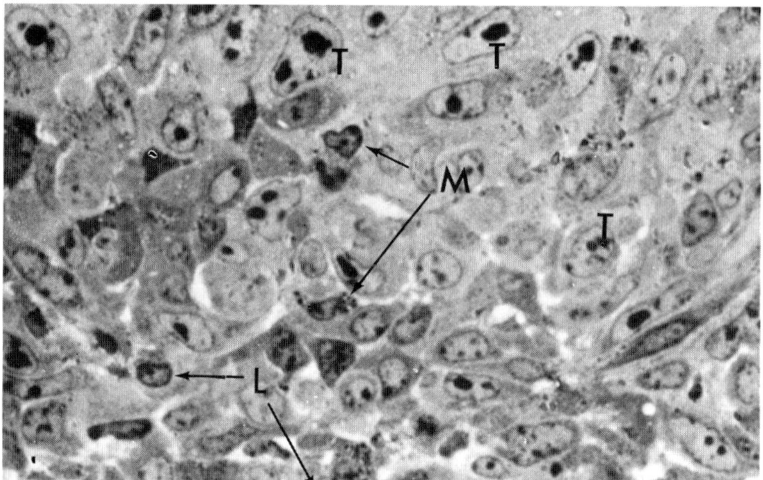

Fig. 1. The edge of a TU-5 tumor nodule induced by SV40-transformed cells growing to a subcutaneous location shows extensive invasion of the tumor mass by lymphocytes (L) and macrophages (M). Tumor cells (T) appear viable.

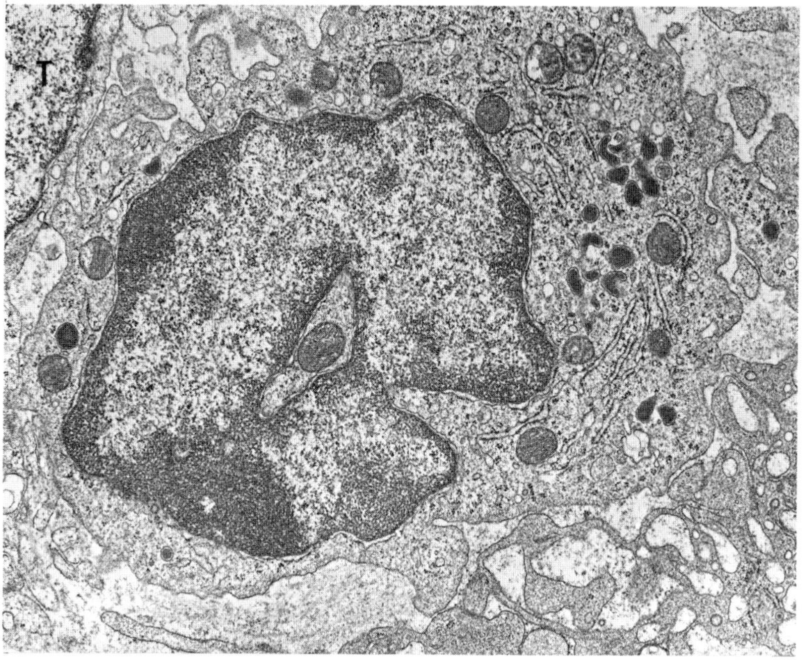

Fig. 2. Electron micrograph of a histiocyte with characteristic reniform nucleus and abundant cytoplasm containing multiple lysosomal elements. Cytoplasmic processes are in contact with an adjacent tumor cell (T).

V. STEPS IN THE DEVELOPMENT OF CELL-MEDIATED IMMUNITY AND THE MECHANISMS OF REJECTION OF DNA VIRUS-INDUCED TUMORS

Some time ago, Habel (1962) and Sjögren *et al.* (1961) postulated that when animals are immunized with polyomavirus, the infected cells synthesize an antigen at their cell surfaces which is identical with the antigen present at the surface of cells derived from the tumor induced by the polyomavirus. Since the tumor cells that are rejected by the virus immunized host were free of both the infectious virus and viral structural antigens, it was presumed that the antigen induced by the virus, which is involved in inducing a rejection response in the host, is a nonvirion antigen and must be synthesized by the transformed cells. The possible steps leading to the development of TSTA in SV40-infected cells and the subsequent sensitization of normal lymphocytes to TSTA are shown in Fig. 3.

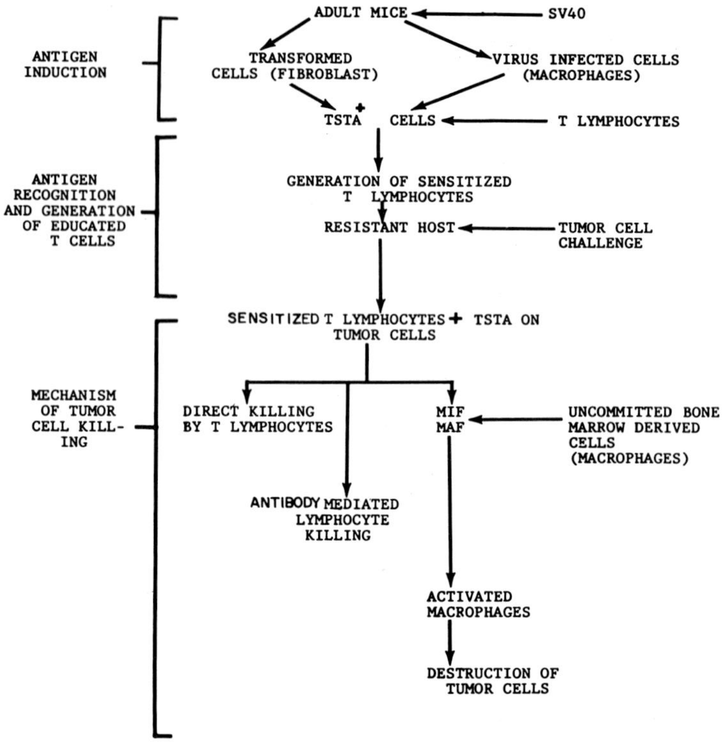

Fig. 3. Steps in the development of cell-mediated immunity and mechanisms of rejection of DNA virus-induced tumors.

When inbred BALB/c mice are inoculated with live SV40, the virus infects host cells. The infected cells develop virus-specific nonvirion antigens but no new virus is synthesized, since the virus undergoes abortive infection in mouse cells. The adult animals inoculated with the virus do not develop tumors but become resistant to the transplantation of syngeneic virus-free SV40 tumor cells. According to Sjögren's and Habel's hypothesis, the target cell for the synthesis of virus-specific TSTA is the cell which upon virus infection will go on to become transformed and proliferate until rejected by the host immune defenses. The kinetic studies on the development of cellular immunity to SV40 TSTA in adult mice inoculated by SV40 have demonstrated that a single immunization of the host with the virus induced a stronger cellular immune response to SV40 TSTA than induced by a large number of X irradiated SV40 tumor cells. Since the number of cells that would be susceptible to transformation by SV40 *in vivo* would be considerably less than the number of transformed cells that are required to induce a rejection immune response in the host, it was postulated that the cells that are infected by the virus but are not the target cell for transformation also synthesize specific TSTA at their cell surface which would greatly amplify the cellular immune response. We now have experimental evidence that the macrophage is such a cell, which after virus infection synthesizes SV40 TSTA (Tevethia and Tevethia, 1975b). We have demonstrated that SV40 virus attaches, penetrates, uncoats, and directs the synthesis of SV40-specific tumor (T) antigen in the nucleus and TSTA at the surface of macrophages. The presence of TSTA at the surface of infected macrophages was demonstrated by sensitizing syngeneic mouse lymphocytes *in vitro* by the method previously described (Cohen *et al.*, 1971). The *in vitro* sensitized lymphocytes specifically inhibited the growth of syngeneic SV40 tumor cells *in vivo* when the sensitized lymphocyte–tumor cell mixture was inoculated *in vivo.* The lymphocytes sensitized with uninfected macrophages had no effect on the growth of SV40 tumor cells *in vivo.* The synthesis of TSTA in SV40-infected mouse embryo fibroblasts was also demonstrated by this method. We have also been able to show that monkey cells in which SV40 induces a lytic response also synthesize specific TSTA at the cell surface, suggesting that the synthesis of TSTA may be an essential step in the virus growth cycle (S. S. Tevethia and M. J. Tevethia, unpublished observations).

The next step in the development of cell-mediated immunity to SV40 TSTA is the recognition of TSTA by lymphocytes and their subsequent proliferation. The details for this process are not known as yet. We do, however, know, as discussed in the previous section, that sensitized lymphocytes are thymus-derived T cells. This was shown by the fact that the generation of sensitized lymphocytes does not take place in mice that lack T cell function and that treatment of sensitized lymphocytes with anti-θ serum and complement abolished the tumor cell inhibiting capacity of the sensitized lymphocytes.

Virus immunized hosts are able to resist the transplantation of 100-fold more tumor cells as compared with the unimmunized animals. Although immunity to allografts and syngeneic plasmacytomas has been shown to be mediated strictly by the T cells both *in vitro* and *in vivo,* it is now apparent that host cells participate in the killing of syngeneic SV40 tumor cells *in vivo.* (For evidence that macrophages can participate in alloimmune reactions, see Lohmann-Matthes, Chapter 18.) The evidence for the participation of host cells (bone marrow derived) has been presented in the previous section. It is conceivable that T lymphocytes can inhibit small numbers of SV40 tumor cells *in vivo* directly. Using an *in vitro* microcytotoxicity assay, we have recently obtained evidence that purified T lymphocytes from animals sensitized to SV40 TSTA play a cytostatic rather than cytotoxic role (S. S. Tevethia and M. J. Tevethia, unpublished observations). The sensitized T lymphocytes, which are cytostatic to SV40 tumor cells *in vitro,* are effective in inhibiting tumor cells *in vivo.* Similar data have been obtained using a ^{51}Cr release assay. The failure of T lymphocytes to destroy syngeneic tumor cells *in vitro* and their ability to inhibit completely the growth of tumor cells *in vivo* at very low numbers coupled with the fact that irradiated immune lymphocytes blocked in DNA synthesis can effectively bring about tumor cell neutralization *in vivo* clearly indicate that host cells participate in the tumor cell killing. Experiments in our laboratory and others have shown that the host cell recruited in the destruction of SV40 tumors *in vivo* is a bone marrow-derived cell and most probably is a macrophage. The evidence presented for the macrophage participation in the rejection of SV40 tumors is consistent with the observations of Alexander and his co-workers on the involvement of macrophages in tumor immunity and has been recently reviewed (Nelson, 1974; Cerottini and Brunner, 1974; Levy and Wheelock, 1974; Evans and Alexander, Chapter 21). The mechanism of the macrophage recruitment and action on the tumor cell is not clear. One way in which macrophages could be involved is by means of cytophilic antibody. This mechanism, however, may not apply in the SV40 tumor system, since specific sensitized lymphocyte population depleted of T cells are ineffective in inhibiting the SV40 tumor cell growth *in vivo* (Tevethia *et al.*, 1974). The most likely possibility is that a mediator or mediators released from the sensitized T lymphocytes as a result of their interaction with TSTA on tumor cells are responsible for the recruitment of macrophages. The possibility that host T lymphocytes are recruited by the sensitized donor T lymphocytes can be ruled out, since sensitized lymphocytes are able to inhibit SV40 tumor cells in recipients that are thymectomized, irradiated, and reconstituted with bone marrow cells (Howell *et al.*, 1974).

The experimental evidence exists showing that the mediators are released from T lymphocytes sensitized to SV40 TSTA as a result of interaction with SV40 TSTA. Specific cellular immune response to SV40 TSTA can be measured by the macrophage migration inhibition test (Blasecki and Tevethia, 1973, 1975). It is not clear at this time whether the migration inhibition factor (MIF) released by the T lymphocytes is also responsible for recruiting and activating host macrophages that can destroy tumor cells. However, in other tumor systems, macrophages have been shown to become activated upon treatment with MIF, and these *in vitro* activated macrophages acquire the ability to kill tumor cells both *in vivo* and *in vitro* (Bernstein *et al.*, 1971; Piessens *et al.*, 1975). If macrophages recruited by the T cells are indeed involved in the rejection of SV40 tumors *in vivo,* as seems to be the case, then it would follow that the activated macrophages might destroy tumor cells nonspecifically. *In vitro* studies have shown that activated macrophages can destroy unrelated tumor cells as well (see reviews by Cerottini and Brunner, 1974; Levy and Wheelock, 1974). Additionally, activated macrophages have been demonstrated to discriminate between malignant and normal cells *in vitro* (Piessens *et al.*, 1975; Hibbs, 1972). There is some evidence for nonspecific killing of tumor cells by activated macrophages *in vivo* (Bernstein *et al.*, 1971). However, the rejection of SV40 tumors by mice immunized either by the live virus or irradiated tumor cells is specific. Preliminary evidence indicates that unrelated tumor cells when mixed with SV40 tumor cells and lymphocytes specifically sensitized to SV40 TSTA are not rejected upon subcutaneous inoculation into normal adult mice. The tumors that appeared did not possess SV40-specific tumor or T antigen in the nucleus of the cells, indicating that only the SV40 tumor cells were rejected (S. S. Tevethia, unpublished observations). The specificity of macrophage killing of SV40 tumor cells could be due to cytophilic factor released by the sensitized T lymphocytes. This factor, known as specific macrophage arming factor (SMAF), has been demonstrated in the supernatant of sensitized lymphocyte–target cell mixtures by Evans and Alexander (1972) and can render normal macrophages specifically cytotoxic to target cells. The synthesis of SMAF was shown to be dependent upon T cells (Evans *et al.*, 1972). It is not clear however, if such a factor is released by T lymphocytes sensitized to SV40 TSTA. The use of *in vitro* techniques for the measurement of cell-mediated immune reactions and the availability of suitable targe cells (SV40-transformed leukemic cells) would be of great help in elucidating the effector mechanisms in tumor immunity to virus-induced tumors.

ACKNOWLEDGMENTS

The authors wish to express their appreciation to Dr. Ronald S. Weinstein for his assistance in providing the electron micrographs. This study was supported in part by research grants CA 14939 and CA 12429 from the National Cancer Institute, National Institutes of Health, Bethesda, Maryland.

REFERENCES

Allison, A. C., Harington, J. S., and Birbeck, M. (1966). *J. Exp. Med.* **124**, 141–154.

Ambrose, K. R., Anderson, N. G., and Coggin, J. H. (1971a). *Nature* (*London*) **233**, 194–195.

Ambrose, K. R., Anderson, N. G., and Coggin, J. H. (1971b). *Nature* (*London*) **233**, 321–324.

Argyris, B. F. (1968). *J. Exp. Med.* **128**, 459–467.

Baur, H. (1974). *Advan. Cancer Res.* **20**, 275–341.

Bernstein, I. D., Thor, D. E., Zbar, B., and Rapp, H. J. (1971). *Science* **172**, 729–731.

Blasecki, J. W., and Tevethia, S. S. (1973). *J. Immunol.* **110**, 590–594.

Blasecki, J. W., and Tevethia, S. S. (1975). *J. Immunol.* **114**, 244–249.

Butel, J. S., Tevethia, S. S., and Melnick, J. L. (1972). *Advan. Cancer Res.* **15**, 1–55.

Cerottini, J. C., and Brunner, K. (1974). *Advan. Immunol.* **18**, 67–132.

Chen, M. G., and Schooley, J. C. (1970). *Radiat. Res.* **41**, 623–636.

Coggin, J. H., and Anderson, N. G. (1974). *Advan. Cancer Res.* **19**, 105–165.

Coggin, J. H., Larson, V. M., and Hilleman, M. R. (1967). *Proc. Soc. Exp. Biol. Med.* **124**, 1295–1302.

Coggin, J. H., Ambrose, K. R., Bellamy, B. B., and Anderson, N. G. (1971). *J. Immunol.* **107**, 520–533.

Cohen, I. R., Globerson, A., and Feldman, M. (1971). *J. Exp. Med.* **133**, 821–833.

deLandazuri, M. Ortiz, Kedar, E., and Fahey, J. L. (1974). *Cell Immunol.* **14**, 193–205.

Diamandopoulos, G. T. (1973). *J. Nat. Cancer Inst.* **50**, 1347–1365.

Drapkin, M. S., Apella, E., and Law, L. W. (1974). *J. Nat. Cancer Inst.* **52**, 259–264.

Eccles, S. A., and Alexander, P. (1974). *Brit. J. Cancer* **30**, 42–49.

Eddy, B. (1964). *Progr. Exp. Tumor Res.* **4**, 1–26.

Evans, R. (1972). *Transplantation* **14**, 468–479.

Evans, R., and Alexander, P. (1970). *Nature (London)* **228**, 620–624.

Evans, R., and Alexander, P. (1972). *Immunology* **23**, 627–636.

Evans, R., Grant, C. K., Cox, H., Steele, K., and Alexander, P. (1972). *J. Exp. Med.* **136**, 1318–1322.

Gershon, R. K., Carter, R. L., and Lane, N. J. (1967a). *Amer. J. Pathol.* **31**, 111–113.

Gershon, R. K., Carter, R. I., and Kondo, D. (1967b). *Nature (London)* **213**, 674–676.

Girardi, A. J. (1965). *Proc. Nat. Acad. Sci. U.S.* **54**, 445–451.

Girardi, A. J., and Roosa R. A. (1967). *J. Immunol.* **99**, 1217–1220.

Girardi, A. J., Reppucci, P., Dierlam, P., Rutala, W., and Coggin, J. H. (1973). *Proc. Nat. Acad. Sci. U.S.* **70**, 183–186.

Gorczynski, R. M. (1974). *J. Immunol.* **112**, 533–539.

Habel, K. (1962). *J. Exp. Med.* **115**, 181–193.

Hellström, K. E., and Hellström, I. (1974). *Advan. Immunol.* **18**, 209–277.

Herberman, R. B. (1974). *Advan. Cancer Res.* **19**, 207–263.

Herberman, R. B., Nun, M. E., Larvin, D. H., and Asosky, R. J. (1973). *J. Nat. Cancer Inst.* **51**, 1509–1512.

Hibbs, J. B. (1972). *Science* **180**, 868–870.

Howell, S. B., Dean, J. H., Esber, E. C., and Law, L. W. (1974). *Int. J. Cancer* **14**, 662–674.

Khera, K. S., Ashkenazi, A., Rapp, F., and Melnick, J. L. (1963). *J. Immunol.* **91**, 604–613.

Kiessling, R., Klein, E., and Wigzell, H. (1975a). *Eur. J. Immunol.* **5**, 112–117.

Kiessling, R., Klein, E., Pross, H., and Wigzell, H. (1975b). *Eur. J. Immunol.* **5**, 117–121.

Kit, S., Kimura, T., and Dubbs, R. (1969). *Int. J. Cancer* **4**, 384–392.

Lamon E. W. (1974). *Biochim. Biophys. Acta* **335**, 149–176.

Lamon, E. W., Skurzak, H. M., Klein, E., and Wigzell, H. (1972). *J. Exp. Med.* **136**, 1072–1079.

Lamon, E. W., Wigzell, H., Klein, E., Andersson, B., and Skurzak, H. M. (1973). *J. Exp. Med.* **137**, 1472–1493.

Leclerc, J. C., Gomard, E., and Levy, J. P. (1972). *Int. J. Cancer* **10**, 589–601.
Levy, J. H., and Wheelock, E. F. (1974). *Advan. Cancer Res.* **20**, 131–163.
Mackaness, G. B. (1971). *Progr. Immunol.* **1**, 413–424.
Nelson, D. S. (1974). *Transplant. Rev.* **19**, 226–254.
Nomoto, K., Gershon, R. K., and Waksman, B. H. (1970). *J. Nat. Cancer Inst.* **44**, 739–747.
Old, L. J., Boyse, E. A., Clarke, D. A., and Carswell, E. (1972). *Ann. N.Y. Acad. Sci.* **101**, 80–106.
Piessens, W. F., Churchill, W. H., and David, J. R. (1975). *J. Immunol.* **114**, 293–299.
Plata, F., Gomard, E., Leclerc, J. C., and Levy, J. (1973). *J. Immunol.* **111**, 667–671.
Salvin, S. B., and Nishio, J. (1972). *J. Exp. Med.* **135**, 985–996.
Simes, R. J., Kearney, R., and Nelson, D. S. (1975). *Immunology* **29**, 343–352.
Sjögren, H. O. (1964). *J. Nat. Cancer Inst.* **32**, 375–393.
Sjögren, H. O., and Borum, K. (1971). *Cancer Res.* **31**, 890–900.
Sjögren, H. O., Hellström, I., and Klein, G. (1961). *Cancer Res.* **21**, 329–337.
Stutman, O. (1975). *Nature (London)* **253**, 142–144.
Tevethia, S. S., and McMillan, V. L. (1974). *Intervirology* **3**, 269–276.
Tevethia, S. S., and Tevethia, M. J. (1975a). *Progr. Med. Virol.* (in press).
Tevethia, S. S., and Tevethia, M. J. (1975b). *In* "A Comprehensive Treatise in Cancer" (F. Becker, ed.), Vol. III. Academic Press, New York.
Tevethia, S. S., Couvillon, L. A., and Rapp, F. (1968a). *J. Immunol.* **100**, 358–362.
Tevethia, S. S., Dreesman, G. R., Lausch, R. N., and Rapp, F. (1968b). *J. Immunol.* **101**, 1105–1110.
Tevethia, S. S., Crouch, N. A., Melnick, J. L., and Rapp, F. (1970). *Int. J. Cancer* **5**, 176–184.
Tevethia, S. S., McMillan, V. L., Kaplan, P. M., and Bushong, S. C. (1971). *J. Immunol.* **106**, 1295–1300.
Tevethia, S. S., Blasecki, J. W., Waneck, G., and Goldstein, A. (1974). *J. Immunol.* **113**, 1417–1423.
Ting, C. C., and Herberman, R. B. (1971). *Int. J. Cancer* **7**, 499–506.
Ting, C. C., Ortaldo, J. R., and Herberman, R. B. (1973). *Int. J. Cancer* **12**, 511–518.
Tubergen, D. G., and Feldman, J. D. (1971). *J. Exp. Med.* **134**, 1144–1154.
Vandeputte, M., Eyssen, H., Sobis, H., and DeSomer, P. (1974). *Int. J. Cancer* **14**, 445–450.
Volkman, A., and Collins, F. M. (1971). *Cell. Immunol.* **2**, 552–566.
Volkman, A., and Gowans, J. L. (1965). *Brit. J. Exp. Pathol.* **46**, 62–70.
Wright, P. W., and Law, L. W. (1971). *Proc. Nat. Acad. Sci. U.S.* **68**, 973–976.
Zarling, J. M., and Tevethia, S. S. (1973a). *J. Nat. Cancer Inst.* **50**, 137–147.
Zarling, J. M., and Tevethia, S. S. (1973b). *J. Nat. Cancer Inst.* **50**, 149–157.
Zarling, J. M., Nowinski, R. C., and Bach, F. H. (1975). *Proc. Nat. Acad. Sci. U.S.* **72**, 2780–2784.
Zbar, B., Wespic, H. T., Borsos, T., and Rapp, H. J. (1970a). *J. Nat. Cancer Inst.* **44**, 473–481.
Zbar, B., Wepsic, A., Rapp, H., Stewart, L., and Borsos, T. (1970b). *J. Nat. Cancer Inst.* **44**, 701–717.
Zembala, M., Ptak, W., and Hanczakowska, M. (1973). *Immunology* **25**, 631–644.

21

Mechanisms of Extracellular Killing of Nucleated Mammalian Cells by Macrophages

R. Evans and P. Alexander

I. Introduction . . . 536
II. Specific Macrophage Cytotoxicity . . . 537
A. Properties of Growth Inhibitory Macrophages . . . 539
B. Properties of Lytic Macrophages . . . 542
C. Mechanisms of Immune Macrophage Cytotoxicity . . . 544
D. Specific Arming of Macrophages with Sensitized Lymphoid Cells . . . 546
E. Specific Arming of Macrophages with Supernatant Factors . . . 548
F. Macrophage Cytotoxicity in the Presence of Antibody . . . 551
III. Nonspecific Macrophage Cytotoxicity . . . 555
A. "Activation" of Macrophages . . . 555
B. Methods of Rendering Macrophages Nonspecifically Cytotoxic . . . 556
C. Mechanisms of Nonspecific Macrophage Cytotoxicity . . . 565
IV. Cytotoxic Macrophages and the Tumor Bearing Host . . . 567
V. *In Vivo* Significance of the Nonspecifically Cytotoxic Macrophage . . . 570
VI. Role of Macrophages in Surveillance . . . 571
VII. Conclusion . . . 572
References . . . 573

I. INTRODUCTION

In his series of lectures on the evolution of the phagocytic cell, Metchnikoff (1891) described how in the case of unicellular organisms phagocytosis fulfilled two basic roles. The first was to provide a means of sustinence, the other, a means of defense. During the course of evolution, the former was abandoned by higher organisms as tissues that digested food developed, but the defensive function was retained and became more refined. Defense in lower organisms is mainly by the phagocytic cell, so defined because in most cases elimination of the invading particule (inert or otherwise) is by phagocytosis. In higher organisms, it is clear that while the basic role of defense by phagocytosis is retained, other specialized mechanisms of defense evolved and, as will be shown, became integrated with the other activities of phagocytic cells. Cooperation between lymphoid cells and macrophages particularly occurs at all levels of the genesis of immune reactions. In this chapter, we deal with the role of macrophages at the effector arm of the immune response. Their role in antigen processing (that is, the afferent arm of the immune response) and in the cooperation between B and T lymphocytes (that is, the central point of the immune response) is dealt with elsewhere.

The nature of the effector cell responsible for the killing in cell-mediated destruction in transplantation and tumor immunity is variable according to the circumstances. The mechanism of destruction is not identical in all cases and may involve rapid lytic events or slower and initially cytostatic events. The recognition of cell-mediated cytotoxicity is frequently obscured by equating cytotoxicity with lysis. To us this is too narrow a use of the term cytotoxicity. By definition, toxicity refers to the extent of virulence of a poison, and a poison is any substance or agent which by its action causes destruction or modification of function. Thus cell-mediated cytotoxicity refers to the extent of damage or modification of function induced by an effector cell on a target cell and may be measured by different assay systems, depending on the nature of the change induced in the target cell. In this chapter we will consider the various mechanisms other than phagocytosis by which macrophages are toxic to tumor cells derived from experimental animals. The primary reaction occurs extracellularly, and phagocytosis, if it occurs at all, is a late event that follows the death and disintegration of cells. The extracellular cytotoxicity for mammalian cells may be expressed in two ways: one resulting in rapid lysis and measured usually by radioisotopic methods, or another involving among other changes the arrest of DNA synthesis, inhibition of growth, and eventual disintegration of tumor cells followed by their phagocytosis. Although cytotoxic macrophages as defined above may be found under a variety of conditions, it is possible to classify them into two broad categories: those that require recognition of specific antigen (whether transplantation, tumor-specific, or bacterial, such as tubercle purified protein derivative) in an immunologically specific way before they express their cytotoxicity and those that require no such antigenic stimulation and express cytotoxicity in a completely nonspecific manner, arresting DNA synthesis in a wide range of lymphoma and sarcoma cells *in vitro*.

II. SPECIFIC MACROPHAGE CYTOTOXICITY

Macrophages obtained from the peritoneal cavity of suitably immunized mice are cytotoxic to tumor cells, and the cytotoxic reaction shows a specificity similar to that of cytotoxic antibodies and cytotoxic T lymphocytes (i.e., the action is directed against the tumor-associated or histocompatibility antigens on the surface of the cells). Gorer (1956) alluded to the infiltration of macrophages during allograft rejection, and later other investigators (Journey and Amos, 1962; Old *et al.*, 1963; Bennett, 1965; Tsoi and Weiser, 1968) showed, by *in vivo* studies, the involvement of macrophages during such rejection. However, apart from these few early reports, the role of macrophages as effector cells in the allograft reaction has been largely neglected. Until recently the emphasis was placed on lymphocytes as effectors of allograft immunity, in spite of the fact that Pearsall and Weiser (1968) showed that silica *in vivo,* a macrophage poison, which does not appear to damage lymphocytes, delayed graft rejection. One reason macrophages have received such scant consideration in the destruction of mammalian cells in immune animals was that the bactericidal activity of macrophages derived from animals immunized with a variety of microorganisms is frequently nonspecific, even though it is immunologically mediated (i.e., via lymphocytes) (Mackaness, 1969). The apparent paradox that nonspecific immunity exerted by macrophages against bacteria can be transferred with immunologically specific lymphocytes is dealt with by Blanden *et al.* (Chapter 15). It was as a result of experiments involving tumor cells as targets that macrophages were first demonstrated to become specifically cytotoxic after cooperation with immune lymphoid cells, but nonspecifically cytotoxic after adding antigen (Takeda, 1969; Evans and Alexander, 1972a).

A role for immunologically specific cytotoxic macrophages in tumor immunity directed against syngeneic or autochthonous tumors by virtue of the recognition of tumor-specific transplantation antigens (TSTA's) present on the surface of cells was reported by Evans and Alexander

(1970). Macrophages taken from the peritoneal cavity of mice that had been immunized against syngeneic tumors (Evans and Alexander, 1970) or from mice that bore a growing subcutaneous tumor (Alexander *et al.*, 1973; Evans, 1973a) were specifically cytotoxic *in vitro* to the tumor cells used. The *in vivo* relevance of such findings was indicated by earlier studies in which mice were immunized with irradiated, syngeneic lymphoma cells, a procedure that rendered them resistant to a subsequent challenge with these cells (Alexander *et al.*, 1966). The lymphocytes from such immunized animals were either not cytotoxic at all or only very feebly cytotoxic *in vitro*. They were, however, capable of mediating the arrest of tumor growth *in vivo* in an immunologically specific manner (Alexander, 1974), as shown by the Winn test (Winn, 1960) in which lymphoid cells are mixed with tumor cells and then injected into normal animals. These data suggested that there was an important effector cell in tumor immunity, one which was not present in the original inoculum of admixed lymphoid and tumor cells. This point was emphasized in experiments reported by Zarling and Tevethia (1973a,b), who showed that injecting normal recipients with a mixture of immune lymphoid cells and tumor cells resulted in death of tumor cells, but if animals were irradiated or treated with silica beforehand, the tumor cells grew. Their data were consistent with the view that another cell type, probably the monocyte or macrophage, was required for tumor rejection. Nevertheless, it was quite clear that immune lymphocytes were necessary in the generation of this effector cell. It is, therefore, necessary to distinguish between three effects, perhaps fundamentally different, of immune lymphocytes: (a) the transference of immunity, as first described by Mitchison (1955); (b) the ability to arrest tumor growth in the Winn test directly or by cooperating with macrophages; and (c) the ability to kill cells *in vitro*.

During the following rejection of syngeneic tumor cells or of allografts, peritoneal macrophages may show two quite different cytotoxic reactions involving either growth inhibition with subsequent disintegration of tumor cells or rapid lysis. The conditions under which either type of cytotoxic macrophage may arise are different, and the situations in which they may be found are summarized in Table I (Evans, 1975c). It is also apparent that the route of injection and method of presentation of tumor cells during immunization is all important. Following intraperitoneal, subcutaneous, or intramuscular injection of irradiated syngeneic or allogenic tumor cells, specifically growth inhibitory macrophages are found in the peritoneal cavity of mice. Intraperitoneal injection of dividing lymphoma cells into allogeneic mice yields a population of strongly cytotoxic macrophages, as reported by a number of investigators (Baker *et al.*, 1962; Granger and Weiser, 1964, 1966; Hoy and Nelson, 1969; McIvor

TABLE I

Cytotoxic Macrophages in Tumor Immunity[a]

Cytolytic macrophage	Mice injected i.p. with allogeneic lymphoma cells
Cytostatic macrophage	Mice injected with irradiated syngeneic lymphoma cells
	Mice or rats bearing subcutaneous tumors
	Macrophages isolated from actively growing fibrosarcomas
	Nonimmune macrophages incubated with sensitized lymphoid cells (syngeneic or allogeneic)
	Nonimmune macrophages incubated with supernates from cultures or sensitized lymphoid cells (syngeneic or allogeneic) and specific antigen [specific macrophage arming factor (SMAF)]
	Rats injected with allogeneic fibrosarcoma cells

[a] From Evans (1975c).

and Weiser, 1971a; Den Otter *et al.*, 1972; Lohmann-Matthes *et al.*, 1972; Zighelboim *et al.*, 1974; Evans and Alexander, 1972). But if the tumor cells are implanted subcutaneous or intramuscularly, the peritoneal macrophages are growth inhibitory. Whether injection of dividing lymphoma cells into syngeneic mice preimmunized with irradiated tumor cells yields lytic macrophages has not been established, but the degree of growth inhibition seen is so high as to suggest this possibility (Den Otter *et al.*, 1974). The relationship between lysis and growth inhibition as mechanisms of cytotoxicity is not clear, and whether different pathways are used to achieve the end point of cell destruction is not known. In some circumstances the two may overlap, particularly since in some *in vitro* systems in which irradiated tumor cells were used as target cells, lysis (^{51}Cr release) was observed (Zembala *et al.*, 1973a), whereas using nonirradiated target cells under our conditions, growth inhibition without rapid release of isotope was seen.

A. Properties of Growth Inhibitory Macrophages

Growth inhibition may be assessed by counting residual cells in a hemocytometer (Evans and Alexander, 1970) or by pulse labeling tumor cells with ^{125}IUdR, a DNA precursor (Boyle and Ormerod, 1975), or [^{3}H]thymidine (Keller, 1973; Krahenbuhl and Remington, 1974). It is initiated by arresting DNA synthesis; hence the reduction in cell numbers compared with control cultures. The reaction becomes irreversible after the target cells have been in contact with the immune macrophages for 24 hours (Evans and Alexander, 1972c). If they are then removed, they can be shown to have lost the capacity to divide, and subsequently the tumor cells disintegrate. Phagocytosis of dead and disintegrating cells was frequently seen by 48–72 hours (Figs. 1 and 2). Cytotoxicity was immunologically specific, and unrelated tumor cells were not inhibited in their growth in the presence of macrophages from mice immunized with other antigens (Table II). Growth inhibition was observed when the ratio of macrophages to target cells was as low as 10 : 1 (Evans and Alexander, 1970), but monolayers of growth inhibitory macrophages progressively lost the capacity to inhibit growth when maintained in culture for a number of days. Moreover, monolayers showed a decrease capacity to inhibit more than one challenge of target cells (Evans and Alexander, 1972c). The capacity to inhibit growth was shown to be extremely radio-

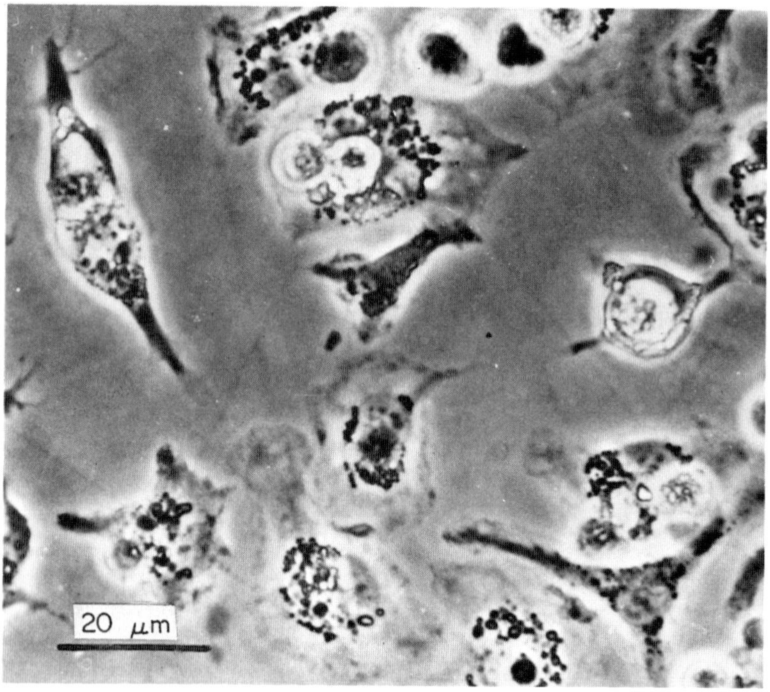

Fig. 1. Immune macrophages 48 hours after challenge with syngeneic DBA/2-L5178Y lymphoma cells. Granulation of cytoplasm pronounced with evidence of phagocytosis of debris. Very few viable lymphoma cells present. Phase contrast, ×450.

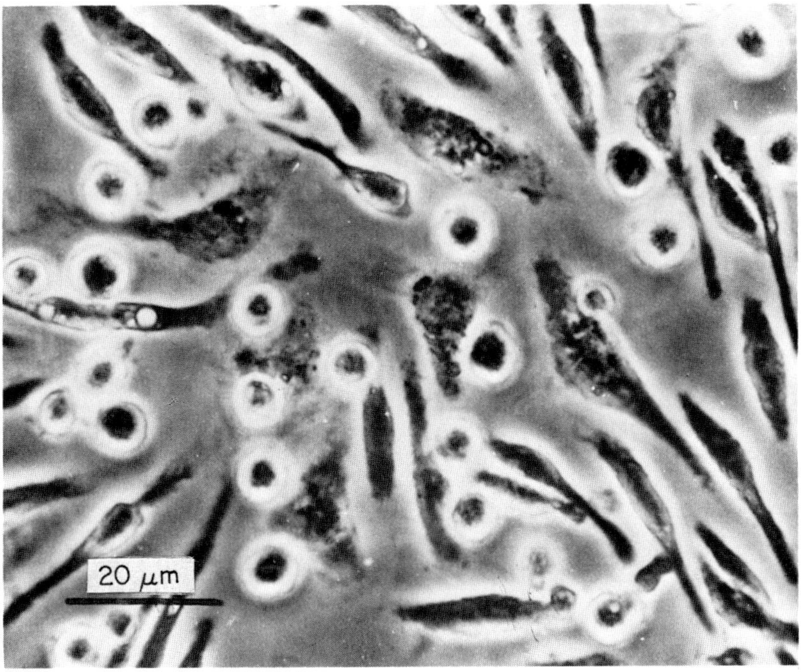

Fig. 2. Nonimmune macrophages 48 hours after challenge with syngeneic DBA/2-L5178Y lymphoma cells. Granulation less marked and no evidence of dead cells or phagocytized debris. Lymphoma cells appear as rounded cells. Phase contrast, ×450.

sensitive, and exposure of immune macrophages to 500 rads of X irradiation completely ablated their growth inhibitory activities if macrophage monolayers were challenged after a period of 5 hours had elapsed (Den Otter *et al.*, 1974). Challenge before this resulted in growth inhibition. X irradiation did not produce any morphologic functionally detectable changes in the macrophages. Immunologically specific growth inhibitory macrophages are not found in mice that have been deprived of T lymphocytes by adult thymectomy followed by whole body irradiation and reconstitution with bone marrow (Evans *et al.*, 1972). Such mice still make low levels of cytotoxic antibodies to the irradiated allogeneic cells with which they have been immunized, possibly because sufficient T lymphocytes are left to cooperate with B cells in the synthesis of antibody. This experiment suggests that T cells are required for the formation of specifically cytotoxic macrophages *in vivo,* and this is confirmed by "arming" experiments referred to below.

TABLE II

Specificity of in Vitro Growth Inhibition by Peritoneal Macrophages from DBA/2 Mice Immunized with Specific Antigens[a]

Macrophages from mice immunized with	Percentage growth inhibition[b] 48 hours after challenge		
	L5178Y	TLX5	TLX9
L5178Y cells (DBA/2)	80	NI[c]	NI
TLX5 cells (CBA)	NI	99	NI
TLX9 cells (C57B1)	NI	NI	99
BCG	NI	NI	NI
Thioglycolate medium	NI	NI	NI
Control	NI	NI	NI

[a] DBA/2 mice immunized with three i.p. injections of irradiated syngeneic L5178Y cells, or allogeneic TLX9 (C57 Black) and TLX5 (CBA) lymphoma cells, or three injections of BCG (Glaxo) or Difco thioglycolate medium. Macrophage cultures were prepared 10 days after the final injection, and challenged with 10^5 lymphoma cells. (From Evans and Alexander, 1972c.)

[b] Growth inhibition

$$= \frac{\text{No. cells in control} - \text{No. cells in test}}{\text{No. cells in control}} \times 100$$

[c] NI, no growth inhibition (less than 20%).

B. Properties of Lytic Macrophages

The properties of the immunologically specific lytic macrophages are quite different in that they induce a rapid release of isotopes, such as ^{51}Cr (Den Otter *et al.*, 1972; Lohmann-Matthes *et al.*, 1972; Zighelboim *et al.*, 1974) or ^{125}I (Boyle and Ormerod, 1975), from the prelabeled tumor cells (Fig. 3). Lytic macrophage monolayers can be exposed to several challenges of tumor cells and still retain their specific cytotoxic capacity (Den Otter *et al.*, 1972; Lohmann-Matthes *et al.*, 1972). Tumor cells become irreversibly damaged within 1 hour of contact with the macrophages. Compared with growth inhibitory macrophages, lytic macrophages retain their lytic capacity after 500 rads, and even after 1000–5000 rads, the level of cytotoxicity was still high (Den Otter *et al.*, 1974) (Table III). Since in these experiments growth inhibition, and not lysis, was measured, it is difficult to assess the effect of irradiation on the lytic macrophage per se, but nevertheless strong growth inhibition was still

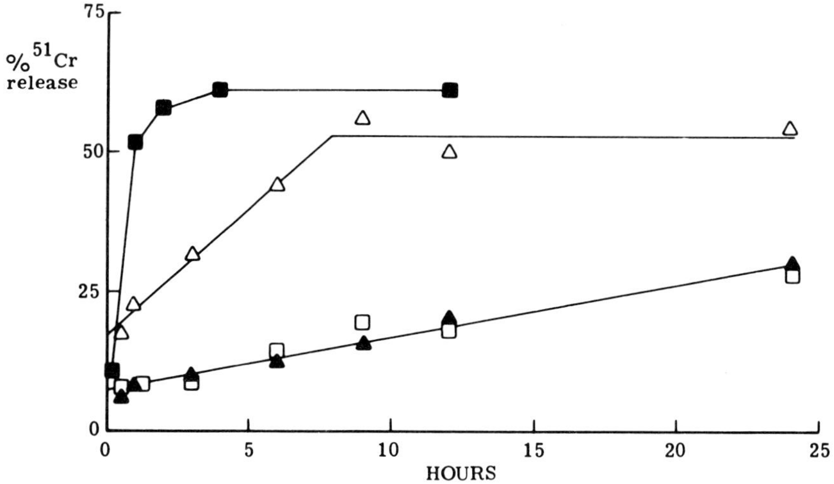

Fig. 3. Release of ^{51}Cr from SL2 cells in the presence of immune macrophages. △——△, immune macrophages; ▲——▲, normal macrophages; □——□, spontaneous release from SL2 cells; ■——■ ^{51}Cr release from SL2 cells after treatment with alloantibody and complement. (From Den Otter *et al.*, 1972.)

detectable after 5000 rads irradiation. Similarly, when mice were preimmunized with irradiated syngeneic lymphoma cells followed by an inoculum of nonirradiated tumor cells, the macrophages retained their cytotoxic potential after 5000 rads, unlike those recovered after immunization only

TABLE III

Effect of Different Doses of X Rays on Cytotoxicity of Alloimmune Macrophages[a]

Dose of X rays to macrophages (rads)	Postirradiation growth inhibition (%) of SL2 cells added to the macrophage monolayer at			
	10 minutes	5 hours	24 hours	48 hours
None	97	96	92	97
500	96	93	90	92
1000	92	64	61	65
3000	90	45	44	46
5000	92	41	40	40

[a] C57B1 mice immunized with living SL2 cells 14 days previously. (From Den Otter *et al.*, 1974.)

TABLE IV

Effect of 500 rads X Irradiation on Macrophage Cytotoxicity

Macrophages[a] from	Percentage growth inhibition of SL2 cells at 48 hours: Unirradiated macrophages	Irradiated macrophages (500 rads)
C57 Black mice immunized with		
Dividing allogeneic SL2 cells × 1	75	78
Irradiated allogeneic SL2 cells × 1	55	<20
Dividing allogeneic SL2 cells × 2	90	85
Irradiated allogeneic SL2 cells × 2	74	29
DBA/2 mice immunized with		
Irradiated syngeneic SL2 cells × 2	78	<20
Irradiated syngeneic SL2 cells × 2 followed by dividing SL2 cells	96	97

[a] Macrophage monolayers washed immediately after X irradiation and before challenge with 10^5 DBA/2 SL2 cells.

with irradiated cells where cytotoxicity was ablated by 500 rads. Table IV summarizes the immunization regimes employed and the sensitivity of macrophage cytotoxicity *in vitro* to 500 rads of X irradiation. Thus there is a difference between the macrophage populations recovered after immunization schedules designed to induce growth inhibitory and lytic macrophages. There is now evidence to suggest that two distinct subpopulations of macrophages occur after immunization of mice with dividing lymphoma cells (Boyle and Ormerod, 1975). This subpopulation of lytic macrophages could be selectively detached from monolayers by EDTA. It was estimated that at the time of harvesting of the peritoneal exudates, less than 15% of the macrophage population were lytic, the rest apparently being specifically growth inhibitory.

C. Mechanisms of Immune Macrophage Cytotoxicity

In spite of these differences between the growth inhibitory and the lytic macrophages, the hypothesis that one acts by inhibiting DNA synthesis and the other by a direct attack on the cell membrane cannot be sustained because cytostatic macrophages will, in fact, lyse target cells after these have been rendered incapable of DNA synthesis by exposure to ionizing radiation (Zembala *et al.*, 1973a). This suggests that for both types of macrophage cytotoxicity, the primary lesion may involve the cell membrane. The lesion induced by the growth inhibitory macrophages may be rapidly repaired and hence is only reflected initially by an effect on DNA synthesis, while the lesion induced by the lytic macrophage may be irreparable. An alternative hypothesis is that close contact between the macrophages and target cells is required for both growth inhibition and lysis, and this close contact is achieved by an immune process possibly similar to antibody-induced mixed agglutination. Electron microscopy (Journey and Amos, 1962; Chambers and Weiser, 1969; Lejeune and Evans, 1972) has demonstrated such close contacts. Once contact is established, toxins (McIvor and Weiser, 1971b) or other "biologically active molecules" released from the macrophages or present in their plasma membranes may attack the targets. Different macrophage toxins may have either cytostatic or lytic effects. Whether these putative toxins act locally at the point of contact between cells or at a distance would depend on thermostability or concentration and also on whether they are denatured in growth medium. However a number of investigators have failed to detect any such humoral factors in both syngeneic (Evans and Alexander, 1972c) and allogeneic (Den Otter *et al.*, 1972; Lohmann-Matthes *et al.*, 1972) combination.

The simplest explanation for the immunologically specific activity of immune macrophages would be to postulate that such macrophages are coated with a specific cytophilic moiety and that immunologically specific interaction between coated macrophages and specific antigen triggers a change in the macrophage, which then manifests its cytolytic or cytostatic potential. Presumably the moiety mediating this effect is not made in mice deprived of T lymphocytes, since such tumor-immunized mice do not have cytotoxic macrophages (Evans *et al.*, 1972). Possibly the avidity of any cytophilic antibody produced is low in these deprived mice, and binding to macrophage Fc receptors is unstable. Immune macrophages were indeed found to have 3–4 times higher concentrations of membrane immunoglobulins (Evans and Alexander, 1972c) than normal macrophages. The effect of trypsin on cytophilic antibody is well documented (Nelson, 1969), and its effect on immune allogeneic and syngeneic cytotoxic macrophages was such that cytotoxicity was abrogated by relatively high concentrations (Evans and Alexander, 1972c; Den Otter *et al.*, 1972; Lohmann-Matthes *et al.*, 1972), although Lohmann-Matthes *et al.* (1972) claimed that specific cytotoxicity reappeared after trypsin treatment. Such findings need clarification. A material with hemagglutinating activity was eluted from alloimmune macrophages (Granger and Weiser, 1966), and this was shown to rearm trypsinized immune macrophages (Granger *et al.*, 1966). Immune serum also showed this property. However, normal macrophages were not armed. This indicated an inherent difference between immune and normal macrophages. Whether this difference is quantitative, in that immune macrophages may have more Fc receptors, remains to be determined. Furthermore, Cruse *et al.* (1973) showed that IgG_2 facilitated macrophage cytotoxicity, which in regard to cell-dependent antibody cytotoxicity studies (see Section II,F) indicates a role for antibody in macrophage-mediated cytotoxicity. These experiments are certainly consistent with the hypothesis that immunologically specific cytotoxic macrophages owe their activity to a molecule that has the capacity to recognize antigens and which carries at least some of the determinants of immunoglobulins.

D. Specific Arming of Macrophages with Sensitized Lymphoid Cells

Following the original observation that lymphoid cells from mice immunized with irradiated syngeneic lymphoma cells protected recipient syngeneic mice against tumor growth (Alexander *et al.*, 1966), experiments carried out *in vivo* and *in vitro* indicated that cooperation between normal macrophages and the immune lymphocytes led to the "arming" of the macrophages against the specific tumor cells (Evans and Alexander, 1970, 1972a,b). These specifically armed macrophages recognized the specific tumor cells and inhibited their growth *in vitro* (Table V).

TABLE V

Specificity of Arming by Immune Spleen Cells[a]

Normal DBA/2 macrophages incubated with spleen cells from DBA/2 mice hyperimmunized with	Percentage growth inhibition 48 hours after challenge[b] with		
	L5178Y	TLX5	TLX9
L5178Y cells	82	NI[c]	NI
TLX5 cells	NI	99	NI
TLX9 cells	NI	NI	99
BCG	NI	NI	NI
Control cultures with or without spleen cells	NI	NI	NI

[a] Immunization regimen as for Table II. From Evans and Alexander (1972c).
[b] Cultures challenges with 10^5 lymphoma cells in 3 ml GM.
[c] NI, no growth inhibition.

Such a cooperative effect was demonstrated in both syngeneic (Evans and Alexander, 1970, 1972b) and allogeneic systems (Evans and Alexander, 1972a; Evans and Grant, 1972; Lohmann-Matthes *et al.*, 1972; Pels and Den Otter, 1974; Zembala *et al.*, 1973a,b) in which monolayers of normal (i.e., completely noncytotoxic) macrophages were rendered cytotoxic after incubation with immune lymphoid cells followed by complete removal of the lymphoid cells by intensive washing. To arm macrophages in this way required that the immune lymphoid cells be in direct contact. Table VI shows that a minimal number of cells was required to arm macrophages, and the optimal ratio for arming was 2–5 lymphocytes to 1 macrophage. There was no need for the specific target cell to be present during arming, and this implies that the arming did not occur by a lymphokine-like factor released when immune lymphoid cells contact antigen (see Section II,E). These *in vitro* experiments appeared to provide a satisfactory explanation for the observed *in vivo* cytotoxicity when immune lymphoid cells were mixed with tumor cells (Alexander *et al.*, 1966; Zarling and Tevethia, 1973a,b). This we attributed to cooperation with host-derived macrophages, and indeed peritoneal macrophages recovered 24 to 48 hours after intraperitoneal injection of immune lymphoid cells were shown to be cytotoxic *in vitro* (Evans and Alexander, 1972b). Indirect evidence to support this concept was obtained when it was shown that tumor bearing mice, which were able to reject an implant of the same tumor material, not only yielded growth inhibiting macrophages but also produced spleen and lymph node cells capable of arming macrophages (Alexander *et al.*, 1973; Evans, 1973a). Since the properties of the macrophages obtained by arming *in vitro* with

TABLE VI

Number of Immune Spleen Cells Required to Arm a Normal Macrophage Monolayer

No. of immune spleen cells incubated with macrophages	Percentage growth inhibition at 48 hours
2×10^7	83 ± 5
2×10^6	89 ± 3
2×10^5	35 ± 4
2×10^4	<20
Control	
2×10^4–2×10^7 normal spleen cells	<20

immune lymphocytes are indistinguishable from the immunologically specific growth inhibitory macrophages isolated from immunized animals, it is tempting to speculate that *in vivo* immune macrophages may be formed by an interaction between normal mononuclear phagocytes and immune lymphocytes.

E. Specific Arming of Macrophages with Supernatant Factors

Specific arming of macrophages by a supernatant factor was demonstrated when immune lymphoid cells from tumor-immunized syngeneic mice were incubated with the specific target cells and the supernatant obtained rendered macrophages specifically cytotoxic (Evans and Alexander, 1971, 1972b). This was later confirmed with allogeneic combinations (Evans and Grant, 1972; Evans *et al.*, 1972; Lohmann-Matthes *et al.*, 1973; Pels and Den Otter, 1974). The specific macrophage arming factor (SMAF) had an affinity for both macrophages and the specific target cell and could be absorbed from solution by both (Evans *et al.*, 1972; Pels and Den Otter, 1974). Target cells that had been exposed to SMAF were growth inhibited when placed on normal macrophage monolayers, and SMAF-treated macrophages (well washed after treatment) were specifically cytotoxic to the target cell used to immunize the animal from which SMAF was derived. Operationally, therefore, SMAF has the properties of a cytophilic antibody, but there is no evidence at the moment to suggest that it belongs to any of the known immunoglobulin classes. Moreover, it would appear to be a product of T lymphocytes and not of B lymphocytes. Detailed investigations have shown that SMAF could not be obtained from lymphoid cells that had been exposed to anti-θ serum (Evans *et al.*, 1972; Grant *et al.*, 1973; Lohmann-Matthes *et al.*, 1973) or from lymphoid cells from T lymphocyte-deprived mice (Evans *et al.*, 1972). Moreover, Grant *et al.* (1972) showed that SMAF could be obtained from thymocytes of immunized animals, and these cells were not cytotoxic, compared with spleen lymphocytes. Thus SMAF-producing T cells are probably distinct from the lytic T cells. Lohmann-Matthes *et al.* (1973) produced SMAF from *in vitro* sensitized cortisone-resistant T cells. The origin of SMAF, therefore, does not indicate that it is a conventional immunoglobulin, but it may be an immunoglobulin-like molecule made or released by T cells. SMAF-containing culture supernatants were fractionated by gel filtration, and activity was mainly found in two fractions (Fig. 4). One of these fractions was in the region of 40,000–100,000 daltons (maximum activity at 50,000–60,000), and the other in the region greater than 300,000 daltons (Evans *et al.*, 1972). Lohmann-Matthes *et al.* (1974) have detected

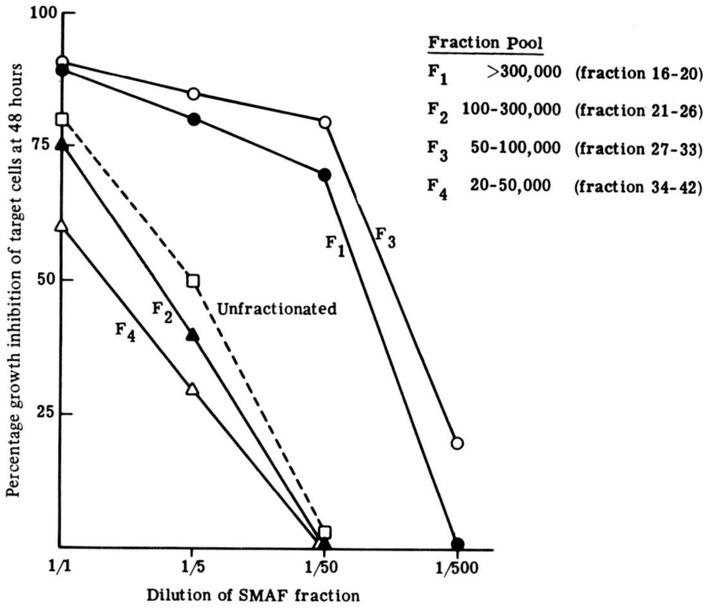

Fig. 4. Growth inhibition of DBA/2 SL2 lymphoma cells by macrophages armed *in vitro* by SMAF. Fractions (F_1–F_4) from a Bio-Gel P-150 polyacrylamide gel column.

SMAF activity in the 25,000–50,000 dalton region. The low molecular weight material cannot be an intact immunoglobulin, but may be part of an immunoglobulin. In this connection it is interesting that Moroz and Hahn (1973) have reported that on the surface of T lymphocytes there are parts of heavy chains having a molecular weight of the order of 40,000. There is evidence that proteins other than immunoglobulins can be cytophilic for macrophages and show antigenic specificity, as reported by Nelson (1970) who showed that γ_1-globulin, cytophilic for macrophages, appeared in serum of mice immunized with sheep red blood cells. The higher molecular weight fraction with SMAF activity could be an immunoglobulin on a molecular weight basis, but the fact that it is made or released by T cells would again indicate that it is not a normal immunoglobulin. It may be an antigen–antibody type complex because in the process of inducing SMAF formation from lymphocytes antigen is present, and this may complex with the antigen-recognizing material. The properties of SMAF are listed in Table VII. Of great interest is the resemblance of SMAF and other T cell products which have an affinity either for antigen or macrophages or both. Cone *et al.* (1974) claimed that T cells released a factor resembling monomeric IgM. This

TABLE VII

Properties of the Specific Macrophage Arming Factor

Product of lymphocytes (probably T cells)
Binds to macrophages from different strains and species
Binds to specific target tumor cells
Stable at 56°C for 30 minutes
Stable at +4°C and −20°C
Nondialysable and readily concentrated
Molecular weight of 50,000–100,000 or >300,000 by gel filtration

T cell product was cytophilic for macrophages and allowed B cells to respond to thymus-dependent antigens. The molecular weight was approximately 200,000 (Marchalonis *et al.*, 1972); thus it is larger than the low molecular weight SMAF and smaller than the high molecular weight material. It is perhaps significant that light chain dimers (MW 50,000?) were occasionally found in their Ig preparations from thymus-derived lymphocytes. Taussig (1974) reported that "educated" mouse T cells released a factor capable of replacing T cells in a cooperation-dependent antibody response *in vivo.* This factor was not an immunoglobulin and could be absorbed out by congenically raised anti-H-2 antibodies (Taussig and Munro, 1974). Moreover, it could be absorbed by specific antigen, and had a molecular weight of about 50,000 (Munro *et al.*, 1974). Whether this factor has an affinity for macrophages is not known. Zembala *et al.* (1975) have shown that lymph node cells from mice previously injected with picryl chloride produced a supernatant factor *in vitro* which depressed the passive transfer of contact sensitivity by immune cells. This factor has a molecular weight of about 50,000, is T cell-dependent, and is absorbed out by specific antigen. Finally, the T cell-dependent, antigen-specific macrophage migration inhibition factor (Amos and Lachman, 1970) is also reported to have a molecular size of about 50,000 as well as having an affinity for macrophages. Only direct testing will determine whether any of these factors is the same as SMAF.

Recently, we have encountered considerable difficulty in preparing SMAF, and many of the supernatants of immune lymphoid cells and target cells have given rise to factors that render macrophages nonspecifically cytotoxic rather than specifically cytotoxic (see Section III,B,3). This nonspecific arming factor may be similar to lymphokines that have been reported to cause increased macrophage aggregation or spreading. We are currently trying to elucidate the conditions under which SMAF and a nonspecific macrophage activator are released when immune lymphocytes are in contact with the specific antigen.

In the above studies, peritoneal macrophages were employed because of the convenience in obtaining them, but clearly extrapolation on a wider scale, such as to the circulating monocytes, may not be valid. However, the relevance of such findings to antitumor effects has recently been strengthened by experiments in a xenogeneic system (Grant *et al.*, 1974). These investigations showed that lymphocytes from the intermediate lymph of sheep immunized with murine lymphoma cells were not cytotoxic to tumor cells but could render cytotoxic bloodborne white cells from normal sheep, as well as macrophages recovered from udders of normal ewes. Moreover, when these lymphocytes were incubated with irradiated lymphoma cells, a supernatant factor was produced which induced cytotoxicity in normal bloodborne sheep white cells. More recently, similar results have been obtained in an allogeneic combination in rats injected with allogeneic fibrosarcoma cells (S. Denham, personal communication). Noncytotoxic thoracic duct lymphocytes from immunized rats were able to render normal rat peripheral blood leukocytes and spleen cells cytotoxic. Whether these cytotoxic effects are mediated by macrophages is not known, but the resemblance to the sheep studies of Grant *et al.* is striking.

F. Macrophage Cytotoxicity in the Presence of Antibody

During recent years much attention has focused on the ability of certain categories of effector cells to lyse target cells in the presence of specific xenogeneic, allogeneic, or syngeneic antibody. The identity of these effectors is frequently confused by lack of appropriate separation techniques. All share basic properties in that they possess Fc receptors capable of binding immune complexes of antibody and antigen which render them cytotoxic in an immunologically specific manner to target cells. The evidence for participation of nonmacrophage effector cells has been critically reviewed by a number of investigators (Perlmann and Holm, 1969; Perlmann *et al.*, 1972; MacLennan, 1972; Cerottini and Brunner, 1974). The involvement of macrophages has received less attention, however, and the number of reports demonstrating specific macrophage-dependent, antibody-mediated cytotoxicity is few (Holm and Hammarström, 1973; Dennert and Lennox, 1973; Zighelboim *et al.*, 1973; Scornik and Cosenza, 1974; Evans, 1974a, 1975a,b). Usually, peritoneal macrophages are used in such tests, since these are readily available and identifiable, although too frequently lack of positive identification of macrophages prevents firm conclusions being drawn in regard to the precise nature of the effector cells responsible. In this laboratory we used a unique source of macrophages which were isolated from actively growing mouse and rat fibrosarcomas and cultivated *in vitro* (Evans, 1972, 1973b). The reason for interest in these macrophages was that if they were potential effector cells they were ideally situated. Monolayers so formed could be shown to consist of up to 100% typical macrophages by morphology, by phagocytosis of opsonized sheep red blood cells, and by lysis by anti-macrophage serum and complement. Figure 5 shows that tumor macrophages in the presence of murine alloantibody and tumor cells could either specifically lyse or inhibit growth of target cells, depending on the antibody dilution employed (Evans, 1974a, 1975a,b). Figure 6 shows the distribution of complement-dependent antibody after gel chromatography of alloimmune serum in relation to the pooled fractions (Fig. 6a) and compares the relative sensitivity of macrophage-dependent growth inhibition with macrophage and complement-dependent lysis (Fig. 6b). It is seen that growth

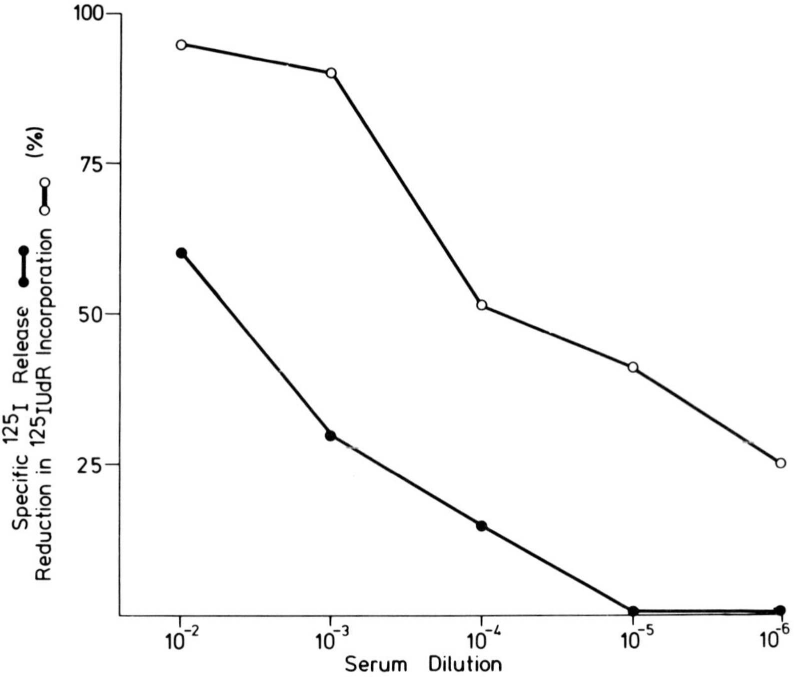

Fig. 5. A comparison of specific macrophage-dependent antibody lysis and growth inhibition. CBA anti-C57 Black serum dilutions 10^5 TLX9 target lymphoma cells (C57 Black) on rat tumor macrophage monolayers (hooded rat A tumor, see Table XII). Lysis was assessed by measuring the level of ^{125}I released from ^{125}IUdR labeled target cells. Growth inhibition was assessed on the basis of reduction of ^{125}IUdR incorporation by target cells. Both lysis and growth inhibition assessed after 18 hours. DBA/2 lymphoma cells as targets grew normally under these conditions. (From Evans, 1975b.)

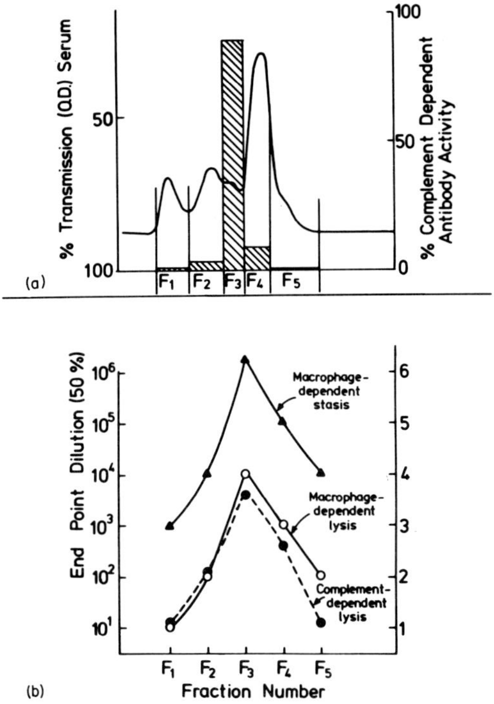

Fig. 6. (a) Fractionation of CBA anti-C57 Black serum by Bio-Gel chromatography in relation to complement-dependent antibody cytotoxicity (hatched areas). Material pooled on molecular weight basis into five fractions (F_1–F_5). (b) Comparison of macrophage-dependent antibody lysis, growth inhibition, and complement-dependent lysis of C57 Black TLX9 lymphoma cells in relation to the distribution of complement-dependent antibody (IgG). (From Evans, 1975a).

inhibition was 100 times more sensitive than lysis in the detection of antibody. Macrophage-dependent lysis was at most three times more sensitive than complement-dependent lysis. On the basis of gel filtration and immunoelectrophoresis, the class of antibody responsible appears to be IgG, in keeping with this reaction induced by the other categories of effector cells. Moreover, at ratios of 2.5 : 1 specific lysis was still detectable, indicating the relative homogeneity of the effector cells. Under the conditions of these experiments, macrophage cytotoxicity toward antibody-coated target cells (murine lymphoma) was difficult to demonstrate, and best results were always obtained by having antibody present throughout. Other investigators have been successful in demonstrating lysis of antibody-coated target cells by macrophages (Dennert and Lennox, 1973; Zighelboim *et al.*, 1973), and we attribute our lack of success to the nature of our target cells. The shedding of surface antigen from these lymphoma cells appears to be rapid in that cultures of antibody-coated cells show a progressive decrease in susceptibility to lysis when complement is added (C. Dean, unpublished data). Thus, the limiting factor in macrophage-dependent antibody-mediated cytotoxicity would appear to be related to the concentration of antibody and antigen–antibody complexes. In the presence of antibody excess, cytotoxicity is detected since an equilibrium is probably established between the amount of antibody binding to the target cells and the concentration of immune complexes in the culture medium. It is of interest that when these cultures of macrophages interact with specific alloantibody and the target cells, both a specific growth inhibitory and a lytic reaction can be detected under appropriate conditions. Whether a subpopulation of macrophages is responsible for lysis, as demonstrated in the allograft situation reported by Boyle and Ormerod (1975), is not known at present. The relationship of this macrophage-dependent antibody-mediated cytotoxic reaction to the immunologically specific cytotoxic action of immune macrophages deserves further investigation.

Earlier experiments had indicated that after incubation of peritoneal macrophages with serum from mice immunized with allogeneic lymphoma cells specific cytotoxicity was observed (Evans and Grant, 1972). However, in the light of the above findings that very little antibody is required to induce growth inhibition of tumors by macrophages, we reexamined these experiments. The overall results indicated that specific arming of macrophages by alloantibody was not seen if the monolayers were washed at least 6 times, but if only 3 washes were employed growth inhibition was detected. This suggests that arming as such might not have actually occurred, and cytotoxicity under these conditions might have been a manifestation of macrophage-dependent antibody-mediated cytotoxicity due to traces of residual antibody. It is also possible that the antibody had only a low binding affinity for macrophages, but such antibody was easily eluted, as demonstrated earlier by Perlmann *et al.* (1972) using a lymphoid line of effector cells. In no experiments have we detected arming by serum from mice immunized with syngeneic tumor cells. Evidence for immunologically specific arming of peritoneal macrophages with serum from tumor bearing mice or rats has been reported (Cox, 1974). Since sera from tumor bearing animals can be demonstrated to contain antibody–antigen complexes at certain stages of tumor growth, it is possible that arming by specific antigen–antibody complexes may occur. However, since we also have data that tumor bearing serum can render macrophages nonspecifically cytotoxic, this whole question requires much more detailed study.

III. NONSPECIFIC MACROPHAGE CYTOTOXICITY

A. "Activation" of Macrophages

Earlier experiments indicated that following addition of the specific antigen to immune or *in vitro* armed macrophage monolayers, a change occurred resulting in the ability of the macrophages to inhibit growth of tumor cells in a nonspecific manner (Evans and Alexander, 1972a). This change was referred to as specific "activation," since it involved a specific immunological stimulus and it alluded solely to the transformation of the specific antigen-recognizing macrophage to the nonspecific growth inhibitory effector cell (Fig. 7). As far as we are aware, such macrophages are not lytic, but are invariably cytostatic. While this term has the advantage of brevity, it has led to a great deal of confusion because "activation" has been used by many other investigators to infer morphological, biochemical, and physiological changes occurring in macrophages after various treatments, which were not necessarily intended to render the macrophages nonspecifically cytotoxic. Nelson (1969) appreciated this difficulty and proposed the use of the term "stimulated" unless there is formal proof of increased intracellular killing of bacteria. While in many cases increased intracellular killing of bacteria and nonspecific tumor cell cytotoxicity may go hand in hand, it is not certain that there is an obligate association between cytotoxicity, as described in this chapter, and antimicrobial activities. Until more is known about the interrelationship between the various changes that can be induced in macrophages,

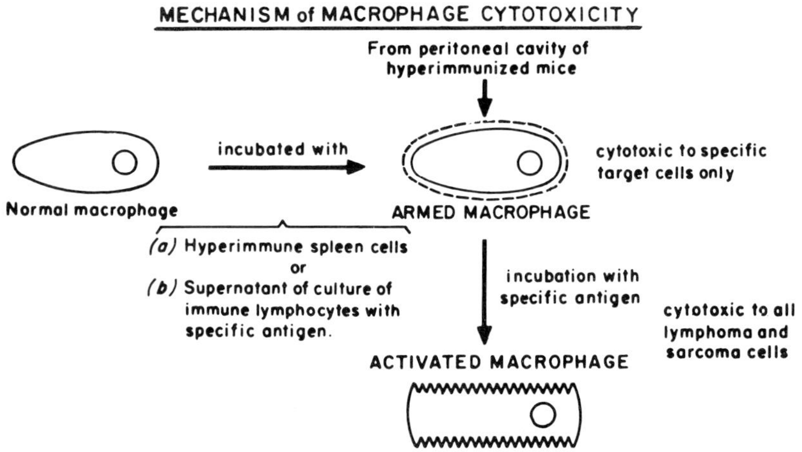

Fig. 7. Mechanism of macrophage cytotoxicity. (From Evans and Alexander, 1972a.)

we feel that if the term activation is to be used at all it should be strictly defined in its context.

When macrophages are rendered nonspecifically cytotoxic *in vivo,* they do not appear to attack any type of normal host cell, but they will kill tumor cells. The degree of discrimination exerted by nonspecifically cytotoxic macrophages may resemble the primitive protective mechanisms of invertebrates, the protection against infective organisms by phagocytic cells, and the clearance of damaged cells by the reticuloendothelial system. The possibility that nonspecifically cytotoxic macrophages may exert surveillance in the body against spontaneously arising malignant cells will be discussed in Section VI.

B. Methods Rendering Macrophages Nonspecifically Cytotoxic

1. Polyanions

Sarcoma and lymphoma cells grow normally on monolayers of peritoneal macrophages taken from control mice, if the mice are free of infection (see below). If such monolayers are exposed to endotoxin, double-stranded RNA (dsRNA), or synthetic poly(I)·poly(C) in minute amounts, they then inhibit the growth of lymphoma and sarcoma cells (Alexander and Evans, 1971; Parr *et al.,* 1973; Evans, 1974b). This effect was not due to a direct toxic action of the endotoxin or dsRNA, which under the conditions used did not influence the growth of the target cells. The essential component of endotoxin needed for activation is not the polysaccharide but the lipid A constitutent (Fig. 8). Neither DNA nor single-stranded RNA rendered macrophages nonspecifically cytotoxic. Since both double-stranded RNA and lipid A are polyanions, we examined a series of polymeric acids (see Table VIII), but none of the compounds studied was as effective as endotoxin or lipid A in rendering macrophages cytotxic. Thus, results of experiments in which the toxicity of various compounds toward tumor cells in culture has been tested should be interpreted with caution, particularly if the compounds are known to activate macrophages and if primary cultures of tumor cells were used, since such cultures frequently contain large numbers of macrophages. The addition of endotoxin to such primary cultures of sarcoma cells was shown to lead to growth inhibition compared with macrophage-free tumor cell cultures whose growth was not affected by endotoxin (Evans, 1974b). Macrophages can also be rendered nonspecifically cytotoxic *in vivo* by injecting endotoxin or double-stranded RNA into the peritoneal cavity and then washing out the macrophages from the animals 3–7 days later (Evans, 1975b). Immediately after injecting these mate-

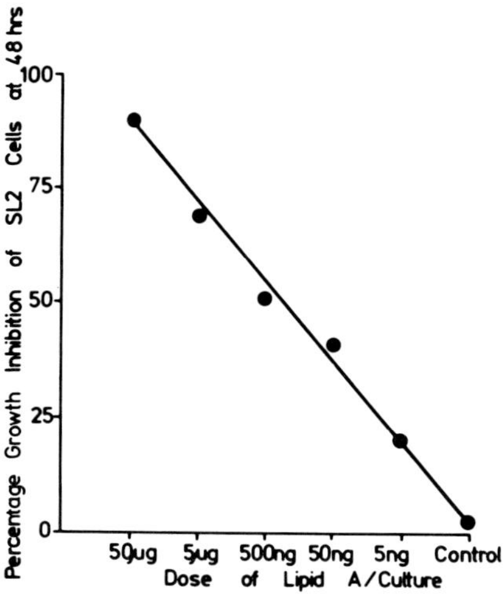

Fig. 8. Macrophages incubated with serial dilutions of lipid A for 1 hour followed by washing of monolayers and challenge with 10^5 DBA/2 SL2 lymphoma cells. (From Evans, 1974b.)

TABLE VIII

***Ability of Various Compounds to Activate Mouse Peritoneal Macrophages*[a]**

Compound	Growth inhibition[b] at 48 hours of					
	200 μg	20 μg	2 μg	200 ng	20 ng	2 ng
Polystyrene sulfuric acid	Toxic	Toxic	−	−	−	−
Polyglutamic acid	−	−	−	−	−	−
Polygalacturonic acid	Toxic	−	−	−	−	−
Polyacrylamide	−	−	−	−	−	−
Polyacrylic acid	Toxic	−	−	−	−	−
Pyran copolymer	−	−	−	−	−	−
CoAM	+	−	−	−	−	−
Poly(I) · poly(C)	+	+	+	+	−	−
Poly(A) · poly(U)	+	+	+	−	−	−
dsRNA	+	+	+	+	−	−
Endotoxin	+	+	+	+	+	+
Lipid A	+	+	+	+	+	+

[a] Each compound incubated for a maximum period of 24 hours with the monolayers followed by extensive washing before challenge with 10^5 lymphoma cells.

[b] +, growth inhibition >20%; −, <20% of control value.

rials i.p., the peritoneal macrophages disappeared. After 3 days macrophages could again be recovered, and these then were nonspecifically cytotoxic when tested *in vitro*. However, maximum cytotoxic activity was not observed until 7 days after injection. The kinetics of *in vivo* activation are similar to those seen after i.p. injection of pyran copolymer (Kaplan *et al.*, 1974). This polyanion also renders macrophages nonspecifically cytotoxic, but unlike endotoxin or dsRNA it does not activate macrophages *in vitro*. Macrophages activated *in vivo* could distinguish between normal and tumor cells (Regelson *et al.*, 1974), although some effect on normal cells was reported later (Kaplan *et al.*, 1974). Whether these macrophage activators *in vivo* exert either a direct effect on macrophages, or an indirect effect by stimulating the synthesis or release of substances capable of activating macrophages, or whether the breakdown products of these compounds activate is not known.

In many ways, the most interesting substance that is capable of rendering macrophages nonspecifically cytotoxic is the simple peptidoglycan (Adam *et al.*, 1974). This substance is a component of the cell wall of all microorganisms and has been found to render macrophages nonspecifically cytotoxic at concentrations of a few μg/ml. The chemical constitution of the three classes of substances, double-stranded RNA, lipid A, and peptidoglycan, able to render macrophages nonspecifically cytotoxic at very low concentrations is quite dissimilar. However, both dsRNA and endotoxin bind complement; thus the possibility exists that binding to macrophages occurs at the C3 receptor. It is not clear whether the action of these agents on macrophages is pharmacological, i.e., via a receptor, or immunological in the sense that the macrophages of all rodents are sensitized to these agents. Hence exposure of "normal" macrophages to endotoxin would be the equivalent of exposing macrophages from immunized animals to the specific antigen. This would explain the disappearance reaction after endotoxin treatment. We found that macrophages from germ-free mice could be rendered nonspecifically cytotoxic by endotoxin, but this does not necessarily exclude the possibility that macrophages were presensitized because even these germ-free mice may have become immune to endotoxin as a result of killed microbial products taken in with the food. While antibodies to endotoxin are common, most of them react via their polysaccharide component, and it is not clear whether antibodies to lipid A are formed.

2. *Specific Immunological Activation by Antigen*

Whatever the mechanism by which endotoxin, double-stranded RNA, and peptidoglycan render macrophages nonspecifically cytotoxic, this same change can be brought about by contacting specifically cytotoxic macrophages described in Section II with the antigen used to immunize the host originally (i.e., by the mechanism shown in Fig. 7). This phenomenon can be demonstrated in two ways: Mice can be immunized to a specific tumor when their macrophages will be cytotoxic only to this tumor as seen in Table I. However, if such macrophages are incubated with the specific tumor, they then undergo a change to nonspecific cytotoxicity (Table IX) (Evans and Alexander, 1972a). Alternatively, mice may be immunized to an antigen such as BCG or sheep red blood cells (Evans *et al.*, 1973) quite unrelated to the tumor target cells. Macrophages from such animals are not cytotoxic in any way, but after being in contact with BCG (or with PPD, the purified protein derivative of tuberculin) or sheep red blood cells (SRBC), they will then acquire the capacity to inhibit the growth of and kill tumor cells nonspecifically. Similarly, if SMAF is prepared from lymphocytes derived from tumor or SRBC-immunized mice, specific arming can be demonstrated (Evans *et al.*, 1973). Addition of the specific antigen leads to activation (Table X). There may be a close relationship between the mechanism by which immunologically specific macrophages inhibit growth and by which nonspecifically cytotoxic macrophages inhibit growth. All the available data are consistent with the hypothesis that the immunological specificity of the immune macrophages resides in the recognition of antigen, contact with which transforms the macrophage into the nonspecifically cytotoxic cell. Furthermore, immune macrophages may be rendered nonspecifically growth inhibitory by rabbit anti-mouse γ-globulin (Evans, 1975a), and in view of the finding that immune macrophages have increased levels of surface immunoglobulins, the hypothesis that immune complexing on

TABLE IX

Specific Immunological Macrophage Activation by Antigen[a]

Macrophage cultures	Cytotoxicity (%) at 48 hours	
	SL2 cells	TLX9 cells
Immune only	85 ± 5	<10
Immune + SL2	82 ± 8	75 ± 6
Immune + TLX9	78 ± 6	<10

[a] DBA/2 mice immunized with three i.p. injections of 10^7 irradiated SL2 cells.

TABLE X

In Vitro Growth Inhibition of Lymphoma Cells by SMAF-Armed and Activated Macrophages[a]

Origin of SMAF used to arm macrophages	Exposure of armed macrophage to antigen	% growth inhibition at 48 hours	
		SL2	TLX9
No SMAF, culture medium alone	None	<10	<10
	SL2	<10	<10
	TLX9	<10	<10
	SRBC	<10	<10
Spleen cells from mice immunized with SL2 cells cultured with SL2 cells for 24 hours	None	79 ± 6	3 ± 2
	SL2	86 ± 4	74 ± 6
	TLX9	78 ± 6	4 ± 3
	SRBC	79 ± 3	7 ± 1
Spleen cells from mice immunized with TLX9 cells cultured with TLX9 cells for 24 hours	None	3 ± 1	78 ± 2
	TLX9	82 ± 8	92 ± 4
	SL2	3 ± 1	83 ± 6
	SRBC	6 ± 2	89 ± 9
Spleen cells from mice immunized with SRBC and cultured with SRBC for 24 hours	None	1 ± 1	NT[b]
	SRBC	78 ± 8	NT
	SL2	4 ± 1	NT
	TLX9	2 ± 3	NT

[a] From Evans *et al.* (1973).
[b] NT, not tested.

the surface of the macrophages leads to activation appears to be supported.

However, in preliminary experiments soluble antigenic membrane fragments derived from tumor cells were shown to inhibit the cytotoxic activity of specifically immune macrophages without inducing the change to nonspecific cytotoxicity (Cox, 1974). The possibility may, therefore, have to be considered that in order for the specific antigen-recognizing macrophage to change into the nonspecifically cytotoxic cell, the antigen may have to be presented in a special form. Possibly the soluble antigen, as opposed to antigen found on intact cells, when it complexes with the antigen receptor (antibody or T cell factor) on the surface of the immune macrophage may form a special type of complex, which may not have the capacity to trigger the macrophage into the activated state. At the same time, the complexes may have blocked the antigen receptor, thus preventing tumor target cell recognition. However, the factors that determine whether an antigen inhibits or converts a macrophage to nonspecific cytotoxicity have yet to be elucidated.

As a working hypothesis, we suggest that one of the ways of rendering macrophages nonspecifically cytotoxic is to bind immune complexes by their modified Fc fragment. Heat-aggregated serum, for example, but not unheated serum, has been shown to activate macrophages (R. Evans, unpublished data). Extending this, it seems feasible to suggest that if the macrophage meets an antibody-coated target cell, the antigen-antibody complex on the surface of the target cell should lead to the transformation of the macrophage into a nonspecific cytotoxic cell. Indeed, following the initiation of macrophage cytotoxicity in the presence of alloantibody and target cells, specific activation occurs (Evans, 1975a). Thus the immunologically specific cytotoxic macrophage, whether produced by arming with intact spleen cells, with SMAF, or when derived from an immune animal, contains on its surface a molecule that has sites showing an affinity for antigen, and binding of this macrophage to the membrane antigen of the tumor cells leads to activation and subsequent nonspecific cytotoxicity.

From the above data, the methods used to activate immune or normal macrophages are now established, but the precise mechanisms are not known. Following antigenic stimulation of immune macrophages or endotoxin treatment of normal macrophages, there is an apparent morphological change in that the macrophages are more spread out. However, since similar changes can be induced by simply replacing the culture medium, they are difficult to evaluate (Evans, 1974b). Cytoplasmic changes occur during specific activation with antigen, including an increase in lysosome numbers; but this is totally nonspecific in that it was apparent that increasing the overall concentration of protein was responsible for this effect (Lejeune and Evans, 1972). Endotoxin treatment of normal macrophages induced the appearance of amorphous material in the cytoplasm as well as an increase in myelin figures (F. Lejeune and R. Evans, unpublished data). Whether the pathway leading to the nonspecific growth inhibitory capacity of activated macrophages is the same is also not known. Endotoxin has been reported to stimulate interferon production by macrophages *in vitro* (Borecky *et al.*, 1974), and dsRNA is a potent interferon inducer *in vivo* (Planterose *et al.*, 1970). Thus, its possible relevance to nonspecific activation of macrophages is clear following endotoxin or dsRNA treatment of mice. Of further interest is the finding that when macrophages from SRBC-immunized mice were activated by SRBC *in vitro* (Evans *et al.*, 1973) very few red cells (less than 1 per

10^3 macrophages) were in fact required. The suggestion currently being investigated is that the red cells triggered the release of a soluble factor from the macrophages, and this activated those macrophages nŏt immediately involved with the red cells. Thus soluble products of macrophage may well play a role in activation, whether this is initiated by a specific or by a nonspecific stimulus.

The process of "activation" of macrophages by contact with specific antigen has a formal similarity to the interaction of antigen with mast cells from specifically immunized donors. Antigen interacts with the IgE on the surface of the mast cells, and during the course of this interaction the conformation of the IgE is altered (Stanworth, 1970). This induces metabolic changes within the mast cell, resulting in the release of amines from it. In this case, the effect of amine release is only produced if a polyvalent antigen is presented to the IgE-coated mast cell.

3. *Nonspecific Lymphoid Supernatants*

In addition to the factors already described, there are also less defined substances that can render macrophages nonspecifically cytotoxic. One of these is obtained when immune spleen cells are cultured with the specific antigen to which the mouse donating the spleen cell has been immunized. A supernatant factor appears which when added to macrophages renders them nonspecifically cytotoxic. It seems likely that in some cases the factor is in fact a lymphokine, perhaps related to lymphokines that induce macrophage aggregation, stimulate macrophage spreading, or inhibit their migration in a nonspecific manner. Under other conditions, the active factor may consist of an antigen-specific macromolecule released from the spleen cell that arms the macrophages. The armed macrophage may then be rendered immediately nonspecifically cytotoxic because antigen is also present, and binding to the macrophage Fc receptors occurs.

4. *Persisting Infections*

Hibbs *et al.* (1971, 1972) and Krahenbuhl and Remington (1974) observed that peritoneal macrophages taken from mice which were carrying an infection of *Toxoplasma gondii, Besnoitia jellisoni,* or *Listeria monocytogenes* were nonspecifically cytotoxic to target cells, and, in subsequent experiments, they showed that the macrophages were cytotoxic to other cell lines with malignant potential. In our laboratory, we found that when mice in our colony had become infected with a strain of *Pasteurella,* they also then acquired nonspecific cytotoxicity (Evans and Alexander, 1972a). The same phenomemon has also been described for rats infected with the nematode *Nippostrongylus brasiliensis* (Keller and Jones, 1971). In all these cases, macrophages were nonspecifically cytotoxic if they were taken from animals that were persistently infected. Variable results have been obtained with mice that have been inoculated with living BCG. In our laboratory, macrophages taken from mice that had been inoculated with BCG 10 days previously were not cytotoxic but could be rendered cytotoxic by exposure to either BCG or PPD (Evans and Alexander, 1972a). In contrast, other investigators (Cleveland *et al.*, 1974; Hibbs, 1973) have found that macrophages from mice that have a chronic BCG infection were cytotoxic. This difference may be attributed to the strain of BCG used, or the strain of mice, or both. The Glaxo strain used by us appear to be less virulent than other strains, which are highly infectious to mice and persist for many weeks. Fortner *et al.* (1974) compared the Glaxo BCG with the Phipps strain of BCG in guinea pigs and found significant difference in terms of growth kinetics and in antitumor effects. The simplest explanation for the presence of nonspecifically cytotoxic macrophages in these situations is that antigen meets specifically sensitized macrophages *in vivo* (whether by direct contact with sensitized lymphocytes or SMAF) and converts them *in situ* to the nonspecifically cytotoxic state. Other possibilities may be that the change was induced by substances resembling endotoxin or peptidoglycan released from these organisms. For example, mice that have been injected with killed *Corynebacterium parvum* have nonspecifically cytotoxic macrophages (Olivotto and Bomford, 1974). This cannot be due to a persisting infection. It is not clear whether cytotoxic macrophages were induced following the release of a factor with the properties of endotoxin or peptidoglycan from *Corynebacterium parvum* itself, acting directly on the macrophages, or whether all the mice had a background immunity to a related organism, such as *C. murium* or to a component of the *Corynebacterium parvum* organism and that the injection of the killed organisms resulted in the interaction of a specific antigen with previously sensitized macrophages. Perhaps parasitization per se may lead to activation. In this context, there is very little information on activation of macrophages following parasitization or infection by bacteria or viruses and whether infection or replication leads to activation. Some viruses are known to infect macrophages. The lactate dehydrogenase elevating virus (LDV), which is known to infect only mice and persists as a life-long viremia (Riley *et al.*, 1960), replicates in macrophage cultures (Evans and Salaman, 1965; Evans, 1970); thus, its presence during macrophage-mediated responses may well be important. The virus is also known to affect various immune responses of the host (Notkins *et al.*, 1966) as well as influencing the incidence of spontaneous mammary tumors (Riley, 1966).

Its presence as a "passenger" virus in very many different murine transplantable tumors (Riley, 1974) is frequently ignored, and its presence might be responsible in part at least for many inconsistences in tumor model systems. One aspect cursorily studied was whether "infection" of peritoneal macrophages resulted in activation. This was shown to be so when LDV and mouse tumor cells were added to mouse peritoneal macrophage cultures, the tumor cells being growth inhibited (Table XI) (Evans, 1975a). To show that replication per se was not required, rat macrophages, in which LDV does not replicate (Evans and Salaman, 1965), were used in place of mouse macrophages. The same effect was noted. Whether LDV mediated this effect directly or by stimulating interferon production, for example, as it does *in vivo* (Evans and Riley, 1968), is not known. However, the principle is established that LDV can activate macrophages. The situation in the virus-infected host has not been explored.

All these findings help to explain one of the major experimental problems that are encountered when studying the cytotoxicity of macrophages: the variable background cytotoxicity of peritoneal macrophages taken from apparently normal animals. Under good conditions, the macrophages are completely noncytotoxic and do not influence the growth of the target cells at all. However, sudden changes may occur in animal colonies such that the macrophages become cytotoxic to varying degrees. This we attribute in part at least to infections that do not necessarily

TABLE XI

Nonspecific Activation of Mouse Peritoneal Macrophage Cultures by LDV[a]

Peritoneal macrophages incubated with[b]	Percentage reduction in ^{125}IUdR incorporation[c] after 24 hours
SL2 cells	<10
FS4 cells	<10
SL2 + LDV	68 – 75
FS4 + LDV	53 – 66

[a] From Evans (1975b).

[b] 10^5 SL2 cells or 5×10^4 DBA/2 fibrosarcoma (FS4) cells in 2 ml of growth medium.

[c] Reduction in ^{125}IUdR incorporation was assessed in relation to uptake by tumor cells in the absence of macrophages ±LDV.

manifest themselves clinically. For several years, mice from our animal colony yielded peritoneal macrophages that were not cytotoxic; but suddenly the macrophages showed a progressive increase in nonspecific cytotoxicity, the effect being more pronounced in some strains than in others. When specific pathogen-free mice were introduced into our animal colony the peritoneal macrophages were quite normal initially; but after a period of 4 or 5 weeks of contact with the conventional mice, the macrophages from these SPF mice showed significant nonspecific cytotoxicity. This was attributed to an airborne cross-infection that was not apparent clinically. The fact that macrophages may be rendered nonspecifically cytotoxic in control untreated animals because of generalized infections or other causes not yet known, frequently makes it difficult to interpret such findings in which, for example, it is reported that "normal" mouse macrophages are cytotoxic to a degree to syngeneic and allogeneic mouse red blood cells (Möller, 1969). Unless the animals are carefully monitored, one cannot decide whether this is a property of normal macrophages or of macrophages that have been rendered nonspecifically cytotoxic due to unknown and unplanned infections.

C. Mechanisms of Nonspecific Macrophage Cytotoxicity

During initial experiments, a number of murine lymphoma and sarcoma cells were used, and the effect of nonspecifically cytotoxic macrophages on these was similar. In all cases, the first effect was growth inhibition, the target cells failing to divide; but rapid lysis as measured by release of isotopes was not seen under these conditions. Disintegration, when it did occur, was a late event. Biochemically, the initial lesion induced in the tumor cells appeared to involve DNA synthesis, and it was tempting to refer to the action of the cytotoxic macrophages as being "radiomimetic," which as in ionizing radiation effects on dividing cells, the initial lesion was on DNA synthesis, and a late consequence of prolonged inhibition of DNA synthesis was the subsequent break up of the cell. While this hypothesis may be partly correct, the situation is certainly more complex, and the nonspecifically cytotoxic macrophages do seem to have a direct action on the membrane of at least some tumor target cells. There are reports that some leukemia and lymphoma lines are lysed within 6–8 hours of coming into contact with nonspecifically cytotoxic macrophages (A. Johnson, personal communication), and moreover tumor cells, such as the lymphomas or sarcomas, used in our experiments are only growth inhibited under our conditions, but may be lysed by macrophages if they have first received a dose of irradiation (Zembala *et al.*, 1973a). In this case, the action of the cytotoxic macrophages and radiation is additive, and this shows clearly that the macrophages induce lesions other than those involving DNA synthesis. The nonspecifically cytotoxic macrophage is extremely radioresistant, unlike the specifically growth inhibitory macrophage (Den Otter *et al.*, 1974). Thus, macrophages can be given 5000 rads of X irradiation before or after treatment with endotoxin or double-stranded RNA and still have the normal cytotoxic capacity. A. Johnson (personal communication), studying macrophages treated with poly(A) · poly(U), found that reagents which inhibited protein synthesis also prevented the induction of nonspecific cytotoxicity, but those reagents which interfered with NA synthesis did not interfere with the induction of nonspecific cytotoxicity.

Although the cytotoxic action has been shown to require cell to cell contact, it is not certain whether cytotoxicity is exerted by a humoral factor released from the "activated" macrophages and acts only in a local manner. In our initial experiments, we were unable to detect a cytotoxic effect from supernatants of endotoxin-treated macrophages (Alexander and Evans, 1971). Other investigators also carried out careful experiments that showed that only tumor cells in actual contact with the macrophages were prevented from growing (Kaplan *et al.*, 1974; Hibbs, 1973; Cleveland *et al.*, 1974). However, there are other reports showing that the supernatants from the culture of endotoxin-treated macrophages inhibited DNA synthesis in lymphoma cells (Boyle, 1974), although the activity of these supernatants was low. Other laboratories have also reported that supernatants from macrophages can affect the growth of cells in culture (Heise and Weiser, 1969; Sintek and Pincus, 1970; McIvor and Weiser, 1971b; Calderon *et al.*, 1974; see Keller, Chapter 19). It is possible that these different experimental results can all be reconciled on the assumption that the active principle of macrophage cytotoxicity is, in fact, a humoral factor, but that this factor has to be present locally at relatively high concentrations. This would explain the apparent need for contact between the target cell and the macrophage. Alternatively, the humoral toxin may be inhibited by components in the culture medium, and this would also explain why close contact is needed. Melsom and Seljelid (1973) showed in earlier studies that lysis of red cells by macrophages required cell to cell contact, but recently these authors (Melsom *et al.*, 1974) demonstrated that a labile macrophage factor was excreted. This appeared to act locally, and therefore permanent cell to cell contact was not required. On the other hand, it is equally possible that while there are humoral factors released by the macrophages which can inhibit DNA synthesis or induce lysis, there may be other cytotoxic mechanisms that require cell to cell contact between the macrophage and the target cell. Hibbs (1974) has produced evidence to show that when the target cell fuses with the nonspecifically cytotoxic macrophage, subcellular components from the macrophage are transferred to the target cell.

Of great interest is the claim made by Hibbs (1973) and by Holterman *et al.* (1973) that only cancer cells and not normal cells are destroyed by macrophages. In the initial experiments, it seemed possible that the difference between the malignant cells and the normal cells lay in the fact that in the former the rate of cell division was rapid and was perhaps responsible for their greater susceptibility to the macrophages. Indeed, the same observation was made by us using embryo fibroblasts, which were not destroyed by the "activated" macrophages, whereas the tumor cells were. However, this did not exclude the possibility that failure to detect destruction of the embryo fibroblasts was due solely to the slower rate of cell division. That this is not the only explanation and that the nonspecifically cytotoxic macrophage can genuinely distinguish between a malignantly transformed cell and a normal cell was demonstrated in experiments with 3T3 cells (which are not malignant but divide rapidly). After exposure to simian virus 40 (SV40), these cells undergo a malignant transformation without any change in their rate of cell division (Hibbs, 1973). The transformed cells but not the normal 3T3 cells were susceptible to the action of the activated macrophages from mice infected with *Toxoplasma* or BCG. The distinction, however, appears not to be absolute. Cleveland *et al.* (1974) reported that macrophages from BCG-infected mice killed syngeneic, allogeneic, and xenogeneic tumor cell lines whether they were proliferating or not, while normal embryo cells were less susceptible. Keller (1974; Chapter 19) reported that rapidly dividing normal cells were inhibited in their growth, but not destroyed, whereas malignant cells were ultimately destroyed. Slowly dividing normal cells were not affected. Kaplan *et al.* (1974) also observed some toxicity toward normal cells. Moreover, it has been suggested that the failure of lymphocytes to divide following PHA stimulation may be due to activated macrophages acting as "suppressor cells" (Kirchner *et al.*, 1974; see Nelson, Chapter 9). Perhaps the issue may resolve itself on the concept that growth inhibition leads ultimately to the death of neoplastic cells but not of normal dividing cells; but clearly further studies are required to elucidate this complex situation.

IV. CYTOTOXIC MACROPHAGES AND THE TUMOR BEARING HOST

Growth inhibitory peritoneal macrophages were demonstrated in the peritoneal cavity of mice bearing subcutaneously implanted fibrosarcomas and lymphomas (Evans, 1973a). Furthermore, to show whether cytotoxic macrophages reached the growing tumors, a technique was devised for the isolation, characterization, and cultivation of tumor-associated macrophages (Evans, 1972, 1973b). Monolayers of relatively pure tumor macrophages were tested against a wide range of tumor cells (lymphoma and sarcoma) *in vitro* (Evans, 1975a). The overall results indicated that the macrophages were indeed activated on isolation from the fibrosarcomas. However, it was seen that some tumor types yielded macrophages that retained nonspecific cytotoxicity for days in culture, others yielding macrophages that lost activity within 24 or 48 hours (Table XII). The reasons for such findings have not been clarified; but recent findings of Keller *et al.* (1974) suggest that loss of activation might be related to the extent of protein synthesis. Other investigators have shown that macrophages isolated from actively growing tumors may be cytotoxic. Haskill *et al.*, (1975) reported that tumor macrophages inhibited colony formation non-specifically, while Van Loveren and Den Otter (1974) claimed that macrophages isolated from a subcutaneously implanted lym-

TABLE XII

The Effect of Macrophages from Different Tumors on Growth of Various Target Cells[a,b]

	Percentage reduction in ^{125}IUdR incorporation by target cells[c]			
Tumor macrophages	SL2	TLX9	ASBP1	FS6
HSN (Hooded rat)	95–99	92–99	90–95	92–99
A (Hooded rat)	0–19	0–22	0–12	NT[d]
ASBP1 (August rat)	93–98	95–99	92–96	NT
FS6 (C57 Black mouse)	8–22	3–15	NT	0–18

[a] From Evans (1975a).

[b] Tumors maintained in syngeneic hosts and excised 2–3 weeks after s.c. trocar implantation. Tumor macrophage monolayers prepared in 3 cm culture dishes, as described previously (Evans, 1972), and maintained in serum-free medium for 24–48 hours before challenge with tumor cells.

[c] Target cells maintained in culture and subcultivated at intervals. Growth medium was Fischer's medium + 10% heated-inactivated fetal bovine serum. 10^5 SL2, TLX9 lymphoma cells and 5×10^4 ASPB1 and FS6 sarcoma cells in 2 ml of growth medium were added to each monolayer. Cultures were pulsed with 0.1 μCi ^{125}IUdR/ml for 4 hours after overnight incubation. The results represent a summary of three different experiments involving three to six dishes per sample.

[d] NT, not tested.

phoma (DBA/2-SL2) were specifically growth inhibitory. Another lymphoma, TLX9 of C57Bl mice, yielded macrophages that were not cytotoxic *in vitro*. In our hands, neither of these lymphomas when implanted subcutaneously yielded sufficient numbers of macrophages for *in vitro* investigation (less than 5% of the total cells compared with 33% for the SL2 lymphoma and 25% for the TLX9 lymphoma reported by Van Loveren and Den Otter). Such marked discrepancies possibly reflect changes in the lymphoma cells since they left our laboratory or differences in the mice used.

It was also shown that transplantable tumor lines contained a constant proportion of macrophages over a number of passage numbers, but that the proportion varied from one tumor to another (Evans, 1972). This suggested a subtle relationship between the tumor type and its macrophage content. Indeed, it was subsequently concluded (Eccles and Alexander, 1974) that the rate or frequency of metastatic spread was directly related to the level of macrophages associated with a given tumor. Further evidence that macrophages may be associated with prevention of metastasis was provided from electron microscopic studies showing that a hamster lymphoma that did not metastasize contained large macrophages with phagosomes containing tumor cells, while another hamster lymphoma that metastasized widely had very small macrophages without phagosomes (Birbeck and Carter, 1972). Eccles and Alexander (1974) also showed that immunosuppression of tumor bearing animals resulted in a marked decrease in the level of tumor macrophages, indicating a relationship between the macrophage level and the lymphoid arm of the immune response. However, the presence of activated macrophages is clearly not sufficient to prevent the growth of the tumor, which ultimately overwhelms the host. This may indicate that specifically activated macrophages do not function under such conditions, cytotoxicity perhaps being blocked or inhibited by excess antigen, as demonstrated for circulating lymphocytes from tumor bearing patients (Currie and Basham, 1972). Nevertheless, tumors usually do not double in size with each division of cells, suggesting that restricting mechanisms occur within the tumor.

The mechanism by which tumor macrophages are activated is not yet known. It is unlikely to be the result of trypsinization or collagenase treatment used to disperse the tumor fragments initially, since peritoneal macrophages similarly treated were not activated. One might expect to find antibody, antigen, and/or antigen–antibody complexes in tumor bearing serum, the proportions of each depending on the tumor load, rate of antigen shedding, as well as the potency of the immune response. Thus the presence and the binding of immune complexes in serum might result in specific activation of circulating monocytes or tumor macrophages. Experiments by Currie and Gage (1973) further indicate the presence of nonspecifically cytotoxic macrophages in the tumor bearing host and the possible involvement of immune complexes. These authors found that draining lymph nodes of tumor bearing rats contained nonspecifically cytotoxic cells, presumably macrophages. Seven days after implanting a tumor in the leg, the cells from the draining lymph node showed immunologically specific cytotoxicity, which was lymphocyte-mediated. However, by 2 weeks, the cells in the lymph node were nonspecifically cytotoxic, although the cells in the distant nodes were specifically cytotoxic for the tumor in the rat. One explanation is that the local node received large quantities of tumor-specific antigen, which combined with specific antibody, whereas distant nodes would receive little or none.

V. *IN VIVO* SIGNIFICANCE OF THE NONSPECIFICALLY CYTOTOXIC MACROPHAGE

Reference has already been made to the fact that macrophages may be rendered nonspecifically cytotoxic *in vivo* by injection of endotoxin or double-stranded RNA, as well as by persisting infections or by injecting the specific antigen PPD into BCG (Glaxo) sensitized mice. At the time when nonspecifically cytotoxic macrophages can be isolated from the peritoneal cavity, mice are much more resistant to an i.p. but not necessarily to an s.c. challenge with tumor cells (I. Parr, personal communication), and it is tempting to correlate this increased resistance to i.p. tumor challenge with the presence of the nonspecifically cytotoxic macrophages. A particularly clear illustration of this is provided by experiments in which PPD was injected into BCG-treated mice. Twenty-four hours after injecting the PPD, the mice were able to withstand a very large challenge dose of both lymphoma and sarcoma cells. Other reports (Hibbs *et al.*, 1971; Lunde and Gelderman, 1971) showed that protozoan parasitization of mice of the AKR strain, which have a very high spontaneous incidence of leukemia, led to much later development of leukemia than in noninfected counterparts. The role of the nonspecifically cytotoxic macrophage in the protection provided to a subsequent challenge with tumor by agents that stimulate the reticuloendothelial system, such as BCG or *Corynebacterium parvum*, is less clear. Protection against both tumor cells and other organisms by inoculation with BCG extends for many weeks, and we have found that this protection is still fully evident when nonspecifically cytotoxic macrophages are absent. The antitumor action of BCG is various and probably relies on several different mechanisms, and the induction of specifically "activated" macrophages is probably confined to the situation where BCG and tumor are injected into the same site. Similarly, the finding by Ashley and Hardy (1973) that the resistance of mice to tumors is increased after infection with *Salmonella* could be explained either by the induction of a state of chronic infection or by providing an antigen to interact with suitably sensitized macrophages always present in the mice. All the experiments show, however, that nonspecifically cytotoxic macrophages can, at least in the peritoneal cavity, arrest tumor growth. They are probably much less active at intramuscular and subcutaneous sites, but it is possible that they may have an important role in protecting the lung. Indeed, one might anticipate that the macrophages in the lung would always be nonspecifically cytotoxic because they are continually being exposed to antigens against which the host may have already been sensitized. It is possible that the relative resistance to animals to intravenously injected tumor cells, the majority of which are destroyed when they reach the lung and only a very few of which survive to give rise to lung tumors, may be ascribed in fact to nonspecifically cytotoxic macrophages.

VI. ROLE OF MACROPHAGES IN SURVEILLANCE

The concept that malignant cells arise much more frequently than indicated by the incidence of tumors in animals and man and that the majority of them are destroyed by an immunological surveillance mechanism is intellectually satisfying and would explain many puzzling observations. This hypothesis has, however, recently run into great difficulties because immunologically suppressed animals, such as genetically athymic mice, do not have a higher rate of spontaneous tumors than do their normally reactive counterparts nor are they more susceptible to chemical or physical carcinogens (Stutman, 1974). The only carcinogenic stimuli to which they respond more readily are the inoculations with oncogenic viruses, which in normal animals only produce tumors if given to newborn animals, but in immunosuppressed animals are oncogenic even in the adult (Allison *et al.*, 1974). Rather than abandoning the whole concept of surveillance, one might assert that the body has a mechanism by which malignant cells, which may occur relatively frequently, are eliminated. It may be that this elimination is carried out by the specific immune reaction (T cell-mediated) directed against the TSTA's. It may also be that the capacity of nonspecifically cytotoxic macrophages to distinguish between normal and malignant cells confers an important role on the macrophage in terms of surveillance, not only against tumor cells but against all invading antigens. It is a property which, on considering the evolutionary development of the phagocytic cell, one would have expected the macrophage to have retained.

VII. CONCLUSION

While the evidence indicates that activated macrophages selectively damage and ultimately destroy malignant cells *in vitro,* an antitumor role for macrophages, or any effector cell, in the tumor bearing host has not been firmly established. As yet there is very little information concerning the conditions that cause the abrogation of specific or nonspecific macrophage cytotoxicity. Hibbs (1975) has reported that trypan blue abrogates the resistance afforded mice after BCG or tumor immunization, suggesting that lysosomal blockade of macrophages induced by the trypan blue is responsible. However, perhaps the major problem is not so much how potent the activated macrophage cytotoxicity may be, as measured by *in vitro* criteria, but what the true nature of the changes occurring in the activated macrophage really is. It is quite clear that our narrow definition of activation covers one particular aspect of macrophage function, but there seems to be little doubt that killing of tumor cells is not their only purpose. The occurrence of activated macrophages in conditions not primarily involved in graft or tumor rejection, such as during persisting infections, and probably in conditions in which one might expect to find immune complexes, such as autoimmune diseases, indicates their ubiquity. Their antibacterial capacity is classical, but the way in which they acquire bactericidal activity may be in some cases identical to the method used to render macrophages nonspecifically cytotoxic to tumor cells.

Of critical importance in the basic understanding of the activated macrophage is the nature and significance of parallel changes occurring in its biochemical, physiological, functional, and morphological characteristics and how these relate to its antitumor activity. In this context one of the most interesting aspects is the synthetic machinery of the macrophage and its capacity to synthesize and excrete numerous different hydrolytic enzymes capable of destroying cartilage matrix, collagen, basement membranes, and probably many other tissues (Allison and Davies, 1974), as well as proteases (such as plasminogen activator) (Gordon *et al.,* 1974) which catalyze other enzymatic reactions (such as the conversion of plasminogen to plasmin). The macrophage shares this capacity to synthesize hydrolytic enzymes with the polymorphonuclear leukocytes, both types of cells being involved in inflammatory lesions of different types and to different degrees. Since these inflammations are frequently a consequence of antigenic stimulation, the occurrence of antigen–antibody complexes, as found, for example, in rheumatoid arthritis (Cracchiolo *et al.*, 1971) may well result in activation of the macrophages. The role of macrophages in diseases such as rheumatoid arthritis is not clear (Evans, 1975a), but the amount of tissue damage involved in this disease suggests that hydrolytic and other enzyme secretions may play an important role in destruction. At present, there is no evidence that such hydrolytic enzymes damage tumor cells, but it seems plausible to suggest that the sequence of biochemical reactions involving hydrolytic enzymes and other components might produce an effect indirectly. If this were so, then the evolution of an extracellular mechanism of killing, as opposed to phagocytosis, has perhaps only rearranged the sequence of events rather than changed the basic components required for destruction.

REFERENCES

Adam, A., Ciobaru, R., Ellouz, F., Petit, J.-F., and Lederer, E. (1974). *Biochem. Biophys. Res. Commun.* **56,** No. 3, 561–567.

Alexander, P. (1974). *In* "Handbuch der allgemeinen Pathologie," pp. 711–746. Springer-Verlag, Berlin and New York.

Alexander, P., and Evans, R. (1971). *Nature (London), New Biol.* **232,** 76–78.

Alexander, P., Connell, D. I., and Mikulska, Z. B. (1966). *Cancer Res.* **26,** 1508–1515.

Alexander, P., Evans, R., and Mikulska, Z. B. (1973). *In* "Chemotherapy of Cancer Dissemination and Metastasis" (S. Garattini and G. Franchi, eds.), pp. 177–185. Raven Press, New York.

Allison, A. C., and Davies, P. (1974). *In* "Activation of Macrophages" (W. H. Wagner and H. Hahn, eds.), Vol. 2, pp. 141–156. Excerpta Med. Found., Amsterdam.

Allison, A. C., Monga, J. N., and Hammond, V. (1974). *Nature (London)* **252,** 746–747.

Amos, H. E., and Lachman, P. J. (1970). *Immunology* **10,** 269–277.

Ashley, M. P., and Hardy, D. (1973). *Aust. J. Exp. Biol. Med. Sci.* **51,** 801–809.

Baker, P., Weiser, R. S., Jutila, J., Evans, C. A., and Blandon, R. J. (1962). *Ann. N.Y. Acad. Sci.* **101,** 46–63.

Bennett, B. (1965). *J. Immunol.* **95,** 656–664.

Birbeck, M. S. C., and Carter, R. L. (1972). *Int. J. Cancer* **9,** 249–257.

Borecky, L., Lackovic, V., Fuchsberger, N., and Hajnicka, V. (1974). *In* "Activation of Macrophages" (W. H. Wagner and H. Hahn, eds.), Vol. 2, pp. 111–122. Excerpta Med. Found., Amsterdam.

Boyle, M. D. P. (1974). Ph.D. Thesis, University of London.

Boyle, M. D. P., and Ormerod, M. G. (1975). *Cell. Immunol.* **17,** 247–258.

Calderon, J., Williams, R. T., and Unanue, E. R. (1974). *Proc. Nat. Acad. Sci. U.S.* **71,** 4273–4277.

Cerottini, J. C., and Brunner, K. T. (1974). *Advan. Immunol.* **18,** 67–132.

Chambers, V. C., and Weiser, R. S. (1969). *Cancer Res.* **32,** 413–419.

Cleveland, R. P., Meltzer, M. S., and Zbar, B. (1974). *J. Nat. Cancer Inst.* **52,** 1887–1894.

Cone, R. E., Feldman, M., Marchalonis, J. J., and Nossal, G. J. V. (1974). *Immunology* **26,** 49–60.

Cox, H. C. (1974). Ph.D. Thesis, University of London.
Cracchiolo, A., Goldberg, L. S., Barnett, E. V., and Bluestone, R. (1971). *Immunology* **20,** 1067–1077.
Cruse, J. M., Whitten, H. D., Lewis, G. K., and Watson, E. S. (1973). *Transplant. Proc.* **5,** 961–967.
Currie, G. A., and Basham, C. (1972). *Brit. J. Cancer* **26,** 427–438.
Currie, G. A., and Gage, J. O. (1973). *Brit. J. Cancer* **28,** 136–146.
Dennert, G., and Lennox, E. S. (1973). *J. Immunol.* **111,** 1844–1854.
Den Otter, W., Evans, R., and Alexander, P. (1972). *Transplantation* **14,** 220–226.
Den Otter, W., Evans, R., and Alexander, P. (1974). *Transplantation* **18,** 421–428.
Eccles, S. A., and Alexander, P. (1974). *Nature (London)* **250,** 667–669.
Evans, R. (1970). *Proc. Soc. Exp. Biol. Med.* **133,** 831–836.
Evans, R. (1972). *Transplantation* **14,** 468–473.
Evans, R. (1973a). *Brit. J. Cancer* **28,** Suppl. 1, 19–25.
Evans, R. (1973b). *J. Nat. Cancer Inst.* **50,** 271–273.
Evans, R. (1974a). *Int. Res. Commun. Syst.* **2,** 1674.
Evans, R. (1974b). *In* "Activation of Macrophages" (W. H. Wagner and H. Hahn, eds.), Vol. 2, pp. 305–317. Excerpta Med. Found., Amsterdam.
Evans, R. (1975a). *Ann. N.Y. Acad. Sci.* **256,** 275–287.
Evans, R. (1975b). *Fogarty Intern. Center Proc. No. 28.* U.S. GPO, Washington, D.C. (in press).
Evans, R. (1975c). *In* "Mononuclear Phagocytes" (R. van Furth, ed.), pp. 827–844. Blackwell, Oxford.
Evans, R., and Alexander, P. (1970). *Nature (London)* **228,** 620–622.
Evans, R., and Alexander, P. (1971). *Transplantation* **12,** 227–229.
Evans, R., and Alexander, P. (1972a). *Nature (London)* **236,** 168–170.
Evans, R., and Alexander, P. (1972b). *Immunology* **23,** 615–626.
Evans, R., and Alexander, P. (1972c). *Immunology* **23,** 627–636.
Evans, R., and Grant, C. K. (1972). *Immunology* **23,** 677–687.
Evans, R., and Riley, V. (1968). *J. Gen. Virol.* **3,** 449–458.
Evans, R., and Salaman, M. H. (1965). *J. Exp. Med.* **122,** 993–1002.
Evans, R., Grant, C. K., Cox, H., Steele, K., and Alexander, P. (1972). *J. Exp. Med.* **136,** 1318–1322.
Evans, R., Cox, H., and Alexander, P. (1973). *Proc. Soc. Exp. Biol. Med.* **143,** 256–259.
Fortner, G. W., Hanna, M. G., and Coggin, J. H. (1974). *Proc. Soc. Exp. Biol. Med.* **147,** 62–67.
Gordon, S., Unkeless, J. C., and Cohn, Z. A. (1974). *J. Exp. Med.* **140,** 995–1010.
Gorer, P. A. (1956). *Advan. Cancer Res.* **4,** 149–186.
Granger, G. A., and Weiser, R. S. (1964). *Science* **145,** 1427–1429.
Granger, G. A., and Weiser, R. S. (1966). *Science* **151,** 97–99.
Granger, G. A., Rudin, J., and Weiser, R. S. (1966). *J. Reticuloendothel. Soc.* **3,** 354 (abstr.).
Grant, C. K., Evans, R., and Alexander, P. (1973). *Cell. Immunol.* **8,** 136–146.
Grant, C. K., Glover, D. J., Hall, J. G., and Alexander, P. (1974). *Transplantation* **17,** 254–264.
Haskill, J., Proctor, J. W., and Yamamura, Y. (1975). *J. Nat. Cancer Inst.* **54,** 387–393.
Heise, E. R., and Weiser, R. S. (1969). *J. Immunol.* **103,** 570–576.
Hibbs, J. B. (1973). *Science* **180,** 868–870.
Hibbs, J. B. (1974). *Science* **184,** 468–471.

Hibbs, J. B. (1975). *RES, J. Reticuloendothel. Soc.* **16,** 12a (abstr.).
Hibbs, J. B., Lambert, L. H., and Remington, J. S. (1971). *J. Infec. Dis.* **124,** 587–592.
Hibbs, J. B., Lambert, L. H., and Remington, J. S. (1972). *Nature (London), New Biol.* **235,** 48–50.
Holm, G., and Hammarström, S. (1973). *Clin. Exp. Immunol.* **13,** 29–43.
Holterman, O. A., Klein, E., and Casale, G. P. (1973). *Cell. Immunol.* **9,** 339–352.
Hoy, W. E., and Nelson, D. S. (1969). *Aust. J. Exp. Biol. Med. Sci.* **47,** 525–539.
Journey, L. J., and Amos, D. B. (1962). *Cancer Res.* **22,** 998–1001.
Kaplan, A. M., Morahan, P. S., and Regelson, W. (1974). *J. Nat. Cancer Inst.* **52,** 1919–1921.
Keller, R. (1973). *J. Exp. Med.* **138,** 625–644.
Keller, R. (1974). *Brit. J. Cancer* **30,** 401–415.
Keller, R., and Jones, V. E. (1971). *Lancet* **2,** 847–849.
Keller, R., Keist, R., and Ivatt, R. J. (1974). *Int. J. Cancer* **14,** 675–683.
Kirchner, H., Chused, T. M., Herberman, R. B., Holden, H. T., and Larvin, D. H. (1974). *J. Exp. Med.* **139,** 1473–1487.
Krahenbuhl, J. L., and Remington, J. S. (1974). *J. Immunol.* **113,** 507–516.
Lejeune, F., and Evans, R. (1972). *Eur. J. Cancer* **8,** 549–555.
Lohmann-Matthes, M. L., Schipper, H., and Fischer, H. (1972). *Eur. J. Immunol.* **2,** 45–49.
Lohmann-Matthes, M. L., Ziegler, F. G., and Fischer, H. (1973). *Eur. J. Immunol.* **3,** 56–58.
Lohmann-Matthes, M. L., Ziegler, F. G., and Ritter, J. (1974). *In* "Activation of Macrophages" (W. H. Wagner and H. Hahn, eds.), Vol. 2, pp. 293–304. Excerpta Med. Found., Amsterdam.
Lunde, M. N., and Gelderman, A. H. (1971). *J. Nat. Cancer Inst.* **47,** 485–488.
McIvor, K. L., and Weiser, R. S. (1971a). *Immunology* **20,** 307–314.
McIvor, K. L., and Weiser, R. S. (1971b). *Immunology* **20,** 315–322.
Mackaness, G. B. (1969). *J. Exp. Med.* **129,** 973–992.
MacLennan, I. C. M. (1972). *Transplant. Rev.* **13,** 67–69.
Marchalonis, J. J., Cone, R. E., and Atwell, J. L. (1972). *J. Exp. Med.* **135,** 956–971.
Melsom, H., and Seljelid, R. (1973). *J. Exp. Med.* **137,** 807–820.
Melsom, H., Kearny, G., Gruca, S., and Seljelid, R. (1974). *J. Exp. Med.* **140,** 1085–1096.
Metchnikoff, E. (1891). "Lectures on the Comparative Pathology of Inflammation" (reprinted by Dover, New York, 1968).
Mitchison, N. A. (1955). *J. Exp. Med.* **102,** 157–177.
Möller, E. (1969). *Immunology* **16,** 609–619.
Moroz, C., and Hahn, Y. (1973). *Proc. Nat. Acad. Sci. U.S.* **70,** 3716–3720.
Munro, A. J., Taussig, M. J., Campbell, R., Williams, H., and Lawson, Y. (1974). *J. Exp. Med.* **140,** 1579–1587.
Nelson, D. S. (1969). "Macrophages and Immunity" North-Holland Publ., Amsterdam.
Nelson, D. S. (1970). *Aust. J. Exp. Biol. Med. Sci.* **48,** 329–341.
Notkins, A. L., Mergerhagen, S. E., Rizzo, A. A., Scheel, C., and Waldmann, T. A. (1966). *J. Exp. Med.* **123,** 347–364.
Old, L. J., Boyse, E. A., Bennett, B., and Lilly, F. (1963). *In* "Cell-Bound Antibodies" (B. Amos and H. Koprowski, eds.), p. 89. Wistar Inst., Philadelphia, Pennsylvania.
Olivotto, M., and Bomford, R. (1974). *Int. J. Cancer* **13,** 478–488.

Parr, I., Wheeler, E., and Alexander, P. (1973). *Brit. J. Cancer* **27,** 370–389.
Pearsall, N. N., and Weiser, R. S. (1968). *J. Reticuloendothel. Soc.* **5,** 107–120.
Pels, E., and Den Otter, W. (1974). *Cancer Res.* **34,** 3089–3094.
Perlmann, R. P., and Holm, G. (1969). *Advan. Immunol.* **11,** 117–193.
Perlmann, P., Perlmann, H., and Wigzell, H. (1972). *Transplant. Rev.* **13,** 91–114.
Planterose, D. N., Birch, P. J., Pilch, P. J., and Sharpe, T. J. (1970). *Nature (London)* **227,** 504–505.
Regelson, W., Morahan, P., Kaplan, A. M., Baird, L. G., and Munson, J. A. (1974). *In* "Activation of Macrophages" (W. H. Wagner and H. Hahn, eds.), Vol. 2, pp. 97–110. Excerpta Med. Found., Amsterdam.
Riley, V. (1966). *Science* **153,** 1657–1658.
Riley, V. (1974). *Cancer Res.* **34,** 1752–1754.
Riley, V. Lilly, F., Huerto, E., and Bardell, D. (1960). *Science* **132,** 545–547.
Scornick, J. C., and Cosenza, H. (1974). *J. Immunol.* **113,** 1527–1532.
Sintek, D. E., and Pincus, W. B. (1970). *RES, J. Reticuloendothel. Soc.* **8,** 508–521.
Stanworth, D. R. (1970). *Clin. Exp. Immunol.* **6,** 1–12.
Stutman, O. (1974). *Science* **183,** 534–536.
Takeda, K. (1969). "Immunology of Cancer," Vol. 2, pp. 10–36. Hokkaido Univ. School of Medicine, Sapporo, Japan.
Taussig, M. J. (1974). *Nature (London)* **248,** 234–236.
Taussig, M. J., and Munro, A. J. (1974). *Nature (London)* **251,** 63–65.
Tsoi, M. S., and Weiser, R. S. (1968). *J. Nat. Cancer Inst.* **40,** 23–30.
Van Loveren, H., and Den Otter, W. (1974). *J. Nat. Cancer Inst.* **53,** 1057–1060.
Winn, H. J. (1960). *Nat. Cancer Inst., Monogr.* **2,** 113–138.
Zarling, J. M., and Tevethia, S. S. (1973a). *J. Nat. Cancer Inst.* **50,** 137–148.
Zarling, J. M., and Tevethia, S. S. (1973b). *J. Nat. Cancer Inst.* **50,** 149–157.
Zembala, M., Ptak, W., and Hanczakowska, M. (1973a). *Immunology* **25,** 631–644.
Zembala, M., Ptak, W., and Hanczakowska, M. (1973b). *Clin. Exp. Immunol.* **15,** 461–466.
Zembala, M., Asherson, G. L., Mayhew, B., and Krejci, K. (1975). *Nature (London)* **253,** 72–74.
Zighelboim, J., Bonavida, B., and Fahey, J. L. (1973). *J. Immunol.* **111,** 1737–1742.
Zighelboim, J., Bonavida, B., and Fahey, J. L. (1974). *Cell. Immunol.* **12,** 280–289.

22

Immunotherapeutic Approaches to Tumors Involving the Skin

O. A. Holtermann, E. Klein, I. Djerassi, J. D. Bernhard, and S. Parmett

I. Introduction 577
II. Clinical Investigations 579
A. Chemically Defined Haptens 580
B. Microbial Antigens 581
C. Tumor Prevention 582
D. Lymphokines 583
III. A Primitive Surveillance Mechanism? 584
IV. Summary 587
References 589

I. INTRODUCTION

Host defense against neoplastic or potentially neoplastic cells represents one of the major areas of inquiry in current cancer research. Several cancer defense mechanisms undoubtedly exist, although they may function with variable degrees of efficiency and specificity. Since these mechanisms are likely to interact and complement each other, they should not necessarily be viewed as being unrelated, but should rather be considered in the overall context of an integrated defense system.

An impressive accumulation of evidence points to a central role of the immune system in cancer resistance. In addition to specific antitumor immunity, it appears that the immune system also indirectly contributes to protection against malignant disease. The chief effectors in immune surveillance of neoplastic cells are considered to be specifically committed lymphocytes. However, both specific (Hellstrom *et al.*, 1969, 1971; Bansal and Sjögren, 1972) and nonspecific (Suciu-Foca *et al.*, 1974; Al-Sarraf and Vaitkevicius, 1971) serum factors may interact or interfere with cell-mediated tumor immunity.

A number of observations indicate that, apart from specific antitumor immunity, the immune system in a broader sense is implicated in cancer resistance. Administration of various agents, such as mycobacteria (Old *et al.*, 1961; Zbar *et al.*, 1971), *Corynebacterium parvum* (Woodruff and Boak, 1966), preparations derived from other bacterial species (Nauts, 1970), nucleic acids (Braun *et al.*, 1963), or synthetic polynucleotides (Levy *et al.*, 1969) have been found to increase resistance to the development of chemically induced and transplanted tumors. A common denominator in the mode of action of these diverse agents seems to be stimulation of the mononuclear phagocytic system (MPS). Stimulation of the MPS may also be responsible for heightened resistance against tumors in animals with chronic parasitic infections (Hibbs *et al.*, 1971). Activated macrophages are likely to play a significant role in increased cancer resistance associated with stimulation of the MPS. An analogous relationship has been proposed to exist between MPS stimulation and host defenses in a number of microbial infections (Mackaness, 1969).

Macrophages appear to be important in both specific and nonspecific resistance against neoplastic cells (Amos, 1960; Baker *et al.*, 1962; Granger and Weiser, 1964; Burnet, 1968; Zbar *et al.*, 1971; Evans and Alexander, 1971; Keller, 1973; Krahenbuhl and Remington, 1974). In animals with specific antitumor immunity, the elimination of tumor cells by macrophages may be mediated by specific antibodies (Evans and Alexander, 1971, 1972). Such antibodies may confer specificity or selectivity to otherwise nonspecifically cytotoxic macrophages.

Besides specificity that may be imparted by antibodies, activated macrophages of nonspecifically stimulated animals seem to possess an inherent recognition mechanism that by itself permits differentiation between certain categories of cells, such as tumor cells and normal cells (Hibbs *et al.*, 1972a,b; Holtermann *et al.*, 1972b, 1973). The relationship of this mechanism to the recognition mechanisms of the adaptive immune system is not clear. It seems that activating factors, which by themselves do not necessarily have antitumor effects, amplify an inherent tumor defense mechanism in which macrophages play a significant role. A group of such factors, the lymphokines (Bloom and Bennett, 1966; David, 1966; Dumonde *et al.*, 1969) may be released by committed lymphocytes during response to challenge with tumor antigens or other sensitizing agents.

An apparently indirect effect of the immune system on resistance against tumors in man is regression of malignant and premalignant neoplasms involving the skin after repeated inductions of delayed-type hypersensitivity challenge reactions to haptens or microbial antigens at the sites of tumors (Klein and Helm, 1963; Helm and Klein, 1965; Klein, 1968, 1969; Stjernsward and Levin, 1971; Klein and Holtermann, 1972; Levis *et al.*, 1973; Holtermann *et al.*, 1975). The wide spectrum of tumors that have been found to respond to such immune challenge regimens suggests the general relevance of these observations to tumor biology.

II. CLINICAL INVESTIGATIONS

Initial clinical studies of malignant and premalignant epidermal neoplasms (Klein and Helm, 1963; Helm and Klein, 1965; Klein, 1967) indicated that local induction of delayed-type hypersensitivity challenge reactions at tumor sites resulted in regression or eradication of neoplastic lesions. Subsequently such challenge reactions were found to have similar effects on other types of tumors involving the skin and subcutaneous tissues (Klein, 1969; Williams and Klein, 1970; Klein and Holtermann, 1972). These observations indicate that local immunological intervention is a feasible approach to the treatment of accessible premalignant and malignant neoplasms. Furthermore, an analogous regimen has proved effective in reducing the incidence of malignant lesions in patients with multiple skin cancer syndromes (Klein, 1967; Klein and Holtermann, 1972). The emergence of neoplastic lesions in patients with these syndromes are undoubtedly discrete oncologic events. It, therefore, appears that prevention of cancer in man by immunologic means may be possible.

The results of extending these investigations to several kinds of metastatic neoplasms involving the skin have indicated the general nature of the principles underlying the antitumor effects of local immune challenge reactions. Elucidation of the mechanisms by which local hypersensitivity challenge reactions result in tumor regression may contribute to the development of improved methods for exploiting immunopotentiation and other immunologic means for the control of cancer. The concomitant regression of neoplasms and reepithelialization at sites of such reactions implies a cytotoxic mechanism with selective effects on neoplastic cells. The comparable clinical results obtained by the use of a number of haptens or microbial antigens indicate that some common components of the delayed hypersensitivity challenge reactions induced by these substances play an essential role in their antitumor effect. Also in support of this point of view are the similar results obtained by local administration of lymphokines at the sites of accessible tumors (Papermaster *et al.*, 1974; Holtermann *et al.*, 1975).

A. Chemically Defined Haptens

During clinical trials of topical chemotherapy of skin neoplasms, it was observed that some of the agents under investigation were potent skin sensitizers (Klein and Helm, 1963; Helm and Klein, 1965; Helm *et al.*, 1965). For instance, the compounds 2,3,5-triethyleneiminobenzoquinone (TEIB) and 5-mercapto-2-deoxyuridine (MUDR) readily induced hypersensitivity reactions of the delayed type after repeated topical applications. Presumably, these compounds acted as haptens, and it became apparent that whenever sensitization occurred their therapeutic effect was considerably enhanced. These observations suggest that in addition to their direct cytotoxic activity, the local immune reactions induced by the topical application of these agents contribute to their clinical effectiveness. In addition to TEIB and MUDR, dinitrochlorobenzene (DNCB) is one of the haptens that has been most extensively investigated with respect to the antitumor effects of induced delayed hypersensitivity reactions. In patients sensitized to DNCB, topical application of this chemical resulted in regression and eradication of premalignant keratoses, superficial basal cell carcinomas, squamous cell carcinomas, and lesions of mycosis fungoides (Klein, 1967, 1969; Ratner *et al.*, 1968; Williams and Klein, 1970; Stjernsward and Levin, 1971; Levis *et al.*, 1973). On the other hand, in patients without sensitivity, topical application of DNCB had no clinically detectable antitumor effect at the concentrations employed (Klein and Holtermann, 1972; Levis *et al.*, 1973).

The procedures used in these studies are outlined below (Klein and Holtermann, 1972).

1. Evaluation of the patient's immunocompetence by skin tests to a number of common microbial antigens.
2. Induction of primary sensitization to one or more haptens, e.g., TEIB or DNCB. For this purpose, the sensitizing agent is applied in a semisolid base at concentrations of 0.1–0.01% under an occlusive dressing until a hypersensitivity reaction is apparent. An alternative method for sensitization to DNCB has been described (Catalona *et al.*, 1972) in which the compound, dissolved in acetone, is used in a single application.
3. The lowest concentration at which the patient shows a reaction is determined by patch tests with serial tenfold dilutions of the sensitizing

agent in a semisolid base. This concentration may range from one part of sensitizing agent per thousand to less than one part per billion of vehicle.

4. The sensitizing agent is applied to the areas of neoplastic involvement at a concentration suitable to induce a reaction of a moderate degree at the tumor sites. This concentration may fluctuate during the course of the treatment. The duration of the immune challenge regimen necessary for induction of a clinically detectable response may vary from a few weeks to several months.

Treatment with delayed-type hypersensitivity challenge to chemically defined haptens was explored over a 5 year period in 24 patients with multiple neoplastic lesions of epidermal origin (Klein, 1974). This group consisted of patients with multiple basal cell nevoid syndrome, late radiation dermatitis with malignant degeneration, xeroderma pigmentosum, arsenical dermatitis, and severe skin damage with multiple premalignant and malignant lesions due to excessive exposure to ultraviolet light. A second group of 54 patients with less severe disease was studied for shorter periods of time. An overall rate of regression of 95% was reported in these 78 patients (Klein, 1974). In another quite comprehensive study on basal cell carcinomas using topical application of DNCB (Levis *et al.*, 1973), a rate of eradication of 32% with an additional rate of regression of 29% was achieved.

B. Microbial Antigens

A possible mechanism for the antitumor effects of topical application of chemically defined haptens could be conjugation of the haptens with tumor antigens resulting in an intensified tumor-specific immune response (Mitchison, 1971). While such a mechanism has not been excluded, hypersensitivity reactions induced by a number of microbial antigens (Klein and Holtermann, 1972; Klein *et al.*, 1974; Holtermann *et al.*, 1975), which are not likely to have the characteristics of haptens, are also effective in eliciting tumor regression. These observations, therefore, suggest that mechanisms other than haptenization of tumor antigens may account for tumor regression at sites of induced hypersensitivity reactions. The antigens under study included purified protein derivative of tuberculin (PPD), mumps vaccine, streptokinase–streptodornase, *Candida* extract, and other microbial antigens. Analogous to the experience with chemically defined haptens, delayed hypersensitivity reactions induced by complete (microbial) antigens at sites of premalignant and malignant lesions resulted in tumor regressions. However, less extensive studies have been carried out with the use of microbial antigens than haptens, and rates of tumor regressions or eradications have not been published. As with chemically defined haptens, a necessary prerequisite for tumor regression after local administration of microbial antigens was sensitivity of the patient to the antigen. In patients without sensitivity to the antigens used, local administration of the antigen was without clinical effect.

Among the neoplasms found to be susceptible to local challenge reactions to microbial antigens were basal cell carcinoma, melanoma, mycosis fungoides, reticulum cell sarcoma, lymphangiosarcoma, and lesions of adenocarcinoma of the breast metastatic to the skin and subcutaneous tissue. Considerable variation was found in the rate and degree of response of different tumors to challenge with microbial antigens. Such variation may be due to different levels of sensitization of individual patients as well as different susceptibility of various types of tumors to the immune challenge regimen.

Immune challenge reactions to microbial antigens or chemical haptens in patients with multiple lesions resulted only in regression of tumors actually undergoing treatment. Although flare reactions at sites of untreated lesions were occasionally observed, clinically detectable regressions were generally not seen in distant, untreated tumors. These observations indicate that the factors responsible for tumor regression at sites of induced delayed hypersensitivity reactions are acting primarily at the local rather than the systemic level.

C. Tumor Prevention

Topical application of chemical haptens has been found to be useful in reducing the incidence of neoplasms in patients with multiple skin cancer syndromes. Such patients continuously develop tumors over extended periods of their lives, and treatment with standard therapeutic procedures can often be difficult. In seven patients with xeroderma pigmentosum requiring repeated surgical procedures, intermittent topical applications to the skin of TEIB or DNCB considerably reduced the number of necessary surgical interventions (Klein and Holtermann, 1972). Clinical trials in which symmetrical, paired areas of the skin were treated or left untreated, respectively, provided clear evidence of the antitumor effects of induced delayed hypersensitivity reactions as a preventive measure. A prophylactic immune challenge regimen has also been of value in the multiple basal cell nevoid syndrome (Klein and Holtermann, 1972).

D. Lymphokines

The experience with induced delayed-type hypersensitivity challenge reactions at tumor sites to a large variety of antigens suggests that some common component of the reactions induced by these antigens was instrumental in the observed antitumor effects. Conceivably, induction of similar inflammatory infiltrates at tumor sites by alternative means might also result in tumor regression. Noncellular mediators of the delayed hypersensitivity reaction, the lymphokines (Bloom and Bennett, 1966; David, 1966; Dumonde *et al.*, 1969), represent in a sense a common final path for the reaction, independent of the antigen used for its induction. Working with guinea pigs, Bernstein and associates (1971) observed suppression of proliferation of transplanted tumor cells by local injections of fractions of fluids of PPD-stimulated lymphocyte cultures derived from PPD-sensitive animals. A fraction that induced tumor suppression also had macrophage migration inhibiting activity. It was, therefore, of interest to explore the potential antitumor effect of local administration of lymphokines to accessible human tumors. Supernatant fluids of primary cultures of normal human lymphocytes stimulated with concanavalin A or phytohemagglutinin were used in limited initial trials (Holtermann *et al.*, 1975). Intradermal administration of such fluids in human skin resulted in reactions that grossly and microscopically resembled accelerated delayed hypersensitivity reactions. Similar reactions have been elicited in guinea pigs by analogous preparations (Schwartz *et al.*, 1971). Repeated intradermal injections of supernatant fluids of mitogen-stimulated human lymphocyte cultures in areas involved by basal cell carcinoma or mycosis fungoides resulted in clinical antitumor responses comparable to those elicited by antigen-induced delayed hypersensitivity challenge reactions (Holtermann *et al.*, 1975).

Since there are practical limitations to the amount of material with lymphokine activity that can be obtained from primary cultures of human lymphocytes, further exploration of the clinical use of lymphokines has been pursued using fractions of supernatant fluids of a tissue culture line of human diploid lymphoid cells. Such supernatants contain substances with lymphokine activity similar to those produced by lymphocytes in contact with specific antigens or mitogens (Glade and Hirschhorn, 1970; Papageorgiou *et al.*, 1972; Tubergen *et al.*, 1972). A crude fraction of intermediate molecular weight (10,000–100,000 daltons) obtained by diafiltration of lymphoid cell culture fluids was used in preliminary clinical trials. Repeated intradermal injections of this material in areas of cutaneous metastases in patients with adenocarcinoma of the breast resulted in partial or complete regression of a number of treated lesions (Papermaster *et al.*, 1974).

III. A PRIMITIVE SURVEILLANCE MECHANISM?

Elucidation of the mechanism by which neoplastic cells are eliminated at sites of induced delayed hypersensitivity challenge reactions is of considerable interest. The large number of different types of tumors that have been found to be susceptible to immune challenge reactions indicates that mechanisms of general relevance to tumor resistance are involved. The similar effects of reactions induced by a number of different antigens as well as by lymphokines point to an important role of some common factor of these reactions in eliciting tumor regression. Elements of delayed hypersensitivity reactions that may be pertinent are local extravasation of plasma proteins and accumulation of a cellular infiltrate. Initially this infiltrate is composed mainly of granulocytes; at later stages mononuclear cells predominate (Turk, 1967). Only a small minority of the leukocytes of the inflammatory infiltrate of the delayed hypersensitivity challenge reaction are cells specifically sensitized to the challenge antigen (Werdelin and McCluskey, 1971). The vast majority of cells of the infiltrate are secondarily recruited from the blood to the site of the reaction, presumably by the action of noncellular mediators. It has been proposed (Holtermann *et al.*, 1972b, 1973) that the cells of this inflammatory infiltrate, with or without the interaction of tumor-specific antibody, are effectors in the selective destruction of neoplastic cells at sites of induced delayed-type hypersensitivity reactions. A direct test of this proposition would encounter technical problems in the isolation of leukocytes from inflammatory infiltrates of delayed hypersensitivity reactions in quantities sufficient to carry out meaningful experiments. However, support for this view has come from investigations employing peritoneal leukocytes of animals (Amos, 1960; Baker *et al.*, 1962; Granger and Weiser, 1964; Bennett, 1965; Hibbs *et al.*, 1972a,b; Holtermann *et al.*, 1972a,b, 1973; Keller, 1973). The composition of such populations of peritoneal leukocytes resembles that of the inflammatory infiltrate of the delayed hypersensitivity challenge reaction. The predominating cells in both populations are large mononuclear leukocytes. Activated peritoneal leukocytes of mice with chronic parasitic infections or rats stimulated by intraperitoneal injection of PPD are highly cytotoxic *in vitro*. This cytotoxicity does not express itself by indiscriminate destruction of any kind of target cell, but rather exhibits a distinct selectivity (Hibbs *et al.*, 1972a,b; Holtermann *et al.*, 1972a,b, 1973; Piessens *et al.*, 1974; Tucker *et al.*, 1974).

Among the target cell types found to be susceptible are neoplastic cells and rapidly replicating cells isolated from normal embryos. Slowly growing cells of normal adult or embryonic tissue origin are quite resistant. Contact inhibited, slowly growing 3T3 mouse fibroblasts, resistant to the cytotoxicity of activated mouse peritoneal macrophages, were rendered susceptible by transformation with SV40 virus (Hibbs, 1974a). Susceptibility was associated with considerable increase in target cell growth rate.

The large mononuclear cells of the peritoneum and other tissues are at least in part derived from the monocytes of the bloodstream (Pearsall and Weiser, 1970). Preliminary investigations indicate that human blood monocytes are cytotoxic toward tumor cells (Holtermann *et al.*, 1974). Increased cytotoxicity of these cells was noted after activation by supernatant fluids of mitogen-stimulated lymphocytes. Whether the cytotoxicity of human blood monocytes exhibits a selectivity comparable to that of peritoneal macrophages of rodents remains to be determined.

The characteristics of cells that are of importance in their recognition and destruction by activated peritoneal leukocytes are not known. Susceptibility or resistance of target cells to the cytotoxic activity of peritoneal macrophages of mice or rats (Hibbs *et al.*, 1972a,b; Holtermann *et al.*, 1972b, 1973) is independent of whether the interacting cells are syngeneic or allogeneic. Antigenic characteristics of target cells may, therefore, not necessarily be decisive in determining susceptibility or resistance. In view of the association between rate of replication of cells obtained from normal embryos and susceptibility to the cytotoxicity of macrophages discussed above, it is conceivable that some unique feature of the cytoplasmic membrane is involved that is shared by neoplastic cells and replicating normal cells. Relevant to this point of view are the findings of Fox and associates (1971) of cytoplasmic membrane receptors for plant lectins which can be detected on normal cells only during mitosis but can be demonstrated at any time on transformed cells derived from the same cell population.

The mechanisms by which nonspecifically activated macrophages destroy other cells remains to a large extent to be clarified (for a discussion, see Keller, Chapter 19). Release of cytotoxic factors by macrophages *in vitro* have been reported (Kramer and Granger, 1971; Melsom *et al.*, 1974). One such factor may be analogous to the lymphotoxin produced by lymphocytes after specific or nonspecific stimulation (Kramer and Granger, 1971). Another cytotoxic factor (Melsom *et al.*, 1974) appears to be extremely labile or masked under ordinary tissue culture conditions in which serum is present in the medium. The role of such toxic factors in the selective cytotoxic activity of macrophages is not clear. Thus, direct transfer of cell-free fluids from tissue cultures, in which extensive destruction of tumor cells by activated macrophages had taken place, to a second set of cultures of the same tumor cells failed to mimic the cytotoxic activity associated with intact macrophages (Holtermann *et al.*, 1973).

As observed by ordinary light microscopy, an intimate contact between macrophage and target cell seems to be an initial step in the cytolytic event (Granger and Weiser, 1964; Hanna *et al.*, 1972; Holtermann *et al.*, 1973; Hibbs, 1974b). This cellular contact may take place across a highly unfavorable energy barrier (Weiss, 1973). Activation of macrophages may result in a reduction of this barrier and thereby facilitate intimate contact between interacting cells. The reduced electrostatic charge of peritoneal macrophages of tuberculin-sensitive guinea pigs after PPD administration (Diengdoh and Turk, 1968) may be of importance in this regard. Cytophilic antibody may serve a similar function in promoting cellular contact in the immunologically specific cytotoxic action of macrophages (Evans and Alexander, 1971, 1972). Possibly related to this mechanism is the antibody-dependent, cell-mediated cytotoxicity described by Perlmann and Holm (1969). Subsequent events may be transfer of lysosomes from macrophage to target cell and destruction of the target cell by lysosomal enzymes or other cytotoxic factors (Hibbs, 1974b). The final cytotoxic mechanism may therefore be the same both in immunologically specific and nonspecific cytotoxic cellular interactions involving macrophages.

Although macrophages may be the principal effector cells in the selective destruction of tumor cells at sites of induced delayed hypersensitivity reactions, other cells of the inflammatory infiltrate (lymphocytes and polymorphonuclear granulocytes) may also participate. Relevant to this possibility is the well-established cytotoxicity of nonspecifically activated lymphocytes (Holm *et al.*, 1964, 1973; Butterworth, 1973). The cytotoxicity of such activated lymphocytes has generally been considered to be nonspecific, but recent observations indicate that it may exhibit some degree of selectivity (Stejskal *et al.*, 1973). A possible role of neutrophilic granulocytes in cancer resistance has received only limited attention. Nonspecific as well as selective cytotoxic effects of such leukocytes on various target cells have been reported (Lundgren *et al.*, 1968; Pickaver *et al.*, 1972). The conspicuous presence of neutrophilic granulocytes in acute inflammatory reactions raises the question of their participation in the regression of skin tumors at the site of irritant reactions induced by local application of croton oil as reported by Levis and associates (1973).

A relationship between the development of an adaptive immune system and an evolutionary need for a surveillance mechanism against neoplastic cells has been proposed by Burnet (1968, 1970). In terms of phylogenetic development, large mononuclear cells (monocytes and macrophages) may be older than the more specialized lymphocytes and plasma cells. Perhaps the large mononuclear cells of vertebrates represent descendants of the hemocytes of lower animals which have the ability to recognize foreign material, but do not appear to possess any memory of previous exposures characteristic of the immunocytes of an adaptive immune system. Possibly the hemocytes of invertebrates function as an effective deterrent against abnormal cells. If so, the targets of "recognition" by hemocytes are probably not classic antigenic properties of neoplastic cells, but rather are some other distinctive physical or chemical features. It has been suggested that large mononuclear cells may be effectors in a primitive surveillance mechanism against aberrent cells (Holtermann *et al.*, 1973). As such this mechanism may represent an evolutionary precursor of the specific immune surveillance mechanism of the adaptive immune system. Regression of tumors after induction of inflammatory infiltrates at tumor sites may be the result of a local amplification of such a primitive surveillance mechanism (Sinkovics, 1970).

Alternative methods for the activation of this surveillance mechanism deserve exploration. Local administration of lymphokines at tumor sites has been used for this purpose in limited trials (Holtermann *et al.*, 1975; Papermaster *et al.*, 1974). The problems of obtaining material with lymphokine activity in quantities sufficient for more extensive studies may be solved by the use of purified preparations from continuous lines of lymphoid cells (Glade and Hirschhorn, 1970; Papageorgiou *et al.*, 1972; Tubergen *et al.*, 1972). Further investigation of the antitumor activity of lymphokines is, therefore, practical and may provide a basis for exploring the systemic effects of these noncellular mediators.

The use of immunologic procedures in the treatment of neoplasms involving the skin as outlined here does not as yet offer practical advantages over already established modalities, except possibly for the control of intractable multifocal cutaneous cancer syndromes. However, the apparent relevance of these procedures to the management of a large number of different types of neoplasms warrants continued exploration of their theoretical implications as well as practical therapeutic potential.

IV. SUMMARY

Tumors involving the skin offer unique opportunities to the clinical investigator. The immediate accessibility of these tumors provides possibilities for direct manipulation and observation. Although current standard methods of treatment for most primary skin cancers yield satisfactory results, the potential applicability of experience acquired from the study of skin tumors to cancer in general warrants continued investigation of new therapeutic modalities.

In the exploration of immunological approaches to the treatment of cancer, skin tumors have proved to be a most valuable model system. Of particular interest is the information gained from studies of the antitumor effect of delayed hypersensitivity challenge reactions when induced at sites of tumor involvement. Repeated inductions of such hypersensitivity reactions have been found to result in regression or eradication of various types of premalignant and malignant lesions. Analogous observations have been made in experimental animals. The similarity of the antitumor effects of challenge reactions elicited by a number of haptens, microbial antigens, or lymphokine preparations indicate that some common components of the reactions induced by these diverse agents are of importance in evoking tumor regression. It has been suggested that activated large mononuclear cells (macrophages) in the cellular infiltrate of delayed hypersensitivity challenge reactions are effectors in the selective eradication of neoplastic cells at sites of induction of such reactions. This implies that activated macrophages are selectively cytotoxic for neoplastic cells.

In vitro studies of the interaction of rodent peritoneal macrophages with neoplastic cells and cells of normal tissue origin support this view. It appears that activated macrophages possess an inherent recognition mechanism that permits distinction between various types of target cells, including neoplastic cells. In addition to an inherent macrophage recognition mechanism, specific antibody can confer specificity to cytotoxic cellular interactions involving macrophages.

The relationship of the intrinsic recognition mechanism of macrophages to that of the adaptive immune system is not clear. Macrophages may be effectors in a surveillance mechanism against aberrant cells which in evolutionary terms is a precursor of the specific immune surveillance mechanism of the adaptive immune system. Tumor regression after induction of a delayed-type hypersensitivity inflammatory infiltrate at the tumor site may be related to a local amplification of such a primitive surveillance mechanism.

ACKNOWLEDGMENTS

The work by E. Klein and O. A. Holtermann quoted in this article was supported by grants No. 9 R01 CA 13599-03 and 1 R01 CA 17205-01 and contracts No. NIH-

NCI-E-71-2137 and N01 CP 33-373 from the National Cancer Institute, National Institutes of Health, the Zelda Radow Weintraub Cancer Fund, Inc., the Cancer Research Institute and the Albert and Mary Lasker Foundation. J. D. Bernhard was supported by a Knox Memorial Fellowship from Harvard University for study at the University of Cambridge, England. S. Parmett was supported by a Rotary Foundation Fellowship for study at the University of Cambridge, England.

REFERENCES

Al-Saraf, M., and Vaitkevicius, V. K. (1971). *Lancet* **2,** 314–315.

Amos, D. B. (1960). *Ann. N.Y. Acad. Sci.* **87,** 273–292.

Baker, P., Weiser, R. S., Jutila, J., Evans, C. A., and Blandau, R. J. (1962). *Ann. N.Y. Acad. Sci.* **101,** 46–63.

Bansal, S. C., and Sjögren, H. O. (1972). *Int. J. Cancer* **9,** 490–509.

Bennett, B. (1965). *J. Immunol.* **95,** 656–664.

Bernstein, D., Thor, D., Zbar, B., and Rapp, H. (1971). *Science* **172,** 729–731.

Bloom, B. R., and Bennett, B. (1966). *Science* **153,** 80–82.

Braun, W., Lampen, J. O., Plescia, O. J., and Pugh, L. (1963). *In* "Conceptual Advances in Immunology and Oncology," p. 450. Harper (Hoeber), New York.

Burnet, F. M. (1968). *Nature (London)* **218,** 426–430.

Burnet, F. M. (1970). *Progr. Exp. Tumor Res.* **13,** 1–27.

Butterworth, A. E. (1973). *Cell. Immunol.* **7,** 357–369.

Catalona, W. J., Taylor, P. T., Rabson, A. S., and Chretien, P. B. (1972). *N. Engl. J. Med.* **286,** 399–402.

David, J. R. (1966). *Proc. Nat. Acad. Sci. U.S.* **56,** 72–77.

Diengdoh, J. V., and Turk, J. L. (1968). *Int. Arch. Allergy Appl. Immunol.* **34,** 297–302.

Dumonde, D. C., Wolstencroft, R. A., Panayi, G. S., Matthew, M., Morley, J., and Howson, W. T. (1969). *Nature (London)* **224,** 38–42.

Evans, R., and Alexander, P. (1971). *Transplantation* **12,** 227–229.

Evans, R., and Alexander, P. (1972). *Nature (London)* **236,** 168–170.

Fox, T. O., Sheppard, J. R., and Burger, M. M. (1971). *Proc. Nat. Acad. Sci. U.S.* **68,** 244–247.

Glade, P. R., and Hirschhorn, K. (1970). *Amer. J. Pathol.* **60,** 483–491.

Granger, G. A., and Weiser, R. S. (1964). *Science* **145,** 1427–1429.

Hanna, M. G., Jr., Snodgrass, M. J., Zbar, B., and Rapp, H. (1972). *Nat. Cancer Inst., Monogr.* **35,** 345–360.

Hellström, I., Hellström, K. E., Evans, C. A., Heppner, G. H., Pierce, G. E., and Yang, J. P. S. (1969). *Proc. Nat. Acad. Sci. U.S.* **62,** 362–368.

Hellström, I., Sjögren, H. O., Warner, G., and Hellström, K. E. (1971). *Int. J. Cancer* **7,** 226–237.

Helm, F., and Klein, E. (1965). *Arch. Dermatol.* **91,** 142–144.

Helm, F., Klein, E., Traenkle, H. L., and Rivera, E. (1965). *J. Invest. Dermatol.* **45,** 152–159.

Hibbs, J. B., Jr., (1974a). *Science* **180,** 868–870.

Hibbs, J. B., Jr. (1974b). *Science* **184,** 468–471.

Hibbs, J. B., Jr., Lambert, L. H., and Remington, J. S. (1971). *J. Infec. Dis.* **124,** 587–592.

Hibbs, J. B., Jr., Lambert, L. H., and Remington J. S. (1972a). *Proc. Soc. Exp. Biol. Med.* **139,** 1049–1052.

Hibbs, J. B., Jr., Lambert, L. H., and Remington, J. S. (1972b). *Science* **177,** 998–1000.

Holm, G., Perlmann, P., and Werner, B. (1964). *Nature (London)* **203,** 841–843.

Holm, G., Stejskal, V., and Perlmann, P. (1973). *Clin. Exp. Immunol.* **14,** 169–179.

Holtermann, O. A., Casale, G. P., and Klein, E. (1972a). *J. Med. Exp. Clin.* **3,** 305–309.

Holtermann, O. A., Lisafeld, B. A., and Klein, E. (1972b). *J. Med. Exp. Clin.* **3,** 359–362.

Holtermann, O. A., Klein, E., and Casale, G. P. (1973). *Cell. Immunol.* **9,** 339–352.

Holtermann, O. A., Djerassi, I., Lisafeld, B. A., Elias, E. G., Papermaster, B., and Klein, E. (1974). *Proc. Soc. Exp. Biol. Med.* **147,** 456–459.

Holtermann, O. A., Papermaster, B., Rosner, D., Milgrom, H., and Klein, E. (1975). *J. Med. Exp. Clin.* **6,** 157–168.

Keller, R. (1973). *J. Exp. Med.* **138,** 625–644.

Klein, E. (1967). *Fed. Proc., Fed. Amer. Soc. Exp. Biol.* **26,** Abstr. No. 430.

Klein, E. (1968). *N. Y. State J. Med.* **68,** 900–911.

Klein, E. (1969). *Cancer Res.* **29,** 2351–2362.

Klein, E. (1974). *N.Y. State J. Med.* **74,** 1384–1387.

Klein, E., and Helm, F. (1963). Presented at the Stephen Rothman Research Meeting, American Academy of Dermatology, Chicago, Illinois.

Klein, E., and Holtermann, O. A. (1972). *Nat. Cancer Inst., Monogr.* **35,** 379–402.

Klein, E., Holtermann, O. A., Case, R. W., Milgrom, H., Rosner, D., and Adler, S. (1974). *Amer. J. Clin. Pathol.* **62,** 281–289.

Krahenbuhl, J. L., and Remington, J. S. (1974). *J. Immunol.* **113,** 507–516.

Kramer, J. J., and Granger, G. A. (1971). *Cell. Immunol.* **3,** 88–100.

Levis, W. R., Kraemer, K. H., Klinger, W. G., Peck, G. L., and Terry, W. D. (1973). *Cancer Res.* **33,** 3036–3040.

Levy, H. B., Law, L. W., and Rabson, A. S. (1969). *Proc. Nat. Acad. Sci. U.S.* **62,** 357–361.

Lundgren, G., Zukoski, C. H. F., and Moller, G. (1968). *Clin. Exp. Immunol.* **3,** 817–836.

Mackaness, G. B. (1969). *J. Exp. Med.* **129,** 973–992.

Melsom, H., Kearny, G., Gruca, S., and Seljelid, R. (1974). *J. Exp. Med.* **140,** 1085–1096.

Mitchison, N. A. (1971). *In* "Immune Surveillance" (R. T. Smith and M. Landy, eds.), p. 246. Academic Press, New York.

Nauts, H. C. (1970). *In* "Host Resistance to Cancer. Review of the Early and Recent Literature," 2nd ed. Monograph No. 5. New York Cancer Research Institute, New York.

Old, L. J., Benacerraf, B., Clarke, D. A. Carswell E. A., and Stockert, E. (1961). *Cancer Res.* **21,** 1281–1300.

Papageorgiou, P., Henley, W. L., and Glade, P. R. (1972). *J. Immunol.* **108,** 494–504.

Papermaster, B., Holtermann, O. A., Rosner, D., Klein, E., and Dao, T. (1974). *Res. Commun. Chem. Pathol. Pharmacol.* **8,** 413–416.

Pearsall, N. N., and Weiser, R. S. (1970). "The Macrophage," Lea & Febiger, Philadelphia, Pennsylvania.

Perlmann, P., and Holm, G. (1969). *Advan. Immunol.* **11,** 117–193.

Pickaver, A. H., Ratcliff, N. A., Williams, A. E., and Smith, H. (1972). *Nature (London), New Biol.* **235,** 186–187.

Piessens, W. F., Churchill, W. H., and David, J. R. (1974). *Fed. Proc., Fed. Amer. Soc. Exp. Biol.* **33,** Abstr. No. 3240.

Ratner, A. C., Waldorf, D. S., and Van Scott, E. J. (1968). *Cancer* **21,** 83–88.
Schwartz, H. J., Catanzaro, P. J., and Leon, M. A. (1971). *Amer. J. Pathol.* **63,** 443–462.
Sinkovics, J. G. (1970). "The Immunology of Malignant Disease," pp. 67–68. Mosby, St. Louis, Missouri.
Stejskal, V., Holm, G., and Perlmann, P. (1973). *Cell. Immunol.* **8,** 71–81.
Stjernsward, J., and Levin, A. (1971). *Cancer* **28,** 628–640.
Suciu-Foca, N., Buda, J., McManus, J., Thiem, T. and Reemtsma K. (1973). *Cancer Res.* **33,** 2373–2377.
Tubergen, D. C., Feldman, J. D., Pollack, E. M., and Lerner, R. A. (1972). *J. Exp. Med.* **135,** 255–266.
Tucker, R., Meltzer, M., and Sanford, K. (1974). *Fed. Proc., Fed. Amer. Soc. Exp. Biol.* **33,** Abstr. No. 2288.
Turk, J. L. (1967). "Delayed Hypersensitivity." North-Holland Publ., Amsterdam.
Weiss, L. (1973). *J. Nat. Cancer Inst.* **50,** 3–19.
Werdelin, O., and McCluskey, R. T. (1971). *J. Exp. Med.* **133,** 1242–1263.
Williams, A. C., and Klein, E. (1970). *Cancer* **25,** 450–462.
Woodruff, M. F. A., and Boak, J. L. (1966). *Brit. J. Cancer* **20,** 345–355.
Zbar, B., Bernstein, I. D., and Rapp, H. J. (1971). *J. Nat. Cancer Inst.* **46,** 831–839.

23

Macrophages and Their Disorders in Man

Mary Territo and Martin J. Cline

I. Metabolism 594
II. Functions 596
A. Immune Responses 597
B. Ingestion of Microorganisms and Other Particles 597
C. Antitumor Activity 600
D. Control of Granulopoiesis and Involvement in Erythropoiesis 600
III. Disorders of the Monocyte–Macrophage System 602
A. Monocytosis 603
B. Reactive Hyperplasia 603
C. Storage Diseases 606
D. Histiocytic Proliferative Disorders of Uncertain Origin 607
E. The Malignant Histiocytic Disorders 608
F. Macrophage Dysfunction Syndromes 610
IV. Summary and Future Perspectives 611
References 612

Our knowledge of the mononuclear phagocyte system has come principally from studies of laboratory animals (Axline, 1970; Cohn, 1968; Karnovsky, 1962; Nelson, 1969; Sutton, 1967). Methods for isolating and cultivating monocytes from human blood were not widely available before 1967, and techniques for the isolation of human tissue macrophages were only rarely applied before 1970. Consequently, our knowledge of the physiology, metabolism, and function of human monocytes and macrophages is still quite fragmentary. Reviewers have generally extrapolated observations made in animal macrophage systems to their human counterparts. Clearly one must guard against too bland an acceptance of such extrapolations. With the introduction of methodology for isolation and cultivation of cells from man, our knowledge has recently expanded at a rapid rate, and, in the past few years, new syndromes of macrophage dysfunction have been recognized. In this review, we shall attempt to indicate where experimental observations relate to human mononuclear phagocytes and where our current concepts are derived from animal studies.

I. METABOLISM

The monocyte–macrophage system in man may be viewed as a continuum of progressively more mature cells beginning with progenitors in the bone marrow (monoblasts and promonocytes), progressing through the blood monocyte and young tissue macrophage, and culminating in the mature tissue macrophage. There are ample observations to suggest that monocytes share a common progenitor with the granulocytic cell line (Chen and Schooley, 1970a,b; Leder, 1966; Metcalf, 1971). It is not known at what level of maturation the cell is irrevocably committed to granulocytic development as opposed to monocyte differentiation, but it is presumably at a stage preceding the promyelocyte (Fig. 1). During this progressive maturation from the bone marrow precursor to the differentiated tissue cell, there is coincident progressive expression of functional characteristics, including phagocytic ability, microbicidal activity,

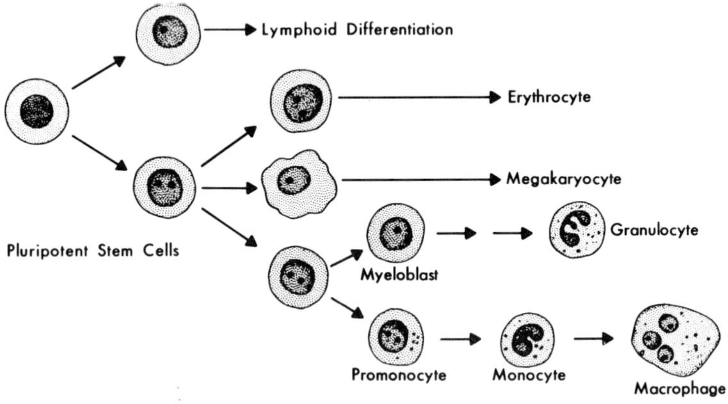

Fig. 1. The relationship between cells of the monocyte–macrophage line and other hematopoietic cells.

adhesiveness to charged surfaces, presence of surface receptors for immunoglobulin, and ability to interact with lymphoid cells in various immune phenomena (Cline, 1970a, 1972; Cohn, 1968; Cohn and Benson, 1965a,b; Hanifin and Cline, 1970) (Fig. 2). Promonocytes, monocytes, and immature macrophages are capable of division; as the cell reaches the mature macrophage stage, it loses its ability to replicate. A corresponding change in mitotic activity and nucleic acid synthetic capacity occurs with maturation of animal macrophages (van Furth and Cohn, 1968; Watts and Harris, 1959).

The metabolic status of mononuclear phagocytes varies with maturational level, with the cellular environment, and with activities such as phagocytosis (Axline, 1970; Cline, 1970a, 1972; Cohn, 1968; Cohn and Benson, 1965a,c). The principal energy source for peritoneal macrophages of animals is glycolysis, even under aerobic conditions (Frei *et al.*, 1961; Karnovsky, 1962; Oren *et al.*, 1963; West *et al.*, 1968), with a relatively small amount of the total glucose being metabolized via the hexose monophosphate shunt (West *et al.*, 1968). The energy for phagocytosis by human monocytes is probably derived principally from glycolysis and is not critically dependent on aerobic mechanisms (Cline and Lehrer, 1968; Cline 1970a). Human monocytes and macrophages increase their oxygen consumption during phagocytosis. This oxygen is used in part to generate hydrogen peroxide during the phagocytic process. The amount of glucose metabolized via the hexose monophosphate shunt also increases during phagocytosis in a manner analogous to granulocytes (Cline and Lehrer, 1968).

In contrast to the behavior of monocytes and peritoneal macro-

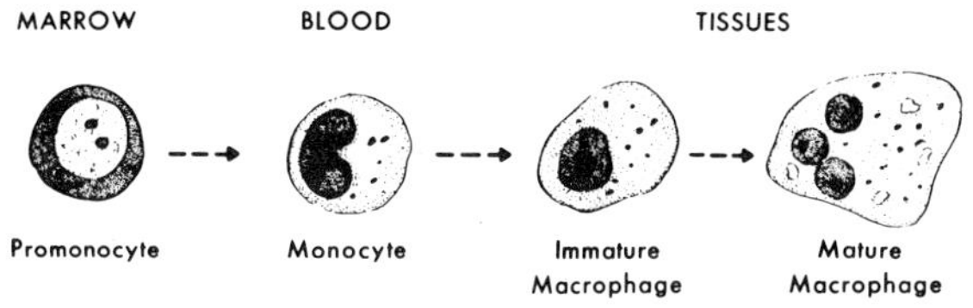

	Promonocyte	Monocyte	Immature Macrophage	Mature Macrophage
Proliferation	++++	+ to +++	++	0
Phagocytosis	±	+	+++	++++
Glass Adherence	+	++	+++	+++
Lysosomes	+	++	++++	++++
IgG Receptors	+	++	+++	+++
Lymphocyte Interaction	?	++	++++	++++

Fig. 2. Changes in cellular functional characteristics with macrophage maturation.

phages, alveolar macrophages of man and animals appear to depend primarily upon aerobic sources of energy production (Karnovsky, 1962; Cline, 1965). Phagocytosis of microorganisms by human alveolar macrophages is severely retarded at low partial pressures of oxygen (Cohen and Cline, 1971). This phenomenon may contribute to the diminished ability to clear bacteria in underventilated lung segments. Furthermore, the metabolic response to phagocytosis appears to differ in alveolar macrophages and other tissue macrophages. A cyanide-insensitive respiratory burst accompanying phagocytosis is not so clearly identifiable in the alveolar cell as in the blood monocyte.

Animal macrophages have an active lipid metabolism. During phagocytosis, phospholipid synthesis is increased—presumably as a consequence of new membrane synthesis (Elsbach, 1967a, 1968). The more mature cells also have a high rate of protein synthesis (consistent with the presence of abundant rough endoplasmic reticulum) (Stecher and Thorbecke, 1967). Much of this synthetic activity is directed toward the production of lysosomal enzymes (Cohn, 1968). There is a paucity of data on these areas of metabolism for human mononuclear phagocytes.

A characteristic feature of human as well as animal monocytes and macrophages is their prominent lysosomal granules, containing acid hydrolases and, in some cases, oxidases (Axline, 1970). The enzymes contained in these granules are made in the endoplasmic reticulum and then packaged in the Golgi apparatus to form the primary lysosomes. The number and contents of the lysosomes vary with the stage of cellular maturation, the extracellular environment, and the activity of the cell. Most of our knowledge of the biochemistry and ultrastructural features of macrophage granulogenesis comes from the studies of murine species (Cohn, 1968; Cohn and Benson, 1965a,c; Cohn *et al.*, 1966a,b), although recent studies indicate that similar events occur in the formation of granules in human mononuclear phagocytes (Nichols and Bainton, 1973; Nichols *et al.*, 1971).

II. FUNCTIONS

A number of functions have been ascribed to cells of the mononuclear phagocyte system. Some of these are well supported by experimental observation: interaction with immunologically active lymphoid cells, antibacterial activity, and removal of damaged or dead cells. Other possible functions, such as wound repair, embryonic remodeling, control of granulopoiesis, tumor cell killing, and anitiviral activity, are less well substantiated and are still under active investigation.

A. Immune Responses

The role of animal macrophages in immune response has been presented in previous chapters. The relatively few studies of the interaction of human mononuclear phagocytes with lymphoid cells have demonstrated phenomena similar to those demonstrable in animal systems. Human macrophages may play a role in lymphocyte blastogenesis (Cline and Swett, 1968; Hanifin and Cline, 1970; Hersh and Harris, 1968) and in production of at least some lymphokines. For example, human macrophages enhance the production of interferon by mitogenically or antigenically stimulated lymphocytes (Epstein *et al.*, 1971). Such evidence as is available suggests that the macrophage is more potent in these interactions than is the less mature monocyte.

The functions of human mononuclear phagocytes, other than immune interactions, have been studied in greater detail and will be considered in subsequent sections of this chapter.

B. Ingestion of Microorganisms and Other Particles

A primary role of monocytes and macrophages is the engulfment and disposal of microorganisms and tissue debris—functions involving the highly developed phagocytic property of the cell line.

1. Phagocytosis

The process of disposal of microorganisms involves a number of steps. The first is the mobilization of the cells into an area of inflammation. The activated fifth component of complement is one serum factor that is known to be chemotactic for monocytes (Snyderman *et al.*, 1971). Other factors probably play a role in the directed movement of monocytes (Hausmian *et al.*, 1972) and macrophages (Wilkinson *et al.*, 1969). The chemotaxis of macrophages is discussed in detail elsewhere in the volume.

Ingestion of the organism is the next step in the process. Opsonization or particle surface coating with immunoglobulin and/or complement is required for the attachment of most microorganisms to the surface of the phagocytic cell (Holland *et al.*, 1972). This attachment is facilitated by the presence of receptors for the Fc portion of the IgG molecule and receptors for C3 on the surface of the mononuclear phagocyte. In the mouse, such cell surface receptors make their appearance by the promonocyte stage of development; in man, such receptors are well developed at the monocyte stage. In both species, the receptors recognize only some of the subclasses of IgG (Cline *et al.*, 1972; Huber and Fudenberg, 1968).

Subsequent to attachment of the opsonized particle, the cell's plasma membrane invaginates and encloses the particle, thus forming a phagocytic vacuole within the cell cytoplasm. The membrane of the phagocytic vacuole then fuses with the membranes of neighboring lysosomes. These in turn discharge their enzymatic contents into the phagocytic vacuole in the process of degranulation. In the neutrophil, and presumptively in the mononuclear phagocyte, the pH falls abruptly within the phagocytic vacuole concurrently with the degranulation process. In neither cell has the acidification mechanism been defined. The metabolic events previously described accompany the ingestion of particles and the degranulation process.

2. *Microbial Killing*

The mononuclear phagocyte system provides a critical tissue defense system against a variety of microorganisms. We generally think of the neutrophil as the primary defense unit against pyogenic organisms, such as the *Staphylococcus* and *Pneumococcus*, and regard the macrophage as a cellular defense unit against intracellular organisms, as *Mycobacterium tuberculosis* and *Mycobacterium leprae*. The mechanisms by which human and animal monocytes and macrophages kill bacteria are largely unknown. The evidence that is available is derived from two sources: studies of genetic defects of host resistance and *in vitro* manipulation of the environment of the mononuclear phagocyte to alter its bactericidal capabilities.

In the absence of oxygen, the ability of human macrophages to kill *Listeria monocytogenes* is impaired (Cline, 1970b). In the presence of oxygen and an agent that stimulates H_2O_2 generation, microbial killing is enhanced (Cline, 1970c; Conalty *et al.*, 1971). Furthermore, monocyte bactericidal capacity is reduced in chronic granulomatous disease, a condition in which phagocytic leukocyte oxygen metabolism is abnormal. In this disorder, neutrophil (and presumably monocyte) generation of hydrogen peroxide and superoxide following phagocytosis is reduced. These observations suggest that the monocyte–macrophage utilizes an oxygen-dependent system as an important bactericidal mechanism. An oxygen-dependent system also comprises a major part of the antibacterial armament of the neutrophil. In the neutrophil, hydrogen peroxide generated during phagocytosis is thought to interact with myeloperoxidase and perhaps intracellular halide to generate a potent antimicrobial system (Klebanoff, 1971).

The enzyme, myeloperoxidase, is present in macrophage precursors up to the stage of the monocyte. It is not present in more mature cells of this series (Cline and Sumner, 1972; van Furth and Cohn, 1968). In the genetic absence of this enzyme, impaired monocyte microbicidal activity is demonstrable, but macrophage killing is normal (Lehrer and Cline, 1969; Salmon *et al.*, 1970). It appears, therefore, that in the monocyte—as in the neutrophil—myeloperoxidase provides an ancillary killing mechanism in conjunction with hydrogen peroxide. In the mature macrophage, however, microbicidal mechanisms are independent of myeloperoxidase. Although it has occasionally been suggested that the abundant catalase of the alveolar macrophage serves the same function as myeloperoxidase, there is little experimental evidence to support such a thesis.

A variety of as yet unidentified mechanisms may exist in the macrophage for microbial killing. As noted elsewhere in this volume, macrophages activated by immune lymphocytes are better killers than nonactivated cells. Whether the enhanced killing capacity of the activated mononuclear phagocyte is based on oxygen-dependent or other mechanisms is not known. It has been suggested that surfactants and other membrane-active substances may be important in the control of *Mycobacterium tuberculosis* by macrophages (D'Arcy-Hart, 1968). Certain monocyte cationic proteins (other than myeloperoxidase) have been shown to be fungicidal (Lehrer, 1975). These probably constitute an important oxygen-independent microbicidal system in mononuclear phagocytes.

3. *Removal of Cell Debris*

The monocyte–macrophage system is important in the removal of damaged or dying cells and cell debris. The appearance of hemosiderin-laden macrophages in diseases characterized by excessive erythrocyte destruction or extravasation of red cells into tissues has been recognized by morphologists and pathologists for many years. Erythrophagocytosis is also a feature of many of the diseases of proliferation of malignant macrophages. The phagocytosis of erythrocytes by macrophages has been studied under a variety of conditions *in vitro*. The phagocyte appears to recognize changes in the erythrocyte surface membrane induced by immunoglobulin coating, chemical injury, or the aging process (Cline and Lehrer, 1968; LoBuglio *et al.*, 1967; Maruta and Mizuno, 1971; Rabinovitch, 1967). In the spleen, mononuclear phagocytes line the walls of the sinusoids. Erythrocytes passing through this organ come into close contact with these lining cells. Isolated inclusions in erythrocytes, such as nuclear remnants or denatured hemoglobin, may be selectively removed by the lining cells. When the erythrocytes are severely damaged. they may be totally phagocytized. Immunoglobulin-coated red cells are also trapped and phagocytized. This process is facilitated by the splenic macrophage receptors for certain IgG subclasses and for C3. Tissue macrophages of animals and presumably of man contain enzymes for catabolizing hemoglobin. The globin moiety is degraded by proteases and the heme by the enzyme heme oxygenase (Pimstone *et al.*, 1971). Heme oxygenase is an inducible enzyme in animal macrophages; its level rises in response to hemoglobin loads. The number of splenic macrophages also increases with exposure to injured erythrocytes. Splenomegaly results. The organism thus has developed adaptive mechanisms for localizing and catabolizing large numbers of damaged red cells.

C. Antitumor Activity

A role for human macrophage in antitumor defense systems has yet to be defined; however, as noted earlier in this volume, abundant animal data suggests that the macrophage does play a role in antitumor activity. Although some evidence indicates that some antitumor activity of macrophages from immunized animals is immunologically specific (Evans and Alexander, 1970; Granger and Weiser, 1964), it is likely that this specificity involves the participation of cytophilic antibody (Fakhri *et al.*, 1973; Mitchell and Mokyr, 1972). This specificity applies to the first phase of tumor antigen recognition. The second phase of the killing reaction appears to be nonspecific (Evans and Alexander, 1972).

"Activated" macrophages appear to have more effective cytotoxic mechanisms; for example, following infection of mice with *Toxoplasma*, the activated macrophages kill L cells more readily than do macrophages from uninfected animals (Hibbs *et al.*, 1972a,b). Additionally, recent observations suggest that macrophages may recognize and subsequently destroy malignantly transformed cells by mechanisms that are nonimmunologic (Hibbs *et al.*, 1972a,b).

The macrophage attack on target cells may be mediated by hydrolytic lysosomal enzymes and perhaps other soluble factors (Heise and Weiser, 1969; Kramer and Granger, 1972); however, relatively little information is available on this interesting subject from animal studies and almost nothing relating to human cells.

D. Control of Granulopoiesis and Involvement in Erythropoiesis

The growth of human bone marrow *in vitro* in semisolid supporting medium requires a factor or factors usually designated colony-stimulating factor (CSF). Under the stimulus of CSF, committed hematopoietic stem cells divide repeatedly to form colonies of several hundred or several thousand cells. Such colonies are comprised of granulocytes or macrophages (Metcalf and Moore, 1971). It is not certain that CSF, which stimulates the growth of granulocytic and mononuclear colonies *in vitro*, is a physiologic regulator of leukopoiesis *in vivo*, but several lines of evidence suggest that this is indeed the case (Dale *et al.*, 1971; Golde and Cline, 1974; Robinson and Mangalik, 1972; Shadduck and Nagabhushanam, 1971; Weiner and Robinson, 1971).

Few sources of CSF, active for human bone marrow, are known. These include peripheral blood leukocytes and certain fetal tissues (Robinson and Mangalik, 1972). When peripheral blood white cells are fractionated into the component subpopulations, and the purified cells cultured *in vitro* without added stimulant, only monocytes produce CSF (Chervenick and LoBuglio, 1972; Golde and Cline, 1972; Golde *et al.*, 1972; Moore *et al.*, 1973). Neither human granulocytes nor unstimulated lymphocytes make detectable CSF. Macrophages derived from blood monocyte cultures *in vitro* as well as tissue macrophages produce CSF (Golde *et al.*, 1972). This production can be enhanced by exposure of the cells to endotoxin (Cline and Golde, 1974; Cline *et al.*, 1974). At the present time, it is a reasonable hypothesis to suggest that mononuclear phagocytes are an important source of CSF in man and that these cells may play a role in the regulation of the production of granulocytes as well as in their own production (Golde and Cline, 1974). Malignant monocytes may retain the capacity to produce CSF, provided they demonstrate some degree of morphologic and functional differentiation (Cline *et al.*, 1972; Cline and Golde, 1973; Golde *et al.*, 1974).

It is clear, however, that human blood cells other than mononuclear phagocytes may produce CSF under some circumstances. Lymphocytes activated by mitogen are also a source of factor or factors that stimulate clonal growth of human bone marrow. CSF levels rise in the serum of animals stimulated by antigen. Whether these lymphocyte factors are identical to monocyte CSF is unknown.

There are occasional reports in the literature suggesting that macrophages and reticulum cells may also be involved in cell interactions leading to bone marrow erythropoiesis. These suggestions that macrophages or reticulum cells may serve as central "nurse" cells in an island of developing normoblasts are based mainly on morphologic, rather than physiologic, observations (Bessis and Breton-Gorious, 1957, 1962). Interestingly, macrophages do have an active transport system for ferritin—an observation consistent with the suggestion that the macrophage may be a source of iron for the developing erythrocyte. Little additional information is available in this interesting area.

III. DISORDERS OF THE MONOCYTE–MACROPHAGE SYSTEM

A variety of human diseases are associated with increased numbers of monocytes and tissue macrophages. Bone marrow hematopoietic cell lines are known to proliferate in response to appropriate stimuli; for example, granulocytic proliferation occurs in response to infection; erythrocytic hyperplasia occurs in response to chronic bleeding; and megakaryocytosis develops in response to increased platelet destruction. Lymphocytosis may be an appropriate response to certain viral and bacterial infections. In addition to these "appropriate" responses, hematopoietic cell lines may proliferate "autonomously" or in response to unidentified stimuli. In such circumstances, we speak of *lymphoproliferative* disorders or *myeloproliferative* disorders. These may be either relatively benign or malignant. In an analogous manner, cells of the monocyte–macrophage series may proliferate appropriately in response to a stimulus, such as *Mycobacterium tuberculosis*. In such a circumstance, the mononuclear leukocyte response is often termed "reactive" hyperplasia. Clinically, reactive hyperplasia is manifested by enlargement of reticuloendothelial organs such as spleen and lymph nodes. On the other hand, mononuclear phagocytes may proliferate "inappropriately" (autonomously) and to an extent that exceeds normal levels as, for example, in monocytic leukemia. A variety of terms has been used to describe neoplastic histiocytic proliferation: reticuloendotheliosis, histiocytic malignancies, reticuloendothlial malignancy. Some of these terms are probably misnomers, since we do not have good evidence that endothelial elements participate in the proliferative process. Perhaps *malignant histiocytic proliferative* disorders would be a more appropriate term to cover this spectrum of diseases.

Another group of disorders in which one observes increased numbers and abnormalities of tissue macrophages is that in which a phagocytizable material accumulates intracellularly more rapidly than it can be disposed of by metabolic processes. For convenience we identify these as storage diseases. Finally, there is a group of diseases in which tissue macrophages are prominent, are probably increased in numbers, and in which the inciting agents have not yet been identified. These disorders do not show the typical characteristics of malignant histiocytic disorders. Examples of such diseases are sarcoidosis and rheumatoid arthritis.

In addition to diseases characterized by mononuclear phagocyte proliferation, there are disorders in which abnormalities of monocyte–macrophage system may be associated with dysfunction of the cells either on a genetic or acquired basis.

A classification of the disorders of the monocyte–macrophage system

TABLE I

Classification of Monocyte–Macrophage System Disorders

Category	Examples
I. Monocytosis	(see Table II)
II. "Reactive" proliferation	
A. Intracellular parasites	Tuberculosis, *Listeria*
B. Chemical	Berylliosis
C. Hemopoietic cell destruction	Hemolytic anemias
III. Storage diseases	Gaucher's disease
IV. Histiocytic proliferation of unknown origin	Sarcoidosis, Felty's syndrome
V. Neoplastic proliferation	Monocytic leukemia, malignant histiocytoses
VI. Monocyte–macrophage dysfunction syndromes	Chronic granulomatous disease

is presented in Table I. It should be stressed that such a classification is tentative and subject to modification as new information becomes available.

A. Monocytosis

The normal relative monocyte count in the adult varies between 1 and 9% of the circulating leukocyte population (Cassileth, 1972; Wintrobe, 1967). The relative monocyte count is significantly elevated when it exceeds 10%. In children, the average relative count is 9%. The normal absolute monocyte count is between 285 and 500/mm^3 in adults and between 750 and 800/mm^3 in children (Bessis, 1956; Miale, 1962; Wintrobe, 1967).

Relative monocytosis is normal in the neonate and may persist for several weeks (Kato, 1935). Causes of monocytosis reviewed in the literature are summarized in Table II. As can be seen, a wide variety of diseases are represented. In general, however, the diseases associated with blood monocytosis also fall into categories II, III and IV of Table I.

B. Reactive Hyperplasia

1. Response to Intracellular Parasites

A variety of intracellular parasites are associated with clinical enlargement of liver, spleen, and sometimes lymph nodes and with microscopic evidence of macrophage hyperplasia. Tuberculosis is still one of the more

TABLE II

Causes of Monocytosis

Infectious and parasitic diseases	Miscellaneous hematologic diseases
Subacute bacterial endocarditis	Polycythemia vera
Tuberculosis	Recovery phase of agranulocytosis
Rickettsial diseases	Postsplenectomy
Syphilis	Myeloid metaplasia
Brucellosis	Hemolytic anemia
Malaria	Collagen vascular diseases
Trypanosomiasis	Rheumatic endocarditis
Leishmaniasis	Systemic lupus erythematosus
Typhoid fever	Rheumatoid arthritis
Following acute infection	Chronic inflammatory gastrointestinal
Neoplastic diseases	diseases
Myelomonocytic leukemia	Ulcerative colitis
Hodgkin's disease and lymphomas	Regional enteritis
"Preleukemia"	Cirrhosis
Multiple myeloma	Miscellaneous disorders
Nonhematological malignant disease	Sarcoidosis
	Drug reactions

common chronic infectious diseases in this country and may be taken as the prototype of histiocytic proliferation in response to an intracellular parasite. Splenomegaly as a feature of reticuloendothelial hyperplasia in generalized tuberculosis is well recognized in the literature (Chapman *et al.*, 1954; Cline, 1967; Englebreth-Holm, 1938). In the early days of human and animal macrophage cultivation, the multinucleate giant cell of the tuberculoid lesion was taken as the prototype of histiocytic response to a facultative intracellular parasite (Sutton, 1967).

In tuberculous lesions of man and animals, one sees macrophages at all stages of development, from the newly arrived monocyte to the mature multinucleated giant cell (Dannenberg, 1968). Many of the phagocytes contain ingested organisms. One of the interesting features of this infection, as well as other infections with facultative and obligate intracellular parasites, is that many organisms survive and even proliferate within the macrophage. The reason that some organisms survive whereas others are killed is uncertain. Armstrong and D'Arcy-Hart (1971) have suggested that surviving organisms are sequestered in phagosomes that do not receive a complement of hydrolytic enzymes from the discharge of primary and secondary lysosomes.

The course of tuberculosis is governed by the overall function of the macrophage system: effectiveness of individual cells and total number of responding cells. Although the organisms may initially multiply intracellularly, with the development of cellular immunity they are destroyed (Dannenberg, 1968; Lurie, 1964). Thus, as noted elsewhere in this volume, the development of delayed hypersensitivity and full expression of macrophage microbicidal function are concomitant phenomena (see Blanden *et al.*, Chapter 15; David and Remold, Chapter 16).

Histiocytic proliferation has been documented in association with a variety of other intracellular infections and parasitic diseases: syphilis (Wintrobe, 1967), brucellosis (Sundberg and Spink, 1947), listeriosis (Khoo and Mackaness, 1964), leprosy (Ptak *et al.*, 1970), malaria (Marsden *et al.*, 1965), schistosomiasis (Rodrigriguez-Molina and Pons, 1936), leishmaniasis (Angevine *et al.*, 1945; Cartwright *et al.*, 1948), cryptococcosis (Sharar, 1968; Sharar *et al.*, 1969), histoplasmosis (Curtis and Grekin, 1947; Simson and Barneston, 1942), and toxoplasmosis (Kalderon *et al.*, 1964).

2. *Response to Chemicals*

Chronic pulmonary disease caused by exposure to beryllium has been known since 1933 (Weber and Engelhardt, 1933). The lesions in berylliosis may be widespread in the reticuloendothelial tissues and may mimic those of sarcoidosis. The lesions are characterized by large macrophages, giant cells, and organized epithelioid cells (Williams, 1958) and appear to be caused by a delayed hypersensitivity reaction (Alekseeva, 1966; Norris and Peard, 1963; Sterner and Eisenbud, 1951).

Lymphocytes from hypersensitive subjects undergo blastogenic transformation when exposed to poorly soluble beryllium salts *in vitro*. Such lymphocytes interact with macrophages in producing clusters of responding cells (Hanifin *et al.*, 1970). The macrophages of such subjects appear to be activated by morphologic criteria in their rate of differentiation from monocytes. However, these macrophages do not show the enhanced ability to kill an intracellular parasite that characterizes the macrophages of patients with active tuberculosis or leprosy (Cline, 1967). These observations indicate that intracellular parasitosis, rather than granulomatous hypersensitivity per se, is necessary for functionally activated macrophages (i.e., those showing enhanced microbicidal activity).

The histiocytic response to zirconium salts appears to be similar, in general, in histologic appearance and pathogenesis to the response to beryllium compounds (Epstein, 1967).

3. *Histiocytic Response to Hematopoietic Cell Destruction*

a. Hemolytic Anemia. In most hemolytic anemias the primary site of destruction of damaged, intrinsically abnormal, or antibody-coated erythrocytes is the reticuloendothelial elements of the spleen and, to a lesser extent, of the liver. Several mechanisms of cell destruction may be operative, including stasis of erythrocytes and subsequent osmotic lysis in the splenic sinusoids and phagocytosis by the reticuloendothelial cells of the spleen, liver, and blood (Ham *et al.*, 1956; Jandl, 1966; Zinkham and Diamond, 1952).

Splenomegaly is clinically apparent in most long-standing hemolytic anemias (Wintrobe, 1967; Young *et al.*, 1951). It is probable that part of this increase in spleen size is the result of hyperplasia of the phagocytic histiocytes. This hyperplasia may also be seen in the liver and to some extent in the lymph nodes. Erythrophagocytosis and its consequence (hemosiderin pigments) may be more or less prominent in histiocytes.

It is probable that the induction of macrophage proliferation by red cells undergoing lysis can take place locally in many areas of the body. Perhaps the best example is the occurrence of large numbers of hemoglobin and hemosiderin-laden alveolar macrophages in a variety of diseases where red cell extravasation into the alveoli occurs, for example, pulmonary hemosiderosis, Goodpasture's syndrome, and severe mitral valve stenosis. There is some evidence that erythrophagocytosis interferes with the ability of macrophages to simultaneously phagocytize and destroy certain intracellular bacteria (Gill *et al.*, 1966). This may be important in the pathogenesis of the frequent infections of sickle cell disease.

b. Destruction of Other Hematopoietic Cells. It is possible that the hyperplasia of histiocytes may occur in disorders in which there is a high turnover and excessive destruction of granulocytes. This is difficult to document, however. Inferential evidence is provided by the observation of large, lipid-laden phagocytes in patients with chronic myelocytic leukemia, where these cells resemble Gaucher's cells (Dosik *et al.*, 1972; Kattlove *et al.*, 1969). Active macrophages in the spleen may be in part responsible for the neutropenia occurring in Felty's syndrome.

C. Storage Diseases

As a generalization one can say that when a phagocytizable organic material accumulates more rapidly than it can be disposed of by normal catabolic or excretory processes, it will accumulate in cells of the reticuloendothelial system and, in particular, in macrophages.

Three causes of accumulation of organic material in mononuclear phagocytes can be identified. (i) Such accumulation occurs in genetic defects of macrophage enzyme function in which a poorly catabolized product accumulates (Gaucher's disease, Niemann-Pick disease). Thus, in Gaucher's disease deficiency of glucocerebrosidase leads to accumulation of glucocerebroside in splenic and liver macrophages. The probable source of glucocerebroside is the membranes of phagocytized erythrocytes and leukocytes. (ii) Accumulation of organic material also occurs in diseases characterized by excessive cell death or turnover (secondary gout and chronic myelogenous leukemia). It is thought that in chronic myelocytic leukemia the macrophages phagocytize dead granulocytes. The phagocytized membranes overwhelm the degradative capacity of the macrophage with the consequent development of a "storage" cell. (iii) In diseases in which the normal excretory pathways for organic materials are blocked, storage macrophages may result. An example is complete bronchial obstruction with formation of foamy macrophages. Clearly in some of the diseases, such as localized bronchial obstruction, more than one mechanism may be operative at inducing histiocytic hyperplasia (Cohen and Cline, 1972).

A common feature of all these storage diseases is the accumulation of tissue macrophages that appear prominent because of their ingested products, for example, lipid-laden macrophages in the lipidoses. Whether there is in addition a true increase in numbers of the histiocytes is not certain.

D. Histiocytic Proliferative Disorders of Uncertain Origin

Histiocytic proliferation, either localized or generalized, occurs in a variety of disease states whose etiologies are unknown. Consequently, the pathogenetic mechanisms leading to cellular proliferation are obscure. These diseases include sarcoidosis, Felty's syndrome, and Wegener's granulomatosis.

There is a rich and complex literature on sarcoidosis that unfortunately provides little insight into thc pathogcncsis of the disease. The important features relevant to the present discussion are that splenomegaly and lymphadenopathy are frequent features of this disease and that monocytosis is an occasional feature. The histologic features of the affected nodes and spleen may resemble those of miliary epithelioid tubercles without necrosis and generally without a surrounding inflammatory zone.

In Felty's syndrome (rheumatoid arthritis, splenomegaly, and leukopenia), Still's disease of childhood, and the more common varieties of rheumatoid arthritis, splenomegaly and hyperplasia of the histiocytic elements of the spleen and lymph nodes are common. Felty's syndrome is generally thought to be a variant of rheumatoid arthritis. The degree of splenomegaly, which may vary from slight to marked, is not generally correlated with the activity of the arthritis or the magnitude of the hematologic changes (Mason and Morris, 1964). Splenectomy often produces a transient improvement in the white blood cell count in this disease (Green and Fromke, 1966).

There are a number of rare diseases in which histiocytic proliferation and granulomatous infiltration occur in the tissues, particularly around damaged blood vessels. These include "allergic" granulomatosis (Churg and Strauss, 1951), Wegener's granulomatosis (Carrington and Liebow, 1966; Fahey *et al.*, 1954; Godman and Churg, 1954), midline granuloma (Williams, 1949), giant cell arteritis (Paulley and Hughes, 1960; Russell, 1962), and Cogan's syndrome (Cody and Williams, 1960; Crawford, 1957). Attempts have been made to analyze and classify these diseases (Alarcon-Segovia and Brown, 1964; Churg, 1963; Sokolov *et al.*, 1962); however, no clear, completely acceptable explanation of the clinical and histologic features of these disorders has yet emerged.

E. The Malignant Histiocytic Disorders (Cline and Golde, 1973)

1. *Monocytic leukemia* is recognized morphologically by the presence in blood, bone marrow, and tissues of immature cells of the monocyte–macrophage cell line. These cells vary from primitive blast forms to morphologically and functionally differentiated monocytes and macrophages. In most cases of monocytic leukemia, there is a variable admixture of myeloblasts and more differentiated granulocytes. This is not surprising in view of the evidence favoring a common stem cell origin for granulocyte and monocyte.

2. *Histiocytic lymphoma* (*reticulum cell sarcoma*) is traditionally classified with lymphoma and the lymphoproliferative disorders. We should, however, distinguish between lymphoid cells and cellular elements of the reticuloendothelial system that are phagocytic, even though the two cell types are intimately related physically in lymphoid tissues and spleen, and function cooperatively in antigen processing and cellular immune responses. Since the proliferating cells in the tissues of patients with reticulum cell sarcoma resemble poorly differentiated histiocytes or reticulum cells more than they resemble lymphocytes, it is logical to classify reticulum cell sarcoma among the histiocytic proliferative disorders (Rappaport, 1966).

The proliferating cells of reticulum cell sarcoma encompass a spectrum ranging between the promonocyte and the immature macrophage.

In occasional patients, the overlap between reticulum cell sarcoma and acute monocytic leukemia is clearly demonstrable. Starting within the lymph nodes, the malignant reticulum cells may subsequently involve the bone marrow and blood, producing a leukemic picture (Ohara *et al.*, 1971; Rosenberg *et al.*, 1961).

3. *Letterer–Siwe disease* is a disease of infancy characterized by hepatosplenomegaly, lymphadenopathy, bleeding diathesis, bone tumors, generalized hyperplasia of non-lipid-storing macrophages in many organs but prominently in skin, and a rapidly fatal downhill course. The major cytologic feature is proliferation of moderately differentiated histiocytes that show some resemblance to the well-differentiated form of histiocytic lymphoma. The possibility of a relationship between Letterer–Siwe disease and other less differentiated histiocytic proliferative disorders is suggested by the report of an illness which began as Letterer–Siwe disease and terminated as monocytic leukemia (Avery *et al.*, 1957; Gray and Taylor, 1953; Imamura *et al.*, 1971).

4. *Histiocytic medullary reticulosis* is a unique form of "lymphoma" with cells resembling moderately well-differentiated histiocytes, with a high proliferative capacity and well-developed phagocytic activity and exhibiting significant erythrophagocytosis. They most closely resemble the immature macrophage. It is a rapidly progressive and fatal disease of adults. Prominent features include hepatosplenomegaly, a lymphadenopathy, fever, and pancytopenia.

5. *Hand–Schuller–Christian disease* is characterized by the focal accumulation within bone, and sometimes within skin and lungs, of masses of tissue macrophages. These lesions may have a variable admixture of lymphocytes, plasma cells, neutrophils, and eosinophils. The disease usually occurs in childhood and has an extremely variable course. The disease rarely, if ever, makes the transition to a more fulminant type of histiocytic proliferation. The clinical pattern is reflected in the histologic changes in tissue. During an active phase of disease, rapidly developing lesions resemble inflammatory histiocytosis with a variable degree of eosinophilic infiltration. With a more chronic illness the histiocytes become lipid-laden and fibrosis appears. Ultimately the lesions are densely fibrotic.

6. *Eosinophilic granuloma* is a disease of children with lesions pathologically resembling Hand–Schuller–Christian disease but localized to bone.

The malignant histiocytic diseases can be viewed as different diseases representing clinically identifiable stopping points along the spectrum of malignant histiocytic proliferative disorders with varying degrees of cellular differentiation (Cline and Golde, 1973). The neoplastic diseases of the histiocytic cells embrace a wide spectrum, from disorders in which there is extensive proliferation of poorly differentiated cells (e.g., acute monocytic leukemia) to disorders in which there is limited and circumscribed proliferation of well-differentiated cells. Clearly, there will be overlap among these diseases, depending on how "tightly" or "loosely" the neoplastic clone is regulated in its differentiation.

It is convenient to catalog these diseases on the basis of cellular differentiation. The grouping proposed here is (a) disease with little cellular differentiation, including acute monocytic leukemia and undifferentiated reticulum cell sarcoma; (b) disease with a moderate degree of histiocytic differentiation, including chronic monocytic leukemia, well-differentiated reticulum cell sarcoma, Letterer–Siwe disease, and histiocytic medullary reticulosis; (c) disease with well-differentiated histiocytes, including Hand–Schuller–Christian disease, unifocal and multifocal eosinophilic granuloma of bone, and localized histiocytoma.

Although there is little dispute about the malignant nature of the disorders in groups (a) and (b), it is not certain that the entities listed group (c) are indeed neoplastic. The clinically chronic disorders characterized by proliferation of well-differentiated histiocytes may represent a reactive response to an unidentified antigen or parasite. In this regard, they may be viewed as having more in common with sarcoidosis than with a true malignancy.

F. Macrophage Dysfunction Syndromes

Several macrophage dysfunction syndromes in man have recently been described. These include genetic abnormalities, such as chronic granulomatous disease (Davis *et al.*, 1968; Rodey *et al.*, 1969), and acquired disorders, such as lymphoma and myelomonocytic leukemia (Cline, 1973) and pulmonary alveolar proteinosis. These disorders are all associated with an increased incidence of opportunistic infection. The mononuclear defect in chronic granulomatous disease is probably related to deficient postphagocytic H_2O_2 and superoxide generation. In acute myelomonocytic leukemia and in some patients with lymphoma, the defective leukocytes phagocytize organisms but fail to inhibit their intracellular replication (Cline, 1973).

In addition to these disorders, high concentrations of adrenocorticosteroids and ionizing irradiation may interfere with the macrophage defense system in animals and probably in man (Donaldson *et al.*, 1956; Dannenberg, 1970; Lurie *et al.*, 1953; Merkow *et al.*, 1968). With high doses of ionizing irradiation, the proliferation of macrophage precursors is impaired, but the metabolic development of the cells appears to be intact (Dannenberg, 1970; Kambara *et al.*, 1970). Thus, the main effect on macrophage defense function of high doses of X ray is against the proliferating cell in the bone marrow rather than the functional cell in the periphery.

In patients receiving adrenocorticosteroids, opportunistic infections are frequent and may carry a grave prognosis (Gray and Killinger, 1966; Johnson and Colley, 1969; Sidransky *et al.*, 1965). Diseases in which such infections occur and in which corticosteroids are used include malignancy (Lehrer and Cline, 1971; Louria *et al.*, 1967), collagen vascular disease (Rosengarten and Bourn, 1959; Schulze *et al.*, 1953), and vasculitis (Buchner and Schneierson, 1968; Johnson and Colley, 1969).

In animal model systems, corticosteroids enhance the susceptibility to opportunistic intracellular infections (Miller and Hedberg, 1965). The mechanism of this enhanced susceptibility is not known with certainty; however, it has been shown that in animals treated with high doses of corticosteroids, the lysosomes of alveolar macrophages fail to fuse properly with phagosomes containing ingested microorganisms (Merkow *et al.*, 1968). This enhanced lysosomal stability may be one mechanism by which corticosteroids promote enhanced susceptibility to opportunistic pathogens. A more important abnormality induced by corticosteroids relates to defective phagocytic leukocyte mobilization into areas of inflammation (Dale *et al.*, 1974).

In addition to these documented macrophage dysfunction syndromes, defective mononuclear cell function has been thought to occur in several other disorders. For obvious reasons, the patients who fail to adequately control intracellular parasitosis must be suspected of having a defective macrophage defense system. Therefore, patients with lepromatous leprosy, miliary tuberculosis, disseminated fungal infections, and Hodgkin's disease may be suspected of having macrophage dysfunction syndromes. However, in these disorders, intrinsic or acquired defects of macrophage function or of macrophage–lymphoid interaction have been inferred, but not proved (Drutz *et al.*, 1974). In many of the putative macrophage dysfunction syndromes, abnormalities of delayed hypersensitivity are a prominent feature of the disease.

IV. SUMMARY AND FUTURE PERSPECTIVES

Our present understanding of the physiology and function of mononuclear phagocytes has been most fully defined in animal systems, usually with rodents as the test animals. When the metabolism and function of human monocytes and macrophages have been examined, they have generally been similar in performance to rodent cells. Nevertheless, many aspects of the activities of human mononuclear phagocytes remain to be studied. Consequently, one must guard against too bland an acceptance of the identity of animal and human macrophages in kinetic behavior and in phagocytic and immunologic properties.

The most promising area for future clinical investigation will be the performance of human mononuclear phagocytes in various disease states. Some such studies have already been undertaken; however, it will be necessary to put our shaky understanding of the role of these cells in man on a more firm physiologic base. The intriguing suggestions that macrophages are involved in the control of leukopoiesis and the modulation of humoral antibody production by lymphoid cells require more detailed examinations in man. In the same manner, one must soon ask for cogent evidence that mononuclear phagocytes constitute a physiological relevant defense against neoplasia in humans. Clearly, an understanding of the normal performance characteristics and function of human monocytes and macrophages must underlie future questions about aberrations of cellular activity in diseases. More importantly, perhaps, knowledge of normal function may permit us to manipulate the mononuclear phagocyte to the advantage of the patient. Macrophage activation by trials of "tumor immunotherapy" with BCG may constitute a first halting step in this direction.

It is now possible to obtain human mononuclear phagocytes in reasonable quantities from the peripheral blood using continuous flow centrifuges or adherence techniques and from the peritoneal cavity and alveolar spaces under appropriate clinical conditions. Preliminary evidence has already shown that microbicidal function of macrophages is impaired in a variety of pulmonary diseases and may be abnormal in certain neoplastic processes. Clearly, examination of the mononuclear phagocyte in human diseases will be an important and fruitful area for future investigation.

REFERENCES

Alarcon-Segovia, D., and Brown, A. L., Jr. (1964). *Mayo Clin. Proc.* **39**, 205–222.

Alekseeva, O. G. (1966). *Fed. Proc.* **25**, Suppl., T843–T846.

Angevine, D. M., Hamilton, T. R., Wallace, F. G., and Hazard, J. B. (1945). *Amer. J. Med. Sci.* **210**, 33–38.

Armstrong, J. A., and D'Arcy Hart, P. (1971). *J. Exp. Med.* **134**, 713–740.

Avery, M. E., McAfee, J. G., and Guild, H. G. (1957). *Amer. J. Med.* **22**, 636–652.

Axline, S. G. (1970). *Semin. Hematol.* **7**, 142–160.

Baehner, R. L., and Johnston, R. B., Jr. (1972). *Blood* **40**, 31–41.

Bessis, M. (1956). "Cytology of the Blood and Blood Forming Organs." Grune & Stratton, New York.

Bessis, M. C., and Breton-Gorious, J. (1957). *J. Biophys. Biochem. Cytol.* **3**, 503–504.

Bessis, M. C., and Breton-Gorious, J. (1962). *Blood* **19**, 635–663.

Buchner, L. H., and Schneierson, S. S. (1968). *Amer. J. Med.* **45**, 904–921.

Carrington, C. B., and Liebow, A. A. (1966). *Amer. J. Med.* **41,** 497–527.
Cartwright, G. E., Chung, H. L., and Chang, A. (1948). *Blood* **3,** 249–275.
Cassileth, P. (1972). *In* "Hematology" (W. J. Williams *et al.,* eds.), Vol. I, pp. 855–858. McGraw-Hill, New York.
Chapman, A. Z., Reeder, P. S., and Baker, L. A. (1954). *Ann. Intern. Med.* **41,** 1225–1231.
Chen, M. G., and Schooley, J. C. (1970a). *J. Cell. Physiol.* **75,** 89–96.
Chen, M. G., and Schooley, J. C. (1970b). *Radiat. Res.* **41,** 623–636.
Chervenick, P. A., and LoBuglio, A. F. (1972). *Science* **178,** 164–166.
Churg, J. (1963). *Ann. Allergy* **21,** 619–628.
Churg, J., and Strauss, L. (1951). *Amer. J. Pathol.* **27,** 277–302.
Cline, M. J. (1965). *Physiol. Rev.* **45,** 674–720.
Cline, M. J. (1967). *Calif. Med.* **106,** 215–221.
Cline, M. J. (1970a). *In* "Third Annual Red Cross Symposium on Formation and Destruction of Blood Cells" (T. J. Greenwalt and G. A. Jamieson, eds.), pp. 222–239. Lippincott, Philadelphia, Pennsylvania.
Cline, M. J. (1970b). *Infec. Immunity* **2,** 156–161.
Cline, M. J. (1970c). *Infec. Immunity* **2,** 601–605.
Cline, M. J. (1972). *In* "Hematology" (W. J. Williams *et al.,* eds.), Vol. I, pp. 741–747. McGraw-Hill, New York.
Cline, M. J. (1973). *J. Clin. Invest.* **52,** 2185–2190.
Cline, M. J., and Golde, D. W. (1973). *Amer. J. Med.* **55,** 49–60.
Cline, M. J., and Golde, D. W. (1974a). *In* "Proceedings of the Second International Conference on Bone Marrow Culture" (W. A. Robinson, ed.), Dept. Health, Education and Welfare Publ. No. (NIH) 74, pp. 200–208.
Cline, M. J., Rothman, B., and Golde, D. W. (1974). *J. Cell Physiol.* **84,** 193–196.
Cline, M. J., and Lehrer, R. I. (1968). *Blood* **32,** 423–435.
Cline, M. J., and Sumner, M. A. (1972). *Blood* **40,** 62–69.
Cline, M. J., and Swett, V. C. (1968). *J. Exp. Med.* **128,** 1309–1325.
Cline, M. J., Warner, N. L., and Metcalf, D. (1972). *Blood* **39,** 326–330.
Cody, D. T. R., and Williams, H. L. (1960). *Laryngoscope* **70,** 447–478.
Cohen, A. B., and Cline, M. J. (1971). *J. Clin. Invest.* **50,** 1390–1398.
Cohen, A. B., and Cline, M. J. (1972). *Amer. Rev. Resp. Dis.* **106,** 69–78.
Cohn, Z. A. (1968). *Advan. Immunol.* **9,** 163–214.
Cohn, Z. A., and Benson, B. (1965a). *J. Exp. Med.* **121,** 153–170.
Cohn, Z. A., and Benson, B. (1965b). *J. Exp. Med.* **121,** 279–287.
Cohn, Z. A., and Benson, B. (1965c). *J. Exp. Med.* **121,** 835–848.
Cohn, Z. A., Hirsch, J. G., and Fedorko, M. E. (1966a). *J. Exp. Med.* **123,** 747–756.
Cohn, Z. A., Fedorko, M. E., and Hirsch, J. G. (1966b). *J. Exp. Med.* **123,** 757–766.
Conalty, M. L., Barry, V. C., and Jina, A. (1971). *Int. J. Lepr.* **39,** 479–492.
Crawford, W. J. (1957). *Pa. Med. J.* **60,** 835–838.
Curtis, A. C., and Grekin, J. N. (1947). *J. Amer. Med. Ass.* **134,** 1217–1224.
Dale, D. C., Brown, C. H., Carbone, P., and Wolff, S. M. (1971). *Science* **173,** 152–153.
Dale, D. C., Fauci, A. S., and Wolff, S. M. (1974). *N. Engl. J. Med.* **291,** 1154–1158.
Dannenberg, A. (1968). *Bacteriol. Rev.* **32,** 85–102.
Dannenberg, A. (1970). *RES, J. Reticuloendothel. Soc.* **7,** 91–108.
D'Arcy-Hart, P. (1968). *Science* **162,** 686–689.
Davis, W. C., Huber, H., Douglas, S. D., and Fudenberg, H. H. (1968). *J. Immunol.* **101,** 1093–1095.
Dosik, H., Rosner, F., and Sawitsky, A. (1972). *Semin. Hematol.* **9,** 309–316.

Donaldson, D. M., Marcus, S., Gyi, K. K., and Perkins, E. H. (1956). *J. Immunol.* **76,** 192–199.

Drutz, D. J., Cline, M. J., and Levy, L. (1974). *J. Clin. Invest.* **53,** 380–386.

Elsbach, P. (1967a). *J. Clin. Invest.* **46,** 1052.

Elsbach, P. (1967b). *J. Lipid Res.* **8,** 359–365.

Elsbach, P. (1968). *J. Clin. Invest.* **47,** 2217–2229.

Englebreth-Holm, J. (1938). *Amer. J. Med. Sci.* **195,** 32–47.

Epstein, L. B., Cline, M. J., and Merigan, T. C. (1971). *J. Clin. Invest.* **50,** 744–753.

Epstein, W. L. (1967). *Progr. Allergy* **11,** 36–88.

Evans, R., and Alexander, P. (1970). *Nature (London)* **228,** 620–622.

Evans, R., and Alexander, P. (1972). *Nature (London)* **236,** 168–170.

Fahey, J. L., Leonard, E., Churg, J., and Godman, G. (1954). *Amer. J. Med.* **17,** 168–179.

Fakhri, O., McLaughlin, H., and Hobbs, J. R. (1973). *Eur. J. Cancer* **9,** 19–23.

Frei, J., Borel, C., Horvath, G., Cullity, B., and Vannotti, A. (1961). *Blood* **18,** 317–327.

Gill, F. A., Kaye, D., and Hook, E. W. (1966). *J. Exp. Med.* **124,** 173–183.

Godman, G. C., and Churg, J. (1954). *AMA Arch. Pathol.* **58,** 533–553.

Golde, D. W., and Cline, M. J. (1972). *J. Clin. Invest.* **51,** 2981–2983.

Golde, D. W., and Cline, M. J. (1974). *N. Engl. J. Med.* **291,** 1388–1395.

Golde, D. W., Finley, T. N., and Cline, M. J. (1972). *Lancet* **2,** 1397–1399.

Golde, D. W., Rothman, B., and Cline, M. J. (1974). *Blood* **43,** 749–756.

Granger, G. A., and Weiser, R. S. (1964). *Science* **145,** 1427–1429.

Gray, J. D., and Taylor, S. (1953). *Cancer* **6,** 333.

Gray, M. L., and Killinger, A. H. (1966). *Bacteriol. Rev.* **30,** 309–382.

Green, R. A., and Fromke, V. L. (1966). *Ann. Intern. Med.* **64,** 1265–1270.

Ham, T. H., Weisman, R., Jr., and Hinz, C. F., Jr. (1956). *AMA Arch. Intern. Med.* **98,** 574–592.

Hanifin, J., and Cline, M. J. (1970). *J. Cell Biol.* **46,** 97–105.

Hanifin, J. M., Epstein, W. L., and Cline, M. J. (1970). *J. Invest. Dermatol.* **55,** 284–288.

Hausman, M. S., Snyderman, R., and Mergenhagen, S. E. (1972). *J. Infec. Dis.* **125,** 595–602.

Heise, E. R., and Weiser, R. S. (1969). *J. Immunol.* **103,** 570–576.

Hersh, E. M., and Harris, J. E. (1968). *J. Immunol.* **100,** 1184–1194.

Hibbs, J. B., Jr., Lambert, L. H., Jr., and Remington, J. S. (1972a). *Nature (London), New Biol.* **235,** 48–50.

Hibbs, J. B., Jr., Lambert, L. H., Jr., and Remington, J. S. (1972b). *Science* **177,** 998–1000.

Holland, P., Holland, N. H., and Cohn, Z. A. (1972). *J. Exp. Med.* **135,** 458–475.

Huber, H., and Fudenberg, H. H. (1968). *Int. Arch. Allergy Appl. Immunol.* **34,** 18–31.

Imamura, M., Sakamoto, S., and Hanazono, H. (1971). *Cancer* **28,** 467–475.

Jandl, J. H. (1966). *Amer. J. Med.* **41,** 657–665.

Johnson, M. L., and Colley, E. W. (1969). *J. Clin. Pathol.* **22,** 465–469.

Kalderon, A. E., Kikkawa, Y., and Bernstein, J. (1964). *Arch. Intern. Med.* **114,** 95–102.

Kambara, T., Chandrasekhar, S., and Dannenberg, A. M., Jr. (1970). *RES, J. Reticuloendothel. Soc.* **7,** 53–78.

Karnovsky, M. L. (1961). *Ciba Found. Study Group* **10**, 60–78.
Karnovsky, M. L. (1962). *Physiol. Rev.* **42**, 143–168.
Kato, K. (1935). *J. Pediat.* **7**, 7–15.
Kattlove, H. E., Williams, J. C., Gaynor, E., Spivack, R., Bradley, R. M., and Brady, R. O. (1969). *Blood* **33**, 379–390.
Khoo, K. K., and Mackaness, G. B. (1964). *Aust. J. Exp. Biol.* **42**, 707–716.
Klebanoff, S. J. (1971). *Annu. Rev. Med.* **22**, 39.
Kramer, J. J., and Granger, G. A. (1972). *Cell. Immunol.* **3**, 88–100.
Leder, L. D. (1966). *Klin. Wochenschr.* **44**, 25–30.
Lehrer, R. I. (1975). *J. Clin. Invest.* **55**, 338–346.
Lehrer, R. I., and Cline, M. J. (1969). *J. Clin. Invest.* **48**, 1478–1488.
Lehrer, R. I., and Cline, M. J. (1971). *Cancer* **27**, 1211–1217.
LoBuglio, A. F., Cotran, R. S., and Jandl, J. H. (1967). *Science* **158**, 1582–1585.
Louria, D. B., Hensle, T., Armstrong, D., Collins, H. S., Blevins, A., Krugman, D., and Buse, M. (1967). *Ann. Intern. Med.* **67**, 261–281.
Lurie, M. B. (1964). "Resistance to Tuberculosis: Experimental Studies in Native and Acquired Defensive Mechanisms." Harvard Univ. Press, Cambridge, Massachusetts.
Lurie, M. B., Zappasodi, P., Dannenberg, A. M., Jr., and Cardona-Lynch, E. (1953). *Ann. N.Y. Acad. Sci.* **56**, 779–792.
Marsden, P. D., Hutt, M. S. R., Wilds, N. E., Voller, A., Blackman, V., Shah, K. K., Connor, D. H., Hamilton, P. J. S., Banwell, J. G., and Lunn, H. F. (1965). *Brit. Med. J.* **1**, 89–92.
Maruta, H., and Mizuno, D. (1971). *Nature (London), New Biol.* **234**, 246–248.
Mason, D. T., and Morris, J. J., Jr. (1964). *Amer. J. Med.* **36**, 463–469.
Merkow, L., Pardo, M., Epstein, S. M., Verney, E., and Sidransky, H. (1968). *Science* **160**, 79–81.
Metcalf, D. (1971). *J. Cell. Physiol.* **77**, 277–280.
Metcalf, D., and Moore, M. A. S. (1971). *In* "Hematopoietic Cells." North-Holland Publ., Amsterdam.
Miale, J. B. (1962). "Laboratory Medicine—Hematology," 2nd ed. Mosby, St. Louis, Missouri.
Miller, J. K., and Hedberg, M. (1965). *Amer. J. Clin. Pathol.* **43**, 248–250.
Mitchell, M. S., and Mokyr, M. B. (1972). *Cancer Res.* **32**, 832–838.
Moore, M. A. S., Williams, N., and Metcalf, D. (1973). *J. Nat. Cancer Inst.* **50**, 591–602.
Nelson, D. S. (1969). "Macrophages and Immunity." North-Holland Publ., Amsterdam.
Nichols, B. A., and Bainton, D. F. (1973). *Lab. Invest.* **29**, 27–40.
Nichols, B. A., Bainton, D. F., and Farquhar, M. G. (1971). *J. Cell Biol.* **50**, 498–515.
Norris, G. F., and Peard, M. C. (1963). *Brit. Med. J.* **1**, 378–382.
Ohara, K., Fried, J., Dowling, M., Bittar, E., and Clarkson, B. (1971). *Cancer* **2**, 862–885.
Oren, R., Franham, A. E., Saito, K., Milofsky, E., and Karnovsky, M. L. (1963). *J. Cell Biol.* **17**, 487–501.
Paulley, J. W., and Hughes, J. P. (1960). *Brit. Med. J.* **3**, 1562–1567.
Pimstone, N. R., Tenhunen, R., Seitz, P. T., Marver, H. S., and Schmid, R. (1971). *J. Exp. Med.* **133**, 1264–1281.
Ptak, W., Gaugas, J. M., and Rees, R. J. (1970). *Clin. Exp. Immunol.* **6**, 117–124.

Rabinovitch, M. (1967). *Proc. Soc. Exp. Biol. Med.* **124,** 396–399.
Rappaport, H. (1966). "Atlas of Tumor Pathology," Sect. III, Fasc. 8. Armed Forces Institute of Pathology, Washington, D. C.
Robinson, W. A., and Mangalik, A. (1972). *Lancet* **2,** 742–744.
Rodey, G. E., Park, B. H., Windhorst, D. B., and Good, R. A. (1969). *Blood* **33,** 813–820.
Rodriquez-Molina, F., and Pons, J. A. (1936). *P. R. J. Publ. Health Trop. Med.* **11,** 369–400.
Rosenberg, S. A., Diamond, H. D., Jaslowitz, G., and Craver, L. F. (1961). *Medicine (Baltimore)* **40,** 31–84.
Rosengarten, R., and Bourn, J. M. (1959). *Neurology* **9,** 704–706.
Russell, R. W. R. (1962). *Ann. Rheum. Dis.* **21,** 171–175.
Salmon, S. E., Cline, M. J., Schultz, J., and Lehrer, R. I. (1970). *N. Engl. J. Med.* **282,** 250–253.
Schulze, M. L., Wahle, G. H., and White, J. B. (1953). *Amer. J. Clin. Pathol.* **23,** 1028–1030.
Shadduck, R. K., and Nagabhushanam, N. G. (1971). *Blood* **38,** **559–568.**
Sharar, A. (1968). *G. Accad. Med. Torino* **81,** 140.
Sharar, A., Kletter, Y., and Aronson, M. (1969). *Isr. J. Med. Sci.* **5,** 1164–1172.
Sidransky, H., Verney, E., and Beede, H. (1965). *Arch. Pathol.* **79,** 299–309.
Simson, F. W., and Barneston, J. (1942). *J. Pathol. Bacteriol.* **54,** 299–305.
Snyderman, R., Shin, H. S., and Hausman, M. S. (1971). *Proc. Soc. Exp. Biol. Med.* **138,** 387–390.
Sokolov, R. A., Rachmaninoff, N., and Kaine, H. D. (1962). *Amer. J. Med.* **32,** 131–141.
Stecher, V. J., and Thorbecke, G. J. (1967). *J. Immunol.* **99,** 643–652.
Sterner, J. H., and Eisenbud, M. (1951). *Arch. Ind. Hyg.* **4,** 123–151.
Sundberg, R. D., and Spink, W. W. (1947). *Blood* **1,** suppl., 7–32.
Sutton, J. S. (1967). *Nat. Cancer Inst., Monogr.* **26,** 71.
van Furth, R., and Cohn, Z. A. (1968). *J. Exp. Med.* **128,** 415–435.
Watts, J. W., and Harris, H. (1959). *Biochem. J.* **72,** 147–153.
Weber, H. H., and Engelhardt, W. E. (1933). *Zentralbl. Gewerbehyg. Unfallverhuet.* **10,** 41.
Weiner, H. L., and Robinson, W. A. (1971). *Proc. Soc. Exp. Biol. Med.* **136,** 29–33.
West, J., Morton, D. J., Esmann, V., and Stjernhom, R. L. (1968). *Arch. Biochem. Biophys.* **124,** 85–90.
Wilkinson, P. C., Borel, J. F., Stecher-Levin, V. J., and Sorkin, E. (1969). *Nature (London)* **222,** 244–247.
Williams, H. L. (1949). *Ann. Otol., Rhinol., & Laryngol.* **58,** 1013–1054.
Williams, W. J. (1958). *Brit. J. Ind. Med.* **15,** 84–91.
Wintrobe, M. M. (1967). *In* "Clinical Hematology," 6th ed. (M. M. Wintrobe, ed.), pp. 279–284 and 1157–1162. Lea & Febiger, Philadelphia, Pennsylvania.
Young, L. E., Izzo, M. J., and Platzer, R. F. (1951). *Blood* **6,** 1073–1098.
Zinkham, W. H., and Diamond, L. K. (1952). *Blood* **7,** 592–601.

24

Macrophages: Perspectives and Prospects

D. S. Nelson

In the office in which I write there are, neatly arranged on a long shelf, the manuscripts produced by more than forty respected colleagues, whose combined invisible presence is more than a little daunting. I find it, indeed, almost impossible to summarize each contribution and it seems not only easier but more equitable to try to sketch an impressionistic picture with a few areas highlighted.

Ten—or even five—years ago it was possible to half-empty a room containing a general immunological audience by beginning to speak about macrophages. By continuing on the same subject, one could induce unconcealed somnolence in at least half the remainder. Macrophages were regarded as cells that were, of course, indispensable and therefore important, but of little more immunological interest than, say, fibroblasts or squamous epithelial cells. They suffered even in comparison with their fellow phagocytes, the polymorphonuclear leukocytes, by moving too slowly, ingesting too much, and thus having all the appeal of Pickwickian fat boys. Now the attention of an audience is less apt to wander; macrophages are seen to be not only important but interesting, and to be important in previously unperceived ways. I shall select four broad areas of importance in illustration.

First, macrophages can play several roles in lymphocyte activation, whether this occurs "naturally" in response to antigens or artificially in response to nonspecific mitogens. They appear to be essential for the activation of T cells. They act as a necessary focusing device for antigen and an optional focusing device for mitogen. Antigen or mitogen constitutes one signal for activation, but macrophages provide an essential second signal in the form of a soluble factor. They are also essential for effective T cell–B cell collaboration in the production of antibodies to thymus-dependent antigens, although the ways in which they mediate this collaboration are not clearly defined. They are, in general, not essential for B cell activation, specific or nonspecific, except in those cases in which they convert an antigen from a tolerogenic into an immunogenic state, either by focusing or by removal of excess molecules. The requirement, or lack of requirement, for macrophages seems to be similar whether the end product is the generation of helper or effector T cells, antibody production, blastogenesis, or lymphokine production.

Macrophages may serve immunoregulatory functions in two senses. They may determine, by the way in which they handle or present antigen, the balance between cell-mediated and humoral immune responses to antigens. In addition, they can inhibit the activation of lymphocytes, especially T cells, perhaps directly but more likely by producing soluble factors with a net depressive effect. This inhibition may be important in determining the extent of development of an immune response, especially to a thymus-dependent antigen, and in limiting the intensity of expression of cell-mediated immunity.

Several interesting questions may be posed. What is it about T cells that causes them to require, for activation, a macrophage-produced signal in addition to direct membrane contact with mitogen or antigen? Precisely what determines the balance between humoral and cell-mediated immune responses to a particular antigen? Do macrophage-derived soluble factors indeed play an important role in immunoregulation? Most important, will the answers to these questions allow the development of biological tools for deliberate immunomanipulation?

The second area in which macrophages are more active than was previously thought is that of secretion. Macrophages are the main, if not the only source of lysozyme, which they produce in surprisingly large quantities. They appear also to be the source of the second and fourth components of complement. Either unstimulated or, more commonly, when subject to various stimuli, they synthesize and release a wide range of biologically active products. Many of these products have a demonstrable role in the genesis of inflammatory lesions. New notions of the roles of macrophages and their products in inflammation—perhaps the commonest of all pathological processes—may lead to new approaches to the pharmacological control of inflammation.

The third area for comment is perhaps an obvious one: the role of macrophages in resistance to infection. Macrophages can become activated to a state in which their capacity to kill intracellular microorganisms in an immunologically nonspecific fashion is grossly increased. In the acquisition of cellular resistance to many infections, this activation occurs as a result of the generation of effector or committed lymphocytes that intereact specifically with microbial antigen, producing lymphokines including macrophage activating factor(s). Other lymphokines presumably contribute in other ways to the expression of resistance in intact hosts; for example, macrophage chemotactic factor may attract cells to sites of infection, and macrophage migration inhibition factor may keep them there. It is obviously desirable to obtain a deeper understanding of the mode of action of lymphokines, especially on macrophage membranes. The receptors for these factors, as well as for immunoglobulins, for complement components, and for a variety of other agents, can now be mapped. Changes in the receptors, especially their movements in relation to each other, can be followed. As with lymphocytes, the establishment of interrelationships between membrane and intracellular events is critical. Now that a substantial outline has been obtained of the events in the expression of cellular resistance to infection, it is possible to pose further questions and, unfortunately, necessary to point to notable gaps in the outline. Chief among the notable gaps is our almost total ignorance of the critical differences between normal and activated macrophages. One could put the unanswered question in two parts: Do activated macrophages utilize the same mechanisms as normal macrophages to kill intracellular microbes, but on a much larger scale, or do they acquire novel mechanisms? And what are the mechanisms by which macrophages can kill such a diverse array of intracellular microbes? Even lacking the answers, however, one can look anew at the problems of diminished resistance to infection in man and animals. In any individual case, one can look for defects in the production of effector lymphocytes, defects in the production of mediators by these cells, the occurrence of inhibitors of mediator production or mediator activity, defects in the capacity of monocytes or macrophages to respond to the mediators, and defects in the capacity of the marrow to respond normally to demands for more monocytes. "Stimulate the phagocytes" has in fact been a sensible enough precept, whatever the sarcastic intent with which Shaw may have put it into the mouth of Sir Ralph Bloomfield Bonington. We possess now a growing armamentarium of substances that will do just that, as well as the means to investigate the failure of phagocytes to be stimulated. As so commonly in the past, our understanding of viral infections lags somewhat; lymphocyte-produced interferon, cytotoxic T cells, and macrophages may all be important in cellular immunity to viruses, but their relative importance seems to vary with the infecting virus.

The fourth large area is currently the most fashionable; as it is of high relevance to malignant disease, it is also the most emotionally charged. Although it has been known for many years that macrophages can participate in the rejection of allografts and tumor isografts, it is only recently that attention has been widely paid to the role of macrophages as effectors of anticellular immunity. This change in perspective has resulted from two developments in particular: demonstrations that effector lymphocytes alone could not suppress certain syngeneic tumor cells without the help of macrophages and demonstrations of quite dramatic nonspecific cytotoxic and/or cytostatic effects of activated macrophages on target tumor cells *in vitro*. The questions prompted by these observations include obvious mechanistic ones. How, for example, do the macrophages exert cytostatic or cytotoxic effects? Is direct contact involved or are soluble mediators of prime importance? How do activated macrophages discriminate, as they appear to do, between normal cells and rapidly proliferating cells often showing malignant growth characteristics in culture? What is the precise mechanism of collaboration between effector lymphocytes and macrophages? Going into more fundamental biological principles, one may well ask whether the antitumor effect of activated macrophages reflects the existence of a primitive surveillance mechanism whose presence might be sought in nonmammalian or even invertebrate species. It is worth noting that pure T cell killing can eliminate a large *allogeneic* tumor mass, whereas macrophage-mediated or macrophage-assisted killing seems inadequate to eliminate large established *syngeneic* tumors. Whether or not this reflects evasion of pure T cell surveillance by successful tumors remains to be established. Finally, in terms of human cancer, the beneficial effects of live BCG vaccine in immunotherapeutic regimes may be due in part to the stimulation of monocyte production and the activation of macrophages by BCG.

The long chain of science begins with the abstractions of pure mathematics and the near-abstractions of fundamental physics. Mankind is arrogant and tends, rather strongly, to see his own benefit as the end of the chain. Certainly, the public justification of biomedical science is not "glorious entertainment" but the prospect of improvement in human well-being. It is now possible to investigate human macrophage function. One can predict with some confidence that this will be done increasingly in the coming years, that important changes in disease states will be discovered, and that manipulation of the immunobiological behavior of macrophages will become more common. Even our current knowledge has deep implications for the management of infectious diseases and cancer.

It was perhaps unfair to entitle this volume "Immunobiology of the Macrophage." Macrophages are heterogeneous; this heterogeneity may reflect a continuum of states of differentiation or the existence of true specialization. It appears quite remarkable that such a large number of functions has devolved upon the cells that began as the most primitive defenders of the body. Not content with their immunological role, they handle iron and fat, remove dead cells, and control fibroblasts. In the evolution of our complex mammalian system they seem almost ubiquitous, emerging from obscurity to make some lysozyme, contribute to the complement system, help a T cell, present a stimulus to a B cell, or quell an unruly mutant. They are the ultimate guardians of our bodily integrity; *sed quis custodiet ipsos custodes?*

Index

A

Acid hydrolases
  chronic inflammation and, 433–434
  immune complexes and, 444
  release of, 435–438, 444–445
  stimulated T lymphocytes and, 444–445
Acid proteinase, 434
Adenylate cyclase, 405–406
Adherence procedures, 9–10
Allogeneic macrophages,
  antigen presentation and, 143–144
  initiation ability of, 153
  lymphocyte activation and, 187–189
  lymphocyte proliferative response, 155
  T cell activation, 153–154
Allograft rejection
  macrophage-mediated cytotoxicity in, 464–469
  in vitro experiments of, 467–469
  in vivo evidence of, 464–467
Alveolar macrophages, 92–95, 98–99, 309
  activity comparison with peritoneal macrophages, 96
  bactericidal activity of, 93
  chemotactic responses of, 93
  Fc receptor of, 94, 98–99
  migration inhibition factor and, 93–94
Antibody-producing cells, *see* B cells
Antibody response, 1–34, 45–90, 136, 236
  alloantisera and, 26–27
  antigen presentation and, 15–20
  B cells and, 2–3
  genetic restrictions and, 24–26
  H-2 linked *Ir* genes and, 22–24
  immunogenetics and, 22–27
  leukocyte alloantigens and, 26–27
  macrophages and, 1–34, 521–554
  Marbrook system and, 4, 9
  methodology of, 4
  Mishell-Dutton system, 4, 9
  requirements of, 7–13
  separation of, 7–9
  suppression of, 26–27
  T cells and, 2–3, 10–13
  T cell-dependent antigens and, 10–12
  T cell-independent antigens and, 12–13
  tissue culture systems in, 4–6
  in vitro, 4–6
  in vivo, 5–6
Antigen
  cell activation by, 38–39
  cell mediated immunity and, 117–123
  characteristics of, 41–42
  chemotaxis and, 361–363
  degradation effects and, 121–123
  differences between, 95, 115
  duration of effects, 122
  histocompatibility and stimulation by, 168
  endocytized distribution of, 103–106
  immunity induction effects, 122
  immunogenicity of, 36–37, 94, 96–97, 123–127
  macrophage and, 79–81, 134–141
  microbial, and immunotherapy, 581–582
  presentation
    allogeneic macrophages and, 144
    cell membranes and, 395–396
    syngeneic macrophages and, 144
  receptors for, 37–38
  recognition of
    cellular and molecular events in, 155–158
    macrophage requirements, 132–134
    T lymphocytes and, 131–160, 155–158
  sensitization effects, 114–117
  signal requirements, 155
  soluble, effects of, 115, 134–141
  specific immunological activation by, 558–562
  stimulation by, 370–371
  T cell-dependent, *see* T cell-dependent antigen
  T cell-independent, *see* T cell-independent antigens

trypsinization effects on, 120
Antimicrobial immunity, 367–400
Anti-tumor activity of macrophages, 600
Asbestos, in chronic inflammation, 442–443

B

Bacterial toxins
macrophages and, 356–358
neutrophils and, 358–360
Bacteriostasis, 408–410
B cells, *see also* T cell-B cell collaboration
activation of, 117, 161–199
antibody responses and, 2–3
cell viability of, 166
chemotaxis and, 334–336
collaboration and, 20–22
function, 214, 334
heterogeneity of, 98
immunogenetics and, 6–7
immunologic function of, 2
lymphokine synthesis and, 190–194
macrophage relationship and, 20–22, 55–57, 113–114, 178–187, 195
monocyte chemotactic factor production and, 193
pathways of, 2
production of, 119
proliferation, 172–187
response, 208, 229
soluble factors and, 177
subpopulations of, 169
T cell presence and, 173–178
thymus-dependent antigen and, 172–178
in vitro responses of, 172–173
Wiskott-Aldrich syndrome and, 345
BCG, immunotherapy and, 240
Blastogenesis, 142, 182, 250, 334
Blood, monocyte in, 302–308
Bone marrow, virus-induced tumors and, 523–525

C

Cancer, immune system and, 577–588
Carbohydrates, migration inhibitory factor action with, 414–418
Carrageenan, in chronic inflammation, 441–442
Cathepsin B1, 434
Cathepsin C, 434
Cathepsin D, 434
Cells, *see also* specific cells
activation of, 42–43
biology of, 141
chemotaxis and, 349–366
chronic inflammation and, 428–430
debris, removal of, 599–600
immunity mediator production, 220–224
lymphotoxin and, 221
macrophage activating factor, 223
migration inhibitory factor, 220–221
monocyte chemotactic factor, 221–223
osteoclast activating factor, 224
kinetics
infection and, 311–319
monocytes, 295–311
theories of, 293
lines, immunobiology of, 275–290
lymphocytes and, 202–203
lymphoid, cytotoxicity of, 546–548
nucleated, 535–573
traffic, 81–83
viability, 134, 210
Cell-mediated immunity, 130
induction, 117–119
Cell membranes
antigen presentation and, 395–396
chemotactic factor interaction and, 356–358
Cell migration, 350
Chemokinesis, chemotaxis and, 352–353
Chemotaxis
antigen-specific, 361–363
bacterial factors and, 337
blastogenesis and, 334
B cell and, 334–336
cellular aspects of, 349–366
chemokinesis, different from, 352–353
complement and, 329–331
conjugation of side groups to proteins and, 354–356
contractile events in, 356–358
definition of, 324, 351
denaturation and, 354

depression of, 339
dysfunctions of, 324
factor recognition and, 353–356
humoral factors in, 329–333
intracellular events in, 356–358
lymphocyte-derived factors in, 333–337
macrophages and, 323–348, 453
measurement of, 328–329
metabolic activation and, 358
molecular aspects of, 349–366
monocyte altering factors and, 337–340
monocyte activity and, 334
peripheral blood monocytes and, 328
peritoneal macrophages, 326–328
phagocyte migration and, 355
plasma activity in, 331–333
quantifying of, 324–329
recognition, 360–361
serum activity and, 331–333
T cell and, 334–336
in vivo activity, 336–337
Collaboration, *see* T cell-B cell collaboration
Collagenase
in activation, 407–408
as macrophage product, 432
in macrophage secretion, 434
neutral proteinases and, 445–446
Colony stimulating factor, 432, 600–601
Corynebacterium parvum, 239
Cytocidal effects
of activated macrophages, 487–507
cloning experiments and, 499–500, 502
correlations of, 502
methods for detecting, 499–500
morphology of, 499–501
nomenclature of, 488
summary of, 505–507
target cell assessment in, 499, 501–503
tumor target alterations in, 500–502
in vitro findings of, 503–505
Cytolytic factor, as macrophage product, 432
Cytostatic effects
of activated macrophages, 487–507
cell to cell contact in, 496
functional requirements for, 498
kinetics of, 494–495
lymphocytes and, 493–494
mechanisms of, 496–499
metabolic requirements for, 498
methods for detecting, 489–491
assessment of, 489–491
in mouse macrophages, 489
procurement of macrophages for, 489
of rat macrophage, 489
target cell lines and, 489–490
nomenclature of, 488
relationship to other agents, 498–499
soluble macrophage factor in, 497–498
summary of, 505–507
target cells and, 489–496
thymus independence of, 496
uniqueness of, 495
in vitro findings of, 503–505
Cytotoxicity
antigen activation and, 558–562
growth inhibitory macrophages and, 539–542
immune macrophage, 544–546
lymphoid cells and, 379, 546–548
lytic macrophages and, 542–544
macrophage-mediated, 463–484
in allograft rejection, 464–469
chemical characterization in, 480–481
cocultivation experiments in, 473–475
culture supernatants in, 475–477
infection with microorganisms and, 472–473
kinetics of, 476–477
macrophage cytotoxicity factor in, 475–481
specificity of, 477–480
syngeneic tumor systems and, 469–472
in vitro induction of, 473–481
in vivo evidence in graft destruction, 464–467
nonspecific lymphoid supernatants and, 562
nonspecific macrophage, 555–567
of nucleated cells, 535–573
persisting infections and, 562–565
specific arming of macrophages in, 546–551
spleen cell activity and, 378
supernatant factors and, 548–551
surveillance and, 571–572
target cells and, 377
T cell, significance of, 380–381
tests, for cytocidal effects, 500–501

tumor bearing host and, 567–570
in vivo significance of, 570–571

D

Delayed hypersensitivity, 123
Dental plaque, homogenates of, 439–441
Diazotized sulfanilic acid (DSA), 420–421
Diisopropyl fluorophosphate (DFP), 418
Dinitrochlorobenzene (DNCB), 580–582
Disorders, macrophage, 593–612
histiocytic, *see* Histiocytic responses
histiocytic proliferation as, 602–603, 607–608
of monocyte-macrophage system, 594, 602–611
monocytosis and, 602–603
reactive hyperplasia and, 603–606
storage disease, 602–603, 606–607
DNA
monocytopoiesis and, 299, 300
synthesis in macrophage, 141
DNA synthesis, 141, 149, 156, 244, 284, 304
DNA virus
immune response to, 512–516
transformed cells and, 509–512
tumor induction, mechanism of, 527–531
DNP-D-GL, immunogencity of, 41
Dysfunction syndromes, 602–603, 610–611

E

Elastase, 434
Enzymes, 51, 427–457
hydrolytic
chronic inflammation, 448–451
secreted by macrophages, 433–435
lysosomal, 407, 443–445
macrophage, secretion of, 427–457
Enzymes, as products of immune reactions 443–445
Eosinophilic granuloma, 609
Erythropoiesis, 600–601
Esterases, 418–421

F

Fibroblasts, in chronic inflammation, 455–456

G

Glucosamine, incorporation by macrophages, 406–407
Glucose oxidation, in macrophage activation, 407
L-Glutamic acid^{60}-L-alanine^{30}-L-tyrosine^{10} (GAT), 277
Glycolysis, macrophage and, 358
Granules, intracellular, 407
Granulopoiesis, macrophages and, 600–601
Graft destruction, 464–467
Growth assay, 277–283
Growth inhibition, 539–542

H

Hageman factor, 454
Hand-Schuller-Christian disease, 609
Haptens, 580–581
Hapten-carrier conjugates, 113–114
H-2 complex, 6–7
H-2-linked *Ir* genes, 22–24
Hematopoietic cell destruction, 602–603, 605–606
Hemolytic anemia, 605–606
Hemopoiesis, 319
Heparin, 419
Heterogeneity, 91–110, 106–107
alveolar macrophages and, 92–95, 98–99
antigen trapping and, 97–98
different tissues and, 92–97
Fc receptors and, 102–103
peritoneal macrophages, 92–95, 99–102
same tissue, in, 97–107
Heterokaryons, 263, 271
Histiocytes, 526–527
Histiocytic responses
eosinophilic granuloma and, 609
Hand-Schuller-Christian disease and, 609
to hematopoietic cell destruction, 602–603, 605–606
Letterer-Siwe disease and, 609
lymphoma and, 608
malignant disorders of, 602–603, 608–610
medullary reticulosis and, 609
monocytic leukemia and, 608

proliferative, disorders of, 602–603, 607–608
Homeostasis and macrophages, 251
Hyaluronidase, 434
Hyperplasia, reactive
clinical response of, 602–603, 605
disorders of macrophages, 603–606
hematopoietic cell destruction and, 602–603, 605–606
response to intracellular parasites, 603–605

I

Immunity
cell-mediated, development of, 219–225, 527–531
of host, to virus-induced tumors, 512–518
macrophage cytotoxicity in, 544–546
macrophage response, 3, 194, 235, 275, 291, 597
to virus-induced tumors, 509–531
Immunization, 116
Immunogenetics
antibody responses and, 22–27, 35–44, 141
B cells and, 6–7
GAT and, 6–7
H-2 complex and, 6–7
introduction to, 6–7
T cells and, 6–7
Immunogenicity
cytophilic antibody effect on, 126
humoral antibody effect and, 124–127
macrophage associated effects and, 124, 127
regulation of, 123–127
soluble antigen effects and, 124
tumors and, 241
Immunological effector mechanisms, 368
Immunoregulation, 235–257, 618
Immunotherapy of tumors, 577–588
chemically defined haptens and, 580–581
clinical investigations of, 579–584
dinitrochlorobenzene and, 580–582
lymphokines and, 583–584
microbial antigens and, 581–582
mononuclear phagocytic system and, 578
prevention and, 582
summary of, 619–621
surveillance of, 584–587
2,3,5-triethyleneiminobenzoquinone and, 580–582
Immunotherapy of skin tumors, 577–588
Infections, 291–322, 618–619
immunity to, 375–395
Inflammation
acid hydrolases and, 433–434
chemotactic factors in, 453
Hageman factor in, 453
kinins in, 453–454
mediators, from macrophage secretions, 453–454
prostaglandins in, 454
Inflammation, chronic, 427–457
acute exacerbations of, 454–455
asbestos in, 442–443
biochemical responses in, 430–431
biologically active secretions in, 432–433
carrageenan in, 441–442
fibroblasts at sites of, 455–456
functional responses in, 430–431
group A streptococcal cell walls and, 438–439
homogenates of dental plaque and, 439–441
hydrolytic enzymes and, 433–435, 448–451
inhaled cytotoxic particles in, 442–443
lysozymes, 432, 435
mediators in, 453–454
modulating factors in, 454–457
neutral proteinases in, 433–435, 448–451
nonimmunological, 438–443
origin and turnover of cells in, 428–430
pathogenesis of, 427–457
pharmacological modifications of, 456–457
silica in, 442–443
in vitro studies of, 430–448
Interferon
definition of, 202
functional macrophage integrity and, 212–214
leukocyte origin of, 225–229
macrophage effects on, 201, 234
mechanisms of action, 202

properties of, 395
response, 209–211
RNA and, 202
sources of, 395
system, 211–212
T and B lymphocytes and, 208–209
Interferon production, 201–234
assay, 206
culture harvesting and, 205–206
experimental conditions of, 204–206
fluorescence activated cell sorter technique and, 204
leukocytes and, 225–229
lymphocytes and, 204, 214–219
macrophage monolayer preparation and, 204
mitogen stimulated lymphocytes, 203–214
nylon fiber column technique and, 204
response, extent of, 206–207

K

Kinetics, T cell, 372–373
Kinins, generation of, 453–454

L

Lactate dehydrogenase elevating virus, (LDV), 563–565
Leprosy, 253
Letterer-Siwe disease, as histiocytic disorder, 609
Leukemia, monocytic, 608
Leukocytes, 225–229, 324, 337
Liver, 95–97
Lymph nodes, 74–79, 97–98, 184
Lymphocytes
activation of, 187–189, 617–618
allogeneic cells and, 187–189
antigen binding by, 146
antigen-stimulated, interferon production by, 214–219
antimicrobial immunity and, 367–400
cellular interactions of, 202–203
chemotactic factors and, 333–337
cytostatic effects and, 493–494
immune cellular mediator production and, 219–225
interferon production and, 201–234
macrophage interaction, 141–144, 151, 367–368, 390–392
mitogen and, 203–204, 207
physical interactions and macrophages, 144–152
proliferative response of, 155
rejection of tumors and, 518–527
stimulated T, acid hydrolases and, 444–445
stimulation and inhibition of, 250–253
traffic, 77–79
Lymphocyte mediators, macrophage activation by, 401–423
adenylate cyclase in, 405–406
bacteriostasis and, 408–410
changes occurring in, 403–411
characterization of, 411–412
collagenase in, 407–408
culture produced, 413–414
glass adherence and, 403
glucosamine incorporation in, 406–407
glucose oxidation in, 407
intracellular granules and, 407
kinetics of, 412
lysosomal enzymes and, 407
phagocytosis in, 405
pinocytosis in, 405
ruffled membrane movement and, 403–405
tumor killing and, 410–411
Lymphocyte responses
macrophage and, 167–168, 243–250
sera effects of, 246
Lymphoid cell supernatants, cytotoxicity and, 562
Lymphoid tissue, cytotoxic T cell activity and, 379
Lymphokines, *see also* Lymphocyte mediators
B and T lymphocytes and, 190–194
definition, 219
production, 336
responses to, 401–423
synthesis, 335
tumor immunotherapy and, 583–584
Lymphoma, histiocytic, 608
Lysis, macrophages in, 542–544
Lysosomal hydrolases, as macrophage products, 432
Lysozymes, 432, 435, 447–448

M

Macrophage
biological properties of, 51, 421–423
capacity of, 117–119
categories of, 162
characteristics of, 9–10
chemokinesis, 351
chemotaxis of, 323–348, 349–366
depletion of, 237
depression of, 238
differences in, 92–95
differentiation, 277
disorders in man, 593–612, *see also* Disorders, macrophage
functions of, 37, 57–60, 91–92, 106–107, 131–160, 212–214, 323, 360–361, 596–601
independence, 178–181
intercellular compartments of, 119–121
lines, 283–288
locomotion of, 350–351, 358–360
metabolism of, 358, 594–596
microbial killing by, 598–599
perspectives and prospects, 617–621
physical interactions of, 144–152
populations of, 96
processing of antigen by, 41–42
products of, 427–457
properties of, 238
protein antigens and, 140
purification of, 7–9, 282–283
putative sites for interaction, 83–85
random migration of, 351
receptor, 49, 51, 261
removal, 179, 239
replacement of, 163–167
responses of, 55–57, 107, 180, 185
separation of, 7–9
source of, 53–54
subclasses of, 101, 107
surface of, 259, 271
compartments of, 119–121
organization and function of, 261–262, 264–266, 272
proteins of, 262–264
synthetic replacement compounds and, 165–167
tolerogenicity and, 35–44
viability requirements of, 119
Macrophage activation, 162–167, 383, 389–394, 396–397
cytocidal effects of, 487–507, *see also* Cytocidal effects
cytostatic effects of, 487–507, *see also* Cytostatic effects
lymphocyte-macrophage interactions in, 367–400, *see also* Lymphocyte-macrophage interaction
by lymphocyte mediators, 401–423, *see also* Lymphocyte mediators
Macrophage and antigen
binding, 102, 103, 146, 177
interactions and, 74–77, 79–81
handling of, 162–163
lymphocyte responses, 167–178
presentation and, 15–20, 144, 335
recognition requirements and, 132–134
Macrophage cytotoxicity factor (MCF), 475–481
Macrophage–lymphocyte collaboration, 367–368
Macrophage–lymphocyte interaction
genetic regulation of, 141–144
histocompatibility requirement of, 151
Macrophage mechanisms, 323–324, 333
B and T lymphocyte proliferation and, 175–178
biochemical basis of, 393
cytotoxicity and, 375–381
H-2 compatibility requirements and, 377–380
interferon and, 394–395
Macrophage membranes, 9–10, 259–273
functions of, 260
antigens and, 51
molecules and, 9–10
and protein transport, control of, 266–271
receptors of, 261, 266–271
Marbrook system, in antibody responses, 4, 9
Medullary reticulosis, histiocytic, 609
Metabolism, of macrophage, disorders, 594–596
Microfilaments, 260
Microtubules, 260, 271, 357, 363
Migration inhibitory factor, 401–428
diazotized sulfanilic acid and, 420–421
diisopropyl fluorophosphate and, 418

L-fucose and, 414–418
heparin and, 419
macrophage interaction with, 401–423
cell surface carbohydrates and, 414–418
L-fucose and, 414–418
macrophage-associated esterases in, 418–421
soybean trypsin inhibitor and, 418–420
target cell interaction with, 401–423
Migration of macrophages, 324, 351–353, 381
Mishell-Dutton system, 4, 9
Mitogens
B and T cell response and, 178–187
and macrophages and, 162–163, 203–204
T lymphocyte proliferation and, 152
Mitosis, 279, 282
Monocyte
antimicrobial mechanism of, 381–389
bacterial effects on, 359
bone marrow source of, 295
cell kinetics of, 295–319
definition, 291
development of, 313
disappearance of, 294
distribution of, 304–306
DNA synthesis and, 304
fate of, 308–311
infectious disease response, mechanism of, 312, 318
interferon system and, 211–212
life span of, 311, 319
locomotion, 363
origin of, 292, 296
oscillation of levels, 306–308
peritoneal macrophages and, 309
population, 291
precursors of, 295–296, 319
recruitment of, 381–389
relationships of, 292
reserve capacity of, 306
role of, 308
stem cells of, 296–298
T cell interaction and, 387
turnover of, 306
viruses and, 338
virus tests, 385, 386, 387, 388
Monocyte chemotaxis, 328, 332, 349–366
cancer and, 341
depression of, 339
human disease abnormalities and, 340–345
immunoglobulin defects and, 344–345
mucocutaneous candidiasis and, 340–341
neoplasm production and, 342–344
tumor removal effects of, 343
Wiskott-Aldrich syndrome and, 344
Monocyte kinetics, 292, 297, 298–303
infection, changes and, 291–322
methodological background of, 293-295
theoretical background of, 293–295
Monocytopoiesis, 299, 300, 319
Monocytosis, 602–604
Mononuclear cell population, 308–311
Mononuclear phagocytic system, 578

N

Neutral proteinases
chronic inflammation and, 433–435 448–451
collagenase, 445–446
plasminogen activator, 447
secretion of, 445–447
Neutrophil locomotion, bacterial toxin effects on, 358–360
Nonantigenic stimulation of macrophages, 152–155

P

Papovavirus, see SV40
Pathogenesis, of chronic inflammation, 427–457, *see also* Inflammation, chronic
Peritoneal macrophages
activity comparison of, 96
antigen-binding activities of, 101
bactericidal activity of, 93, 99–100
chemotaxis of, 93, 326–328
endocytized antigen and, 103–106
Fc receptor of, 94, 101–102
immunogenic RNA activities of, 101
migration effects on, 362
migration inhibition factor response and, 93–94
monocytes and, 309
RNA and, 100–102
subclasses of, 100–101

Phagocytosis, 264–265, 271, 279, 360–361, 383, 405, 597–601
Pinocytosis, in macrophage activation, 405
Plasminogen activator
as macrophage product, 432
in macrophage secretion, 434
neutral proteinase secretion and, 447
Polyanion method, for nucleated cells, 556–558
PPG (C-mucopolysaccharide-peptidoglycan complex), 438–440
Promonocytes, 296
Prostaglandins
as inflammatory mediator, 454
as macrophage product, 432, 451–453
Pyrogen
in macrophage secretion, 451
as macrophage product, 432

R

RNA
immunogenicity of, 100–102
interferon and, 202
synthesis, 211, 262
in tumor induction, 512
RNA virus, immune response to, 516–518
Ruffled membrane movement, 403–405

S

Silica, in chronic inflammation, 442–443
Skin tumors, immunotherapy for, 577–588, *see also* Immunotherapy of tumors
Soluble macrophage factor
cytostatic effects of, 497–498
replacement of macrophages by, 163–167
Specific macrophage arming factor (SMAF), 531
Spleen, 79–83, 95–98
cytotoxic activity and, 378
functional anatomy of, 79–83
Soybean trypsin inhibitor, migration inhibitory factor action and, 418–420
Specific arming of macrophages, 546–548
virus-induced tumors and, 520–523
Storage diseases, of monocyte-macrophage system, 602–603, 606–607
Streptococcal cell walls, 438–439
Supernatant factors, 243–250, 548–551
SV40
development of, 527–531
in induction of tumors, 509–516
rejection of tumors, 518–527
tumor-specific transplantation antigen and, 511–516
Syngeneic macrophages, 143–144
antigen presentation and, 144
lymphocyte proliferative response, 155
Syngeneic tumor systems, *see* Tumor systems
Synthetic compounds, macrophage replacement by, 163–167

T

T cells (thymus-derived lymphocytes), *see also* T cell—B cell collaboration
antibody production and, 112
activation of, 119, 161–199
aldehyde-induced proliferation of, 154–155
alloantigens and, 153–154
antibody responses and, 2–3, 115
antigen dose and, 371
antigen recognition and, 131–160
antigen stimulation of, 370–371
antimicrobial mechanism of, 381–389
cell-mediated immunity factors and, 368
chemotaxis and, 334–336
collaboration with macrophage, 20–22
cytoxicity significance of, 380–381
defects of, 213
effector generation of, 369–375
function, 214, 334, 381
generation, 396
immunogenetics and, 6–7
immunologic role of, 2, 112, 369
immunoprophylaxis and, 370
induction of, 370, 396
infection control and, 369
interferon production and, 229
macrophage and, 20–22, 54–55, 113–114, 133, 184, 185, 387
mitogens, 152, 169–172, 178, 181–187
monocyte recruitment and, 381–389, 387

nonantigenic stimulation of, 152–155
pathways of, 2
production of, 369
proliferation *in vitro,* 169–172, 185
receptor interaction of, 134
receptors, 396
recovery process, importance of, 370
recruitment, importance of, 382
replacing factors, 236
subpopulations of, 169
T cell–B cell collaboration, 45–90, 113, 131–132, 158
antigen focusing in, 61
antigen receptor in, 46–48
B cell in, 46, 49–50
biological properties of, 51
C3 activation model and, 68–69, 73
components of, 46
cytophilic antibody model and, 66–68, 73
deblocking and protection model, 71–72, 73
enzymes and, 51
Fc receptors in, 48–49, 50
functions in, 57–60
IgT–antigen complex model of, 65–67, 73
immunobiology of, 46–52
information transfer in, 60–61
Ir-CI gene complex model and, 69–70, 73
macrophage factor model and, 70–71, 73
macrophages in, 46, 50–52
mechanisms of, 60–73
membrane associated antigens and, 51
pre-T cell (induction) in, 57–59
receptors of, 51
soluble mediator in, 62–65
theories of, 60–65
three-cell models of, 65–72, 73
in vivo, 73–85
T cell–dependent antigens
antibody responses to, 10–12
macrophages and, 10–12
T cell-independent antigens and, 3
T cell-independent antigens, 12–13
antibody responses to, 12–13
T cell-dependent antigens and, 3
macrophages and, 12–13
T cell mechanisms, 360
antigen, recognition of, 389, 392, 393
antiviral, restrictions of, 390
biochemical, basis of, 393
cytotoxicity and, 375–381
H-2 compatibility requirements and, 377–380, 393
infection immunity and, 375–395
interferon and, 394–395
macrophage activation and, 389–394
production
fate of, 374
kinetics of, 372–373
memory and, 375
migration of, 374–375
regulation and, 373
proliferation, 175–178
Tetanus toxoid, immunogenicity of, 118
Thymocytes, 146–152
interaction with macrophage, 147
Thymus, cytostatic effects and, 496
Thymus-derived lymphocytes, *see* T cells
Thymus-independent antigens, 178, 181
Tissue culture systems, 4–6
2,3,5-Triethyleneiminobenzoquinone, 580–582
Trypsinization, immune response and, 138–139
Tumor-specific transplantation antigen (TSTA)
development of, 527–531
SV40 and, 511–516
TU-5 cells, virus-induced tumors and, 518–527
Tumors
clinical investigations of, 579–584
cytocidal effects on, 500–502
destruction of, 509–531
host, cytotoxic macrophages and, 567–570
immunotherapy, 577–588, *see also* Immunotherapy of tumors
killing, in macrophage activation, 410–411
macrophages and, 241, 287–288, 342–344
prevention, 582
rejection, 469–472, 518–527
RNA virus induced, 512
surveillance of, 584–587

SV40 induced, 509–516
systems
morphology of, 469–471
syngeneic, cytotoxic macrophages in, 469–472
in vitro experiments, 471–472
virus-induced, 509–531
bone marrow and, 523–525
cell-mediated immunity to, 527–531
DNA, immune response to, 512–516, 527–531
histiocytes and, 526–527
immunity to, 509–531
macrophages and, 225–229, 509–531
RNA, immune response to, 516–518
specific macrophage arming factor and, 531
spleen cells and, 520–523
SV40 and, 518–527
T lymphocytes and, 518–527
TU-5 cells and, 518–527

V

Virus, oncogenic, 509–512
DNA virus-transformed cells and, 509–512
RNA tumor virus-transformed cells and, 512
Vitamin E, macrophage replacement and, 166

W

Wiskott-Aldrich syndrome, 344–345

7
C 8
D 9
E 0
F 1
G 2
H 3
I 4
J 5